SPINE
SECRETS PLUS

SECOND EDITION

VINCENT J. DEVLIN, MD
ORTHOPAEDIC SURGEON
SILVER SPRING, MARYLAND

ELSEVIER
MOSBY

3251 Riverport Lane
St. Louis, Missouri 63043

SPINE SECRETS PLUS, SECOND EDITION

ISBN: 978-0-323-06952-6

Notices

Knowledge and best practice in this field are constantly changing. As new research and experience broaden our understanding, changes in research methods, professional practices, or medical treatment may become necessary.

Practitioners and researchers must always rely on their own experience and knowledge in evaluating and using any information, methods, compounds, or experiments described herein. In using such information or methods they should be mindful of their own safety and the safety of others, including parties for whom they have a professional responsibility.

With respect to any drug or pharmaceutical products identified, readers are advised to check the most current information provided (i) on procedures featured or (ii) by the manufacturer of each product to be administered to verify the recommended dose or formula, the method and duration of administration, and contraindications. It is the responsibility of practitioners, relying on their own experience and knowledge of their patients, to make diagnoses, to determine dosages and the best treatment for each individual patient, and to take all appropriate safety precautions.

To the fullest extent of the law, neither the Publisher nor the authors, contributors, or editors assume any liability for any injury and/or damage to persons or property as a matter of products liability, negligence or otherwise, or from any use or operation of any methods, products, instructions, or ideas contained in the material herein.

ISBN: 978-0-323-06952-6

Senior Acquisitions Editor: James Merritt
Developmental Editor: Barbara Cicalese
Publishing Services Manager: Anne Altepeter
Senior Project Manager: Doug Turner
Designer: Steven Stave

Printed in the United States of America

Last digit is the print number: 9 8 7 6 5 4 3 2 1

To my wife, Sylvia.
Without her support and encouragement,
completion of this book would not have been possible.

PREFACE

Appropriate diagnosis and treatment of spinal disorders remain a challenge for both patient and physician. Rapid advances in the field of spinal disorders have opened new avenues for diagnosis and treatment. A wide range of medical specialties—orthopedic surgery, neurosurgery, anesthesiology, physical medicine, pain management, radiology, internal medicine, family practice, pediatrics, neurology, emergency medicine, pathology, and psychiatry—are involved in the evaluation and treatment of patients with spinal problems on a daily basis. Knowledge of current concepts relating to spinal disorders is crucial to provide appropriate evaluation, referral, and treatment.

The goal of *Spine Secrets Plus* is to provide broad-based coverage of the diverse field of spinal disorders at an introductory level, using the proven and time-tested question-and-answer format of the Secrets Series®. The book covers the common conditions encountered during evaluation and treatment of spinal problems. Topics are arranged to provide the reader with a sound knowledge base in the fundamentals of spinal anatomy, clinical assessment, spinal imaging, and nonoperative and operative treatment of spinal disorders. The full spectrum of disorders affecting the cervical, thoracic, and lumbar spine in pediatric and adult patients is covered, including degenerative disorders, fractures, spinal deformities, tumors, infections, and systemic problems, such as osteoporosis and rheumatoid arthritis. The detailed information will benefit the reader during patient rounds, as well as in the clinic and the operating room. The book is not intended to provide comprehensive coverage of specific topics, which is more appropriately the domain of major textbooks. However, it is hoped that readers will be stimulated to further their knowledge of spinal disorders through additional study, as directed by the Internet resources and references listed at the end of each chapter.

The intended audience is wide-ranging and includes all physicians interested in furthering their knowledge and understanding of spinal disorders: medical students, residents, fellows, and practicing physicians. The book may also be of interest to nurses, physical therapists, chiropractors, hospital administrators, attorneys, worker compensation professionals, and medical device professionals, as well as patients with spinal problems.

I wish to acknowledge the numerous people who have provided guidance over the years and contributed to my development as a physician and spinal surgeon. I am especially grateful to Dr. Marc A. Asher, Dr. Thomas R. Haher, Dr. Behrooz A. Akbarnia, Dr. Oheneba Boachie-Adjei, Dr. David S. Bradford, Dr. James W. Ogilvie, Dr. Ensor E. Transfeldt, Dr. Paul A. Anderson, Dr. Dale E. Rowe, Professor Jürgen Harms, Dr. Arthur D. Steffee, Dr. Joseph Y. Margulies, and Dr. William O. Shaffer. I also thank the staff at Elsevier, especially Barbara Cicalese, for bringing this project to completion. Finally, I thank my practice colleagues during the past 2 decades for their support and efforts in helping me treat patients with challenging spinal problems.

—Vincent J. Devlin, MD
Date Submitted: 8/1/2010

CONTRIBUTORS

Behrooz A. Akbarnia, MD
Clinical Professor, Orthopedics, University of California–
San Diego; Medical Director, San Diego Center for Spinal
Disorders, La Jolla, California

Todd J. Albert, MD
Richard Rothman Professor and Chair, Orthopaedics, and
Professor, Neurosurgery, Thomas Jefferson University
Hospital, Philadelphia, Pennsylvania

D. Greg Anderson, MD
Associate Professor, Department of Orthopaedic Surgery,
Thomas Jefferson University; Orthopaedic Surgery,
Thomas Jefferson University Hospital, Philadelphia,
Pennsylvania

Paul A. Anderson, MD
Professor, Department of Orthopedics and Rehabilitation,
University of Wisconsin, Madison, Wisconsin

Carlo Bellabarba, MD
Associate Professor and Spine Fellowship Director,
Department of Orthopaedics and Sports Medicine,
University of Washington, Harborview Medical Center;
Director, Orthopaedic Spine Service, Harborview
Medical Center, Seattle, Washington

Darren L. Bergey, MD
Director, Spinal Surgery, Rancho Specialty Hospital, Rancho
Cuccomonga; Owner/Director, Bergey Spine Institute,
Colton, California

Richard J. Bransford, MD
Assistant Professor, Department of Orthopaedics and Sports
Medicine, University of Washington; Assistant Professor,
Department of Orthopaedics and Sports Medicine,
Harborview Medical Center, Seattle, Washington

Keith H. Bridwell, MD
Asa C. and Dorothy W. Jones Professor of Orthopaedic
Surgery, Washington University, St. Louis, Missouri

Thomas N. Bryce, MD
Associate Professor, Department of Rehabilitation Medicine,
Mount Sinai School of Medicine; Medical Director, Spinal
Cord Injury Program, Mount Sinai Medical Center, New
York, New York

R. Carter Cassidy, MD
Assistant Professor, Department of Orthopaedic Surgery,
University of Kentucky, Lexington, Kentucky

Jens R. Chapman, MD
Professor, Acting Chair, and Director, Spine Service,
Department of Orthopaedics and Sports Medicine;
Joint Professor, Neurological Surgery, University of
Washington, Seattle, Washington

Charles H. Crawford, III, MD
Fellow, Adult and Pediatric Spinal Surgery, Washington
University, St. Louis, Missouri

Gina Cruz, DO
Orthopaedic Surgeon, Riverside County Regional Medical
Center, Moreno Valley, California

Jeffrey E. Deckey, MD
Orthopaedic Spine Surgeon, Orthopaedic Specialty Institute,
Orange, California

Stephen L. Demeter, MD, MPH
Independent Medical Evaluation Examiner, Honolulu Sports
Medical Clinic, Honolulu, Hawaii

Vincent J. Devlin, MD
Orthopaedic Surgeon, Silver Spring, Maryland

Maury Ellenberg, MD, FACP
Clinical Professor, Physical Medicine and Rehabilitation,
Wayne State University; Section Chief, Physical Medicine
and Rehabilitation, Sinai Grace Hospital, Detroit, Michigan

Michael Ellenberg, MD
Spine and Musculoskeletal Fellow, Physical Medicine
and Rehabilitation, Rehabilitation Physicians PC,
Novi, Michigan

Paul Enker, MD, FRCS, FAAOS
Long Island Arthritis and Joint Replacement, Lake Success,
New York

Avital Fast, MD
Professor and Chair, Physical and Rehabilitation Medicine,
Montefiore Medical Center and Jack D. Weiler Hospital
of Albert Einstein College of Medicine, Bronx, New York

Winston Fong, MD
Clinical Instructor, Department of Orthopaedic Surgery,
University of California–Los Angeles, Los Angeles,
California

Robert W. Gaines, Jr., MD
Professor, Orthopaedic Surgery, University of Missouri;
Orthopaedic Surgeon, Columbia Regional Hospital;
Director, Spine Fellowship Program, Columbia
Orthopaedic Group, Columbia, Missouri

Jaspaul S. Gogia, MD
Chief Resident, Department of Orthopaedic Surgery,
University of California–Davis, Davis Medical Center,
Sacramento, California

John M. Gorup, MD
Director, Indiana Spine Center, Lafayette, Indiana

Munish C. Gupta, MD
Professor and Chief, Spine Surgery, Department of
    Orthopaedic Surgery, University of California–Davis,
    Sacramento, California

Thomas R. Haher, MD
Adjunct Professor, Orthopaedic Surgery, New York Medical
    College, Valhalla, New York; Syracuse Orthopedic
    Specialists, Syracuse, New York

Richard T. Holt, MD
Spine Surgery, PSC, Louisville, Kentucky

Mary Hurley, MD
Clinical Professor, Orthopaedics, Loma Linda University,
    Loma Linda; Chief, Orthopaedic Surgery, Kaiser
    Permanente Medical Group, Fontana Medical Center,
    Fontana, California

Darren L. Jacobs, DO
Associate Physician and Clinical Clerkship Director,
    Department of Neurosurgery, Geisinger Medical Center,
    Danville, Pennsylvania

Lawrence I. Karlin, MD
Assistant Professor, Orthopaedic Surgery, Harvard Medical
    School; Associate, Orthopaedic Surgery, Children's
    Hospital, Boston, Massachusetts

Anna M. Lasak, MD
Attending Physician, Clinical Assistant Professor, and
    Medical Director, Outpatient Rehabilitation Clinic,
    Physical and Rehabilitation Medicine, Montefiore Medical
    Center and Jack D. Weiler Hospital of Albert Einstein
    College of Medicine, Bronx, New York

Mohammad E. Majd, MD
Spine Surgery, PSC; Orthopedic and Spine Surgery, Floyd
    Memorial Hospital, New Albany, New York

Steven Mardjetko, MD, FAAP
Associate Professor, Department of Orthopaedic Surgery,
    Rush Medical College, Chicago; Orthopaedic Surgeon,
    Advocate Lutheran General Hospital, Park Ridge;
    Orthopaedic Surgeon, Illinois Bone and Joint Institute,
    Morton Grove, Illinois

Joseph Y. Margulies, MD, PhD
Orthopedic Spine Surgeon, Pleasantville, New York

Scott C. McGovern, MD
Co-Director, Peninsula Spine Center, Peninsula Regional
    Medical Center; Orthopaedic Spine Surgeon, Peninsula
    Orthopaedic Associates, PA, Salisbury, Maryland

Ronald Moskovich, MD, FRCS
Assistant Professor, Orthopaedic Surgery, New York
    University School of Medicine; Associate Chief, Spine
    Surgery, New York University Hospital for Joint Diseases,
    New York, New York

Gregory M. Mundis, Jr., MD
Orthopedic Spine Surgeon, San Diego Center for Spinal
    Disorders, La Jolla, California

Justin Munns, MD
Resident Surgeon, Orthopaedic Surgery, Ohio State
    University, Columbus, Ohio

Douglas H. Musser, DO
Assistant Clinical Professor of Orthopaedic Surgery, Ohio
    University, Athens; Assistant Clinical Professor of
    Orthopaedic Surgery, Northeastern Ohio Universities,
    Rootstown; Orthopaedic and Spine Surgery, Humility
    of Mary Health Partners and Forum Health System,
    Youngstown, Ohio

John W. Nelson, MD, FIPP
Private Practice, Oklahoma City, Oklahoma

Brian A. O'Shaughnessy, MD
Fellow, Adult and Pediatric Spinal Surgery, Washington
    University, St. Louis, Missouri

Daniel K. Park, MD
Fellow, Spine Surgery, Emory University, Atlanta, Georgia

Ashit C. Patel, MD
Spine Surgeon, Department of Orthopedics, Overlake
    Hospital, Bellevue, Washington

Thomas A. Schildhauer, MD
Professor and Chair, Universitätsklinik für Unfallchirurgie
    und Sporttraumatologie, Medizinische Universität Graz,
    Graz, Austria

Jerome Schofferman, MD
Director, Research and Education, San Francisco Spine
    Institute, SpineCare Medical Group, Daly City, California

William O. Shaffer, MD
Orthopaedic and Spine Surgery, Northwest Iowa Bone,
    Joint and Sports Surgeons, Spencer, Iowa

Adam L. Shimer, MD
Assistant Professor, Orthopaedic Surgery, University of
    Virginia, Charlottesville, Virginia

Edward D. Simmons, MD, MSc, FRCS(c)
Clinical Professor, Department of Orthopaedic Surgery,
    State University of New York at Buffalo; Department of
    Orthopaedic Surgery, Buffalo General Hospital, Buffalo,
    New York

Kern Singh, MD
Assistant Professor, Orthopaedic Surgery, Rush University
    Medical Center, Chicago, Illinois

Edward A. Smirnov, MD
Bucks County Specialty Hospital, Bensalem, Pennsylvania

John C. Steinmann, DO
Associate Clinical Professor, Department of Orthopaedic
    Surgery, Loma Linda University, Loma Linda, and Western
    University of Health Sciences, Pomona; Medical Staff,
    Department of Orthopaedic Surgery, Arrowhead Regional
    Medical Center, Colton; Medical Staff, Department of
    Orthopaedic Surgery, St. Bernardines Medical Center,
    San Bernardino, and Redlands Community Hospital,
    Redlands, California

Brian W. Su, MD
Orthopaedic Spine Surgeon, Mt. Tam Orthopedics, Spine
    Center, Larkspur, California

Mark A. Thomas, MD
Associate Professor, Physical Medicine and Rehabilitation, Albert Einstein College of Medicine; Attending Faculty, Physical Medicine and Rehabilitation, Montefiore Medical Center, Bronx, New York

Eeric Truumees, MD
Director, Spinal Research, and Attending Spine Surgeon, Seton Spine Center, Seton Brain and Spine Institute, Austin, Texas

Alexander R. Vaccaro, MD, PhD
Everett J. and Marion Gordon Professor of Orthopaedic Surgery, Professor of Neurosurgery, Co-Director of the Delaware Valley Spinal Cord Injury Center, Co-Chief Spine Surgery, Co-Director Spine Surgery, Thomas Jefferson University and the Rothman Institute, Philadelphia, Pennsylvania

Robin H. Vaughan, PhD, DABNM
Neurophysiology, Department of Surgery, Scripps Memorial Hospital–La Jolla, San Diego, California

Sayed E. Wahezi, MD
Assistant Professor, Department of Rehabilitation Medicine, Albert Einstein College of Medicine; Assistant Professor, Department of Rehabilitation Medicine, Montefiore Medical Center, Bronx, New York

Jeffrey C. Wang, MD
Professor, Department of Orthopaedic Surgery and Neurosurgery, UCLA Spine Center, UCLA School of Medicine; Department of Orthopaedic Surgery and Neurosurgery, UCLA Medical Center, Los Angeles, California

Robert G. Watkins, III, MD
Co-Director, Marina Spine Center, Marina del Rey Hospital, Marina del Rey, California

Robert G. Watkins, IV, MD
Co-Director, Marina Spine Center, Marina del Rey Hospital, Marina del Rey, California

Burt Yaszay, MD
Assistant Clinical Professor, Orthopaedic Surgery, University of California San Diego; Staff, Orthopedics, Rady Children's Hospital, San Diego, California

Yinggang Zheng, MD
Attending Physiatrist, Desert Institute of Spine Care, Phoenix, Arizona

CONTENTS

TOP 100 SECRETS

These secrets are 100 of the top board alerts. They summarize the concepts, principles, and most salient details of spinal disorders.

1. The typical spinal column is composed of 33 vertebrae: 24 pre-sacral vertebrae (7 cervical, 12 thoracic, and 5 lumbar); the sacrum (5 fused vertebrae); and the coccyx (4 fused vertebrae).

2. There are eight pairs of cervical nerve roots but only seven cervical vertebrae. The cervical nerve roots exit the spinal canal above the pedicle of the corresponding vertebrae. The thoracic and lumbar nerve roots exit beneath the pedicle of the corresponding vertebrae.

3. The thoracic spinal cord between T4–T9 is poorly vascularized. This region is termed the critical vascular zone of the spinal cord and corresponds to the narrowest region of the spinal canal.

4. The spinal cord normally terminates as the conus medullaris at the L1–L2 level in adults. The cauda equina occupies the thecal sac distal to the L1–L2 level.

5. The posterior spinal musculature maintains normal sagittal spinal alignment through application of dorsal tension forces against the intact anterior spinal column (tension band principle). The posterior spinal musculature can function as a tension band only if the anterior spinal column is structurally intact. In the normal lumbar spine approximately 80% of axial load is carried by the anterior spinal column and the remaining 20% is transmitted through the posterior spinal column (load-sharing concept).

6. Pedicle dimensions are smallest in the mid-thoracic region (T4–T6), widen slightly in the upper thoracic region (T1–T3), and widen markedly in the lower thoracic region (T10–T12). The lower thoracic pedicles are typically larger than the upper lumbar pedicles. L1 is generally the narrowest pedicle in the lumbar spine. Pedicle dimensions gradually increase between L2 and S1.

7. There is a poor correlation between the severity of degenerative changes on spinal imaging studies and the severity of spine-related symptoms.

8. MRI is the best initial advanced spinal imaging study to evaluate non-traumatic spinal conditions because it provides the greatest amount of information regarding a single spinal region. MRI provides excellent visualization of pathologic processes involving the disc, thecal sac, epidural space, neural elements, paraspinal soft tissue, and bone marrow.

9. Multiplanar CT is the imaging study of choice for evaluating the osseous anatomy of the spine and is the preferred initial advanced imaging study for evaluation of spinal trauma. CT myelography is useful for evaluation of patients with contraindications to MRI and for evaluation of the spinal canal in patients with extensive metallic spinal implants. The radiation dosage associated with CT is an important concern and may be minimized by following appropriate protocols.

10. A technetium-99m bone scan detects regions of increased blood flow or osteoblastic activity. It plays a role in the diagnosis of spondylolysis, spinal infection, metastatic disease, and fractures and is useful for evaluation of patients with contraindications to MRI.

11. A major goal in the initial evaluation of a patient with axial pain is to differentiate common non-emergent spinal conditions (e.g. acute non-specific axial pain, spondylosis) from serious disorders such as spinal infections, spinal tumors, or myelopathy.

12. Impairment reflects an alteration from normal bodily functions, can be assessed using traditional medical means, and can be objectively determined. Disability results from impairment, is task specific, and is measured in the context of the system to which an injured worker has applied for relief. Disability determination is an administrative determination that uses both medical and non-medical information.

13. Cervical spondylotic myelopathy is the most common cause of spinal cord dysfunction in patients older than 55 years of age. Diagnosis is based on a history of myelopathic symptoms, the presence of myelopathic signs on physical examination, and imaging findings that demonstrate cervical cord compression.

14. The standard straight-leg raise test and its variants increase tension along the sciatic nerve and are used to assess the L5 and S1 nerve roots. The reverse straight leg raise test increases tension along the femoral nerve and is used to assess the L2, L3, and L4 nerve roots.

15. Identification and resolution of psychosocial barriers to recovery is critical for successful treatment of chronic spinal pain syndromes.

16. It is important to differentiate nociceptive pain (due to a structural disorder that stimulates small nerve endings) from neuropathic pain (due to nerve damage or injury). Analgesics are the most effective medications for nociceptive pain and include peripherally-acting analgesics (e.g. acetaminophen, aspirin, NSAIDS) and centrally-acting analgesics (e.g. opioids). The drugs of choice for neuropathic pain are anticonvulsants and noradrenergic antidepressants.

17. Options for lumbar epidural injections include translaminar, transforaminal, and caudal approaches.

18. Use of provocative discography in the management of axial pain syndromes remains controversial. False-positive results are reported in a high percentage of patients with psychologic distress, chronic pain syndromes, and anular disruption and in individuals involved in litigation or workman's compensation cases.

19. Electrodiagnostic evaluation is useful to differentiate whether extremity symptoms are due to radiculopathy, peripheral nerve entrapment neuropathy, or polyneuropathy.

20. The TLSO provides effective motion restriction between T8 and L4 but paradoxically increases motion at the L4–L5 and L5–S1 levels. If motion restriction is required above T8, a cervical extension is added. If motion restriction is required at L4–L5 and L5–S1, a thigh cuff is necessary.

21. Surgical treatment is indicated for moderate or severe cervical spondylotic myelopathy unless medically contra-indicated, because there is no good non-surgical treatment

22. Anterior cervical plates are the most commonly used implants in the C3–C7 spinal region. Cervical plates may be classified as static (constrained) plates or dynamic (semi-constrained) plates.

23. C5 nerve root dysfunction is the most common nerve root problem after cervical laminectomy or laminoplasty. Nerve root dysfunction may be noted immediately after surgery or may develop 1–5 days following surgery.

24. Cervical laminoplasty and laminectomy are contraindicated in patients with cervical kyphosis.

25. Spinal degeneration occurs in all individuals but remains asymptomatic in many patients. Mechanical, traumatic, nutritional, biochemical, and genetic factors interact and contribute to development of spinal degeneration.

26. The clinical manifestations of degenerative spinal disorders include axial pain syndromes, radiculopathy, myelopathy, spinal instabilities, and spinal deformities

27. LBP is ubiquitous in the human race and is not a disease. LBP is a symptom and not a diagnosis.

28. Acute LBP and chronic LBP are completely different disorders and require different treatment algorithms.

29. General indications for surgical intervention for spinal disorders include decompression, stabilization, and spinal deformity correction.

30. By providing evidence-based information on surgical options and outcomes, surgeons can partner with patients through *shared decision making* to determine the preferred treatment course for spine pathologies having multiple potential treatment options.

31. Inappropriate patient selection guarantees a poor surgical result despite how expertly a surgical procedure is performed.

32. The nerve roots of the lumbar spine exit the spinal canal beneath the pedicle of the corresponding numbered vertebrae and above the caudal intervertebral disc. A posterolateral L4–L5 disc herniation compresses the L5 nerve root (the traversing nerve root of the L4–L5 motion segment). An L4–L5 foraminal or extraforaminal disc herniation compresses the L4 nerve root (the exiting nerve root of the L4–L5 motion segment).

33. Relief of leg pain is the primary goal of lumbar discectomy.

34. Cauda equina syndrome manifests as a constellation of symptoms including bladder and bowel dysfunction, perineal anesthesia, and lower extremity radicular symptoms resulting from a space-occupying lesion (e.g. disc herniation) within the lumbosacral canal. Treatment is urgent surgical decompression within 48 hours of symptom onset.

35. Evidence-based treatment options for symptomatic lumbar degenerative disc disease include a structured outpatient physical rehabilitation program, spinal fusion, and artificial disc replacement.

36. Patients with *neurogenic claudication* report tiredness, heaviness, and discomfort in the lower extremities with ambulation. The distance walked until symptoms begin and the maximum distance that the patient can walk without stopping varies from day to day and even during the same walk. Patients report that leaning forward relieves symptoms while activities performed in extension (e.g. walking down hill) exacerbate symptoms. Patients with *vascular claudication* describe cramping or tightness in the calf region associated with ambulation. The distance walked before symptoms occur is constant and is not affected by posture.

37. Surgical treatment options for lumbar spinal stenosis include insertion of an interspinous spacer, lumbar decompression (laminotomy or laminectomy), and lumbar decompression combined with fusion with or without the use of spinal instrumentation.

38. Radiculopathy most commonly involves the exiting nerve root in isthmic spondylolisthesis, while the traversing nerve root is most commonly involved in degenerative spondylolisthesis.

39. For degenerative spondylolisthesis patients, surgical outcomes are improved when decompression is combined with posterior fusion compared with patients treated with decompression without fusion.

40. Spinal arthrodesis and spinal instrumentation are indicated in conjunction with decompression in the presence of spinal deformity, spinal instability, or when decompression results in destabilization at the surgical site.

41. Successful posterior fusion is dependent on meticulous preparation of the graft bed, decortication of the osseous elements, and application of sufficient and appropriate graft material.

42. Posterior spinal instrumentation most commonly involves the use of rod-screw systems. Screws may be placed in the occiput, C1 (lateral mass screws), and C2 (pedicle, pars, or translaminar screws). In the subaxial cervical region, lateral mass screws are most commonly used at the C3–C6 levels, while pedicle screws are typically used at C7 and distally in the thoracic and lumbar region.

43. Reconstruction of the load-bearing capacity of the anterior spinal column is critical for successful application of spinal instrumentation. Options for anterior column reconstruction include autogenous bone grafts (iliac or fibula), allograft bone grafts, or synthetic materials (e.g. titanium mesh cages, carbon fiber cages, PEEK cages).

44. Although short-term stabilization of the spine is provided by spinal implants, long-term stabilization of the spine occurs only if fusion is successful.

45. For *high-risk* fusions to the sacrum, using bilateral S1 pedicle screws supplemented with iliac fixation and structural interbody support is the most reliable surgical technique.

46. Multimodality intraoperative neurophysiologic monitoring permits assessment of the functional integrity of the spinal cord and nerve roots during spinal surgery. Intraoperative assessment of spinal cord function is optimally achieved with a combination of transcranial electric motor-evoked potentials (tceMEPs) and somatosensory-evoked potentials (SSEPs). Nerve root function is assessed via electromyographic (EMG) monitoring techniques.

47. The optimal anesthetic protocol to permit successful intraoperative neurophysiologic monitoring of spinal cord function is a total intravenous anesthesia regimen (TIVA) with avoidance of muscle relaxation, nitrous oxide, and inhalational agents.

48. Complications following spine surgery are unavoidable, but their negative effects can be lessened by prompt diagnosis combined with appropriate and expedient intervention.

49. Selection of appropriate candidates for revision spinal surgery depends on comprehensive assessment to determine the factors that led to a less than optimal outcome. For poor surgical outcomes due to errors in *surgical strategy* or *surgical technique*, appropriate revision surgery may offer a reasonable chance of improved outcome. For surgical failures due to *errors in diagnosis* or *inappropriate patient selection* for initial surgery, revision surgery offers little chance for improved outcome. In the absence of relevant and specific anatomic and pathologic findings, pain itself is not an indication for revision surgery.

50. Spinal cord stimulation is a minimally invasive treatment appropriate for select patients with persistent pain following spinal surgery, chronic regional pain syndromes, and other neuropathic pain syndromes. Implantable drug delivery systems are considered for patients with nociceptive and/or neuropathic pain syndromes who do not experience relief with medication, spinal cord stimulation, or neuroablative procedures.

51. Scoliosis presenting in adulthood may represent *idiopathic scoliosis* that initially developed in adolescence or scoliosis that developed in adulthood secondary to asymmetric disc degeneration and is termed *de novo* or *degenerative scoliosis*.

52. Consequences of untreated spinal deformity include poor cosmesis, pain, neurologic deficit, postural difficulty, pulmonary compromise, and impairment in activities of daily living.

53. Sagittal imbalance syndrome (originally termed "flatback syndrome") is a postural disorder characterized by low back pain, forward inclination of the trunk, and difficulty in maintaining an erect posture. This syndrome results from decreased lumbar lordosis, which leads to global sagittal imbalance. Patients report back pain and fatigue due to the inability to stand without flexing their hips and knees.

54. Appropriate surgical treatment for adult scoliosis often requires structural interbody support, osteotomies, segmental pedicular fixation, use of osteobiologics, and iliac fixation.

55. Important techniques for the prevention of postoperative sagittal imbalance following spinal instrumentation and fusion include appropriate patient positioning, use of an operating table that enhances lumbar lordosis, appropriate sagittal rod contouring and restoration of segmental sagittal alignment using interbody fusion, wide posterior releases, and posterior osteotomies as needed.

56. Surgical options for treatment of sagittal imbalance in the previously fused spine include Smith-Petersen osteotomy, Ponte osteotomy, pedicle subtraction osteotomy, combined anterior and posterior osteotomy, and vertebral column resection.

57. The American Spinal Injury Association Impairment Scale (AIS) is a five-category scale (A–E) used to specify the severity of neurologic injury. It includes definitions of complete and incomplete injuries.

58. Incomplete spinal cord syndromes include: 1) central cord syndrome, 2) anterior cord syndrome, 3) Brown-Séquard syndrome, 4) conus medullaris syndrome, and 5) cauda equina syndrome.

59. Complications of spinal cord injury (SCI) that may manifest within the first several days following injury include hypotension, bradycardia, hypothermia, hypoventilation, gastrointestinal bleeding, and ileus. Pneumonia is the most common cause of early death in tetraplegics. Venous thromboembolism occurs in up to 75% of patients with traumatic SCI who are not receiving anticoagulant prophylaxis.

60. In a patient with spinal cord injury, the combination of hypotension and bradycardia is consistent with the diagnosis of neurogenic shock. Hypotension and tachycardia support the diagnosis of hemorrhagic shock.

61. Central cord syndrome is the most common incomplete spinal cord injury syndrome. It is frequently associated with a hyperextension injury mechanism in patients with preexistent cervical stenosis. Clinical presentation includes bilateral sensory and motor deficits with greater upper extremity weakness than lower extremity weakness. Lower extremity hyperreflexia and sacral sparing are present. The prognosis is good for a partial recovery of motor function, but return of hand function is generally poor.

62. Brown-Séquard syndrome is caused by hemisection of the spinal cord. Clinical presentation includes ipsilateral motor and proprioception loss combined with contralateral pain and temperature loss distal to the level of injury. Prognosis for recovery is good, with most patients recovering some degree of ambulatory capacity, as well as bowel and bladder function.

63. Immediate traction reduction of subaxial cervical facet dislocations can be performed safely in alert, awake, and cooperative patients whose neurologic status can be clinically monitored. MRI should be obtained prior to attempting reduction in uncooperative or unconscious patients to guide treatment. Cervical MRI should be obtained following closed reduction of a subaxial cervical facet dislocation and prior to operative intervention.

64. Direct fracture osteosynthesis is an option for surgical treatment of select type 2 odontoid fractures and C2 pars interarticularis fractures.

65. The most common athletic-related injury in the cervical region is a *stinger* or *burner* (burner syndrome). This peripheral nerve injury typically results from an ipsilateral shoulder depression and contralateral neck flexion mechanism. Patients present with *unilateral* dysesthetic pain and paresthesia, which may be accompanied by weakness, most often in the muscle groups supplied by the C5 and C6 nerve roots. Normal painless cervical motion is usually present and distinguishes a "stinger" from other types of cervical pathology.

66. Cervical cord neurapraxia is characterized by an acute transient episode of *bilateral* sensory and/or motor abnormalities involving the arms, legs, or both. Neck pain is generally absent. An episode of cervical cord neurapraxia generally resolves in less than 10–15 minutes. The most commonly described mechanism of injury is axial compression with a component of either hyperflexion or hyperextension. Subsequent imaging studies typically show findings of cervical spinal stenosis.

67. Classification of a thoracolumbar fracture involves a description of the injury morphology, neurologic status, and integrity of the posterior ligamentous complex. The use of an injury severity score to guide treatment has been popularized.

68. Thoracolumbar flexion-distraction spinal injuries are frequently accompanied by abdominal visceral injuries, and a high index of suspicion for this injury combination is warranted.

69. Denis classification of sacral fractures uses the *most medial fracture extension* to distinguish three types of fractures. *Zone 1* fractures remain lateral to the sacral foramina and are the most frequent fracture type. This fracture type is associated with the lowest rate of neurologic injury (5%). These injuries involve the L5 root or sciatic nerve. *Zone 2* injuries extend through the sacral foramina and are the second most frequent fracture type. Associated lumbosacral root injuries occur in 25% of patients. *Zone 3* injuries involve the central sacral spinal canal. These are the least common injury type but have the highest rate of neurologic injuries (50%). Neurologic injuries range from sacral root deficits to cauda equina transection with associated bowel and bladder dysfunction.

70. The majority of pediatric patients presenting with back pain do not have an identifiable diagnosis.

71. Children younger than eight years of age are predisposed to upper cervical injury due to their high head to body ratio and horizontal facet orientation.

72. Evaluation of C1–C2 instability should include assessment of the atlantodens interval (ADI) and the space available for the spinal cord (SAC).

73. The presence of a Klippel-Feil anomaly should prompt investigation for associated organ system anomalies involving the genitourinary, cardiovascular, auditory, gastrointestinal, skeletal, and neurologic systems.

74. Pediatric patients with spondylolysis usually respond to nonsurgical treatment including activity restriction and orthotic treatment. Surgical treatment options include intertransverse fusion or direct repair of the pars interarticularis.

75. Spondylolisthesis may be classified into two main types: developmental and acquired.

76. Circumferential fusion provides the highest likelihood of successful arthrodesis in patients with high-grade spondylolisthesis.

77. Idiopathic scoliosis has traditionally been categorized according to the age at diagnosis as *infantile* (birth to 3 years), *juvenile* (age 3 to 10 years), or *adolescent* (age beyond 10 years). An alternative classification recognizes two categories: *early onset* (birth to 5 years) and *late onset* (beyond 5 years of age). This alternative classification is intended to reflect the physiologic stages of thoracic development, because growth of the thorax and lungs is greatest in the first five years of life.

78. The management options for patients diagnosed with idiopathic scoliosis include observation, orthoses, and operative treatment.

79. Multilevel spinal fusion in infantile and juvenile spinal deformity patients limits future increase in spinal height and restricts development of the thoracic cage and lung parenchyma. Growth-preserving surgical treatment options include dual growing rods and a vertically expandable prosthetic titanium rib (VEPTR).

80. Common causes of pediatric kyphotic deformities include Scheuermann's disease, postural roundback, trauma, postlaminectomy deformity, congenital anomalies, infection, and achondroplasia.

81. Evaluation of the patient with a neuromuscular spinal deformity requires assessment of the underlying disease process in combination with the spinal deformity. Surgical treatment is challenging and is associated with a high complication rate. Surgery has the potential to improve a patient's functional ability and quality of life, as well as provide improved caregiver satisfaction.

82. The prognosis for a congenital spinal deformity depends on three factors: type of anomaly, patient age, and location of the defect. A wide range of intraspinal and extraspinal anomalies are associated with congenital spinal deformities. Comprehensive work-up is critical and includes an MRI of the entire spine.

83. Children younger than 8 years of age have a large cranium in relation to their thorax, which must be accommodated when they are immobilized on a spine board in order to prevent excessive cervical flexion.

84. Odontoid fractures are the most common pediatric cervical spine fracture.

85. Skeletally immature patients who sustain a spinal cord injury require surveillance for the development of spinal deformities.

86. Primary tumors of the spine arise de novo in the bone, cartilage, neural or ligamentous structures of the spine and are classified as extradural or intradural. Primary spine tumors are extremely rare. Secondary tumors are either metastatic to the spine from distant origins or grow into the spine from adjacent structures (e.g. Pancoast tumor from the upper lobe of the lung). Metastatic lesions involving the spine are the most common type of spinal tumor and account for 95% of all spinal tumors.

87. En bloc resection with tumor-free surgical margins provides the best possible local control for malignant primary tumors of the spinal column and is the procedure of choice when technically feasible.

88. The differential diagnosis of a spinal tumor is determined by the anatomic compartment in which it occurs: extradural, intradural-extramedullary, or intramedullary. The most common extradural spinal tumor is a metastatic tumor. The most common tumors occurring in the intradural-extramedullary compartment are schwannomas, neurofibromas, or meningiomas. The most common types of intramedullary tumors are ependymomas, astrocytomas, and hemangioblastomas.

89. The most common primary osseous malignant process is multiple myeloma.

90. Treatment strategies for metastatic spine tumors include orthoses, bisphosphonates, steroids, radiotherapy, chemotherapy, hormonal therapy, vertebroplasty, kyphoplasty, surgical decompression and stabilization, or combinations of these options.

91. Vertebral compression fracture is the most common fracture due to osteoporosis. Vertebral fractures are two to three times more prevalent than hip fractures or wrist fractures. A person who suffers a vertebral fracture is five times more likely to suffer an additional fracture when compared with a control patient without a fracture.

92. The disc is nearly always involved in pyogenic vertebral infections. In contrast, granulomatous infections typically do not involve the disc space.

93. Initial treatment of pyogenic vertebral osteomyelitis is culture-guided antibiotic therapy and orthotic immobilization. Surgical intervention is considered for: 1) failure of medical management, 2) open biopsy following non-diagnostic closed biopsies, 3) drainage of a clinically significant abscess, 4) neurologic deficit, or 5) progressive spinal deformity.

94. Three types of cervical deformities develop secondary to rheumatoid disease: atlantoaxial subluxation, atlantoaxial impaction (vertical migration of the odontoid), and subaxial subluxation.

95. A classic feature of ankylosing spondylitis is inflammation at the attachments of ligaments, tendons, and joint capsules to bone and is termed *enthesopathy*. Reactive bone formation leads to formation of marginal syndesmophytes and ossification of the spinal column, resulting in the characteristic "bamboo spine" picture. Surgical intervention in ankylosing spondylitis patients may be required for atlantoaxial instability, spondylodiscitis, fractures, and sagittal plane spinal deformities.

96. Diffuse idiopathic skeletal hyperostosis (DISH or Forestier's disease) affects the ligaments along the anterolateral aspect of the spine that become ossified. DISH typically affects four or more vertebrae, is most common in the thoracic region, and typically spares the lumbar spine and sacroiliac joints. The radiographic hallmark of DISH is the presence of asymmetric non-marginal syndesmophytes, which appear as flowing anterior ossification originating from the anterior longitudinal ligament.

97. Minimally invasive spine procedures intend to limit approach-related surgical morbidity through use of smaller skin incisions and targeted muscle dissection but do not eliminate the potential for serious and life-threatening complications.

98. Cervical total disc arthroplasty is indicated for treatment of radiculopathy and/or myelopathy due to neural compression caused by a disc herniation or spondylosis between C3–C7, which is refractory to non-operative treatment.

99. Lumbar total disc arthroplasty is indicated for treatment of isolated discogenic low back pain (usually without radiculopathy) caused by degenerative disc disease between L3 and S1 without instability and which is refractory to non-operative treatment.

100. The ideal graft material for spine fusion is cost-effective, osteoinductive, osteogenic, biocompatible and possesses favorable structural properties analogous to autogenous bone.

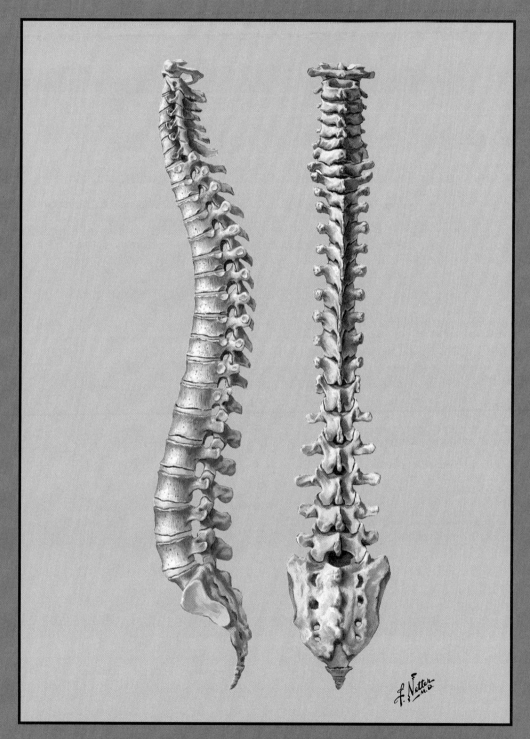

CLINICALLY RELEVANT ANATOMY OF THE CERVICAL REGION

Vincent J. Devlin, MD, and Darren L. Bergey, MD

OSTEOLOGY

1. Describe the bony landmarks of the occiput.

The occiput forms the posterior osseous covering for the cerebellum. The **foramen magnum** is the opening through which the spinal cord joins the brainstem. The anterior border of the foramen magnum is termed the **basion** (clivus), and the posterior border is termed the **opisthion**. The **inion** or **external occipital protuberance** is the midline region of the occiput where bone is greatest in thickness. The **superior and inferior nuchal lines** extend laterally from the inion. The transverse sinus is located in close proximity to the inion (Fig. 1-1). The occipital area in the midline below the inion is the ideal location for screw insertion for occipitocervical fixation as it is the thickest portion of the occiput.

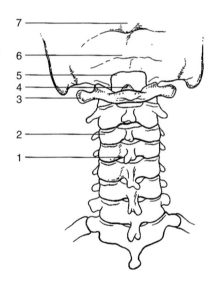
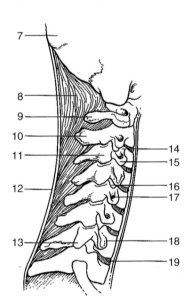

Figure 1-1. Posterior and lateral views of the occiput and cervical spine showing the basic bony anatomy. 1, Spinous process; 2, Lateral articular process or lateral mass; 3, Transverse process of C1; 4, Odontoid process of C2; 5, Foramen magnum; 6, Inferior nuchal line; 7, Inion; 8, Ligamentum nuchae; 9, Posterior arch of C1; 10, Spinous process of C2; 11, Lateral mass; 12, Supraspinous ligament; 13, Lateral articular process; 14, Uncinate process; 15, Anterior tubercle of transverse process; 16, Neural foramen; 17, Transverse foramen; 18, Carotid tubercle; 19, Intervertebral disc. (From An HS, Simpson JM. Surgery of the Cervical Spine. Baltimore: Williams & Wilkins; 1998, with permission.)

2. What is meant by typical and atypical cervical vertebrae?

C3, C4, C5, and C6 are defined as typical cervical vertebrae because they share common structural characteristics. In contrast, C1 (atlas), C2 (axis), and C7 (vertebra prominens) possess unique structural and functional features and are therefore termed atypical cervical vertebrae.

3. Describe a typical cervical vertebra.

The components of a typical cervical vertebra (C3–C6) include an **anterior body** and a **posterior arch** formed by **lamina** and **pedicles**. The lamina blend into the **lateral mass**, which comprises the bony region between the superior and inferior articular processes. The paired superior and inferior articular processes form the **facet joint**. The **uncovertebral (neurocentral) joints** are bony ridges that extend upward from the lateral margin of the superior surface of the vertebral body. The **intervertebral foramina** protect the exiting spinal nerves and are located behind the vertebral bodies between the pedicles of adjacent vertebra. The **transverse processes** of the lower cervical spine are directed anterolaterally and composed of an anterior costal element and a posterior transverse element. The **transverse foramen**, located at the base of the transverse process, permits passage of the vertebral artery. The **spinous process** originates in the midsagittal plane at the junction of the lamina and is bifid between C2 to C6 (Fig. 1-2).

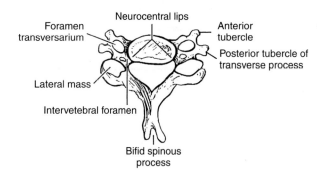

Figure 1-2. Typical cervical vertebra (superior view). (From Raiszadeh K, Spivak JM. Spine. In: Spivak JM, DiCesare PE, Feldman DS, et al., editors. Orthopaedics: A Study Guide. New York: McGraw-Hill; 1999, p. 63–72, with permission.)

4. What are the distinguishing features of C1 (atlas)?

The ring-like atlas (C1) is unique because during development its body fuses with the axis (C2) to form the odontoid process. Thus, the atlas has no body. It is composed of two thick, load-bearing lateral masses, with concave superior and inferior articular facets. Connecting these facets are a relatively straight, short anterior arch and a longer, curved posterior arch. The anterior ring has an articular facet on its posterior aspect for articulation with the dens. The posterior ring has a grove on its posterior-superior surface for the vertebral artery. The weakest point of the ring is at the narrowed areas where the anterior and posterior arches connect to the lateral masses (location of a Jefferson fracture). The transverse process of the atlas has a single tubercle, which protrudes laterally and can be palpated in the space between the tip of the mastoid process and the ramus of the mandible (Fig. 1-3).

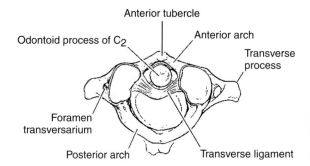

Figure 1-3. Atlas (superior view). (From Raiszadeh K, Spivak JM. Spine. In: Spivak JM, DiCesare PE, Feldman DS, et al., editors. Orthopaedics: A Study Guide. New York: McGraw-Hill; 1999, p. 63–72, with permission.)

5. What are the distinguishing features of C2 (axis)?

The axis (C2) receives its name from its **odontoid process (dens)**, which forms the axis of rotation for motion through the atlantoaxial joint (Fig. 1-4). The dens is a bony process extending cranial from the body of C2, formed from the embryologic body of the atlas (C1). The dens has an anterior hyaline articular surface for articulation with the anterior arch of C1 as well as a posterior articular surface for articulation with the transverse ligament. The C2 superior articular processes are located anterior and lateral to the spinal canal while the C2 inferior articular processes are located posterior and lateral to the spinal canal. The articular processes are connected by the **pars interarticularis**.

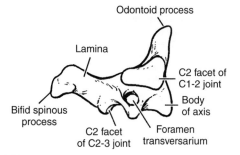

Figure 1-4. Axis (lateral view). (From Raiszadeh K, Spivak JM. Spine. In: Spivak JM, DiCesare PE, Feldman DS, et al., editors. Orthopaedics: A Study Guide. New York: McGraw-Hill; 1999. p. 63–72, with permission.)

Hyperflexion or hyperextension injuries may subject the axis to shear stresses, resulting in a fracture through the pars region (termed a *hangman's fracture*). The **C2 pedicle** is defined as that portion of the C2 vertebra connecting the dorsal elements with the vertebral body. This is a narrow area between the vertebral body and the pars articularis. The atlantodens interval is the space between the hyaline cartilage surfaces of the anterior tubercle of the atlas and the anterior dens. Normal adult and childhood measurements are 3 mm and 5 mm, respectively.

6. What are the distinguishing features of C7 (vertebra prominens)?

The unique anatomic features of the C7 vertebra reflect its location as the transitional vertebra at the cervicothoracic junction:

- Long non-bifid spinous process, which provides a useful landmark
- Its foramen transversarium usually contains vertebral veins but usually does not contain the vertebral artery, which generally enters the cervical spine at the C6 level
- The C7 transverse process is large in size and possesses only a posterior tubercle
- The C7 lateral mass is the thinnest lateral mass in the cervical spine
- The inferior articular process of C7 is oriented in a relatively perpendicular direction (like a thoracic facet joint)

ARTICULATIONS, LIGAMENTS, AND DISCS

7. Describe how normal range of motion is distributed across the cervical region.

Facet joint orientation, bony architecture, intervertebral discs, uncovertebral joints, and ligaments all play a role in determining range of motion at various levels of the cervical spine. Approximately 50% of cervical flexion-extension occurs at the occiput–C1 level. Approximately 50% of cervical rotation occurs at the C1–C2 level. Lesser amounts of flexion-extension, rotation, and lateral bending occur segmentally between C2 and C7.

8. What are the key anatomic features of the atlantooccipital (O–C1) articulation?

The atlantooccipital joints are synovial joints comprised of the convex occipital condyles that articulate with the concave lateral masses of the atlas. Motion at the O–C1 segment is restricted primarily to flexion-extension due to bony and ligamentous constraints and absence of an intervertebral disc. The most important ligaments are the paired alar ligaments (extend from the tip of the dens to the medial aspect of each occipital condyle and restrict rotation of the occiput on the dens). The tectorial membrane is also important (continuous with the posterior longitudinal ligament and extends from the posterior body of C2 to the anterior foramen magnum and occiput). Less important ligaments include the anterior and posterior atlanto-occipital membrane, the O–C1 joint capsules, and the apical ligament (Fig. 1-5).

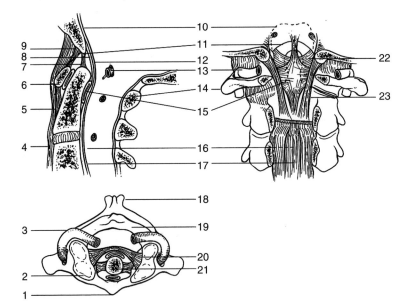

Figure 1-5. Ligamentous and bony anatomy of the upper cervical region. 1, Anterior tubercle; 2, Superior articular facet; 3, Vertebral artery; 4, Anterior longitudinal ligament; 5, Anterior atlas–axis membrane; 6, Anterior arch of atlas; 7, Apical ligament; 8, Vertical cruciform ligament; 9, Anterior atlas–occipital membrane; 10, Attachment of tectorial membrane; 11, Anterior edge of foramen magnum; 12, Tectorial membrane; 13, Vertebral artery; 14, Atlas; 15, Transverse ligament; 16, Origin of tectorial membrane; 17, Posterior longitudinal ligament; 18, Spinous process (axis); 19, Atlas; 20, Transverse ligament; 21, Dens (odontoid process); 22, Alar ligament; 23, Deep tectorial membrane. (From An HS, Simpson JM. Surgery of the Cervical Spine. Baltimore: Williams & Wilkins; 1998, with permission.)

9. What are the key anatomic features of the atlantoaxial (C1–C2) articulation?

The atlantoaxial articulation is composed of three synovial joints—paired lateral mass articulations and a central articulation between the dens and the anterior C1 arch and transverse ligament (see Fig. 1-5). The primary motion at the atlantoaxial joint is rotation with approximately 50% of rotation of the cervical spine occurring at the C1–C2 joints. The approximation of the odontoid against the anterior arch of C1 resists translation of C1 relative to C2.

The transverse atlantal ligament, the major stabilizer at the C1–C2 level, attaches to the medial aspect of the lateral masses of the atlas (see Fig. 1-5). This ligament has a wide middle portion where it articulates with the posterior surface of the dens. Superior and inferior longitudinal fasciculi extend to insert on the anterior foramen magnum and the posterior body of the axis respectively. These structures are collectively named the cruciform ligament. This ligament holds the dens firmly against the anterior arch of the atlas. Other important ligaments attaching to C2 include:

- *Anterior atlantoaxial ligament*—continuous with the anterior longitudinal ligament in the lower cervical spine
- *Posterior atlantoaxial ligament*—continuous with the ligamentum flavum in the subaxial spine

- *Apical ligament*—extends from the tip of the dens to the foramen magnum
- *Alar ligaments*—extend from the lateral dens and attach to the medial border of the occipital condyles

10. Name the arrangement of ligaments at the craniovertebral junction as the spine is sectioned in an anterior to posterior direction.
1. Anterior atlantooccipital membrane (continuous with anterior longitudinal ligament)
2. Apical ligament (extends from tip of the dens to anterior edge of foramen magnum)
3. Alar ligaments (extend from the tip of the dens to the medial aspect of each occipital condyle)
4. Cruciform ligament
5. Tectorial membrane (continuous with the posterior longitudinal ligament)
6. Posterior atlantooccipital membrane (continuous with the ligamentum flavum)

11. Describe the ligament anatomy of the subaxial spine.
The major ligaments of the subaxial cervical spine are:
- *Anterior longitudinal ligament (ALL)*—this strong ligament extends from the body of the axis to the sacrum binding the anterior aspect of the vertebral bodies and intervertebral discs together. It resists hyperextension of the spine and gives stability to the anterior aspect of the disc space. It is continuous with anterior atlanto-occipital membrane.
- *Posterior longitudinal ligament (PLL)*—this is a weaker ligament, which extends from the axis to the sacrum. It is thicker and wider in the cervical spine than in the thoracolumbar segments. It serves to protect from hyperflexion injury and reinforces the intervertebral discs from herniation. It is continuous with tectorial membrane.
- *Ligamentum flavum*—this structure may be considered to be a segmental ligament which attaches to adjacent lamina. This structure attaches to the ventral aspect of the superior lamina and the dorsal aspect of the inferior lamina. Laterally, the ligamentum flavum is in continuity with the facet capsules.
- *Interspinous and supraspinous ligaments*—these ligaments lie between or dorsal to the spinous processes, respectively. The supraspinous ligament is in continuity with the ligamentum nuchae, which runs from C7 to the occiput and acts as a posterior tension band to maintain an upright neck posture.

12. Describe the articulations between vertebrae in the subaxial cervical spine (C3–C7).
The anatomy of the lower cervical spine (C3–C7) can be described in terms of a functional spinal unit consisting of two adjacent vertebrae, an intervertebral disc, and related ligaments and joint capsules. The anterior elements include the vertebral body and intervening intervertebral disc. Paired lateral columns consist of pedicles, lateral masses, and facet joints. The posterior structures include the laminae, spinous processes, and posterior ligamentous complex. Various theories have conceptualized the functional anatomy of the cervical spine in terms of a columnar structure. (Fig. 1-6).

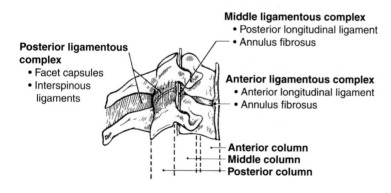

Middle ligamentous complex
- Posterior longitudinal ligament
- Annulus fibrosus

Posterior ligamentous complex
- Facet capsules
- Interspinous ligaments

Anterior ligamentous complex
- Anterior longitudinal ligament
- Annulus fibrosus

Anterior column
Middle column
Posterior column

Figure 1-6. Components of the three columns of the cervical spine. (From Stauffer ES, MacMillan M. Fractures and dislocations of the cervical spine. In: Rockwood CA, Green DP, Bucholz RW, et al., editors. Fractures in Adults, vol. 2. 4th ed. Philadelphia: Lippincott-Raven; 1996, p. 1473–1628, with permission.)

13. What are the unique features of the subaxial cervical facet joints?
At each cervical level (C3–C7) there are paired superior and inferior articular processes. The superior articular process is positioned anterior and inferior to the inferior articular process of the adjacent cranial vertebra. These articulations are covered with hyaline cartilage and form synovial zygapophyseal (facet or Z) joints. The orientation of the facet joints is a major factor in the range of motion of the cervical spine. The typical cervical facet joints are oriented 45° in the sagittal plane and 0° in the coronal plane. These are the most horizontally oriented regional facet joints in the spinal column. Laxity of the joint capsule permits sliding motion to occur and explains why unilateral or bilateral dislocation without fracture may occur. The orientation of these facets allows flexion and extension, lateral bending, and rotation of the lower cervical spine. Flexion and extension are greatest at the C5–C6 and C6–C7 levels. This has been postulated to be responsible for the relatively high incidence of degenerative changes noted at these two cervical levels.

14. What are the uncovertebral joints (joints of Luschka)?

When viewed anteriorly, the lateral margin of the superior surface of each subaxial cervical vertebral body extends cranially as a bony process called the **uncinate process**. These processes articulate with a reciprocal convex area on the inferolateral aspect of the next cranial vertebral body. This articulation is named the uncovertebral joint or neurocentral joint of Luschka. It is believed to form as a degenerative cleft in the lateral part of the annulus fibrosus. The uncinate process, unique to the cervical spine, serves as a "rail" to limit lateral translation or bending and as a guiding mechanism for flexion and extension.

15. What are the components of the intervertebral disc?

Each intervertebral disc is composed of a central gel-like nucleus pulposus surrounded by a peripheral fibrocartilaginous annulus fibrosus. The endplates of the vertebral bodies are lined with hyaline cartilage and bind the disc to the vertebral body. The **annulus fibrosus** (predominantly type 1 collagen) attaches to the cartilaginous endplates via collagen fibers, which run obliquely at a 30° angle to the surface of the vertebral body and in a direction opposite to the annular fibers of the adjacent layer. The **nucleus pulposus** is composed primarily of glycosaminoglycans and type 2 collagen, which have the capacity to bind large amounts of water. In a normal healthy disc, loads acting on the disc are transferred to the annulus by swelling pressure (intradiscal pressure) generated by the nucleus. With aging, biochemical changes occur which limit the ability of the nucleus pulposus to bind water. Dehydration of the nucleus and increased loading of the annulus occurs. Fissuring and disruption of the annulus develops and migration of nuclear material through the annulus may occur.

NEURAL ANATOMY

16. Describe the cross-sectional anatomy of the spinal cord and the location and function of the major spinal cord tracts.

A cross-sectional view of the spinal cord demonstrates a central butterfly-shaped area of gray matter and peripheral white matter (Fig. 1-7). The central gray matter contains the neural cell bodies. The peripheral white matter contains the axon tracts. Tracts are named with their point of origin first. Ascending (afferent tracts) carry impulses toward the brain, whereas the descending (efferent tracts) carry nerve signals away from the brain. The axon tracts may receive and transmit signals to the same side of the body (uncrossed tracts) or may transmit or receive signals from the opposite side (crossed tracts). The major spinal tracts important to the clinician include:

- **Corticospinal tracts:** The lateral corticospinal tract (pyramidal tract) is a descending tract located in lateral portion of the cord that transmits ipsilateral motor function. The tract is anatomically organized with efferent motor axons to the cervical area located medially and sacral efferent axons located laterally. The anterior corticospinal tract is a crossed tract, which facilitates skilled movements.
- **Spinothalamic tracts:** Ascending tracts located in the anterior and lateral portion of the cord that transmit sensations of pain and temperature. Light touch sensation is carried primarily in the ventral spinothalamic tract. These tracts cross shortly after entering the spinal cord and therefore transmit sensations from the contralateral side of the body.
- **Dorsal column tracts:** Ascending tracts that convey proprioception, vibration, and discriminative touch sensation from the ipsilateral side of the body.

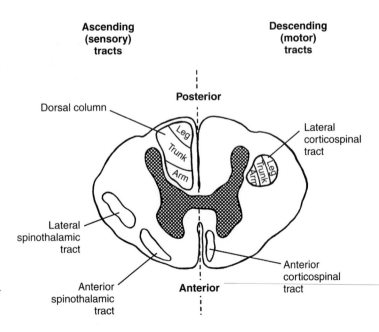

Figure 1-7. Cross-sectional anatomy of the spinal cord. (From Raiszadeh K, Spivak JM. Spine. In: Spivak JM, DiCesare PE, Feldman DS, et al., editors. Orthopaedics: A Study Guide. New York: McGraw-Hill; 1999, p. 63–72, with permission.)

17. How many spinal nerves exit from the spinal cord?

The spinal nerves exit from the spinal cord in pairs. There are 31 pairs of spinal nerves: 8 cervical, 12 thoracic, 5 lumbar, 5 sacral, and 1 coccygeal nerve root pairs.

18. What structures contribute to the formation of a spinal nerve? What are the branches of a spinal nerve?

Each spinal nerve (Fig. 1-8) is composed of both sensory and motor fibers. The collection of sensory fibers is termed the **dorsal root**. The cell bodies for these sensory fibers are located in the **dorsal root ganglion**. The collection of motor fibers is termed the **ventral or anterior root**. A typical spinal nerve is formed by the union of the dorsal and ventral roots, which occurs just distal to the dorsal root ganglion. The spinal nerve becomes covered by a common dural sheath and gives off the following branches:

- **Dorsal ramus:** Provides sensation to the medial two-thirds of the back, the facet joint capsules, and the posterior ligaments. The dorsal ramus also innervates the deep spinal musculature.
- **Ventral ramus:** Supplies all other skin and muscles of the body. In the cervical and lumbar regions the ventral rami form plexuses (cervical plexus, brachial plexus, lumbar plexus, lumbosacral plexus). In the thoracic levels ventral rami form the intercostal nerve.
- **Recurrent meningeal branch (sinuvertebral nerve):** Innervates the periosteum of the posterior aspect of the vertebral body, basivertebral and epidural veins, epidural adipose tissue, posterior annulus and posterior longitudinal ligament, and anterior aspect of the dural sac.

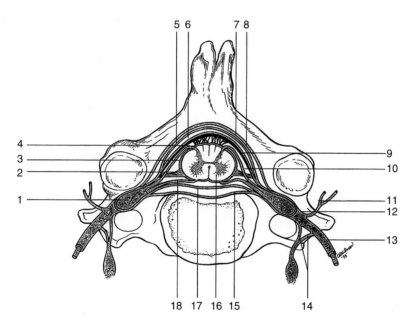

Figure 1-8. Components of a spinal nerve. 1, Spinal ganglion; 2, Dentate ligament; 3, Pia mater; 4, Dorsal root of spinal nerve; 5, Dura mater; 6, Subdural space; 7, Periosteum; 8, Epidural space; 9, Arachnoid membrane; 10, Subarachnoid space; 11, Dorsal ramus; 12, Spinal nerve; 13, Ventral ramus of spinal nerve; 14, Ramus communicans; 15, Periosteum; 16, Medulla spinalis; 17, Dura mater; 18, Ventral root of spinal nerve. (From An HS, Simpson JM. Surgery of the Cervical Spine. Baltimore: Williams & Wilkins; 1998, with permission.)

19. Describe the relationship of the exiting spinal nerve to the numbered vertebral segment for each spinal region.

In the cervical region there are eight cervical nerve roots and only seven cervical vertebra. The first seven cervical nerve roots exit the spinal canal above their numbered vertebra. For example, the C1 root exits the spinal column between the occiput and the atlas (C1). The C5 nerve root passes above the pedicle of the C5 vertebra and occupies the intervertebral foramen between C4 and C5. The C8 nerve root is atypical because it does not have a corresponding vertebral element and exits below the C7 pedicle and occupies the intervertebral foramen between C7 and T1. In the thoracic and lumbar spine, the nerve roots exit the spinal canal by passing below the pedicle of their named vertebra. The T12 nerve passes below the T12 pedicle and exits the neural foramen between T12 and L1. The L4 nerve root passes beneath the L4 pedicle and exits the neural foramen between L4 and L5.

20. How does the course of the recurrent laryngeal nerve differ from left to right?

The recurrent laryngeal nerve originates from the vagus nerve and enters the tracheoesophageal groove. On the right side, it passes around the subclavian artery; on the left side, it passes under the aortic arch. Anterior surgical exposure of the lower cervical spine must be carefully performed in the interval between the tracheoesophageal sheath and carotid sheath to avoid injury to this nerve. The right recurrent laryngeal nerve is at greater risk of injury than the left nerve during surgical exposure because it reaches the tracheoesophageal groove at a higher cervical level and has a less predictable course

VASCULAR STRUCTURES OF THE CERVICAL REGION

21. Describe the course of vertebral artery.

The vertebral artery (Fig. 1-9) is the first branch off the subclavian artery and provides the major blood supply to the cervical spinal cord, nerve roots, and vertebrae. It can be divided into **four segments**. During its first segment, the vertebral artery passes from the subclavian artery anterior to C7 to enter the C6 transverse foramen. In the second segment, it continues from the C6 transverse foramina along its course through the cephalad transverse foramina to the level of the atlas. During its course it lies lateral to the vertebral body and in front of the lateral mass. During its upward course between C6 and C2, the vertebral artery gradually shifts to an anterior and medial position, thereby placing the artery at greater risk of injury during anterior decompressive procedures at the upper cervical levels. In its third segment, the artery exits C1 and curves around the C1 lateral mass, running medially along the cranial surface of the posterior arch of C1 in its sulcus, before passing through the atlantooccipital membrane and entering the foramen magnum. The artery stays at least 12 mm lateral from midline of C1, making this a safe zone for dissection. In its fourth segment, the vertebral artery joins the contralateral vertebral artery to form the basilar artery.

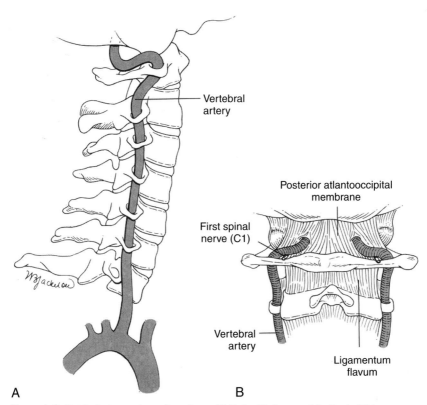

Vertebral artery

Posterior atlantooccipital membrane

First spinal nerve (C1)

Vertebral artery

Ligamentum flavum

A   B

Figure 1-9. Vertebral artery anatomy. (From Emery SE, Boden SD. Surgery of the Cervical Spine. Philadelphia: Saunders; 2003, p. 6.)

22. Describe the blood supply to the spinal cord.

The anterior median spinal artery and the two posterior spinal arteries supply the spinal cord. The anterior spinal artery supplies 85% of the blood supply to the cord throughout its length. Radicular or segmental arteries feed these arteries. In the cervical spine, the majority of radicular arteries arise from the vertebral artery. These arteries enter the spinal canal through the intervertebral foramina and divide into anterior and posterior radicular arteries. The most consistent radicular artery in the cervical spine is located at the C5–C6 level. On average, there are 8 radicular feeders to the anterior spinal artery and 12 to the posterior spinal arteries throughout the length of the spinal cord. The basilar artery also anastomoses with the anterior spinal artery, variably supplying the cord to the fourth cervical level.

FASCIA AND MUSCULATURE OF THE CERVICAL SPINE

23. What are the fascial layers of the anterior neck?
The fascial layers of the neck consist of a superficial layer and a deep layer. The superficial layer of the cervical fascia surrounds the platysma muscle. The deep cervical fascia consists of three layers:
1. **Superficial layer:** Surrounds the sternocleidomastoid and trapezius muscles.
2. **Middle layer:** Consists of the pretracheal fascia, which surrounds the strap muscles, trachea, esophagus, and thyroid gland. This layer is continuous with the lateral margin of the carotid sheath.
3. **Deep layer:** Consists of the prevertebral fascia, which surrounds the posterior paracervical and anterior prevertebral musculature.

24. Describe the muscular triangles of the neck.
The anterior aspect of the neck is divided by the sternocleidomastoid into an anterior and posterior triangle. The **posterior triangle** borders are the trapezius, sternocleidomastoid, and middle third of the clavicle. The inferior belly of the omohyoid further divides this space into subclavian (lower) and occipital (upper) triangles. The **anterior triangle** is bounded by the sternocleidomastoid, the anterior median line of the neck, and lower border of the mandible. It is further subdivided into the submandibular, carotid, and muscular triangles. The posterior belly of the digastric separates the carotid from the submandibular triangles. The superior belly of the omohyoid separates the carotid from the muscular triangles (Fig. 1-10). The standard anterior approach to the midcervical spine is done through the muscular triangle.

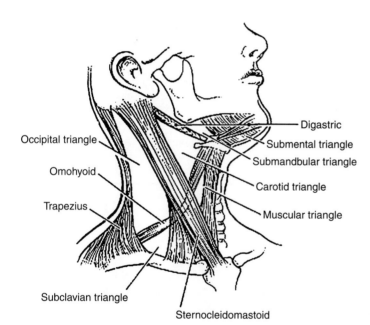

Figure 1-10. Muscular triangles of the neck. (From Raiszadeh K, Spivak JM. Spine. In: Spivak JM, DiCesare PE, Feldman DS, et al., editors. Orthopaedics: A Study Guide. New York: McGraw-Hill; 1999, p. 63–72, with permission.)

25. Name the muscles most commonly encountered during anterior and posterior cervical spine procedures.
- *Anterior muscles:* platysma, sternocleidomastoid, strap muscles of the larynx, omohyoid, longus colli
- *Posterior muscles:* superficial layer—trapezius; middle layer—splenius capitis, splenius cervicis; deep layer—semispinalis capitis, longissimus capitis; muscles of the suboccipital triangle—rectus capitis posterior major and minor, obliquus capitis superior and inferior

Key Points

1. Appreciation of the distinguishing features of typical (C3–C6) and atypical (C1, C2, C7) vertebrae is important for understanding cervical spinal anatomy.
2. There are eight pairs of cervical nerve roots but only seven cervical vertebra.

Websites

1. Spinal cord, topographical and functional anatomy:
   http://emedicine.medscape.com/article/1148570-overview
2. See cervical spine anatomy:
   http://www.orthogate.org/patient-education/cervical-spine/cervical-spine-anatomy.html
3. See spine anatomy index section:
   http://www.spineuniverse.com/displayarticle.php/article1297.html

BIBLIOGRAPHY

1. Aebi M, Arlet V, Webb JK. AO Spine Manual. New York: Thieme; 2007.
2. An HS, Simpson JM. Surgery of the Cervical Spine. Baltimore: William & Wilkins; 1998.
3. Clark CR. The Cervical Spine. 4th ed. Philadelphia: Lippincott; 2005.
4. Emery SE, Boden SD. Surgery of the Cervical Spine. Philadelphia: Saunders; 2003.
5. Kim DH, Henn JS, Vaccaro AR, et al., editors. Surgical Anatomy and Techniques to the Spine. Philadelphia: Saunders; 2006.

CHAPTER 2

CLINICALLY RELEVANT ANATOMY OF THE THORACIC REGION

Vincent J. Devlin, MD, and Darren L. Bergey, MD

OSTEOLOGY

1. Describe a typical thoracic vertebra.

T1 and T10 to T12 possess unique anatomic features due to their transitional location between the cervicothoracic and thoracolumbar spinal regions, respectively. Thoracic vertebra two through nine are termed typical thoracic vertebra because they share common structural features (Fig. 2-1):

- **Vertebral body:** Heart-shaped in cross-section. Posterior vertebral height exceeds anterior vertebral height, resulting in a wedged shape of the vertebral body when viewed in the lateral plane. This wedge shape is responsible for the kyphotic alignment in the thoracic region.
- **Costovertebral articulations:** The lateral surface of the vertebral body has both superior and inferior facets for articulation with adjacent ribs.
- **Costotransverse articulation:** Rib articulation with the transverse process of vertebra.
- **Vertebral arch:** formed by lamina and two pedicles, which support seven processes:
  Spinous process (1)
  Transverse processes (2)
  Superior facets (2)
  Inferior facets (2)

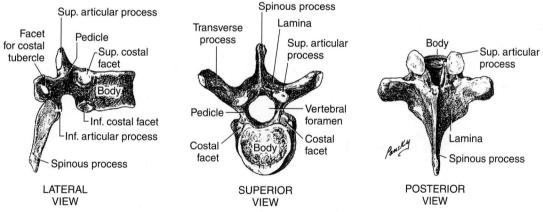

Figure 2-1. Typical thoracic vertebra. (From Pansky B: Review of Gross Anatomy. 4th ed. New York, Macmillan, 1979, with permission.)

2. What are the unique anatomic features of the first thoracic vertebra?

T1 vertebral body dimensions resemble a cervical vertebra more closely than a typical thoracic vertebra. The T1 vertebral body possesses a well-developed superior vertebral notch. The T1 spinous process is very prominent and may be larger than the C7 spinous process. The first rib articulates with T1 vertebral body via a costal facet.

3. What are the unique anatomic features of T10, T11, and T12?

- Lack of costotransverse articulations (T11 and T12)
- Ribs articulate with vertebral bodies and do not overlie the disc space
- Vertebral body dimensions increase and approximate lumbar vertebral dimensions
- Facet morphology transitions from thoracic to lumbar in function and appearance
- T12 transverse process consists of three separate projections

4. What anatomic relationships are useful in determining the level of a thoracic lesion on a thoracic spine radiograph?

The first rib attaches to the T1 vertebral body. The second rib attaches to the T2 vertebral body. The third rib articulates with both the second and third vertebral bodies and overlies the T2–T3 disc space. This latter pattern continues until the tenth vertebral body. The tenth, eleventh, and twelfth ribs articulate only with the vertebral body of the same number and do not overlie a disc space.

5. Describe the anatomy of the thoracic pedicles.

The paired pedicles arise from the posterior-superior aspect of the vertebral bodies. The superior-inferior pedicle diameter is consistently larger than the medial-lateral pedicle diameter. Pedicle widths are narrowest at the T4 to T6 levels, with medial-lateral pedicle diameter increasing both above (T1–T3) and below this region. The medial pedicle wall is two to three times thicker than the lateral pedicle wall across all levels of the thoracic spine. The medial angulation of the pedicle axis decreases from T1 to T12. The site for entry into the thoracic pedicle from a posterior spinal approach is in the region where the facet joint and transverse process intersect and varies slightly, depending on the specific thoracic level.

ARTICULATIONS, LIGAMENTS, AND DISCS

6. What anatomic structures provide articulations between the thoracic vertebral bodies? Between the vertebral arches?

The structures that provide articulations between the thoracic vertebral bodies are:
1. The anterior longitudinal ligament
2. Posterior longitudinal ligament
3. Intervertebral disc
   Five anatomic elements provide articulations between the adjacent vertebral arches:
1. Articular capsules: Thin capsules attach to the margins of the articular processes of adjacent vertebra.
2. Ligamentum flavum: Yellow elastic tissue that connects laminae of adjacent vertebrae and attaches to the ventral surface of lamina above and to the dorsal surface and superior margin of the lamina below.
3. Supraspinous ligaments: Strong fibrous cord that connects the tips of the spinous processes from C7 to sacrum.
4. Interspinous ligaments: Interconnect adjoining spinous processes. Attachment extends from base of each spinous process to the tip of the adjacent spinous process.
5. Intertransverse ligaments: Interconnect the transverse processes.
   The pattern described above continues in the lumbar region as well.

7. What are the two types of articulations between the ribs and the thoracic vertebra?

The two types of articulations between thoracic vertebra and ribs are costovertebral and costotransverse. The **costovertebral articulation** is the articulation between the head of the rib (costa) and the vertebral body. The articular capsule, radiate ligaments, and intraarticular ligaments stabilize this articulation.

The **costotransverse articulation** occurs between the neck and tubercle of the rib (costa) and the transverse process. The ligaments that stabilize this articulation include the superior and lateral costotransverse ligaments (Fig. 2-2). The T11 and T12 transverse processes do not articulate with their corresponding ribs.

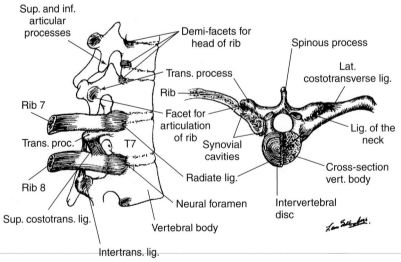

Figure 2-2. Extrinsic ligaments of the thoracic spine. (From Johnson RM, Murphy MJ, Southwick WD: Surgical approaches to the spine. In Herkowitz HN, Garfin SR, Balderston RA, et al., editors. Rothman-Simeone The Spine. 4th ed. Philadelphia: Saunders; 1999, with permission.)

8. Describe the anatomy of the facet joints in the thoracic region.

The facet joints are located at the junction of the vertebral arch and the pedicle. The paired superior articular processes face posterolaterally, and the paired inferior articular processes face anteromedially. The thoracic facets are oriented 60° in the sagittal plane and approximate the coronal plane with a slight medial inclination (20°). Flexion-extension is minimal at T1–T2 and maximal at T12–L1, where facet joint orientation transitions to a lumbar pattern. Axial rotation is maximal at T1–T2 and minimal at the thoracolumbar junction. Lateral bending is more equally distributed across the thoracic region. Motion of the thoracic vertebrae is limited by anatomic constraints, including the rib cage and its attachment to the sternum, ligamentous attachments at the costovertebral and costotransverse joints, narrow intervertebral discs, and overlap of the adjacent lamina and spinous processes.

NEURAL ANATOMY

9. Describe the contents of the spinal canal in relation to the vertebral segments in the thoracic and thoracolumbar spinal regions.

During childhood, the distal end of the spinal cord migrates proximally due to more rapid longitudinal growth of the osseous spinal elements and generally reaches the lower border of L1 by 8 years of age. In the adult, the spinal cord occupies the upper four-fifths of the vertebral canal. It extends from the foramen magnum and ends distally at the level of the L1–L2 disc space (Fig. 2-3). The inferior region of the spinal cord, named the **conus medullaris**, is characterized by

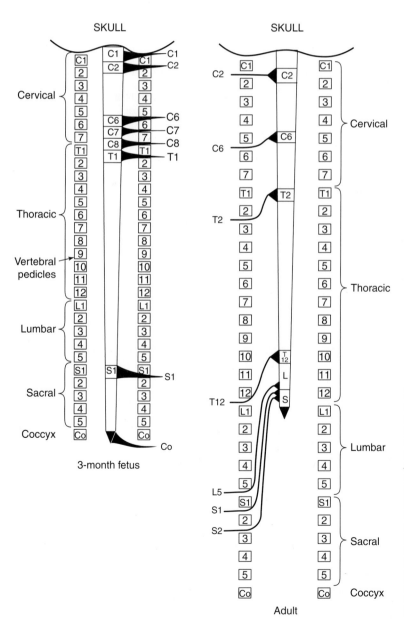

Figure 2-3. Relationships between vertebral levels, spinal nerves, and spinal cord segments in the three month fetus and adult (dorsal view). In the fetus, the spinal cord extends the full length of the vertebral column, the spinal cord segments and vertebral levels correspond, and the spinal nerves course horizontally to exit from their intervertebral foramina. However, in adults the spinal cord ends at the L1–L2 vertebral level, only upper cervical cord segments correspond to their vertebral levels with lower cord segments at progressively higher vertebral levels, and lower spinal nerves pursue increasingly more vertical courses. (From Shenk C: Functional and clinical anatomy of the spine. Phys Med Rehabil State Art Rev 1995;9(3):577.)

the presence of both spinal cord and spinal nerve elements within the dural sac. Distal to the termination of the spinal cord (conus), the lumbar, sacral, and coccygeal roots continue as a leash of nerves termed the **cauda equina**. The **filum terminale** is a fibrous band extending from the distal tip of the spinal cord and attaching to the first coccygeal segment. Enlargements of the spinal cord between C3 and T2 (cervical enlargement) and between T9 and T12 (lumbar enlargement) correlate with the origin of nerves supplying the upper and lower extremities. The spinal cord possesses a trilayered covering termed **meninges** and consisting of dura mater, arachnoid mater, and pia mater. The dura mater is the only meningeal layer that extends the entire length of the vertebral column from the foramen magnum to S2. Between the arachnoid and pia mater is the subarachnoid space, a large interval filled with cerebrospinal fluid.

10. Describe the anatomy of thoracic spinal nerves.

Dorsal (sensory) and ventral (motor) roots originate from the spinal cord to form a spinal nerve in the region of the intervertebral foramen. The spinal nerve divides in the region of the foramen into a posterior (dorsal) primary ramus (innervates the posterior aspect of the associated dermatome and myotome) and an anterior (ventral) primary ramus, which continues as the intercostal nerve. The thoracic spinal nerves are numbered according to the pedicle of the vertebral body that the nerve contacts. For example, the T6 nerve root passes beneath the pedicle of the T6 vertebra.

11. Describe the contents of a thoracic neurovascular bundle.

Each neurovascular bundle is composed of a posterior intercostal vein, posterior intercostal artery, and anterior primary ramus of a spinal nerve (mnemonic: **VAN** superior to inferior). The neurovascular bundle lies immediately below the inferior edge of each rib in the neurovascular groove.

12. Where is the thoracic portion of the sympathetic trunk located?

The thoracic portion of the sympathetic trunk is located along the anterior surface of the rib head. The sympathetic chain or trunk consists of a series of **ganglia** that extend from the skull to the coccyx. There are two sympathetic chains, located on each of the anterolateral surfaces of the vertebral column. Each consists of approximately 22 ganglia. Each ganglia gives off a **gray ramus communicans** that joins the adjacent spinal nerve just distal to the junction of the anterior and posterior roots.

13. What is the innervation of the diaphragm?

Innervation of the diaphragm is provided by the phrenic nerve, which originates from the C2 to C4 segments. Because the diaphragm receives its innervation and blood supply centrally, it can be incised and retracted from its insertion along the thoracic wall to permit surgical exposure of the thoracolumbar vertebral bodies without compromising its neurovascular supply.

VASCULAR STRUCTURES

14. Describe the vascular supply of the thoracic spinal cord.

As in the cervical region, single anterior and paired posterior spinal arteries supply the spinal cord. Radicular (segmental) arteries enter the vertebral canal through the intervertebral foramina and divide into anterior and posterior radicular arteries, which supply the anterior and posterior spinal arteries, respectively. The majority of the vascular supply of the spinal cord is supplied by the anterior spinal artery. In the thoracic spine, the radicular arteries originate from intercostal arteries. The intercostal arteries arise segmentally from the aorta and course along the undersurface of each rib. Segmental arteries supplying the spine branch off from the intercostal arteries at the level of the costotransverse joint and enter the spinal canal via the intervertebral foramen. The number of radicular arteries is variable throughout the thoracic spine. The **radicular artery of Adamkiewicz** is the largest of these segmental arteries and is a major blood supply to the lower spinal cord. It originates from the left side in 80% of people and usually accompanies the ventral root of thoracic nerves 9, 10, or 11. However, it may originate anywhere from T5 to L5. Careful dissection near the intervertebral foramen and costotransverse joints is necessary to prevent injury to this vascular supply.

15. Explain the *watershed region* and *critical supply zone* of the thoracic spinal cord.

The blood supply of the spinal cord is not entirely longitudinal. It is partly transverse and dependent on a series of radicular arteries that feed into the anterior and posterior spinal arteries at various levels. The limited number of radicular arteries supplying the thoracic spinal cord results in a less abundant blood supply in this region compared with the cervical and lumbar regions. Branches of the anterior median spinal artery supply the ventral two-thirds of the spinal cord, whereas branches of the posterior spinal arteries supply the dorsal third of the cord. The region where these two zones meet is relatively poorly vascularized and is termed the **watershed region**. The zone located between the fourth and ninth thoracic vertebrae has the least profuse blood supply and is termed the **critical vascular zone of the spinal cord**. This region corresponds to the narrowest region of the spinal canal. Interference with circulation in this zone during surgery is most likely to result in paraplegia. Surgical dissection in this region of the spine requires added care. Segmental vertebral arteries should be divided as far anteriorly as possible. Dissection in the region of the intervertebral foramen and costotransverse joint should be limited, and electrocautery should not be used in this area.

FASCIA, MUSCULATURE, AND RELATED STRUCTURES

16. Describe the anatomy of the posterior muscles of the thoracic and lumbar spinal regions.

The anatomy of the posterior muscles of the back is confusing because of the multiple overlapping muscle layers and the fact that distinct muscle layers are not seen during posterior surgical dissection. It is helpful to divide the back muscles into three main layers:

- **Superficial layer:** Consists of muscles that attach the upper extremity to the spine. The trapezius (innervated by spinal accessory nerve), latissimus dorsi (thoracodorsal nerve), and levator scapulae muscles (dorsal scapular nerve) overlie the deeper rhomboid major and minor muscles (dorsal scapular nerve) (Fig. 2-4).
- **Intermediate layer:** Consists of the serratus posterior superior and inferior. These muscles of accessory respiration are innervated by the anterior primary rami of segmental nerves (Fig. 2-5).
- **Deep layer:** Consists of the intrinsic back muscles, which function in movement of the spinal column. These muscles are innervated by the posterior rami of segmental thoracic and lumbar spinal nerves (Fig. 2-6).

The muscles comprising this deep layer can be subdivided into three layers:
1. Splenius capitis and splenius cervicis
2. Sacrospinalis (erector spinae), subdivided into spinalis, longissimus, and iliocostalis portions in the thoracic region
3. Semispinalis, multifidi, rotatores, intertransversari, and interspinales

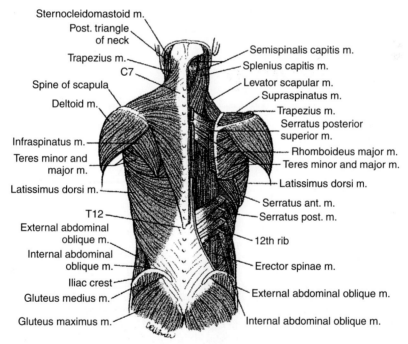

Figure 2-4. Superficial layer of the muscles of the back. (From An HS. Principles and Techniques of Spine Surgery. Baltimore: Williams & Wilkins; 1998, with permission.)

17. Why should a spine specialist understand the anatomy of the thoracic cavity?

There are two important reasons why a spine specialist must possess a working knowledge of anatomy and pathology relating to the thoracic cavity. First, extraspinal pathologic processes within the thoracic cavity (e.g. aneurysm, malignancy) may mimic the symptoms of thoracic spinal disorders. Second, surgical treatment of many types of spinal problems involves exposure of the anterior aspect of the thoracic spine.

The thoracic cavity contains the pleural cavities and the mediastinum. The pleural cavities contain the lungs. The **mediastinum** is the intrapleural region that separates the pleural cavities and is subdivided into four regions that contain the following structures:
1. Superior mediastinum (thymus gland, aortic arch and great vessels, trachea, bronchi, esophagus)
2. Anterior mediastinum (thymus gland, sternopericardial ligaments)
3. Middle mediastinum (pericardial cavity and related structures)
4. Posterior mediastinum (esophagus, thoracic aorta, inferior vena cava, azygos system, sympathetic chain)

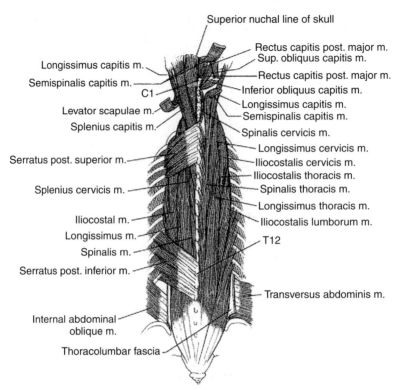

Superior nuchal line of skull

Rectus capitis post. major m.
Sup. obliquus capitis m.

Longissimus capitis m.
Semispinalis capitis m.
C1

Rectus capitis post. major m.
Inferior obliquus capitis m.
Longissimus capitis m.
Semispinalis capitis m.

Levator scapulae m.
Splenius capitis m.

Spinalis cervicis m.

Serratus post. superior m.

Longissimus cervicis m.
Iliocostalis cervicis m.
Iliocostalis thoracis m.
Spinalis thoracis m.

Splenius cervicis m.

Longissimus thoracis m.
Iliocostalis lumborum m.

Iliocostal m.
Longissimus m.
Spinalis m.

T12

Serratus post. inferior m.

Transversus abdominis m.

Internal abdominal oblique m.

Thoracolumbar fascia

Figure 2-5. Intermediate layer of the muscles of the back. (From An HS: Principles and Techniques of Spine Surgery. Baltimore: Williams & Wilkins; 1998, with permission.)

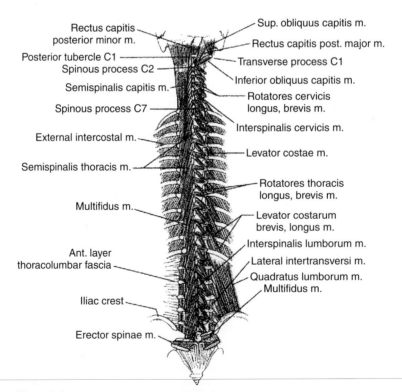

Rectus capitis posterior minor m.

Sup. obliquus capitis m.
Rectus capitis post. major m.

Posterior tubercle C1
Spinous process C2

Transverse process C1

Semispinalis capitis m.

Inferior obliquus capitis m.
Rotatores cervicis longus, brevis m.

Spinous process C7

Interspinalis cervicis m.

External intercostal m.

Levator costae m.

Semispinalis thoracis m.

Rotatores thoracis longus, brevis m.

Multifidus m.

Levator costarum brevis, longus m.
Interspinalis lumborum m.

Ant. layer thoracolumbar fascia

Lateral intertransversi m.
Quadratus lumborum m.
Multifidus m.

Iliac crest

Erector spinae m.

Figure 2-6. Deep layer of the muscles of the back. (From An HS: Principles and Techniques of Spine Surgery. Baltimore: Williams & Wilkins; 1998, with permission.)

Key Points

1. Thoracic spinal motion is limited by multiple anatomic constraints.
2. The blood supply to the thoracic spinal cord is less abundant than in the cervical or lumbar region.
3. The third through ninth ribs overlap the posterolateral aspect of the adjacent disc space.
4. The intercostal artery and vein are located along the inferior surface of the rib.

Websites

1. See spine anatomy index section, thoracic spine:
   http://www.spineuniverse.com/displayarticle.php/article1397.html
2. See thoracic spine anatomy:
   http://www.orthogate.org/patient-education/thoracic-spine/thoracic-spine-anatomy.html

BIBLIOGRAPHY

1. An HS: Principles and Techniques of Spine Surgery. Baltimore: Williams & Wilkins; 1998.
2. Herkowitz HN, Garfin SR, Eismont FJ, et al. Rothman-Simeone The Spine. 5th ed. Philadelphia: Saunders; 2006.
3. Hoppenfeld S, deBoer P: Surgical Exposure of the Spine and Extremities. 3rd ed. Philadelphia, Lippincott; 2003.
4. Schneck C: Functional and clinical anatomy of the spine. Phys Med Rehabil State Art Rev 1995;9(3).
5. Vaccaro AR: Spine Anatomy. In Garfin SR, Vaccaro AR, editors. Orthopaedic Knowledge Update—Spine, Vol. 1. Rosemont, IL: American Academy of Orthopaedic Surgeons; 1997, pp 3–18.

CLINICALLY RELEVANT ANATOMY OF THE LUMBAR AND SACRAL REGION

3 CHAPTER

Vincent J. Devlin, MD, and Darren L. Bergey, MD

OSTEOLOGY

1. Describe a typical lumbar vertebra.

The vertebral bodies are kidney-shaped with the transverse diameter exceeding the anteroposterior diameter (Fig. 3-1). The vertebral body may be divided by an imaginary line passing beneath the pedicles into an upper and lower half. Six posterior elements attach to each lumbar vertebral body. Three structures lie above this imaginary line (superior facet, transverse process, pedicle) and three structures lie below (lamina, inferior facet, spinous process). The pars interarticularis is located along this imaginary dividing line. The transverse processes are long and thin except at L5, where they are thick and broad and possess ligamentous attachments to the pelvis. The five lumbar vertebral bodies increase in size from L1 to L5.

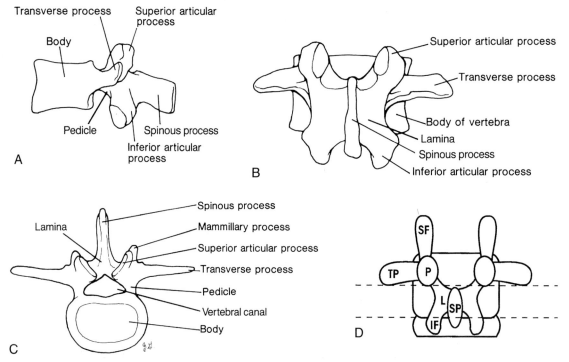

Figure 3-1. Typical lumbar vertebra. Lateral (**A**), posterior (**B**), and cranial (**C**) views. **D**, The six named posterior elements: SF, superior facet; IF, inferior facet; L, lamina; SP, spinous process; P, pedicle; TP, transverse process. (A, B, C, From Borenstein DG, Wiesel SW, Boden SD. Anatomy and biomechanics of the lumbosacral spine. In: Low Back Pain: Medical Diagnosis and Comprehensive Management. 2nd ed. Philadelphia: Saunders; 1995. D, From McCulloch JA, Young PH. Musculoskeletal and neuroanatomy of the lumbar spine. In: McCulloch JA, Young PH, editors. Essentials of Spinal Microsurgery. Philadelphia: Lippincott-Raven; 1998. p. 250.)

2. What region of the posterior elements of the spine is prone to failure when subjected to repetitive stress?

The **pars interarticularis** is an area of force concentration and is subject to failure with repetitive stress. A defect in the bony arch in this location is termed **spondylolysis**. The pars interarticularis is the concave lateral part of the lamina that connects the superior and inferior articular facets. The medial border of the pedicle is in line with the lateral border of the pars between L1 and L4. At L5 the lateral border of the pars marks the middle of the pedicle.

3. Describe the anatomy of the lumbar pedicles.

The pedicle connects the posterior spinal elements (lamina, transverse processes, facets) to the vertebral body. Lumbar pedicle widths are largest at L5 (18 mm) and smallest in the upper lumbar region (6 mm at L1). The pedicles in the lumbar spine possess a slight medial inclination, which decreases from distal to proximal levels. The pedicles angle medially 30° at L5 and 12° at L1.

4. What are the key anatomic features of the sacrum?

The sacrum is a triangular structure formed from five fused sacral vertebrae (Fig. 3-2). The S1 pedicle is the largest pedicle in the body. The **sacral promontory** is the upper anterior border of the first sacral body. The **sacral ala** (lateral sacral masses) are bilateral structures formed by the union of vestigial costal elements and the transverse processes of the first sacral vertebra. Four intervertebral foramina give rise to ventral and dorsal sacral foramina. The median sacral crest is formed by the fused spinous processes of the sacral vertebrae. The sacral cornu (horn) is formed by the S5 pedicles and is a landmark for locating the sacral hiatus. The **sacral hiatus** is an opening in the dorsal aspect of the sacrum due to absence of the fourth and fifth sacral lamina.

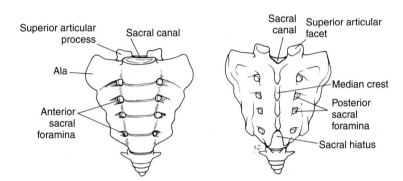

Figure 3-2. Anatomy of the sacrum and coccyx. Left, Anterior view. Right, Posterior view. (From Borenstein DG, Wiesel SW, Boden SD. Anatomy and biomechanics of the lumbosacral spine. In: Low Back Pain: Medical Diagnosis and Comprehensive Management. 2nd ed. Philadelphia: Saunders; 1995.)

5. What are the key anatomic features of the coccyx?

The coccyx is a triangular structure that consists of three, four, or five fused coccygeal vertebrae. The coccyx articulates with the inferior aspect of the sacrum.

ARTICULATIONS, LIGAMENTS, AND DISCS

6. Describe the anatomy of the facet joints of the lumbar spine.

The inferior articular process of the cephalad vertebra is located posterior and medial to the superior articular process of the caudad vertebrae. The upper and mid-lumbar facet joints are oriented in the sagittal plane. This orientation allows significant flexion-extension motion in this region but restricts rotation and lateral bending. The facets joints at L5–S1 oriented in the coronal plane, thereby permitting rotation and resisting anterior-posterior translation.

7. What anatomic structures provide articulations between the lumbar vertebral bodies? Between the vertebral arches? Between L5 and the sacrum?

The structures that provide articulations between the lumbar vertebral bodies are the same as in the thoracic region: (1) anterior longitudinal ligament, (2) posterior longitudinal ligament, and (3) intervertebral disc.

The anatomic elements that provide articulations between the adjacent lumbar vertebral arches are the same as in the thoracic region: (1) articular capsules, (2) ligamentum flavum, (3) supraspinous ligaments, (4) interspinous ligaments, and (5) intertransverse ligaments.

Specialized ligaments connect L5 and the sacrum:
1. Iliolumbar ligament, which arises from the anteroinferior part of the transverse process of the fifth lumbar vertebra and passes inferiorly and laterally to blend with the anterior sacroiliac ligament at the base of the sacrum as well as the inner surface of the ilium.
2. Lumbosacral ligament, which spans from the transverse processes of L5 to the anterosuperior region of the sacral ala and body of S1.

8. Describe the alignment of the normal lumbar spine in reference to the sagittal plane.

The normal lumbar spine is lordotic (sagittal curve with its convexity located anteriorly). Normal lumbar lordosis (L1–S1) ranges from 30° to 80° with a mean lordosis of 50°. Normal lumbar lordosis generally begins at L1–L2 and gradually increases at each distal level toward the sacrum. The apex of lumbar lordosis is normally located at the L3–L4 disc space. Normally two-thirds of lumbar lordosis is located between L4 and S1 and one-third between L1 and L3 (Fig. 3-3).

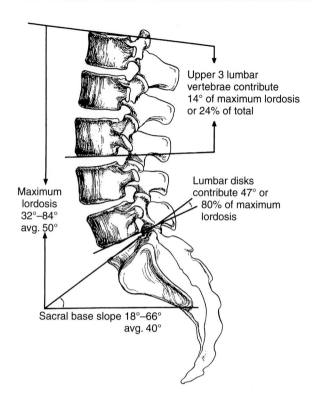

Figure 3-3. Sagittal alignment of the lumbar spine. Average maximum lordosis as measured from superior L1 to superior S1. (Reproduced with permission from DeWald RL: Revision surgery for spinal deformity. In: Eilert RE, editor. Instructional Course Lectures, vol. 41. Rosemont, IL: American Academy of Orthopaedic Surgeons; 1992.)

9. **Which contributes more significantly to the normal sagittal alignment of the lumbar region—the shape of the intervertebral discs or the shape of the vertebral bodies?**

Eighty percent of lumbar lordosis occurs through wedging of the intervertebral discs, and 20% is due to the lordotic shape of the vertebral bodies. The wedge shape of the lowest three discs is responsible for one-half of total lumbar lordosis.

10. **Describe the anatomy of the sacroiliac joint.**

The sacroiliac joint is a small, auricular-shaped synovial articulation located between the sacrum and ilium (Fig. 3-4). The complex curvature and strong supporting ligaments of the sacroiliac joint minimizes motion. Ligamentous support is provided by anterior sacroiliac ligaments, interosseous ligaments, and posterior sacroiliac ligaments (most important). Other supporting ligaments in this region include the sacrospinous ligaments (ischial spine to sacrum) and sacrotuberous ligaments (ischial tuberosity to sacrum). Functionally, the sacrum and pelvis can be considered as one vertebra (pelvic vertebra), which functions as an intercalary bone between the trunk and lower extremities.

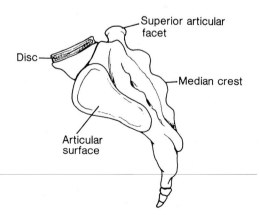

Figure 3-4. Lateral view showing the articular surface of the sacrum. (From Borenstein DG, Wiesel SW, Boden SD. Anatomy and biomechanics of the lumbosacral spine. In: Low Back Pain: Medical Diagnosis and Comprehensive Management. 2nd ed. Philadelphia: Saunders; 1995.)

NEURAL ANATOMY

11. Describe the contents of the spinal canal in the lumbar region.
The spinal cord terminates as the conus medullaris at the L1–L2 level in adults. Below this level, the **cauda equina**, composed of all lumbar, sacral, and coccygeal nerve roots, occupies the thecal sac. The lumbar nerves exit the intervertebral foramen under the pedicle of the same numbered vertebral body.

12. What structures comprise a lumbar anatomic segment?
The vertebral body, its associated posterior elements, and the disc below comprise an anatomic segment.

13. What is the difference between an exiting nerve root and a traversing nerve root?
Each lumbar anatomic segment can be considered to possess an exiting nerve root and a traversing nerve root. The **exiting nerve root** passes medial to the pedicle of the anatomic segment. The **traversing nerve root** passes through the anatomic segment to exit beneath the pedicle of the next caudal anatomic segment. For example, the exiting nerve root of the fifth anatomic segment is L5. This nerve passes beneath the L5 pedicle and exits the anatomic segment through the neural foramen of the L5 anatomic segment. The S1 nerve is the traversing nerve root and passes over the L5–S1 disc to exit beneath the pedicle of S1, which is located in the next caudad anatomic segment (Fig. 3-5).

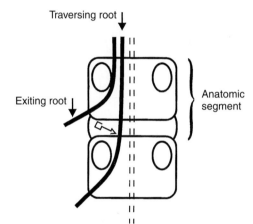

Figure 3-5. The exiting nerve root and traversing root(s) of an unnumbered spinal segment. At the open arrow, the traversing nerve root becomes the exiting root of the anatomic segment below. (From McCulloch JA, Young PH. Musculoskeletal and neuroanatomy of the lumbar spine. In: McCulloch JA, Young PH, editors. Essentials of Spinal Microsurgery. Philadelphia: Lippincott-Raven; 1998. p. 249–327, http://www.lww.com.)

14. What analogy is commonly used to localize spinal pathology from caudad to cephalad within a lumbar anatomic segment?
The analogy of a house with three floors is most commonly used to localize spinal pathology (Fig. 3-6A). The first story of the anatomical house is the level of the disc space. The second story is the level of the neural foramen and lower vertebral body. The third story is the level of the pedicle and includes the upper vertebral body and transverse process.

15. How is the spinal canal subdivided into zones from medial to lateral to precisely locate compressive spinal pathology within a lumbar anatomic segment?
Neural compression may affect the thecal sac, nerve roots, or both structures. **Central spinal stenosis** refers to neural compression in the region of the spinal canal occupied by the thecal sac. **Lateral stenosis** involves the nerve root and its location is described in terms of **three zones** (see Fig. 3-6B and C) using the pedicle as a reference point. **Zone 1** (also called the subarticular zone, entrance zone, or lateral recess) includes the area of the spinal canal medial to the pedicle and under the superior articular process. **Zone 2** (also called the foraminal or midzone) includes the portion of the nerve root canal located below the pedicle. **Zone 3** (also called the extraforaminal or exit zone) refers to the nerve root in the area lateral to the pedicle.

16. An L4–L5 posterolateral disc protrusion located entirely within zone 1 results in compression of which nerve root?
The most common location for a disc protrusion is *posterolateral*. This type of disc herniation impinges on the traversing nerve root of the L4 anatomic segment. This nerve is the L5 nerve root.

17. An L4–L5 lateral disc protrusion located entirely within zone 3 results in compression of which nerve root?
This describes the so-called *far lateral* disc protrusion. This type of disc protrusion impinges on the exiting nerve of the L4 anatomic segment. This nerve is the L4 nerve root.

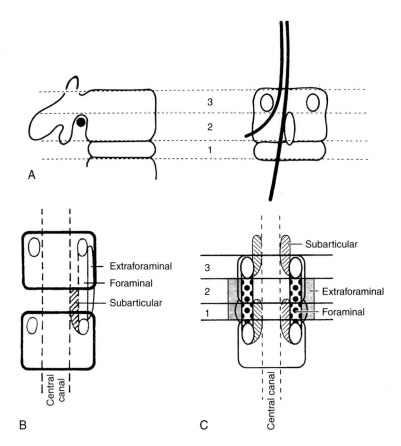

Figure 3-6. **A,** Conceptualization of the lumbar anatomic segment as a house. **B and C,** Zone concept of the lumbar spinal canal. (From McCullough JA. Microdiscectomy: The gold standard for minimally invasive disc surgery. Spine State Art Rev 1997;11(2):382.)

18. Describe the location and significance of the superior hypogastric plexus. What can happen if it is injured during exposure of the anterior aspect of the spine?

The superior hypogastric plexus is the sympathetic plexus located along the anterior prevertebral tissues in the region of the L5 vertebral body and anterior L5–S1 disc. This sympathetic plexus is at risk during anterior exposure of the L5–S1 disc space. Disruption of this plexus in men may cause retrograde ejaculation and sterility. Erection would not be affected because it is a parasympathetically mediated function (Fig. 3-7).

VASCULAR STRUCTURES

19. Describe the blood supply to the lumbar vertebral bodies.

Each lumbar vertebra is supplied by paired lumbar segmental arteries. The segmental arteries for L1 to L4 arise from the aorta. The origin of the segmental arteries for L5 is variable and may arise from the iliolumbar artery, fourth lumbar segmental artery, middle sacral artery or aorta. As the segmental artery courses toward the intervertebral foramen, it divides into three branches:

1. The anterior branch (supplies the abdominal wall)
2. The posterior branch (supplies paraspinous muscles and facets)
3. The foraminal branch (supplies the spinal canal and its contents)

The venous supply of the lumbar region parallels the arterial supply. It consists of an anterior and posterior ladder-like configuration of valveless veins that communicate with the inferior vena cava.

20. What is Batson's plexus?

Batson's plexus is a system of valveless veins located within the spinal canal and around the vertebral body. It is an alternate route for venous drainage to the inferior vena cava system. Because it is a valveless system, any increase in abdominal pressure (e.g. secondary to positioning during spine surgery) can cause blood to flow preferentially toward the spinal canal and surrounding bony structures. Batson's plexus also serves as a preferential pathway for metastatic tumor and infection spread to the lumbar spine.

21. Where is the bifurcation of the aorta and vena cava located?

Most commonly, the bifurcation is over the L4–L5 disc or L5 vertebral body (Fig. 3-7).

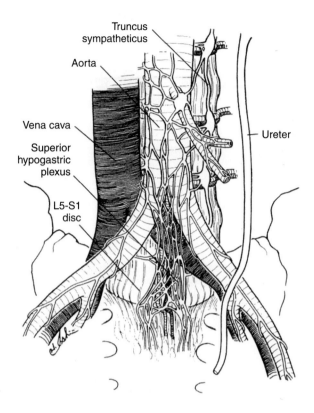

Figure 3-7. Bifurcation of aorta and vena cava in relation to the spine. The superior hypogastric plexus. (From Hanley EN, Delmarter RB, McCulloch JA. Surgical indications and techniques. In: Wiesel SW, Weinstein JN, Herkowitz H. The Lumbar Spine. 2nd ed. Philadelphia: Saunders; 1996. p. 492–524.)

22. What is the significance of the iliolumbar vein?

The iliolumbar vein is a branch of the iliac vein that limits mobilization of the iliac vessels off of the anterior aspect of the spine (Fig. 3-8). This vein should be carefully isolated and securely ligated before attempting to expose the anterior aspect of the spine at the L4–L5 disc level.

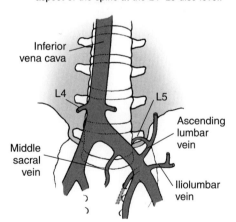

Figure 3-8. Anatomy of the iliolumbar vein and environs. (From Canale ST, Beaty J. Campbell's Operative Orthopedics. 11th ed. Philadelphia: Mosby; 2007.)

FASCIA, MUSCULATURE, AND RELATED STRUCTURES

23. Why should a spine specialist be knowledgeable about the anatomy of the abdominal and pelvic cavities?

There are many important reasons why a spine specialist must possess a working knowledge of anatomy and pathology relating to the abdominal and pelvic cavities. Extraspinal pathologic processes within the abdominal and pelvic cavities (e.g. aneurysm, infection, tumor) may mimic the symptoms of lumbosacral spinal disorders. Surgical treatment of many spinal problems involves exposure of the anterior lumbar spine and/or sacrum through a variety of surgical approaches. Evaluation of complications after spinal procedures requires assessment not only of the vertebral and neural structures but also of vascular and visceral structures (e.g. bladder, intestines, spleen, kidney, ureter).

24. What muscles of the posterior abdominal wall cover the anterolateral aspect of the lumbar spine?

Psoas major and minor. These muscles originate from the lumbar transverse processes, intervertebral discs, and vertebral bodies and insert distally at the lesser trochanter and iliopectineal region, respectively. They must be mobilized during exposure of the anterior lumbar spine, taking care to avoid nerves that cross the psoas muscles (genitofemoral nerve, sympathetic trunk) as well as the lumbar plexus, which passes within the substance of these muscles.

Key Points

1. Lumbar lordosis begins at L1–L2 and gradually increases at each distal level toward the sacrum.
2. Six named posterior osseous elements attach to each lumbar vertebral body.
3. The spinal cord normally terminates as the conus medullaris at the L1– L2 level in adults.
4. The cauda equina occupies the thecal sac distal to the L1–L2 level in adults.

Websites

1. See lumbar spine anatomy: http://www.orthogate.org/patient-education/lumbar-spine/lumbar-spine-anatomy.html
2. See spine anatomy section, lumbar spine: http://www.spineuniverse.com/displayarticle.php/article1286.html

BIBLIOGRAPHY

1. Borenstein DG, Wiesel SW, Boden SD: Anatomy and biomechanics of the lumbosacral spine. In: Low Back Pain: Medical Diagnosis and Comprehensive Management, 2nd ed. Philadelphia: Saunders; 1995, pp 1–16.
2. Daubs, MD: Anterior lumbar interbody fusion. In Vaccaro AR, Baron EM, editors. Spine Surgery. Philadelphia: Saunders; 2008, pp 391–400.
3. Herkowitz HN, Dvorak J, Bell G, et al., editors. The Lumbar Spine. 3rd ed. Philadelphia: Lippincott; 2004.
4. Herkowitz HN, Garfin SR, Eismont FJ, editors. The Spine. 5 ed., Philadelphia: Saunders; 2006.
5. McCulloch JA, Young PH Musculoskeletal and Neuroanatomy of the Lumbar Spine. In: McCulloch JA, Young PH, editors. Essentials of Spinal Microsurgery. Philadelphia: Lippincott-Raven; 1998, p. 249–327.
6. Wong DA: Open lumbar microscopic discectomy. In: Vaccaro AR, Albert TJ, editors. Spine Surgery, Tricks of the Trade. 2nd ed. New York: Thieme; 2009, p. 119–121.

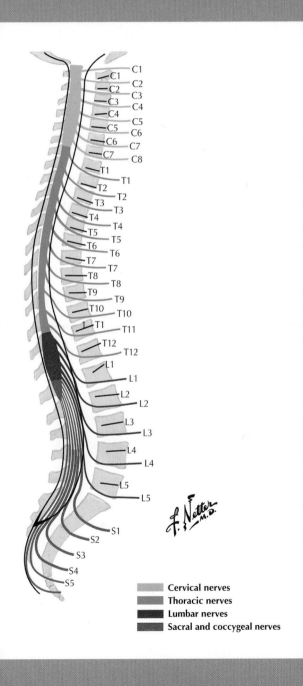

C1
C1
C2
C2
C3
C3
C4
C4
C5
C5
C6
C6
C7
C7
C8
T1
T1
T2
T2
T3
T3
T4
T4
T5
T5
T6
T6
T7
T7
T8
T8
T9
T9
T10
T10
T11
T11
T12
T12
L1
L1
L2
L2
L3
L3
L4
L4
L5
L5
S1
S2
S3
S4
S5

F. Netter
M.D.

Cervical nerves
Thoracic nerves
Lumbar nerves
Sacral and coccygeal nerves

4 CHAPTER

EVALUATION OF CERVICAL SPINE DISORDERS

Winston Fong, MD, Scott C. McGovern, MD, and Jeffrey C. Wang, MD

1. How does the evaluation of a patient with a spine complaint begin?
A complete history and physical exam are performed. The purpose of the history and physical exam is to make a provisional diagnosis that is confirmed by subsequent testing as medically indicated.

2. What are some of the key elements to assess in the history of any spine problem?
- *Chief complaint:* Pain, numbness, weakness, gait difficulty, deformity
- *Symptom onset:* Acute vs. insidious
- *Symptom duration:* Acute vs. chronic
- *Pain location:* Is the pain primarily axial neck pain, arm pain, or a combination of both?
- Pain quality and character: Sharp vs. dull, radiating vs. stabbing vs. aching
- *Temporal relationship of pain:* Night pain, rest pain, or constant unremitting pain suggests systemic problems such as tumor or infection. Morning stiffness that improves throughout the day suggests an arthritic problem or an inflammatory arthropathy.
- *Relation of symptoms to neck position:* Increased arm pain with neck extension suggests nerve root impingement.
- *Aggravating and alleviating factors:* Is the pain mechanical (activity-related) or nonmechanical (not influenced by activity) in nature?
- *Family history:* Inquire about diseases such as ankylosing spondylitis or rheumatoid arthritis.
- *Concurrent medical illness:* Diabetes, peripheral neuropathy, peripheral vascular disease
- *Systemic symptoms:* A history of weight loss or fever suggests possibility of tumor or infection.
- *Functional impairment:* Loss of balance, gait or balance difficulty, loss of fine motor skills in the hands
- *Prior treatment:* Include both nonoperative and operative measures.
- *Negative prognostic factors:* Pending litigation, Workers' Compensation claim

3. What disorders should be considered in the differential diagnosis of neck/arm pain?
- *Degenerative spinal disorders:* discogenic pain, radiculopathy, myeloradiculopathy, myelopathy
- *Soft tissue disorders:* sprains, myofascial pain syndromes, fibromyalgia, whiplash syndrome
- *Inflammatory disorders:* rheumatoid arthritis, ankylosing spondylitis
- *Infections:* discitis, osteomyelitis
- *Tumors:* metastatic vs. primary tumors
- *Intraspinal disorders:* tumors, syrinx
- *Systemic disorders with referred pain:* angina, apical lung tumors (Pancoast tumor)
- *Shoulder and elbow pathology:* rotator cuff disorders, medial epicondylitis
- *Peripheral nerve entrapment syndromes:* radial, ulnar or median nerve entrapment, suprascapular neuropathy
- *Thoracic outlet syndrome*
- *Psychogenic pain*

4. What are the basic elements of an examination of any spinal region?
- Inspection
- Palpation
- Range of motion (ROM)
- Neurologic exam
- Evaluation of related areas (e.g. shoulder joints)

5. What should the examiner look for during inspection of the cervical region?
During the initial encounter, much can be learned from observing the patient. Assessment of gait and posture of the head and neck is important. Patients should undress to allow inspection of anatomically related areas, including the shoulders, back muscles, and scapulae.

6. What is the purpose of palpation during assessment of the cervical region?
To examine for tenderness and locate bone and soft tissue pathology. Specific areas of palpation correspond to specific levels of the spine:
- Hyoid bone C3
- Thyroid cartilage C4–C5
- Cricoid membrane C5–C6
- First cricoid ring C6

Spinous processes should be palpated and checked for alignment. If tenderness is detected, it should be noted whether the tenderness is focal or diffuse and the area of maximum tenderness should be localized.

7. In which three planes is ROM assessed for the cervical spine?
- Flexion/extension
- Right/left rotation
- Right/left bending

8. What is normal range of motion of the cervical spine?
- Flexion 45°
- Right/left bending 40°
- Extension 55°
- Right/left rotation 70°

Clinical estimates of motion are more commonly used in office practice. Flexion may be reproducibly measured using the distance from the chin to the sternum. For extension, the distance from the occiput to the dorsal spine may be helpful. Distances can be described in terms of fingerbreadths or measured with a ruler. The normal patient, for example, can nearly touch chin to chest in flexion and bring the occiput to within three or four fingerbreadths of the posterior aspect of the cervical spine in extension. Normal rotation permits the chin to align with the shoulder.

9. Describe an overview of the approach to the neurologic exam for cervical disorders.
The goal of examination is to determine the presence or absence of a neurologic deficit. If present, the level of a neurologic deficit is determined through testing of sensory, motor, and reflex function. The neurologic deficit may arise from pathology at the level of the spinal cord, nerve root, brachial plexus, or peripheral nerve. Examination of the cervical region is focused on the C5 to T1 nerve roots because they are responsible for supplying the upper extremities. For each nerve root, the examiner tests sensation, strength, and, if one exists, the appropriate reflex. (Table 4-1).

Table 4-1. Testing Sensory, Motor, and Reflex Function

LEVEL	SENSATION	MOTOR	REFLEX
C5	Lateral arm (axillary patch)	Deltoid	Biceps
C6	Lateral forearm	Wrist extension, biceps	Brachioradialis
C7	Middle finger	Triceps, wrist flexion, finger extension	Triceps
C8	Small finger	Finger flexion	None
T1	Medial arm	Interossei	None

10. How is sensation examined?
Sensation can be assessed using light touch, pin prick, vibration, position, temperature, and two-point discrimination. In assessing sensation, it is helpful to assess both sides of the body simultaneously. In this manner, sensation that is intact but subjectively decreased compared with the contralateral side can be easily documented.

11. What are the neural pathways tested during sensory examination?
- Spinothalamic tracts: transmit pain and temperature sensation
- Posterior columns: transmit two-point discrimination, position sense and vibratory sensation

12. How is motor strength graded? How are reflexes graded?

Table 4-2. Grading Motor Strength and Reflexes

MOTOR GRADE	FINDINGS
5	Full range of motion against full resistance
4	Full range of motion against reduced resistance
3	Full range of motion against gravity alone
2	Full range of motion with gravity eliminated
1	Evidence of contractility
0	No contractility
REFLEX GRADE	**FINDINGS**
4+	Hyperactive
3+	Brisk
2+	Normal
1+	Diminished
0	Absent

13. What is the significance of hyperreflexia? An absent reflex?

Hyperreflexia signifies an upper motor neuron lesion. An **absent reflex** implies pathology at the nerve root level(s) that transmits the reflex (in the lower motor neuron).

14. What is radiculopathy?

Radiculopathy is a lesion that causes irritation of a nerve root (lower motor neuron). It involves a specific spinal level with sparing of levels immediately above and below. The patient may report pain, a burning sensation, or numbness that radiates along the anatomic distribution of the affected nerve root. Other signs include severe atrophy of muscles and loss of the reflex supplied by the nerve. Severe radiculopathy may result in the flaccid paralysis of muscles supplied by the nerve.

15. What symptoms are associated with a C5–C6 disc herniation? Explain.

A disc herniation at the C5–C6 level causes compression of the C6 nerve root. Thus, weakness of biceps and wrist extensors, loss of the brachioradialis reflex, and diminished sensation of the radial forearm into the thumb and index finger are expected. As there are eight nerve roots and seven cervical vertebrae, the C1 nerve root exits above the C1 vertebra, the C2 nerve root below it, and so on. Thus, the C2 nerve root exits through its neuroforamen adjacent to the C1–C2 disc. The nerve root of the inferior vertebra of a given motion segment (e.g. C3 for C2–C3 disc, C7 for C6–C7 disc) is the one typically affected by a herniated disc.

16. Describe testing of the cervical nerve roots.

Table 4-3. Testing the Cervical Nerve Roots

ROOT	DISC LEVEL	SENSATION	REFLEX	MOTOR LEVEL
C3	C2–C3	Posterior neck to mastoid	None	Nonspecific
C4	C3–C4	Posterior neck to scapula ± anterior chest	None	Nonspecific
C5	C4–C5	Lateral arm (axillary patch) to elbow	± Biceps	Deltoid ± biceps
C6	C5–C6	Radial forearm to thumb	Biceps, brachioradialis	Biceps, wrist extensors
C7	C6–C7	Midradial forearm to middle finger ± index/ring fingers	Triceps	Triceps, wrist flexors, finger extensors
C8	C7–T1	Ulnar forearm to little and ring fingers	None	Finger flexors ± intrinsics
T1	T1–T2	Medial upper arm	None	Hand intrinsics

17. What provocative maneuvers are useful in examining a patient with a suspected radiculopathy? Explain how each is carried out.

Spurling's test (Fig. 4-1) is used to assess cervical nerve roots for stenosis as they exit the foramen. The patient's neck is extended and rotated toward the side of the pathology. Once the patient is in this position, a firm axial load is applied. If radicular symptoms are worsened by this maneuver, the test is said to be positive. It is thought that the extended and rotated position of the neck decreases the size of the foramen through which the nerve roots exit, thereby exacerbating symptoms when an axial load is applied.

- **Axial cervical compression test:** Arm pain that is elicited by axial compressive force on the skull and relieved by distractive force suggests that radicular symptoms are due to neuroforaminal narrowing
- **Valsalva maneuver:** This maneuver may increase radicular symptoms. Increased intraabdominal pressure simultaneously increases cerebrospinal pressure, which, in turn increases pressure about the cervical roots.
- **Shoulder abduction test:** Patients with cervical radiculopathy may obtain relief of radicular symptoms by holding the shoulder in an abducted position, which decreases tension in the nerve root (Fig. 4-2)

18. What is Adson's test?

Adson's test helps to distinguish thoracic outlet syndrome from cervical radiculopathy. The affected arm is abducted, extended, and externally rotated at the shoulder while the examiner palpates the radial pulse. The patient turns the head toward the affected side and takes a deep breath. In a positive Adson's test, the radial pulse on the affected side is diminished or lost during the maneuver. A positive test suggests thoracic outlet syndrome (compression of the subclavian artery by a cervical rib, scalenus anticus muscle, or other cause).

19. What is cervical myelopathy? How does it present?

Myelopathy is the manifestation of cervical spinal cord compression. **Cervical myelopathy** arising from spinal cord compression due to cervical degenerative changes is the most common cause of spinal cord dysfunction in patients

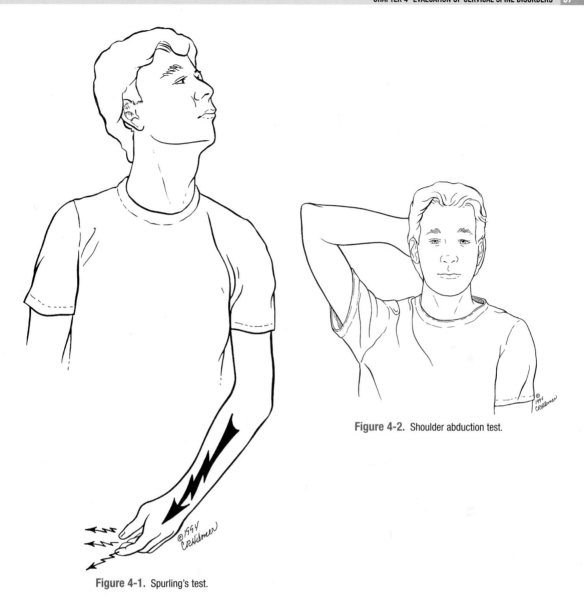

Figure 4-2. Shoulder abduction test.

Figure 4-1. Spurling's test.

older than 55 years. Vague sensory and motor symptoms involving the upper and/or lower extremities are common. **Lower motor neuron changes** occur at the level of the lesion, with atrophy of upper extremity muscles, especially the intrinsic muscles of the hands. **Upper motor neuron findings** are noted below the level of the lesion and may involve both the upper and lower extremities. Lower extremity spasticity and hyperreflexia are common. There may be relative hyperreflexia in the legs compared with the arms. Hoffmann's sign and Babinski's sign may be present. Additional findings may include neck pain and stiffness, spastic gait, loss of manual dexterity, or problems with sphincter control.

20. What reflexes or signs should be assessed when evaluating a patient with suspected cervical myelopathy? How are they evaluated?
- **Babinski's test** is performed by stroking the lateral plantar surface of the foot from the heel to the ball of the foot and curving medially across the heads of the metatarsals. It is termed positive if there is dorsiflexion of the big toe and fanning of the other toes (Fig. 4-3).
- **Hoffmann's sign** is performed on the patient's pronated hand while the examiner grasps the patient's middle finger (Fig. 4-4). The distal phalanx is forcefully and quickly flexed (almost a flicking motion) while the examiner observes the other fingers and thumb. The test is termed positive if flexion is seen in the thumb and/or index finger. Hoffmann's sign implies an upper motor lesion in the cervical spinal region as it is an upper extremity reflex. In contrast, pathology anywhere along the entire spinal cord can lead to a positive Babinski sign.

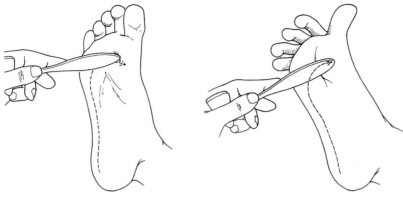

Figure 4-3. Babinski's test.

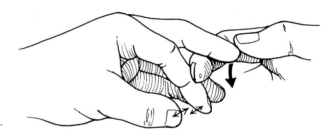

Figure 4-4. Hoffmann's sign.

- **Finger escape sign (finger adduction test)** is performed by asking the patient to hold all digits of the hand in an extended and adducted position. With myelopathy, the two ulnar digits will fall into flexion and abduction usually within 30 seconds.
- **Inverted radial reflex** is elicited by tapping the distal brachioradialis tendon. The reflex is present when the tapping produces spastic contraction of the finger flexors and suggests cord compression at the C5–C6 level.
- The **scapulohumeral reflex** is performed by tapping the tip of the spine of the scapula. If the scapula elevates or the humerus abducts, it is termed a hyperactive reflex suggesting upper motor neuron dysfunction above the C4 cord level.
- **Lhermitte's sign** is a generalized electric shock sensation that involves the upper and lower extremities as well as the trunk and it is elicited by extreme flexion or extension of the head and neck.
- **Clonus.** Upward thrusting of the ankle joint leads to rhythmic, repetitive motion of the ankle joint due to reflex contraction of the gastrocnemius-soleus complex due to lack of central nervous system inhibition.

Key Points

1. A comprehensive patient history and physical examination is the first step in diagnosis of a spine complaint.
2. A major goal of the initial patient evaluation is to differentiate common nonemergent spinal conditions such as acute nonspecific neck pain and cervical spondylosis from serious disorders such as spinal infections, spinal tumors, or cervical myelopathy.
3. Nonspinal pathology may mimic the symptoms of spinal disorders and must be considered in the differential diagnosis.

Websites

1. Cervical spine exam for neck and shoulder conditions (video): http://www.hss.edu/conditions_13653.asp
2. Provocative tests in cervical spine examination: historical basis and scientific analyses: http://www.painphysicianjournal.com/2003/april/2003;6;199-205.pdf
3. Demonstration of a patient with ankle clonus (video):
   http://en.wikipedia.org/wiki/Clonus

BIBLIOGRAPHY

1. Albert TJ: Physical Examination of the Spine. London, Thieme, 2004.
2. Hoppenfeld S: Physical Exam of the Spine and Extremities. 1st ed. New York: Appleton & Lange, 1976.
3. Macnab I, McCulloch J. Neck Ache and Shoulder Pain. 1st ed. Baltimore: Lippincott Williams & Wilkins; 1994.
4. Rainville J, Noto DJ, Jouve C, et al., Assessment of forearm pronation strength in C6 and C7 radiculopathies. Spine 2007; 32:72–75.
5. Scherping SC. History and Physical Examination. In: Frymoyer JW, Wiesel SW, editors. The Adult Spine: Principles and Practice. 3rd ed. Philadelphia: Lippincott Williams & Wilkins; 2004, p. 49–68.
6. Standaert CJ, Herring SA, Sinclair JD. Patient history and physical examination—cervical, thoracic and lumbar. In: Herkowitz HN, Garfin SR, Eismont FJ, et al., Rothman-Simeone The Spine. 5th ed. Philadelphia: Saunders; 2006, p. 169–186.
7. Zeidman SM. Evaluation of patients with cervical spine lesions. In: Clark CR, editor. The Cervical Spine. 4th ed. Philadelphia: Lippincott Williams & Wilkins; 2005, p. 149–165.

5 CHAPTER

EVALUATION OF THORACIC AND LUMBAR SPINE DISORDERS

Winston Fong, MD, Scott C. McGovern, MD, and Jeffrey C. Wang, MD

1. **What are the most common reasons for referral to evaluate the thoracic spinal region?**
   Pain and spinal deformity. The differential diagnosis of thoracic pain is extensive and includes both spinal and nonspinal etiologies. Spinal deformities (e.g., scoliosis, kyphosis) are generally painless in children but may become symptomatic in adult life.

2. **What are some common spinal causes of thoracic pain?**
   - *Degenerative disorders:* spondylosis, spinal stenosis, disc herniation
   - *Fracture:* traumatic, pathologic
   - *Neoplasm*
   - *Infection*
   - *Metabolic:* osteoporosis, osteomalacia
   - *Deformity:* kyphosis, scoliosis, trauma
   - *Neurogenic:* spinal cord neoplasm, arteriovenous malformation, inflammatory (e.g., herpes zoster)

3. **What are some common nonspinal causes of thoracic pain?**
   - **Intrathoracic**
     - Cardiovascular (angina, aortic aneurysm)
     - Pulmonary (pneumonia, carcinoma)
     - Mediastinal (mediastinal tumor)
   - **Intra-abdominal**
     - Hepatobiliary (hepatitis, cholecystitis)
     - Gastrointestinal (peptic ulcer, pancreatitis)
     - Retroperitoneal (pyelonephritis, aneurysm)
   - **Musculoskeletal**
     - Post-thoracotomy syndrome
     - Polymyalgia rheumatica
     - Fibromyalgia
     - Rib fractures
     - Intercostal neuralgia

4. **What should an examiner assess during inspection of the thoracic spinal region?**
   The patient should be undressed, and posture should be evaluated in both frontal and sagittal planes. Shoulder or rib asymmetry suggests the presence of scoliosis. A forward-bending test should be performed to permit assessment of rib cage and paravertebral muscle symmetry. If increased thoracic kyphosis is noted, it should be determined whether the kyphotic deformity is flexible or rigid. Leg lengths should be assessed. Look for any differences in height of the iliac crests. Note any skin markings such as café-au-lait spots, hairy patches, or birthmarks that may suggest occult neurologic or bony pathology.

5. **What is the usefulness of palpation during examination of the thoracic spine?**
   Palpation allows the examiner to locate specific areas of tenderness, which aids in localization of pathology. Tenderness over the paraspinal muscles should be differentiated from tenderness over the spinous processes.

6. **How precisely is range of motion assessed in the thoracic region?**
   Range of motion is limited in the thoracic region, and precise assessment is not an emphasized component of the thoracic spine exam. Nevertheless, thoracic range of motion is tested in all planes. Flexion-extension is limited by facet joint orientation, rib cage stability, and small intervertebral disc size. Thoracic rotation is typically greater than lumbar rotation due to facet orientation. Testing of lateral bending is relevant in assessing the flexibility of thoracic scoliosis. Asymmetric range of motion, especially in forward-bending, suggests the presence of a lesion that irritates neural structures, such as a tumor or disc herniation.

7. How is the neurologic examination of the thoracic spinal region performed?

Sensory levels are assessed by testing for light touch and pin-prick sensation. The exiting spinal nerves create band-like dermatomes (T4, nipple line; T7, xiphoid process; T10, umbilicus; T12, inguinal crease) (Fig. 5-1). **Motor function** is assessed by having the patient perform a partial sit-up and checking for asymmetry in the segmentally innervated rectus abdominis muscle. Weakness causes the umbilicus to move in the opposite direction and is termed **Beevor's sign.** Reflex testing consists of evaluation of the **superficial abdominal reflex.**

8. What is the superficial abdominal reflex? What does it signify?

The superficial abdominal reflex is an upper motor neuron reflex. It is performed by stroking one of the four abdominal quadrants. The umbilicus should move toward the quadrant that was stroked. The reflex should be symmetric from side to side. Asymmetry suggests intraspinal pathology (upper motor neuron lesion) and is assessed with magnetic resonance imaging (MRI) of the spine.

9. What findings in the history and physical exam suggest the presence of a thoracic disc herniation?

Clinically significant thoracic disc herniation is rare. It is difficult to reach an accurate diagnosis from history and physical exam alone. Thoracic disc herniations may cause thoracic axial pain, thoracic radicular pain, myelopathy, or a combination of these symptoms. Neurologic findings may include nonspecific lower extremity weakness, ataxia, spasticity, numbness, hyperreflexia, clonus, and bowel or bladder dysfunction.

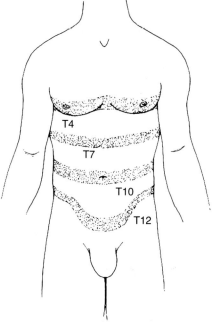

Figure 5-1. Dermatomes of the trunk.

LUMBAR SPINE EXAM

10. What pathologies should be considered in the differential diagnosis of low back pain?
- *Soft tissue disorders* (sprains, myofascial pain syndromes, fibromyalgia)
- *Degenerative spinal disorders* (disc herniation, spinal stenosis, facet joint arthritis)
- *Spinal instabilities* (e.g. spondylolisthesis)
- *Rheumatologic disorders* (rheumatoid arthritis, Reiter's syndrome, psoriatic arthritis, ankylosing spondylitis)
- *Infection* (bacterial, tuberculosis, fungal, HIV)
- *Tumor* (primary spine tumors, metastatic tumors)
- *Trauma* (fractures)
- *Metabolic disorders* (osteoporosis, osteomalacia, Paget's disease)
- *Hematologic disorders* (sickle-cell disease)
- *Systemic disorders with referred pain* (peptic ulcers, cholecystitis, pancreatitis, retrocecal appendicitis, dissecting abdominal aortic aneurysm, pelvic inflammatory disease, endometriosis, prostatitis)
- *Psychogenic pain*

11. Does the age of the patient with low back pain or lower extremity radicular symptoms suggest an etiology?

Yes. Although no diagnosis is unique to a single age group, some generalizations apply:
- **Less than 10 years:** consider spinal infection or tumor
- **10 to 25 years:** disorders involving repetitive loading and trauma: spondylolysis, isthmic spondylolisthesis, Scheuermann's disease, fractures, apophyseal ring injury
- **25 to 55 years:** annular tear, disc herniation, isthmic spondylolisthesis
- **Over 60 years:** spinal stenosis, degenerative spondylolisthesis, metastatic disease

12. What factors in the patient history should prompt the examiner to consider further diagnostic testing, such as laboratory tests or imaging studies, during evaluation of symptoms of acute low back pain?

Factors that may indicate serious underlying pathology are termed **red flags** and include fever, unexplained weight loss, bowel or bladder dysfunction, cancer history, significant trauma, osteoporosis, age older than 50 years, failure to improve with standard treatment, and a history of alcohol or drug abuse.

13. **What is a simple method for differentiating spinal symptoms due to physical disease from symptoms due to inappropriate illness behavior before the patient is examined?**

Important clinical information can be obtained by having the patient complete a **pain diagram**. Pain diagrams completed by patients with physical disease (e.g. disc herniation, spinal stenosis) tend to be localized, anatomic, and proportionate. Pain diagrams completed by patients with magnified or inappropriate illness behavior tend to be regional, nonanatomic, and highly exaggerated.

14. **What are the basic elements of a physical examination directed at the lumbar spine?**

Examination should address the lumbar region, pelvis, hip joints, lower limbs, gait, and peripheral vascular system. A complete exam should include:
1. Inspection
2. Palpation
3. Range of motion (lumbar spine, hips, knees)
4. Neurologic exam (sensation, muscle testing, reflexes)
5. Assessment of nerve root tension signs
6. Vascular exam

15. **What is looked for during inspection?**

During the initial encounter, much can be learned from observing the patient. Abnormalities of gait (e.g. a *drop foot* gait or Trendelenburg gait) and abnormal posturing of the trunk are important clues for the examiner. It is also helpful to watch patients undress to observe how freely and easily they are able to move the trunk and extremities. In addition, the base of the spine should be inspected for a hairy patch or any skin markings that may be associated occult intraspinal anomalies. Waistline symmetry should be noted as asymmetry suggests lumbar scoliosis. The overall alignment and balance of the spine should be assessed by dropping a plumb line from the C7 spinous process to see that it is centered on the sacrum. If it is not, the lateral distance from the gluteal cleft should be noted.

16. **What is the purpose of palpation?**

To examine for tenderness and localize pathology. Palpation must include the spinous processes as well as the adjacent soft tissues. The area of the sciatic notch should be deeply palpated to look for sciatic irritability. Specific areas of palpation correspond to specific levels of the spine (e.g. iliac crest, L4–L5; posterior superior iliac spine, S2).

17. **How is range of motion assessed?**

In the spine, motion is assessed in three planes: flexion/extension, right/left bending, and right/left rotation. Range of motion can be estimated in degrees or measured with an inclinometer. It is important to note that a significant portion of lumbar flexion is achieved through the hip joints. The normal range of motion for forward flexion is 40° to 60°; for extension, 20° to 35°; for lateral bending, 15° to 20°; and for rotation, 3° to 18°.

18. **What is Schober's test?**

Schober's test is a simple clinical test useful to evaluate spinal mobility. This test is based on the principle that the skin over the lumbar spine stretches as a person flexes forward to touch the toes. A tape measure is used to mark the skin at the midpoint between the posterior superior iliac crests and at points 10 cm proximal and 5 cm distal to this mark while the patient is standing. The patient is then asked to bend forward as far as possible, and the distance between the two marked points is measured with the patient in the flexed position. In 90% of asymptomatic persons, there is an increase in length of at least 5 cm. This maneuver eliminates hip flexion and is a true indication of lumbar spine movement.

19. **How is the neurologic examination of the lumbar region performed?**

Neurologic examination of the lumbar region focuses primarily on a sequential examination of nerve roots. For each nerve root, the examiner tests sensation, motor strength, and, if one exists, the appropriate reflex (see Table 5-1).

Table 5-1. Neurologic Examination of the Lumbar Region

LEVEL	SENSATION	MOTOR	REFLEX
L1	Anterior thigh	Psoas (T12, L1, L2, L3)	None
L2	Anterior thigh, groin	Quadriceps (L2, L3, L4)	None
L3	Anterior and lateral thigh	Quadriceps (L2, L3, L4)	None
L4	Medial leg and foot	Tibialis anterior	Patellar
L5	Lateral leg and dorsal foot	Extensor hallucis longus	None
S1	Lateral and plantar foot	Gastrocnemius, peroneals	Achilles
S2--S4	Perianal	Bladder and foot intrinsics	None

20. What provocative maneuvers are used to assess a patient with a suspected lumbar radiculopathy?

The **standard straight-leg raise test** and its variants increase tension along the sciatic nerve and are used to assess the L5 and S1 nerve roots. The **reverse straight leg raise test** increases tension along the femoral nerve and is used to assess the L2, L3, and L4 nerve roots.

21. Describe how the straight leg raise test and the femoral nerve stretch test are performed.

The straight-leg raise test is a tension sign that may be performed with the patient supine (Lasegue's test; Fig. 5-2) or sitting (flip test; Fig. 5-3). The leg is elevated with the knee straight to increase tension along the sciatic nerve, specifically the L5 and S1 nerve roots. If the nerve root is compressed, nerve stretch provokes radicular pain. Back pain alone does not constitute a positive test. The most tension is placed on the L5 and S1 nerve roots during a supine straight-leg raise test between 35° and 70° of leg elevation. A variant of this test is the bowstring test, in which the knee is flexed during the standard supine straight-leg raise test to reduce leg pain secondary to sciatic nerve stretch. Finger pressure is then applied over the popliteal space at the terminal aspect of the sciatic nerve in an attempt to reestablish radicular symptoms.

The femoral nerve stretch test (or reverse straight-leg raise test) increases tension along the femoral nerve, specifically the L2, L3, and L4 nerve roots (Fig. 5-4). It may be performed with the patient in the prone position or in the lateral position with the affected side upward. The test is performed by extending the hip and flexing the knee. This is exactly opposite to the standard straight-leg raise test. The femoral nerve stretch test is considered positive if radicular pain in the anterior thigh region occurs.

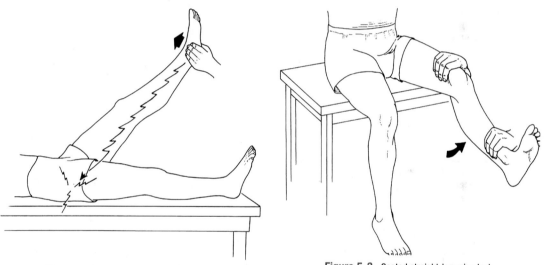

Figure 5-2. Supine straight-leg raise test.

Figure 5-3. Seated straight-leg raise test.

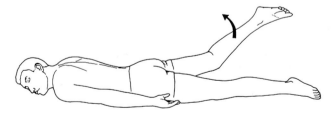

Figure 5-4. Femoral nerve stretch test.

22. What is the contralateral straight-leg raise test? Why is it a significant test?

This test is performed in the same fashion as the standard straight-leg raise test except that the asymptomatic leg is elevated. If this test reproduces the patient's sciatic symptoms in the opposite extremity, it is considered positive. A positive test is strongly suggestive of a disc herniation medial to the nerve root (in the axilla of the nerve root). The combination of a positive straight-leg raise test on the symptomatic side and a positive contralateral straight-leg raise test is the most specific clinical test for a disc herniation, with accuracy approaching 97%.

23. What nerve root is affected by a posterolateral disc herniation?

The nerve roots of the lumbar spine exit the spinal canal beneath the pedicle of the corresponding numbered vertebra and above the caudad intervertebral disc. The most common location for a lumbar disc herniation is posterolateral. This type of disc herniation compresses the traversing nerve root of the motion segment. For example, a posterolateral disc herniation at the L4–L5 level would compress the traversing nerve root (L5).

24. What nerve root is affected by a disc herniation lateral to or within the neural foramen?

A disc herniation lateral to or within the neural foramen compresses the exiting nerve root of the motion segment. For example, a disc herniation at the L4–L5 level located in the region of the neural foramen compresses the exiting L4 nerve root and spares the traversing L5 nerve root.

25. What nerve roots are affected by a central disc herniation?

A central disc herniation can compress one or more of the caudal nerve roots. A large central disc herniation is a common cause of a cauda equina syndrome.

26. What is cauda equina syndrome?

Cauda equina syndrome is a symptom complex that includes low back pain, unilateral or bilateral sciatica, lower extremity motor weakness, sensory abnormalities, bowel or bladder dysfunction, and saddle anesthesia. Cauda equina syndrome may result from acute or chronic compression of the nerve roots of the cauda equina. Causes of cauda equina syndrome include massive central lumbar disc protrusion, spinal stenosis, epidural hematoma, spinal tumor, and fracture. The syndrome can result in permanent motor deficit and bowel and bladder incontinence. Once identified, cauda equina syndrome constitutes a true surgical emergency because it can be irreversible if not treated promptly with surgical decompression.

27. What are Waddell's signs?

Waddell described five categories of tests that are useful in evaluating patients with low back pain. These signs do not prove malingering but are useful to highlight the contribution of psychologic and/or socioeconomic factors to spinal symptoms. Presence of three of more of the signs is considered significant. Isolated positive signs are not considered significant. Waddell's tests include:

1. **Superficial tenderness**: Nonorganic tenderness with light touch over a wide lumbar area or deeper tenderness in a nonanatomic distribution.
2. **Simulation**: Maneuvers that should not be uncomfortable are performed. If pain is reported, nonorganic pathology is suggested. Examples of such tests include production of low back pain with axial loading of the head or when the shoulders and pelvis are passively rotated in the same plane.
3. **Distraction**: The examiner performs a provocative test in the usual manner and rechecks the test when the patient is distracted. For example, a patient with a positive straight-leg raise test in the supine position can be assessed with a straight-leg raise test in the seated position under the guise of examining the foot or another part of the lower extremity. If the distraction test is negative but a formal straight-leg raise test in the supine position is positive, this finding is considered a positive sign.
4. **Regionalization**: Presence of findings that diverge from accepted neuroanatomy. For example, entire muscle groups, which do not have common innervation, may demonstrate *giving way* on strength testing or sensory abnormalities may not follow a dermatomal distribution.
5. **Overreaction**: Disproportionate response to examination may take many forms such a collapsing, inappropriate facial expression, excessive verbalization, or any other type of overreaction to any aspect of the exam.

28. During assessment of a lumbar spine problem, what two nonspinal pathologies should be ruled out during the physical exam?

Degenerative arthritis of the hip joint and vascular disease involving the lower extremities. The presentation of these pathologies and common spinal problems can overlap. Anterior thigh pain may be due to either nerve impingement involving the upper lumbar nerve roots (L2, L3, L4) or hip arthritis. Range-of-motion testing of the hip joints can rule out hip pathology. Lower extremity claudication may be due to either vascular disease or lumbar spinal stenosis (neurogenic claudication). Assessment of peripheral pulses is helpful in diagnosing these problems.

29. How is the sacroiliac joint assessed?

Sacroiliac pain is difficult to confirm on clinical assessment and generally requires a diagnostic joint injection under radiographic control for confirmation. Clinical tests that have been described to assess this joint include:

- **Patrick's test**: With the patient supine, the knee on the affected side is flexed and the foot placed on the opposite patella. The flexed knee is then pushed laterally to stress the sacroiliac joint. This is also called the FABER test (flexion-abduction-external rotation).
- **Pelvic compression test**: With the patient supine, the iliac crests are pushed toward the midline in an attempt to elicit pain in the sacroiliac joint.

Key Points

1. A comprehensive patient history and physical examination is the first step in diagnosis of a spine complaint.
2. A major goal of the initial patient evaluation is to differentiate common non-emergent spinal conditions such as acute nonspecific thoracic or lumbar pain and degenerative spinal disorders from serious and urgent problems such as spinal infections, spinal tumors or cauda equina syndrome.
3. Nonspinal pathology (e.g., osteoarthritis of the hip joint, peripheral vascular disease) may mimic the symptoms of lumbar spinal disorders and must be considered in the differential diagnosis.

Websites

1. Low back exam (video):http://www.hss.edu/conditions_14639.asp
2. Physical examination of the cervical, thoracic, and lumbar spine (video): http://videos.med.wisc.edu/videoInfo.php?videoid=3121
3. Key points related to physical examination of the lumbar spine: http://www.wheelessonline.com/ortho/exam_of_the_lumbar_spine
4. United States Disability Examination Worksheets: http://www.vba.va.gov/BLN/21/Benefits/exams/disexm53.htm

BIBLIOGRAPHY

1. Albert TJ. Physical Examination of the Spine. London: Thieme; 2004.
2. Apeldoorn AT, Bosselaar H, Blom-Luberti T, et al. The reliability of nonorganic sign-testing and the Waddell score in patients with chronic low back pain. Spine 2008;33:821–6.
3. Hoppenfeld S. Physical Exam of the Spine and Extremities. 1st ed. New York: Appleton & Lange; 1976.
4. Rainville J, Jouve C, Finno M, et al. Comparison of four tests of quadriceps strength in L3 or L4 radiculopathies. Spine 2003;28:2466–71.
5. Scherping SC. History and physical examination. In: Frymoyer JW, Wiesel SW, editors. The Adult Spine: Principles and Practice. 3rd ed. Philadelphia: Lippincott Williams & Wilkins; 2004, p. 49–68.
6. Standaert CJ, Herring SA, Sinclair JD. Patient history and physical examination—cervical, thoracic and lumbar. In: Herkowitz HN, Garfin SR, Eismont FJ, et al., editors. Rothman-Simeone The Spine. 5th ed. Philadelphia: Saunders; 2006, p. 169–86.

EVALUATION OF THE SPINE TRAUMA PATIENT

John Steinmann, DO, and Gina Cruz, DO

1. What are the incidence and leading causes of spinal cord injuries?

It is estimated that 12,000 new cases of spinal cord injury occur each year in the United States. This equates to approximately 40 cases per million population. There is a distinct predominance of male patients, representing 81% of patients enrolled in the spinal cord injury database. The average age of spinal cord injury in the United States for the years 2000 through 2005 was 37.6 years with the past 30 years showing a slow steady increase in the average age of patients sustaining spinal cord injuries. The leading causes of spinal cord injury are:

- Vehicular accidents (45%)
- Falls (20%)
- Acts of violence (15%)
- Sport-related injuries (15%)
- Miscellaneous causes (5%)

2. What are the goals in treating a patient with spinal cord injury?

- Safe extrication and transport
- Maintenance of airway, breathing, and circulation
- Prevention of hypoxemia and hypotension
- Accurate identification and classification of spinal injury
- Identification of associated injuries (head, pulmonary, abdominal, long bone injuries)
- Rapid reduction of fractures and dislocations
- Timely stabilization of unstable spinal segments
- Early transfer to an appropriate acute spinal cord rehabilitation center

3. Summarize the important aspects of the prehospital care of the potentially spine-injured patient.

Patients with high-energy mechanisms or altered mental status should be assumed to have sustained a spinal injury and undergo extrication and transport using strict spinal precautions. Treatment begins with ensuring an adequate airway, breathing, and circulation. Prevention of hypoxemia and hypotension through the use of supplemental oxygen, intravenous fluids, and vasopressors helps limit the zone of spinal cord injury. Transport to a facility prepared to manage acute spinal cord injury is essential.

4. Discuss the role of steroids in the treatment of acute spinal cord injury.

Proponents have reported enhanced neurologic recovery in patients with incomplete motor lesions when methylprednisolone is administered within 8 hours of injury. A loading dose of 30 mg/kg is followed by 5.4 mg/kg for 23 hours if administered within 3 hours of injury or for 48 hours if administered between 3 and 8 hours after injury. Contraindications to steroid administration include:

- Patients presenting more than 8 hours following injury
- Injuries limited to the cauda equina or individual nerve roots
- Gunshot wounds
- Age <13 years
- Pregnancy
- Uncontrolled diabetes
- Patients on steroid maintenance

Opponents of the use of methylprednisolone in acute spinal cord injury dispute the benefits of this practice, citing risks of steroid administration in polytrauma patients including wound infection, pulmonary embolus, and sepsis. As a result, the use of methylprednisolone in spinal cord injuries is no longer considered standard of care but remains a treatment option.

5. A patient presents with acute quadriplegia following a C5-6 bilateral facet dislocation. The patient has associated minor closed fractures of the extremities and no evidence of injury to any other organ system. The emergency department physician reports that the patient is hypotensive (blood pressure is 78/50 mm Hg)

and bradycardic (pulse is 48 beats/minute). What is the likely etiology of this patient's hypotension?

Both neurogenic and hypovolemic etiologies (as well as a combination of both) should be considered in the trauma setting. In a patient with a severe spinal cord injury who exhibits the combination of hypotension and bradycardia, the more likely etiology is neurogenic shock. A temporary generalized sympathectomy effect decreases cardiac output and peripheral vascular resistance. Treatment often requires the use of vasopressors, and, in severe cases, cardiac pacing is needed. It is important not to confuse this picture with hemorrhagic shock, which presents with hypotension and an increased pulse rate. Increasing fluids will not raise blood pressure in neurogenic shock and instead may cause serious fluid overload and pulmonary edema.

6. **In evaluating the conscious patient with spinal injury, what are the important aspects of the history?**

The history should establish the mechanism of injury, time of injury, location of pain, loss of consciousness, and, very importantly, the presence of transient or persistent neurologic complaints (sensory and/or motor). In addition, the history should seek to understand the patient's relevant past medical history.

7. **What is the importance of a transient neurologic deficit following high-energy trauma?**

A stable spine maintains appropriate alignment and protects the neural elements under physiologic loads. A transient neurologic deficit indicates a moment during the injury when the spine failed to protect the neural elements. Although this may be the result of preexistent stenosis, when associated with a high-energy mechanism one must assume an injury has occurred that has rendered the spine unstable.

8. **Describe the essential elements of the physical exam in the spine-injured patient.**

The *primary survey* should focus on establishing the presence of adequate airway, breathing, and circulation. The *secondary survey* involves a general inspection of the entire body, including detailed examination of the spine. The patient is log-rolled, and the spine is inspected and palpated. One should note localized tenderness, bruising, and interspinous widening or displacement. The neurologic examination should follow the *Standard Neurological Classification of Spinal Cord Injury form* established by the American Spinal Injury Association (ASIA) (Figs. 6-1 and 6-2). A detailed motor, sensory, and reflex exam must include a rectal exam to assess for sacral sparing and the bulbocavernosus reflex.

9. **What is sacral sparing? What is its significance in patients with spinal cord injury?**

Sacral sparing refers to the presence of perianal sensation after an acute spinal cord injury that has otherwise rendered the patient with complete motor deficit below the level of injury. This finding indicates some degree of transmission of neural impulses across the level of spinal cord injury and signifies that the patient has sustained a partial spinal cord injury, with the potential for some degree of neurologic recovery. Sacral sparing is due to the topographic cross-sectional organization of the spinal cord in which the sensory and motor fibers supplying caudad regions are located laterally and closer to the surface of the spinal cord. Spinal cord contusion and ischemia typically result in greater damage to centrally located tracts than tracts located in the periphery of the spinal cord.

10. **Define spinal shock and explain its significance after an acute spinal cord injury.**

Spinal shock refers to the period after spinal cord injury (usually 24 hours) when the reflex activity of the entire spinal cord becomes depressed. During this period the reflex arcs below the level of spinal cord injury are not functioning. The return of reflex activity below the level of a spinal cord injury signifies the end of spinal shock. The significance of spinal shock lies in the determination of whether a patient has sustained a complete vs. incomplete spinal cord injury. This cannot be determined until spinal shock has ended. Bulbocavernosus reflex is used to assess the end of spinal shock.

11. **What is the bulbocavernosus reflex? What is its significance?**

The *bulbocavernosus reflex* is a spinal reflex mediated by the S2 to S4 cord segments. It is tested by application of digital pressure on the penis or clitoris or gently pulling on the Foley catheter to cause reflex anal sphincter contraction. Absence of this reflex indicates spinal shock. Return of this reflex signifies the end of spinal shock. At this point, the patient with complete loss of motor and sensory function below the level of injury and absence of sacral sparing is considered to have a complete spinal injury.

12. **How is the degree of neurologic injury described following an osteoligamentous injury to the spine?**

Patients are stratified into the following categories:

Neurologically intact. The patient is awake, alert, and demonstrates normal motor, sensory, and reflex function

Root injury. There is evidence of peripheral nerve injury as exhibited by painful dysesthesias and/or motor deficits along an individual nerve root without evidence of sensory, motor, or reflex changes at cord levels below the level of this injury. As a root injury is a peripheral nerve injury, it has potential for recovery

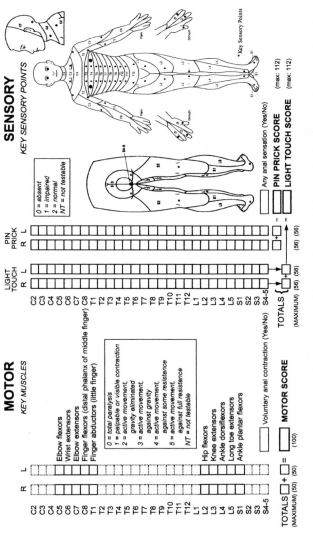

Figure 6-2. American Spinal Injury Association impairment scale.

Figure 6-1. American Spinal Injury Association classification of spinal cord injury.

Incomplete spinal cord injury. Partial preservation of neural function is noted below the level of injury. Recovery may vary from minimal to complete, depending on the type of incomplete spinal cord injury. Six incomplete spinal cord injury syndromes have been described: (1) central cord, (2) Brown-Sequard, (3) anterior cord, (4) posterior cord, (5) conus medullaris, and (6) cauda equina

Complete spinal cord injury: Absent sensory and motor function more than three segments below the level of injury

13. Describe the Frankel classification of spinal cord injury.

The Frankel classification has been used to separate patients with spinal cord injuries into five functional grades:

Grade A: Absent motor and sensory function

Grade B: Absent motor function with sensory sparing

Grade C: Very weak motor function (not useful); sensation present

Grade D: Weak but useful motor functions; sensation present

Grade E: Normal motor and sensory function

14. What is the ASIA Impairment Scale for assessing the spinal cord injured patient?

The American Spinal Injury Association (ASIA) Impairment Scale provides a more detailed method for classifying the neurologic status of patients with spinal injuries:

ASIA A: Complete injury. No motor or sensory function distal to the level of injury including the sacral segments S4–S5

ASIA B: Incomplete injury. Sensory but not motor function is preserved below the neurologic level and includes the sacral segments S4–S5

ASIA C: Incomplete injury. Motor function is preserved below the neurologic level, and more than half of key muscles below the neurologic level have a muscle grade less than 3

ASIA D: Incomplete injury. Motor and sensory incomplete (motor functional) with at least half of key muscles below the neurologic level having a muscle grade 3 or 4

ASIA E: Normal; sensory and motor function intact

15. Name the location and function of the major spinal cord tracts important in the assessment of the patient with spinal cord injury.

Corticospinal tracts: Descending tracts originate in the primary motor cortex, cross within the brainstem, descend within the anterior and lateral portion of the cord, and terminate directly on motor neurons in the ventral gray matter of the spinal cord. These tracts transmit ipsilateral fine motor movement. Injury to the corticospinal tracts leads to loss of fine motor function ipsilateral to the cord injury

Spinothalamic tracts: Ascending tracts located in the anterolateral portion of the cord that transmit sensations of pain and temperature. These tracts cross shortly after entering the spinal cord and, therefore, transmit sensation from the contralateral side of the body

Dorsal column tracts: Ascending tracts that convey proprioceptive, vibratory, and discriminative touch sensation. Fibers originate in the dorsal root ganglion, ascend the ipsilateral dorsal column, and cross within the brainstem. Lesions to the dorsal column tracts result in loss of proprioception and vibratory sense ipsilateral to the injury

16. Briefly explain the mechanism and clinical presentation of the incomplete spinal cord injury syndromes involving the cervical spinal cord.

Central cord syndrome is the most common incomplete spinal cord injury syndrome. It is often seen in elderly patients with preexisting cervical stenosis who sustain a hyperextension injury. The clinical presentation includes bilateral sensory and motor deficits with upper extremity weakness greater than lower extremity weakness. Lower extremity hyperreflexia and sacral sparing are noted. The prognosis is good for a partial recovery. Recovery of hand function is generally poor. Typical management of central cord syndrome is initiated with traction and immobilization for a period to allow early recovery and diminish spinal cord edema followed by decompression of the preexisting stenosis and stabilization of the injured level.

Brown-Sequard syndrome is caused by a hemisection of the spinal cord. The clinical presentation includes ipsilateral motor and proprioception loss with contralateral pain and temperature loss distal to the level of injury. The prognosis for recovery is good, with most patients recovering some degree of ambulatory capacity and bowel and bladder function. Common causes include knife wounds, missile wounds, and asymmetrically located spinal cord tumors.

Anterior cord syndrome results from vascular ischemia or compression of the anterior spinal artery and anterior spinal cord. Typically, neural function is absent in the anterior two-thirds of the spinal cord. Findings include complete loss of motor function and pain and temperature sensation distal to the site of injury with preservation of vibration and proprioception. The prognosis for recovery is poor. A common causes is a vertebral body fracture associated with spinal cord injury secondary to retropulsed bone. Intraoperative hypotension during complex spinal procedures for cervical myelopathy is an additional potential cause.

Posterior cord syndrome presents with loss of discriminative touch as well as position and vibratory sense. However, motor function and pain and temperature sensations are intact. Patients typically ambulate with a foot-slapping gait. This syndrome is uncommon. Potential causes include vitamin B_{12} deficiency and syphilis.

17. What is SCIWORA?

SCIWORA refers to **s**pinal **c**ord **i**njury **w**ith**o**ut **r**adiographic **a**bnormality. This syndrome is seen in young children and older adults. In children, the elasticity of the immature spine permits neurologic injury without a fracture. In older adults with preexistent central spinal stenosis, an acute central cord syndrome may develop after a fall despite the absence of a spinal fracture.

18. What initial imaging studies should be obtained in spine-injured patients?

Traditionally, imaging assessment of the polytraumatized patient began with plain radiographs: anteroposterior (AP) chest, anteroposterior (AP) pelvis, and cervical spine (AP, lateral, and open mouth odontoid views). The advent of high-speed spiral computed tomography (CT) scanning has largely replaced routine plain radiographic imaging of the cervical spine. In addition, high-speed CT scanning of the chest, abdomen, and pelvis has largely eliminated the need for AP chest and pelvic radiographs. All polytrauma patients require adequate imaging of the spine (cervical, thoracic, and lumbar), chest, and pelvis, either via plain x-rays or preferably, if facilities allow, high-speed spiral CT imaging. Helical CT imaging of the traumatized spine has greatly increased the sensitivity for identification of spinal injuries.

19. Describe how to evaluate a lateral cervical spine radiograph in a patient following spinal trauma.

Count the number of vertebral bodies that are clearly seen. The lateral view must visualize from the occiput to the superior endplate of T1. Inability to visualize T1 necessitates traction view, a swimmer's view, or a cervical CT scan.

Evaluate the thickness of the retropharyngeal soft tissues. Normal retropharyngeal swelling is up to 3 to 5 mm at C3 and less than 15 mm at C6. Increased soft tissue thickness may indicate a serious injury but absence of swelling does not rule out a significant injury.

Assess subaxial cervical alignment by constructing four parallel lines: anterior vertebral line, posterior vertebral line, spinolaminar line, and posterior spinous process line. Check the relationship of adjacent vertebra at the level of the spinous processes, facet joints, disc spaces, and vertebral margins for potential asymmetry, subluxation, or distraction.

Examine C1–C2 and occiput–C1 alignment. Check the atlantodens interval (normally 3.5 mm in adults and 5 mm in children) as increase in this interval signifies rupture of the transverse ligament. Look for signs of injury involving the atlanto-occipital articulation by checking the dens-basion interval, Wackenheim's line, and Harris lines (see Chapter 55).

20. What are indications for magnetic resonance imaging (MRI) in patients with spinal injury?

- Unexplained neurologic deficit
- Incomplete neurologic deficit
- Neurologic deterioration
- Before reduction of the cervical spine in neurologically intact patients
- Preoperatively in patients scheduled for posterior cervical, thoracic, or lumbar reduction and stabilization
- To assess the degree of spinal cord or ligamentous injury

21. When are cervical flexion-extension views indicated?

Flexion-extension views are to be avoided in the acute setting. In a patient who has normal radiographs and spinal tenderness, a rigid collar should be used for the first two weeks. If tenderness persists, controlled flexion-extension views under physician supervision may help to rule out a ligamentous injury.

22. What are the criteria necessary to clear the cervical spine?

- Conscious, mentally alert, and oriented patient
- Negative, adequate plain radiographs or cervical CT scan
- Absence of localized posterior spinal tenderness
- Intact neurologic status

Key Points

1. Patients with high-energy injury mechanisms or altered mental status should be assumed to have sustained a significant spinal injury and undergo immediate spinal immobilization during extrication, transport, and initial evaluation.
2. The potentially spinal-injured patient is assessed according to Advanced Trauma Life Support (ATLS) protocols.
3. Patients with neurologic injury are assessed according to the Standards for Neurologic Classification established by the American Spinal Injury Association (ASIA).
4. Hypotension and hypoxemia require aggressive treatment in the spinal cord injured patient.
5. The clinical syndromes resulting from spinal cord injury depend on the level of injury and the anatomic tracts involved by the injury.

Websites

1. General trauma evaluation: http://www.fpnotebook.com/ER/Trauma/TrmEvltn.htm
2. Steroids for spinal cord injury: http://www.trauma.org/index.php/main/article/394/
3. American Spinal Injury Association classification worksheet:
   http://www.asia-spinalinjury.org/publications/2006_Classif_worksheet.pdf
4. Guidelines for diagnosis of suspected spine trauma:
   http://www.guideline.gov/summary/summary.aspx?ss=15&doc_id=11597&nbr=6010

BIBLIOGRAPHY

1. American Spinal Injury Association, International Medical Society of Paraplegia. International Standards for Neurological and Functional Classification of Spinal Cord Injury, Revised 1996. Chicago: American Spinal Injury Association; 1996.
2. Bracken NB, Shepard MJ, Collins WF, et al. A randomized controlled trial of methylprednisolone and naloxone in the treatment of acute spinal cord injury: Results of the Second National Acute Spinal Cord Injury Study. N Engl J Med 1990;322:1405–11.
3. Gupta MC, Benson DR, Keenen TL. Initial evaluation and emergency treatment of the spine-injured patient. In: Browner BD, Jupiter JB, Levine AM, et al., editors. Browner: Skeletal Trauma. 4th ed. Philadelphia: Saunders; 2008.
4. Hurlbert RJ. Methylprednisolone for acute spinal cord injury: an inappropriate standard of care. J Neurosurg 2000;93(1 Suppl):1–7.
5. Kim DH, Ludwig SC, Vacarro AR, et al. Atlas of Spine Trauma. Philadelphia: Saunders; 2008.
6. McCulloch PT, France J, Jones DL, et al. Helical computed tomography alone compared with plain radiographs with adjunct computed tomography to evaluate the cervical spine after high energy trauma. J Bone Joint Surg 2005;87A:2388–94.
7. Mirza SK, Bellabarba C, Chapman JR. Principles of spine trauma care. In: Bucholz RW, Hechman JD, editors. Rockwood and Green's Fractures in Adults. 6th ed. Philadelphia: Lippincott Williams & Wilkins; 2006. p. 1401–34.
8. White AA III, Panjabi MM, editors. Clinical Biomechanics of the Spine. 2nd ed. Philadelphia: Lippincott; 1990.

CHAPTER 7

EVALUATION OF SPINAL DEFORMITIES

Robert W. Gaines, Jr., MD, and Vincent J. Devlin, MD

1. What are the most common spinal deformities that require recognition by the clinician?

Traditionally spinal deformities have been classified into those that affect predominantly the coronal plane (e.g. idiopathic scoliosis) and those affecting the sagittal plane (e.g. Scheuermann's kyphosis). In reality, spinal deformities are complex and simultaneously affect the sagittal, coronal, and axial plane alignment of the spinal column and its relationship to pelvis and thoracic cage. A spinal deformity may result from a pathologic process at a single vertebra level (e.g. spondylolisthesis), or multiple spinal levels (e.g. Scheuermann's kyphosis), or it may involve the entire spinal column and pelvis due to compromised postural support mechanisms (e.g. neuromuscular scoliosis).

2. Why does the assessment of spinal deformities require a comprehensive assessment of the patient's health status?

Every facet of human disease is associated with spinal deformities. The etiology of spinal deformities is wide ranging and includes congenital disorders, developmental disorders, degenerative disorders, trauma, infection, tumor, metabolic disorders, neuromuscular disorders, and conditions whose precise etiology remains elusive (e.g. idiopathic scoliosis). Clinical examination is critical for detection of spinal deformities and makes subsequent detailed assessment possible. Radiographs and higher-level imaging studies are required to document the severity and extent of a specific spinal deformity. A spinal deformity may be only one manifestation of an underlying systemic disorder that may affect multiple organ systems.

3. What are the potential consequences of untreated spinal deformities?

The consequences depend on many factors, including age, underlying health status, deformity etiology, deformity magnitude, and the potential for future progression of the deformity during the patient's lifespan. Potential consequences of untreated spinal deformity may include cosmetic problems, pain, neurologic deficit, postural difficulty, and impairment in activities of daily living. Severe thoracic deformity may impair respiratory mechanics with resultant hypoxemia, pulmonary hypertension, cor pulmonale, or even death.

4. Describe the basic components of the clinical assessment of a patient with spinal deformity.

1. Detailed history:

    What is the presenting complaint? (deformity? pain? neurologic symptoms? impaired function in activities of daily living? cardiorespiratory symptoms?)

    When was the deformity first noticed?

    Is there a family history of spinal deformity?

    Were there any abnormalities during development?

    What is the patient's maturity and growth potential?

    Has prior treatment been performed?

    Are there any associated general medical problems?

2. Comprehensive physical exam

    Inspection. The patient must be undressed to fully assess the trunk and extremities. Assess for asymmetry of the neckline, shoulder height, rib cage, waistline, flank, pelvis, and lower extremities. The patient should be assessed in the standing position and bent forward to 90°. The patient should be inspected from both anterior and posterior aspects as well as from the side. Note any skin lesions (e.g. midline hair patch, sinus tract, hemangiomas, café-au-lait pigmentation). Observe the patient's gait. Observe body proportions and height.

    Palpation. Palpate the spinous processes and paraspinous region for tenderness, deviation in spinous process alignment, or a palpable step-off.

    Spinal range of motion. Test flexion-extension, side-bending, and rotation. Any restriction or asymmetry with range of motion is noted.

    Neurologic exam. Assess sensory, motor, and reflex function of the upper and lower extremities, including abdominal reflexes.

    Spinal alignment and balance in the coronal plane. Normally the head should be centered over the sacrum and pelvis. A plumb line dropped from C7 should fall through the gluteal crease.

Spinal alignment and balance in the sagittal plane. When the patient is observed from the side, assess the four physiologic sagittal curves (cervical and lumbar lordosis, thoracic and sacral kyphosis). When the patient standing with the hips and knees fully extended, the head should be aligned over the sacrum. The ear, shoulder, and greater trochanter of the hip should lie on the same vertical line.

Extremities. Measurement of leg lengths and assessment of joint flexibility is performed. Note any contractures or deformities involving the extremities (e.g. cavus feet).

Examination of related body systems. A detailed medical assessment should be performed. Some spinal deformities are associated with abnormalities in other organ systems, especially the nervous system and renal system. Screening for cardiac disorders, vision problems, hearing problems, and learning disorders may be required.

5. What are the most common types of scoliosis?

Scoliosis refers to a spinal deformity in the coronal (frontal) plane. The commonly described causes of scoliosis include:

- Idiopathic
- Neuromuscular (e.g. cerebral palsy, muscular dystrophy, myelomeningocele, Friedreich's ataxia)
- Congenital: failure of formation (e.g. hemivertebra), failure of segmentation (e.g. congenital bar)
- Neurofibromatosis
- Mesenchymal (e.g. Marfan syndrome, Ehlers-Danlos syndrome)
- Trauma
- Secondary to extraspinal contracture (e.g. after empyema)
- Osteochondrodystrophies (e.g. Morquio's syndrome, diastrophic dwarfism)
- Infection
- Metabolic (e.g. osteoporosis, rickets)
- Tumor (spinal cord or vertebral column)
- Related to anomalies of the lumbosacral joint (e.g. spondylolisthesis)

6. Describe the assessment of an adolescent referred for evaluation for possible scoliosis.

The patient should be examined with the back exposed (Fig. 7-1). First the patient is examined in the standing position. Then the patient is examined as he or she bends forward at the waist with the arms hanging freely, the knees straight, and the feet together. Findings that suggest the presence of scoliosis include:

- Shoulder height asymmetry
- Scapula or rib prominence
- Chest cage asymmetry
- Unequal space between the arm and the lateral trunk on side to side comparison
- Waist line asymmetry
- Asymmetry of the paraspinous musculature

7. What is a scoliometer? How is it used?

In North America, it is common for children in the 10- to 14-year age group to undergo a screening assessment at school for detection of scoliosis. The *Adams test* (assessment for spinal asymmetry with the patient in the forward-bending position) is typically used to assess for possible scoliosis. The use of an *inclinometer (scoliometer)* has been popularized to quantitate trunk asymmetry and help decide whether radiographs should be obtained to further evaluate a specific patient. The scoliometer is used to determine the *angle of trunk rotation (ATR)*. The ATR is the angle formed between the horizontal plane and the plane across the posterior aspect of the trunk at the point of maximal deformity when a region of the spine is evaluated with the patient in the forward-bending position. According to its developer, an ATR of 5° is correlated with an 11° curve and an ATR of 7° is correlated with a 20° curve.

8. How is scoliosis due to leg-length discrepancy distinguished from other types of scoliosis?

Performing the forward-bend test with the patient in the sitting position eliminates the effect of leg-length discrepancy on the spine. Alternatively, evaluation of the patient after placing wood blocks beneath the shortened extremity eliminates the contribution of leg-length discrepancy to pelvic obliquity and scoliosis. Finally, leg-length inequality should be directly quantitated with a tape measure by determining the distance from anterior-superior iliac spine to medial malleolus.

9. What is the significance of painful scoliosis in pediatric patients?

The presentation of painful scoliosis is atypical in the pediatric patient. If pain is present in the pediatric patient with idiopathic scoliosis, it is typically mild, nonspecific, intermittent, and nonradiating. It is typically mechanical (improves with rest), does not awaken the patient from sleep, and does not limit activity. Persistent severe back pain should prompt the physician to further investigate the cause of the patient's symptoms. Workup (e.g. lateral spinal radiograph, magnetic resonance imaging [MRI], bone scan) is needed to rule out etiologies such as spinal tumor, spinal infection, spondylolisthesis, or Scheuermann's disease.

Clinical Evaluation of Scoliosis

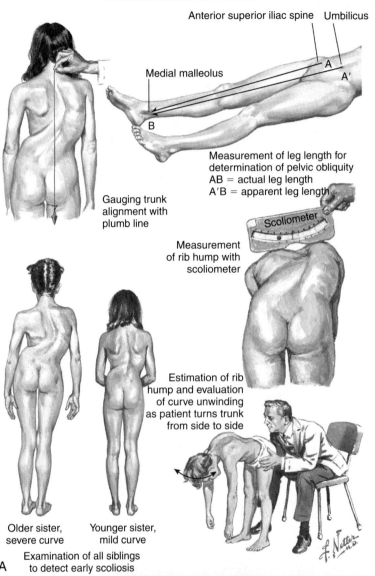

Anterior superior iliac spine   Umbilicus

Medial malleolus

Measurement of leg length for
determination of pelvic obliquity
AB = actual leg length
A'B = apparent leg length

Gauging trunk
alignment with
plumb line

Scoliometer

Measurement
of rib hump with
scoliometer

Estimation of rib
hump and evaluation
of curve unwinding
as patient turns trunk
from side to side

Older sister,
severe curve

Younger sister,
mild curve

Examination of all siblings
A   to detect early scoliosis

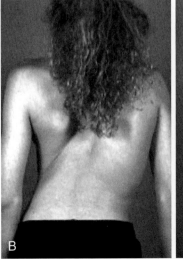

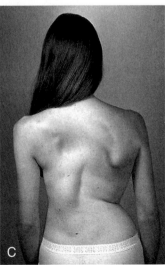

Figure 7-1. A, Clinical evaluation of
scoliosis. **B,** Thoracic scoliosis. **C,** Thoracic and lumbar scoliosis. (**A.** Reprinted
from The Netter Collection of Medical
Illustrations – Musculoskeletal System,
Part II, Developmental Disorders, Tumors,
Rheumatic Diseases and Joint Replacements, p. 34. ©Elsevier Inc. All Rights
Reserved.)

B

C

10. **What conditions should be considered in the differential diagnosis of neckline asymmetry or shoulder height asymmetry?**
In addition to an upper thoracic curvature secondary to idiopathic scoliosis, other conditions that may be responsible for this clinical finding include torticollis, Klippel-Feil syndrome, and congenital vertebral anomalies.

11. **What is Klippel-Fell syndrome?**
Klippel-Feil syndrome refers to a congenital fusion of the cervical spine associated with the clinical triad of a short neck, low posterior hairline, and limited neck motion.

12. **What condition should be considered in a child with limited lumbar flexion and a fixed lumbar lordosis?**
Lumbar lordosis that is rigid and does not correct when the patient is asked to perform a forward-bend test suggests the possibility of an intrathecal mass (tumor). A workup should be initiated to rule out this possibility, including an MRI of the spine.

13. **What should an examiner assess in the evaluation of an adult patient with scoliosis?**
In contrast to pediatric patients, it is not uncommon for adult patients with scoliosis to present with back pain. However, the incidence of back pain in the adult population is significant regardless of the presence of a spinal deformity. Thus, it cannot be assumed that symptoms of back pain are necessarily related to the presence of a spinal deformity. Examination of the adult patient should be directed at localizing the painful areas of the spine. Is the pain localized to an area of deformity, or is it localized to the lumbosacral junction? Does the patient have symptoms consistent with spinal stenosis or radiculopathy that warrant further workup with spinal canal imaging studies (MRI and/or computed tomography [CT]-myelography)? Is there evidence of deformity progression or cardiopulmonary dysfunction? There are no short cuts in the evaluation of spinal deformity, and a complete history and physical exam are mandatory.

14. **What is sciatic scoliosis?**
Pain as a result of lumbar nerve root irritation secondary to a disc herniation or spinal stenosis may lead to a postural abnormality that mimics scoliosis. This condition has been termed *sciatic scoliosis*.

15. **Define gibbus.**
The term *gibbus* derives from the Latin word for hump. It refers to a spinal deformity in the sagittal plane characterized by a sharply angulated spinal segment with an apex that points posteriorly (Fig. 7-2).

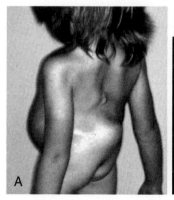
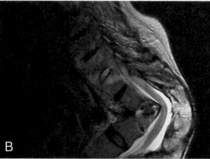

Figure 7-2. **A,** Congenital kyphosis with gibbus. **B,** Magnetic resonance imaging demonstrates sharply angulated kyphotic deformity secondary to congenital kyphosis.

16. **What are the common causes of increased thoracic kyphosis?**
Thoracic kyphosis is one of the four physiologic sagittal curves in normal people. Many different spinal pathologies can lead to an abnormal increase in thoracic kyphosis. In the pediatric population, increased thoracic kyphosis is commonly associated with Scheuermann's disease or congenital spinal anomalies. In the adult population, a wide range of pathology can manifest as increased thoracic kyphosis. A common cause is osteoporotic compression fractures, which lead to an increased thoracic kyphotic deformity termed *dowager's hump* (Table 7-1).

17. **How are postural kyphosis and kyphosis due to Scheuermann's disease distinguished clinically?**
Postural kyphosis (postural roundback) and Scheuermann's kyphosis are common causes of abnormal sagittal plane alignment in teenagers (Fig. 7-3). They can be distinguished on clinical assessment by performing a forward-bend test and observing the patient from the side. With postural kyphosis, the sagittal contour normalizes because the deformity is flexible. In kyphosis due to Scheuermann's disease, the deformity is rigid (structural) and does not normalize on forward bending.

Table 7-1. Causes of Kyphotic Spinal Deformities

Postural disorders	Metabolic (osteoporosis, osteomalacia, osteogenesis imperfecta)
Scheuermann's kyphosis	Skeletal dysplasia
Congenital disorders (failure of formation, failure of segmentation)	Collagen diseases
Neuromuscular disorders	Tumor
Myelomeningocele	Infection
Trauma (acute, chronic)	Rheumatologic disorders (e.g. ankylosing spondylitis)
Prior Surgery	
Irradiation	

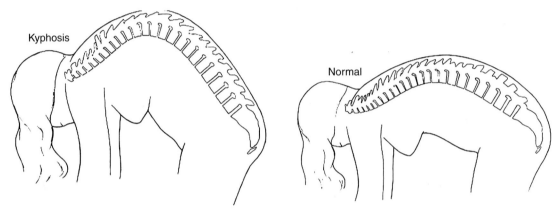

Kyphosis

Normal

Figure 7-3. Normal and kyphotic sagittal spine profile.

18. **What is sagittal imbalance syndrome? What are the most common causes?**
    Sagittal imbalance syndrome is a disabling postural disorder characterized by low back pain, forward inclination of the trunk, and difficulty in maintaining an erect posture. The patient attempts to compensate for this abnormal posture by either hyperextending the hips or standing with the hips and knees flexed. This syndrome results from decreased lumbar lordosis with subsequent global imbalance in the sagittal plane. The disorder was initially termed *flatback syndrome* and described in association with the surgical treatment of scoliosis, in which a fusion was performed into the lower lumbar spine in association with distraction instrumentation resulting in loss of normal lumbar lordosis. When a patient with a sagittal imbalance syndrome attempts to stand with the hips and knees fully extended, the head is no longer aligned over the sacrum. The reference line connecting the ear, shoulder, and greater trochanter of the hip lies anterior to an imaginary line drawn upward from the patient's feet. (Fig. 7-4) Additional causes of sagittal imbalance syndrome include hypolordotic lumbar fusions, deterioration of motion segments proximal or distal to a previous fusion mass, and pseudarthrosis.

19. **What additional evaluation is indicated for a patient who presents with a congenital spinal deformity?**
    Congenital spinal deformities are associated with abnormalities in other organ systems in a significant number of patients. Assessment for associated anomalies is part of the workup of a patient with congenital scoliosis. Associated anomalies of the neural axis (spinal dysraphism) are evaluated with an MRI of the spine. Nonspinal anomalies most frequently involve the renal system may be evaluated with renal ultrasound or intravenous pyelography.

20. **Describe the key points to assess during examination of a patient with spinal deformity secondary to neuromuscular disease (Fig. 7-5).**
    * Assessment of level of function. Can the patient sit independently? Is the patient ambulatory?
    * Assessment of general health status. Is there a history of seizures, frequent pneumonia, or poor nutrition?

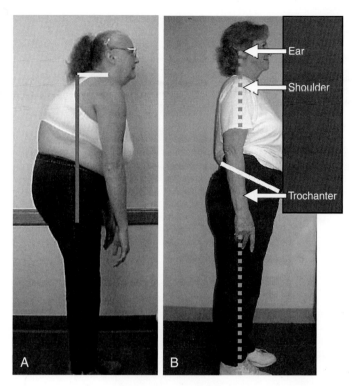

Figure 7-4. **A,** Flatback syndrome. **B,** Normal sagittal plane alignment.

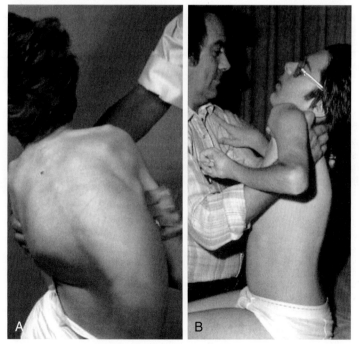

Figure 7-5. Neuromuscular scoliosis. **A,** Long sweeping curve with associated pelvic obliquity and loss of sitting balance. **B,** Assessment of curve flexibility.

- Evaluation of head control, trunk control, and motor strength. Does the underlying neuromuscular problem result in a spastic, flaccid, or athetoid picture?
- Assessment of curve flexibility. Curve flexibility can be assessed by grasping the head in the area of the mastoid process and lifting the patient from the sitting or standing position.
- Is pelvic obliquity present? Is it correctable with traction and positioning?
- Evaluation of the hip joints for coexistent pathology, including contractures.
- Is the patient's underlying neuromuscular disorder associated with any other organ system problems? For example, Duchenne muscular dystrophy is associated with cardiomyopathy.
- Documentation of pressure sores and areas of skin breakdown.

21. What findings may be noted in a pediatric patient with spondylolisthesis?

Spondylolisthesis in children may present with a variety of symptoms and physical findings, depending on the degree of slippage and the degree of kyphosis at the level of the slip. Low back pain and buttock pain are the most common presenting symptoms. Physical exam typically reveals localized tenderness with palpation at the level of slippage. Hamstring tightness is a commonly associated finding. In the most severe cases, the patient is unable to stand erect because of sagittal plane decompensation associated with compensatory lumbar hyperlordosis and occasionally neurologic deficit (Fig. 7-6).

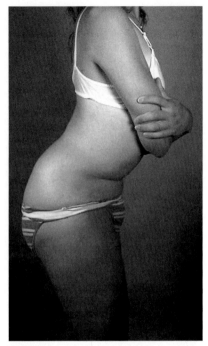

Figure 7-6. Severe spondylolisthesis associated with sagittal plane decompensation.

Key Points

1. The key components of the evaluation of a spinal deformity patient are a detailed patient history, comprehensive physical examination, appropriate diagnostic imaging studies, and assessment for potential abnormalities in other organ systems (e.g. renal, cardiac, gastrointestinal, pulmonary).
2. Consequences of untreated spinal deformity include cosmetic problems, pain, neurologic deficit, postural difficulty, pulmonary compromise, and impairment in daily living activities.

Websites

1. Scoliosis Research Society: http://www.srs.org/professionals/
2. Scoliosis Resources: http://www.nlm.nih.gov/medlineplus/scoliosis.html
3. Spondylolisthesis Resources: http://www.nlm.nih.gov/medlineplus/ency/article/001260.htm
4. Overview of resources for spinal diseases: http://www.nlm.nih.gov/medlineplus/spinaldiseases.html

BIBLIOGRAPHY

1. Gaines RW. Clinical evaluation of the patient with spine deformity. In DeWald RL, editor. Spinal Deformities: The Comprehensive Text. New York: Thieme; 2003. p. 267–71.
2. Lonner BS. Spinal deformity in the clinical setting. In: Errico TJ, Lonner BS, Moulton AW, editors. Surgical Management of Spinal Deformities. Philadelphia: Saunders; 2009. p. 61–70.
3. Lonstein JE. Patient evaluation. In: Lonstein JE, Winter RB, Bradford DS, et al., editors. Moe's Textbook of Scoliosis and Other Spinal Deformities. 3rd ed. Philadelphia: Saunders; 1995. p. 45–86.
4. McCarthy RE. Evaluation of the patient with deformity. In: Weinstein SL, editor. The Pediatric Spine - Principles and Practice. 2nd ed. Philadelphia: Lippincott Williams & Wilkins; 2001. p. 133–160.
5. Tolo VT. Clinical evaluation for neuromuscular scoliosis and kyphosis. In: DeWald RL, editor. Spinal Deformities: The Comprehensive Text. New York: Thieme; 2003. p. 272–83.
6. Winter RB. Evaluation of the patient with congenital spine deformity. In: DeWald RL, editor. Spinal Deformities: The Comprehensive Text. New York: Thieme; 2003. p. 258–66.

DISABILITY EVALUATION

Stephen L. Demeter, MD, MPH

CHAPTER 8

1. What are the definitions of impairment, disability, and handicap?

- An **impairment** is the "deviation of an anatomic structure, physiologic function, intellectual capability, or emotional status from that which the individual possessed prior to an alteration in those structures or functions or from that expected from population norms."
- A **disability** is the "inability to complete a specific task successfully that the individual was previously capable of completing or that most members of a society are capable of completing owing to a medical or psychological deviation from prior health status or from the status expected of most members of a society." In other words, a disability is the inability to perform a specified task because of an impairment.
- An impaired individual is considered to have a handicap if there are obstacles to accomplishing life's basic activities that can be overcome only by compensating in some way for the effects of the impairment. In this context, a **handicap** is an assistive device or a task modification that allows an individual with an impairment to complete a task.

An example contrasting impairment and disability serves well. A person who sustains a thoracic fracture associated with a complete spinal cord injury has an impairment. Loss of motor and sensory function in the lower extremities and bowel/bladder dysfunction result from the anatomic deficit. If the person is an accountant, this medical impairment may or may not translate into disability, as the person may be able to perform accounting duties at work. On the other hand, if the person is a professional basketball player, the same medical impairment creates total disability. Thus, *disability* is *task-specific*, whereas *impairment* merely reflects an *alteration from normal body functions*. However, disability must be considered in the context of the system in which the individual has applied for relief. In certain systems, a person with lower extremity paraplegia may be presumed to be totally disabled. In this example, use of a wheelchair and specialized van may permit the accountant to travel to work and would be considered a *handicap*.

2. What is an impairment evaluation?

An *impairment evaluation* is a medical evaluation. Its purpose is to define, describe, and measure the differences in a particular person compared with either the average person (e.g. an IQ of 86 compared with the normal expected average of 100) or that person's prior capability (e.g. a preinjury IQ measured at 134 compared with the current level of 100). Such differences may take the form of anatomic deviations (e.g. amputations), physical abnormalities (e.g. decreased motion of a joint, decreased strength surrounding that joint, or abnormal neurologic input), physiologic abnormalities (e.g. diminished ability to breathe, electrical conduction disturbances in the heart), or psychological (e.g. diminished ability to think, reason, or remember).

3. Who performs an impairment evaluation?

Impairment evaluations should be performed only by professionals with a background in medical practice. Doctors of medicine and osteopathy are the logical choices. However, other professionals also possess such training and background and often perform impairment evaluations. Examples include chiropractic doctors, dentists, optometrists, psychologists, and physical therapists. Further, an impairment evaluation should be performed only by professionals qualified by training or experience to assess the organ system that needs to be evaluated. Ideally, a neurologist should evaluate neurologic impairment. However, many specialties cross boundaries so that an occupational medicine specialist or physiatrist will also be able to evaluate orthopaedic impairment, not just orthopedic surgeons.

4. How does an impairment evaluation differ from a normal history and physical examination?

Several important differences are seen when these types of examinations are contrasted: the goal of the evaluation is different, the patient may be defined differently, and the opportunity for reevaluation is limited in impairment examinations.

The goal of an impairment evaluation is to define deviations from normalcy. Having or arriving at a specific diagnosis/diagnoses is often useful and helpful. However, a specific diagnosis is not the end result in an impairment evaluation as it is in the standard history and physical examination. Both evaluations require appropriate educational background, skill, thoroughness, and dedication. In a normal history and physical exam, there is a doctor-patient relationship and the physician attempts to diagnose and determine what treatment is required. In an impairment examination, the evaluator attempts to determine deviations in the examinee's health status and to quantify those deviations in a passive manner and does not enter into an active doctor-patient relationship.

The results of the standard history and physical belong to the person being evaluated (although not always, as in the case of a child). The results of an impairment evaluation are usually provided to the requesting source, such as an attorney, insurance company, or governmental agency (e.g. workers' compensation boards or the Social Security Department). This point often raises an interesting legal concept. Physicians are not allowed to disclose medical information to anyone but the patient. To whom does such confidentiality apply in an impairment evaluation? Usually it exists between the physician and the referring agency or party as opposed to the person evaluated.

Another basic distinction is that the impairment evaluation report focuses on and addresses the questions asked by the referring party. For example, if the physician is asked to evaluate a person for a specific injury, such as an amputation or dysfunction of an arm, the entire evaluation focuses on the arm. The end result is a report that describes the injury and the differences in the function of the injured arm from a normal person's arm (or the individual's arm function prior to the injury) and provides a prognosis for future recovery. This information is then used by other parties to determine appropriate compensation. Other diagnoses discovered during the evaluation may be irrelevant. Other issues, such as causation, apportionment, and diagnostic or therapeutic recommendations, may or may not be desired. If these issues are not requested, they are not included in the report.

Lastly, impairment evaluations are generally limited to a single encounter with the examinee.

5. How does a disability evaluation differ from an impairment evaluation?
A disability is defined as a medical impairment that precludes a specific task. Generally, during a disability evaluation, that task is the examinee's job. Thus, the disability evaluation is comprehensive and based on various factors. One of these factors is the medical impairment. Other factors may include a person's age, educational background, educational capabilities, and other social factors. Such elements are used by the system to which the worker has applied for relief. For example, a person whose right arm has been amputated may be capable of entering the work force in some other capacity. If the person is young enough, smart enough, and sufficiently motivated, he or she may be capable of performing remunerative activities in some other job market. The referring agency uses such factors when determining whether a person is totally or partially disabled and which benefits are applicable. Thus, in a disability evaluation, the physician must not only quantify impairment but address additional issues such as:
- What tasks is the examinee capable of performing?
- Can the examinee attend work?
- Are job modifications an option?
- When will the examinee reach maximum medical improvement (MMI)?

6. What is workers' compensation?
According to Elisburg, "Workers' compensation is a disability program to provide medical economic support to workers who have been injured or made ill from an incident arising out of and in the course of employment. It is a complex $70 billion a year program in the United States that involves nearly sixty different systems." This program originated as a social experiment by Bismarck in Germany in the 1880s. It is a *no-fault compensation system* designed to replace the traditional *tort system*, under which an injured worker had to sue his employer to get benefits. In a tort system, the employee was at a disadvantage for various reasons. To rectify this problem, many states developed workers' compensation systems. The last state to do so was Mississippi in 1949. The federal government has similar systems. These systems often are industry-specific and have their own rules regarding impairment, disability, and compensation.

7. What is Social Security Disability (SSD)?
According to the Social Security Administration (SSA), disability is defined as "the inability to engage in any substantial gainful activity by reason of any medically determinable physical or mental impairment(s) which can be expected to result in death or which has lasted or can be expected to last for a continuous period of not less than 12 months." In addition, for a person under the age of 18, disability can exist "if he or she has a medically determinable impairment(s) that is of comparable severity" to the impairment in an adult. To comply with these definitions, a person may have a single medical impairment or multiple impairments that, when combined, are of such severity that the person can no longer perform his or her previous occupation or sustain any remunerative activity after age, education, and prior work experience are considered.

Two groups of people are eligible for SSD:
- Under Title II, Social Security Disability Insurance (SSDI) provides cash benefits for disabled workers and their dependents who have contributed to the Social Security Trust Fund through taxes.
- Under Title XVI (Supplemental Security Income [SSI]) provides a minimum income level for the needy, aged, blind, and disabled. People qualify for SSI because of financial need. Under SSI, financial need is said to exist when a person's income and resources are equal to or below an amount specified by law ($637/month in 2009).

8. What is the cost of disability?
This question is difficult to answer. For example, if a worker is injured on the job, what defines the cost of the disability? Is it the cost of time off work? Is it the worker's medical expenses (e.g. physician's fees, operative costs, prescription costs, physical therapy, rehabilitation costs)? Is it the cost of paying the worker while he or she is out of work? Is it offset by money earned when a spouse had to return to work? Is it the money to fund the social programs and human resource departments needed to fill out the forms and provide the benefits? Ultimately, of course, all of these factors must be considered.

Medical expenditures related to disability in 1987 totaled $336 billion. Approximately 6.5% of the gross domestic product is used in this process. Approximately 51% of disability costs is for medical care and other goods and services provided to the disabled. Approximately 39% of the overall cost comes from lost earnings and approximately 10% from the labor market losses of household members or persons with disabilities.

9. Who wrote the rules for impairment evaluation?

Disability is a big business in the United States and other countries. Various institutions pay the costs, such as state governments (workers' compensation), the federal government (e.g. for veterans or longshoremen), insurance companies, and self-insured employers. Many systems that pay for disability have their own rules and regulations, including rules about the performance and rating of the impairment. The most commonly used system is a formal set of rules developed by the American Medical Association, which is constantly updated (*The Guides to the Evaluation of Permanent Impairment*). Another system is the Social Security Administration Disability Program whose rules are explained in *The Blue Book*. The rules and regulations found in these sources are vastly different. For example, the SSA recognizes only total impairment. The AMA *Guides* fractionates impairment from 1% to 100%. Highly specific rules are applied to these impairments in each set of guidelines. The impairment evaluator must be thoroughly familiar with the system that he or she is required to use.

10. Define the concept *whole person impairment.*

In the AMA *Guides,* an individual who is totally dependent of others for care is considered 90+% impaired with 100% impairment reserved for those who are *approaching death*. Using the AMA *Guides*, a person whose right arm was amputated at the shoulder has a 60% impairment of the whole person; a leg amputation at the hip is equivalent to a 40% whole person impairment. A person with coronary disease may have whole person impairment ranging from 0% to 65%. The precise amount of whole person impairment depends on the degree of deviation from normalcy that can be found by history and physical examination and the diagnostic tests performed.

11. What is *maximum medical improvement* (MMI)?

This concept, when is used in impairment evaluations, states that a person has achieved MMI if no further substantial improvement is anticipated with time and/or additional treatment. Treatment may include medications, surgery, or physical therapy or other types of rehabilitation. Most impairment systems require that the person achieve MMI before a final impairment rating can be given. This rating is then used as a basis for the final disability settlement. Note that this concept does not consider whether the individual will worsen with time. Further, the concept of MMI usually allows for an individual to accept further treatment (with MMI determined after an appropriate recovery time following that treatment) or to decline further treatment (in which case, they have attained MMI). In other words, an individual may decline treatment that might mitigate the current level of impairment (as well as the impairment rating).

12. What is *apportionment*?

Apportionment refers to a division of responsibility. Apportionment can be applied to the impairment rating based on causative factors. For example, if a worker applies for disability benefits because of a toxic gas inhalation, some states take into consideration the fact that this person was a two-pack a day smoker for the past 20 years. The final amount of the loss of lung function is thus apportioned into the various contributing/causative factors.

Apportionment can also refer to the division of payment responsibility. A man had a back injury while at work but also had a similar back injury at work two years ago with ongoing symptoms and treatment. The current treatment costs can be apportioned to both the old and the new injury, as can the impairment rating. Most jurisdictions have their own rules as to whether apportionment is used and in which circumstances. A great deal of skill and expertise are needed for an examiner to apportion an individual's current condition to all the causative factors, including the normal aging process.

13. How does one perform an impairment evaluation?

The examiner starts with the questions that are asked by the referring party and directs the evaluation based on those questions. For example, if the examinee's right arm has been amputated, the examiner focuses on the amputation. One does not perform a complete history and physical examination if it is not requested, called for, or appropriate. On the other hand, the body part that was injured and/or specified in the referral is evaluated thoroughly. This evaluation may take the form of a history and physical examination, specialized physical examination techniques, radiographs and other types of body imaging studies, physiologic testing, and other types of examinations. The examiner must answer the specific questions asked in the report. Additionally, the report is tempered by the specifics of the evaluating system used for that particular examination. For example, some evaluating systems require certain tests to be performed and ignore the results from other types of testing. The impairment evaluator must thoroughly understand the system to be used for each evaluation so that the appropriate examinations can be performed and appropriate answers provided.

14. What is a functional capacity assessment?

A functional capacity assessment or evaluation (FCE) is a test that assesses how well a particular organ system is working. Thus, any stress test (cardiac, pulmonary, heat tolerance) is a functional capacity assessment. On a more global level, an FCE measures the body as a whole and determines how much work a person is capable of doing. This concept, the idea of testing how much work a person is able to perform, was derived from work performed by ergonomists and physical therapists.

When used as a descriptive phrase, an FCE describes a test of work capacity. It must be appreciated that testing for a person's ability to work assesses many organ systems at one time. Generally, it is assumed that organ systems such as the cardiac, pulmonary, and neurologic systems are functioning normally. However, dysfunction in any other organ systems is a sufficient cause for an abnormal FCE.

Most FCEs assess the ability to work. There are many components to this test, and it is common for an FCE to take 4 to 6 hours. Tests that take 2 or 3 days to perform are not unusual. The end result is a list of body regions and both the maximum and the sustainable levels of physical exertion that the examinee is capable of performing in each body region. For example, the test will describe how much weight can be lifted, how many times it can be lifted, or for how long the examinee can perform the activities. The results can be linked to the specifics of a job. For example, if a person is capable of lifting, on a sustained basis, only 20 pounds (although on a rare basis he is capable of lifting as much as 50 pounds) and the job entails lifting 60 to 80 pounds on a frequent basis, one might conclude that he is not fit or qualified for the job. While this type of evaluation might seem ideal when determining if a person is able to do a job (for a new hire) or return to his or her normal job (for a recently injured individual who is deemed to have attained MMI), it must always be remembered these types of tests only measure how much the examinee is willing to do, not necessarily how much he or she can do.

15. What is the American with Disabilities Act (ADA)?

In 1990 Congress passed the ADA. This law protects people with disabilities from discrimination and mandates accommodations for disabled employees, customers, clients, patients, and others. It prohibits discrimination in public or private employment, governmental services, public accommodations, public transportation, and telecommunication. The ADA defines a person with a disability in three ways:

1. Any person who has a physical or mental impairment that substantially limits one or more of the individual's major life activities
2. Any person who has a *record of* a substantially limiting impairment
3. Any person who is *regarded as* having a substantially limiting impairment, regardless of whether the person is in fact disabled.

According to the ADA, before a job offer, an employer may not inquire about an applicant's impairment or medical history. In addition, inquiries about past injuries and/or workers' compensation claims are expressly prohibited. An employer may offer a position conditionally, based on completion of a medical examination or medical inquiry—but only if such examinations or inquiries are made of all applicants for the same job category and the results are kept confidential. A post-offer medical evaluation is also permissible and may be more comprehensive. The job offer may be withdrawn only if the findings of the medical examination show that a person is unable to perform the essential functions of a job, even with a reasonable accommodation, or if the person poses a direct threat to his or her own health or safety or to the health and safety of others, even with reasonable accommodation. Obviously, it is important to have the list of the essential functions of a job for comparison.

Over the years, the intent of the ADA became diluted based on a variety of judicial rulings. On July 26, 2008, President Bush signed into law the ADA Amendments Act of 2008 (ADAAA) that clarified and extended the original law. Among other things, the ADAAA added "major life activities" to the ADA to include issues, such as "caring for oneself, performing manual tasks, seeing, hearing, eating, sleeping, walking, standing, lifting," and others. It specified the operation of several "major bodily functions." It overturned two U.S. Supreme Court decisions that held that an employee was not disabled if the impairment could be corrected by some device and that an impairment that limits one major life activity must also limit other life activities to be considered a disability.

16. How do I fill out back-to-work forms?

Functional capacity assessment(s) are often useful when determining if an individual can return to his or her normal occupation. Some of the basic principles from the ADA are also applicable. One starts with a description of the job, primarily its essential functions, although peripheral functions may sometimes be important and be included. For an assembly-line worker, the job description may include where the worker has to stand, how many times the worker has to bend over, whether the worker has to pick up a part, how heavy the part is, how often the worker does this activity, and various other ergonomic issues. Ideally, one then matches the worker's capability with the requirements of the job. For example, if we can measure how long workers can stand, how often they can bend, how much bending they are capable of doing, and what strength they have while performing various tasks, we should be able to say whether they are capable of returning to their job or whether they need to be assigned to modified and/or restricted duties.

In most circumstances, we do not achieve this perfect state of knowledge and blending of the worker with the job. Also, in most circumstances, we do not need this level of evaluation. When physicians approach the issue of whether their patient can or cannot return to one's normal job, they have two choices: they can either refer the person for appropriate testing, or they can make an *educated guess* based on their experience, knowledge, and background. The more educated the examiner and the better his or her understanding of the job requirements, the more valid his or her determination will be.

17. How do I fill out the forms from the SSA?

Social Security forms frequently cross a physician's desk. They are often multipaged documents asking many questions. They can be daunting for those who do not understand the process of how the SSA determines disability. The completed forms are intended to provide background information to the impairment and disability evaluator in the Social Security system. An independent impairment examination also may be performed on such patients. The attending physician's report is used to provide background information so that a decision can be made whether or not a person qualifies for Social Security disability. If the information provided does not allow the decision makers to answer the questions regarding qualifications, then a separate examination, paid for and scheduled by the SSA, will be performed. It is not the attending physician's job to perform an impairment evaluation, obtain consultation with other physicians, or perform additional diagnostic testing. On occasions, the SSA will ask the attending physician to provide an opinion regarding his or her patient's ability to perform remunerative employment, but these opinions are not to be provided unless asked for.

18. **During work hours, a man slips on ice while delivering packages for his job. He has the sudden onset of pain and discomfort in his lower back. He has pain and numbness and tingling in his right leg. After treatment with analgesics and physical therapy, he recovers. Two years later, he has a similar injury. A magnetic resonance imaging (MRI) discloses a herniated disc at the L4–L5 interspace. He has surgery because of persistent, severe symptoms. He has a successful outcome and returns to the work force. He is asymptomatic except for mild discomfort in the lower back after a long day. Does the man have an impairment? If so, how much?**
Certainly the man has an impairment based on the anatomic deviation from normalcy. Using the *AMA Guides,* he has 10% impairment of the whole person because of the herniated disc and neurologic abnormalities, despite the fact that he has had a successful operation and is now relatively asymptomatic.

19. **The same man returns to work and slips and falls again. His symptoms are now severe. He has constant low back pain. He can no longer participate in sports activities, which he enjoyed in the past. He cannot go back to work in his heavy manual labor job. These symptoms have persisted for the past 4 years, and he has been told that he is not a surgical candidate. Does he have an impairment? If so, how much?**
This man continues to have impairment caused by the first and second injuries and has been made worse (exacerbated) by the third. However, no further impairment is awarded. The 10% impairment that he received originally (although he was essentially asymptomatic at that time) was given because of the known risk for further problems as time passes. Thus, there is no increase in the impairment rating.

Key Points

1. Impairment reflects an alteration from normal bodily functions, can be assessed using traditional medical means, and can be objectively determined.
2. Disability results from impairment, is task-specific, and is measured in the context of the system to which the worker has applied for relief. Disability determination is an administrative determination that uses both medical and nonmedical information.
3. One individual can be impaired significantly and have no disability, while another person can be severely disabled with only a limited impairment.

Websites

1. Help for health professionals to understand the Social Security Disability determination process: http://www.ssa.gov/disability/professionals/index.htm
2. Impairment rating and disability determination: http://emedicine.medscape.com/article/314195-overview
3. Information and technical assistance relating to The Americans with Disabilities Act: http://www.ada.gov/
4. Musculoskeletal disorders and workplace factors: http://www.cdc.gov/niosh/docs/97-141/
5. Social Security Administration, U.S. Department of Health and Human Services: Disability Evaluation under Social Security. Available only online: http://www.ssa.gov/disability/professionals/bluebook

BIBLIOGRAPHY

1. American Medical Association. Guides to the Evaluation of Permanent Impairment. 5th ed. Chicago: American Medical Association; 2000. p. 2–5.
2. American Medical Association. Guides to the Evaluation of Permanent Impairment. 6th ed. Chicago: American Medical Association; 2008. p. 572.
3. Barth PS. Economic costs of disability. In: Demeter SL, Anderson GBJ, Smith GM, editors. Disability Evaluation. St. Louis: Mosby; 1996. p. 13–9.
4. Barth PS. Economic costs of disability. In: Demeter SL, Andersson GBJ, editors. Disability Evaluation. 2nd ed. St. Louis: Mosby; 2003. p. 20–7.
5. Bell C, Judy B. Overview of the Americans with Disabilities Act and the Family and Medical Leave Act. In: Demeter SL, Andersson GBJ, editors. Disability Evaluation. 2nd ed. St. Louis: Mosby; 2003. p. 664–71.
6. Demeter SL. Appendix B. In: Demeter SL, Andersson GBJ, editors. Disability Evaluation. 2nd ed. St. Louis: Mosby; 2003. p. 871–91.
7. Demeter SL. Contrasting the standard, impairment, and disability examination. In: Demeter SL, Andersson GBJ, editors. Disability Evaluation. 2nd ed. St. Louis: Mosby; 2003. p. 101–10.
8. Elisburg D. Workers' compensation. In: Demeter SL, Andersson GBJ, Smith GM, editors. Disability Evaluation. St. Louis: Mosby; 1996. p. 36–44.

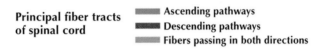

Principal fiber tracts of spinal cord

- Ascending pathways
- Descending pathways
- Fibers passing in both directions

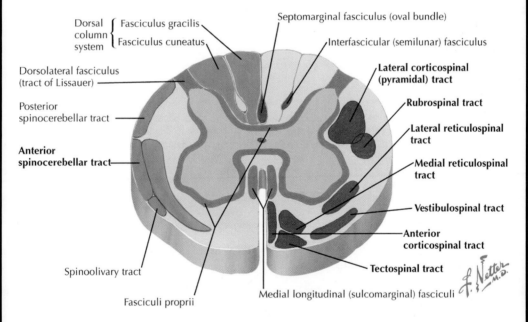

Dorsal column system
- Fasciculus gracilis
- Fasciculus cuneatus

Dorsolateral fasciculus (tract of Lissauer)

Posterior spinocerebellar tract

Anterior spinocerebellar tract

Spinoolivary tract

Fasciculi proprii

Septomarginal fasciculus (oval bundle)

Interfascicular (semilunar) fasciculus

Lateral corticospinal (pyramidal) tract

Rubrospinal tract

Lateral reticulospinal tract

Medial reticulospinal tract

Vestibulospinal tract

Anterior corticospinal tract

Tectospinal tract

Medial longitudinal (sulcomarginal) fasciculi

STRATEGIES FOR IMAGING IN SPINAL DISORDERS

Joseph Y. Margulies, MD, PhD, and Vincent J. Devlin, MD

1. What are the major objectives of spinal imaging tests?

Spinal imaging studies are an adjunct to the process of establishing a diagnosis. Imaging studies should be performed to address a specific diagnostic question and not as screening tests. Common reasons to order spinal imaging studies are to:

1. Rule out serious spinal pathology such as tumor or infection
2. Evaluate spinal morphology in patients presenting with symptoms due to neural compression, spinal deformity, or mechanical insufficiency of the spinal column
3. Identify the level(s) of a spinal lesion
4. Create a topographic map to guide surgical intervention
5. Evaluate the results of operative and nonoperative treatment

2. What are the most common diagnostic imaging tests used to evaluate spinal disorders?

- Plain radiographs
- Magnetic resonance imaging (MRI)
- Computed tomography (CT)
- CT-myelography
- Bone scan

3. What additional tests may play a role in the diagnosis of spinal disorders?

- **Bone densitometry.** Dual energy x-ray absorptiometry (DEXA) is widely used to assess bone density.
- **Discography.** This provocative test involves injecting lumbar discs in an attempt to determine whether a degenerated lumbar disc is a pain generator.
- **Facet joint injections.** Local anesthetic or steroid may be injected in the facet region to provide diagnostic information or an anesthetic effect.
- **Selective spinal nerve blocks.** Local anesthetic or steroid may be injected around a segmental spinal nerve to provide diagnostic information or an anesthetic effect.
- **Angiography.** Vascular structures in proximity to the spine may be visualized with CT angiography or magnetic resonance angiography.
- **Biopsy.** CT-guided biopsies are commonly used to obtain tissue for diagnostic study in cases of tumor and infection as well as lesions whose diagnosis has yet to be determined.

4. What is the greatest challenge facing both patients and physicians regarding the use of spinal imaging tests?

Both patients and physicians tend to overestimate the ability of modern imaging tests to detect symptomatic spinal pathology and guide treatment. Each imaging modality—radiographs, CT, MRI, bone scan—is extremely sensitive but relatively nonspecific. Many studies have documented that spinal imaging studies reveal abnormalities in at least one-third of asymptomatic patients. One of the major challenges in utilization of imaging tests is to determine the clinical relevance of abnormal spinal morphology. This determination is especially challenging in attempts to distinguish imaging abnormalities likely to have clinical significance from those that are part of the normal aging process or part of a normal sequence of postoperative healing. In the absence of clinical assessment, imaging tests cannot determine whether a specific spinal structure is responsible for symptoms. Excessive emphasis on imaging tests without clinical correlation is hazardous to both patient and physician and may lead to inappropriate treatment.

5. What steps can the clinician take to minimize the inappropriate use of diagnostic imaging tests?

1. Perform a detailed history and physical exam before ordering any imaging tests.
2. Formulate a working diagnosis to explain symptoms and guide testing.
3. Order the imaging study best suited to evaluate the suspected pathologic process based on the working diagnosis.
4. Order imaging tests only when the information obtained from the test will affect medical decision-making.

6. Into what major etiologic groups can patients presenting with spinal symptomatology be classified?
1. Degenerative disorders
2. Trauma
3. Tumor
4. Infections
5. Spinal deformities
6. Congenital disorders
7. Inflammatory disorders
8. Metabolic disorders
9. Extraspinal conditions that mimic spinal pathology

7. When should I order a spine radiograph?
Plain radiographs should be the initial imaging study of the spine. Because of the favorable natural history of acute cervical and lumbar pain syndromes, it is not necessary to order initial spine radiographs for every patient who presents with neck or low back pain. Indications for obtaining spine radiographs in patients presenting with cervical, thoracic, or lumbar pain include:
- Patients younger than 20 years or patients older than 50 years
- Patients who fail to respond to conservative management within 6 to 8 weeks
- Patients with a history of trauma (to rule out fracture)
- Complaints of pain at rest or night pain, history of cancer, fever, unexplained weight loss (to rule out tumor or infection)

8. What are the major advantages of using plain radiographs to assess spinal disorders?
- Plain radiographs are inexpensive and readily available.
- Rapid assessment of a specific spinal region (cervical, thoracic, lumbar) or the entire spinal axis (occiput to sacrum) in orthogonal planes is possible.
- Weight-bearing (standing) and dynamic studies (flexion-extension views, side-bending views) may be obtained.
- Plain radiographs are useful to confirm normal osseous structure, vertebral alignment, and structural integrity of the spine.

9. What are the major disadvantages of using plain radiographs to assess spinal disorders?
- Radiographs have a low sensitivity and specificity in identifying symptomatic spinal pathology. Age-related degenerative changes are present equally in symptomatic and asymptomatic populations.
- Radiographs cannot visualize neural structures and other soft tissue lesions (e.g. disc herniation).
- Radiographs cannot diagnose early-stage tumor or infection because significant bone destruction (40–60% of bone mass) must occur before a radiographic abnormality is detectable.

10. When should I order a spine MRI?
An MRI is indicated if the clinical history and physical exam suggest a serious spinal problem and initial plain radiographs do not provide sufficient diagnostic information. The clinician should consider how the information obtained from a spinal MRI will affect the decision-making process for a specific patient before ordering this study.

11. What are the major advantages of using MRI to assess spinal disorders?
- Avoids ionizing radiation
- Provides imaging in orthogonal planes
- Visualizes an entire spinal region and avoids missed pathology at transition zones between adjacent spinal regions
- Provides excellent visualization of pathologic processes involving the disc, thecal sac, epidural space, neural elements, paraspinal soft tissue, and bone marrow

12. What are the major disadvantages of using MRI to assess spinal disorders?
- MRI does not define osseous anatomy as well as CT.
- Many implanted devices are contraindications to MRI (e.g., pacemakers, drug pumps, spine stimulators)
- Claustrophobic patients may have difficulty with the test.

13. When should I order a CT scan?
CT is most helpful when osseous abnormality is suggested. Common disorders for which CT is helpful include fractures, facet arthrosis, spondylolysis, and spondylolisthesis.

14. What are the major advantages of using CT to assess spinal disorders?
- CT is the best test for assessment of bone anatomy.
- Multiple cross-sectional images can be reconstructed to provide images in orthogonal planes (e.g. coronal, sagittal, and three-dimensional images).
- CT is useful when MRI is contraindicated (e.g. cardiac pacemaker).

15. What are the major disadvantages of using CT to assess spinal disorders?
- Exposure to ionizing radiation.
- CT provides poor delineation of the neural elements.
- Significant pathology can be missed. For example, standard lumbar CT visualizes the L3 to S1 region and fails to detect pathology in the upper lumbar region

16. When should I order a myelogram?
Rarely. Myelography is no longer used as a stand-alone test to evaluate spinal pathology. However, myelography has a role in spinal imaging when it is combined with a CT scan. CT- myelography plays an important role in the assessment of complex spine problems such as lumbar spinal stenosis associated with scoliosis or cervical spinal stenosis associated with ossification of the posterior longitudinal ligament (OPLL). CT-myelography plays an important role in the assessment of patients requiring revision spinal surgery, especially when metallic spinal implants are present following prior surgical procedures.

17. What are the main advantages of myelography in the assessment of spinal disorders?
Myelography is the only widely available test that can provide dynamic information about the spine and its relation to the neural elements. Upright weight-bearing views as well as flexion-extension views are possible. Such views are especially helpful in assessing patients whose symptoms are exacerbated in the erect position as myelography permits imaging of the spine in the symptomatic position. Other advanced imaging tests such as CT and MRI are generally performed with the patient in the supine position. Standing MRI scanner technology is evolving and will play an increasingly important role in the future.

18. What are the main disadvantages of using myelography as an isolated test to assess spinal disorders?
- Myelography is an invasive test.
- Complications and unpleasant side effects may occur (e.g. adverse reaction to contrast, spinal fluid leak, spinal headache).
- Myelography is less accurate than CT or MRI in evaluating disc pathology.
- Myelography cannot detect pathology below the level of a complete block to contrast.
- Myelography provides only indirect evidence of neural compression by demonstrating changes in contour of contrast-filled neural structures.
- Myelography cannot differentiate whether extradural compression is due to disc, osteophyte, tumor, or infection.
- Myelography cannot visualize pathology in the lateral zone of the spinal canal because the contrast-filled dural sac ends in the region of the pedicle.
- Pathology may be missed at the L5–S1 level, where the spinal canal is very wide, and a large disc protrusion or osteophyte may not deform the dye column.

19. When should I order a CT-myelogram?
For many complex spinal problems, high-quality MRI and CT scans may be used as complementary studies to define the clinical problem. Nevertheless, in certain situations, a CT-myelogram remains the test of choice. Some of these situations include:
- Evaluation of the neural elements in a postoperative patient with stainless steel spinal implants
- Patients with significant symptoms and equivocal MRI findings
- Patients with cervical or lumbar spinal stenosis problems in whom MRI is contraindicated
- Preoperative planning for surgery in patients with symptomatic spinal stenosis and severe lumbar scoliosis
- Preoperative planning for revision spinal stenosis surgery, especially if symptoms suggest a relation to postural change
- Preoperative planning for surgical treatment of specific complex spinal deformities

20. What are the major advantages of CT-myelography to assess spinal disorders?
The use of CT and myelography together exceeds the value of either test performed alone. The addition of contrast to the CT scan improves delineation of neural structures, permitting distinction between disc margin, thecal sac, and ligamentum flavum. As a result, the accuracy of CT-myelography is comparable to MRI for a wide range of spinal disorders. An advantage of CT-myelography is that it can provide useful diagnostic information when MRI is contraindicated.

21. What are the major disadvantages of using CT-myelography to assess spinal disorders?
The disadvantages of CT-myelography include its invasive nature, need for contrast administration, and use of ionizing radiation.

22. When should I order a bone scan?
1. To screen the skeletal system for metastatic disease
2. To screen the spinal column for metastatic tumor, primary bone tumor, disc space infection, or vertebral osteomyelitis

3. To assess the relative biologic activity of bone lesions, such as pars interarticularis defects or facet joint degenerative changes
4. To aid in diagnosis of sacroiliac joint pathology, such as infection or arthritis
5. To diagnose fractures in areas difficult to visualize with plain radiographs (e.g. sacral insufficiency fractures)

23. What are the major advantages of using a bone scan to assess spinal disorders?
- Bone scans provide an excellent method for rapidly screening the entire skeleton for osseous abnormalities; they are especially useful for tumors and infections.
- Bone scans are an effective method for determining the relative biologic activity of a bone lesion. For example, differentiation is possible between acute vs. chronic vertebral fractures or acute vs. chronic pars defects.
- Both planar and cross-sectional images (single-photon emission computed tomography ([SPECT]) may be obtained.

24. What are the major disadvantages of using bone scans to assess spinal disorders?
- Bone scans are highly sensitive but not highly specific.
- Bone scans do not have sufficient resolution for surgical planning.
- Certain tumors, such as multiple myeloma or some purely lytic metastases, may not demonstrate increased activity on bone scan as they do not stimulate a significant osteoblastic response.

25. Describe the sequence of ordering spinal imaging studies in terms of an algorithm.
Plain radiographs are generally the first imaging study obtained in the evaluation of patients with a spinal problem. If radiographs do not provide sufficient information, MRI is generally the next best study to evaluate most clinical conditions because it provides the greatest amount of information regarding a single spinal region. CT may be obtained to complement the information obtained with MRI, especially when additional information is required about osseous anatomy. CT-myelography and radionuclide studies have limited indications but play a crucial role in specific situations. An exception to this algorithm occurs in the assessment of acute spine fractures. CT is preferred over MRI as an initial test in this setting because of its superior depiction of bone detail and fracture anatomy.

Key Points

1. One of the major challenges in utilization of spinal imaging tests is to determine the clinical relevance of abnormal spinal morphology.
2. Plain radiographs are inexpensive, readily available, and can provide valuable information but have a low sensitivity and specificity in identifying symptomatic spinal pathology.
3. MRI is generally the best initial advanced spinal imaging study to evaluate nontraumatic clinical conditions because it provides the greatest amount of information regarding a single spinal region.
4. CT is obtained to complement MRI, especially when additional information is required regarding osseous spinal anatomy.

Websites

Diagnostic tests and procedures:
http://www.spineuniverse.com/displayarticle.php/article2422.html
MRI of the spine: http://www.radiologyinfo.org/en/pdf/spinemr.pdf
Neuroradiology teaching file database: http://spinwarp.ucsd.edu/NeuroWeb/TF.html

BIBLIOGRAPHY

1. Boden SD, Davis DO, Dina TS. Abnormal lumbar spine MRI scans in asymptomatic subjects: a prospective investigation. J Bone Joint Surg 1990;72A:403–8.
2. Boden SD, McCowin PR, David DO, et al.: Abnormal cervical spine MR scans in asymptomatic individuals: A prospective and blinded investigation. J Bone Joint Surg 1990;72A:1178–84.
3. Carragee EJ, Hannibal M. Diagnostic evaluation of low back pain. Ortho Clin North Am 2004;35:7–16.
4. France JC. Radiographic imaging of the traumatically injured spine: plain radiographs, computed tomography, magnetic resonance imaging, angiography, clearing the cervical spine in trauma patients. In: Kim DH, Ludwig SC, Vaccaro AR, et al., editors. Atlas of Spine Trauma. Philadelphia: Saunders, Elsevier; 2008, p. 37–67.
5. Ross JS, Bell GR. Spine imaging. In: Herkowitz HN, Garfin SR, Eismont FJ, et al., editors. The Spine. Philadelphia: Saunders, Elsevier; 2006, p. 187–217.
6. Shafaie FF, Wippold FJ II, Gado M, et al. Comparison of computed tomography myelography and magnetic resonance imaging in patients with degenerative disorders. Spine 1999;24:1781–85.

10 CHAPTER | RADIOGRAPHIC ASSESSMENT OF THE SPINE

Vincent J. Devlin, MD

CERVICAL SPINE

1. What radiographic views are commonly used to assess the cervical spinal region?

Standard cervical spine views include: anteroposterior (AP) view (Fig. 10-1), lateral view (Fig. 10-2), right and left oblique views (Fig. 10-3), and open-mouth AP odontoid view (Fig. 10-4).

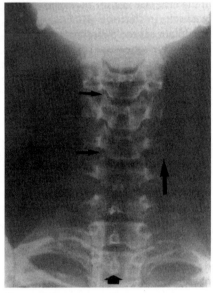

Figure 10-1. Normal anteroposterior cervical radiograph. The joints of Luschka are sharply defined and uniform (*thin arrow*). The spinous processes are midline and aligned (*short thick arrow*). The lateral margins of the articulating masses are smooth and undulating (*long thick arrow*). (From Schwartz AJ. Imaging of degenerative cervical disease. Spine State Art Rev 2000;14:545–69, with permission.)

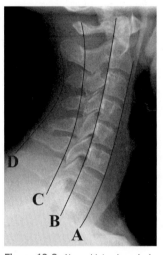

Figure 10-2. Normal lateral cervical radiograph. All cervical vertebra and the superior aspect of T1 are visualized. Four parallel lines used for assessment of alignment are drawn: A. anterior vertebral; B. posterior vertebral; C. spinolaminar; D. posterior spinous process. The atlantodens interval is within normal limits. (From Pretorious ES, Solomon JA, editors. Radiology Secrets. 2nd ed. Philadelphia: Elsevier; 2006.)

2. What important parameters require assessment on each cervical radiographic view?

AP VIEW
- Confirm that spinous processes align with each other
- Assess distance between adjacent spinous processes and vertebral endplates
- Assess facet joint margins and uncinate processes

LATERAL VIEW
- Assess prevertebral and retropharyngeal soft tissue shadows
- Assess alignment via anatomic lines along anterior and posterior vertebral margins, spino-laminar junctions, and spinous processes
- Measure the distance from the posterior margin of the anterior C1 arch to the anterior aspect of the odontoid (atlantodens interval)
- Assess intervertebral disc space heights
- Confirm that the superior aspect of T1 is well visualized

OBLIQUE VIEW
- Assess facet joint alignment
- Assess neural foramina and their bony boundaries

OPEN-MOUTH VIEW
- Check symmetry of the odontoid in relation to the lateral masses
- Assess the atlantoaxial joints

70

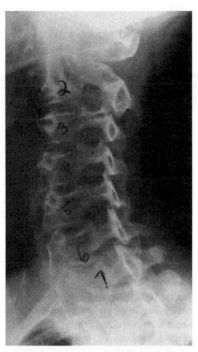

Figure 10-3. Normal 45° oblique cervical radiograph. The foramina are oval spaces and the facet joints are well defined. (From Katz DS, Math KR, Groskin SA, editors. Radiology Secrets. Philadelphia: Hanley & Belfus; 1998.)

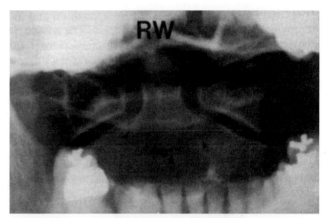

Figure 10-4. Open-mouth anteroposterior (AP) view. Note the relationship of the odontoid process and adjacent C1–C2 facet joints. (From Heller JG, Carlson GC. Odontoid fractures. Spine State Art Rev 1991;5:217–34, with permission.)

3. What are the options if the C7–T1 level cannot be visualized?

A swimmer's view may be obtained when the C7–T1 level cannot be visualized on a lateral cervical spine radiograph. This view is obtained in the supine position by raising the patient's arm overhead and directing the x-ray beam obliquely cephalad through the axilla. An alternative is to obtain a cross-table radiograph with traction applied to the patient's arms. Another option is to obtain bilateral oblique views of the C7–T1 level. Alternatively, a computed tomography (CT) scan of the cervical spine with sagittal reconstructions through the C7–T1 spinal level can be obtained.

4. When are flexion-extension views of the cervical spine indicated?

- To assess potential spinal instability due to soft tissue disruption when static radiographs show no significant bony injury or malalignment but clinical findings suggest a significant injury
- To determine healing of a cervical fusion
- To assess integrity of the C1–C2 articulation in patients at high risk for C1–C2 instability (e.g. rheumatoid arthritis, Down syndrome)

Lateral flexion-extension cervical views should be obtained only in neurologically intact, cooperative and alert patients. Neck motion must be voluntary and there is no role for passive or assisted range of motion during these views. Because of protective muscle spasm, flexion-extension views are rarely of value in the acute postinjury period.

5. What is the significance of the prevertebral soft tissue shadow distance?

Increased thickness of the prevertebral soft tissue space may be a tip-off to the presence of a significant soft tissue injury to the bony or ligamentous structures of the anterior cervical spine. This finding is less reliable in infants and children because of the wide normal variation in the pediatric population. The normal prevertebral soft tissue shadow distance in adults is 7 mm at C2 and 22 mm at the C6 vertebral level. In general, prevertebral soft tissue thickness should not exceed 50% of the sagittal diameter of the vertebral body at the same level.

6. What is the significance of an abnormal atlantoaxial interval?

Abnormal widening of the space between the posterior aspect of the anterior arch of C1 and the anterior aspect of the odontoid (dens) defines an atlantoaxial subluxation and implies laxity of the transverse ligament. This space should not be greater than 3 mm in adults or 5 mm in children. Common causes of atlantoaxial subluxation include trauma, rheumatoid arthritis, and Down syndrome.

7. **What radiographic criteria are used to define instability of the spine in the region from C2 to T1?**
Commonly accepted radiographic criteria for diagnosing clinical instability in the middle and lower cervical spine (C2–T1) include sagittal plane translation greater than 3.5 mm or sagittal plane angulation greater than 11° in relation to an adjacent vertebra.

THORACIC SPINE

8. **What radiographic views are used to assess the thoracic spinal region?**
Standard thoracic spine views include an AP view and lateral view (Fig. 10-5).

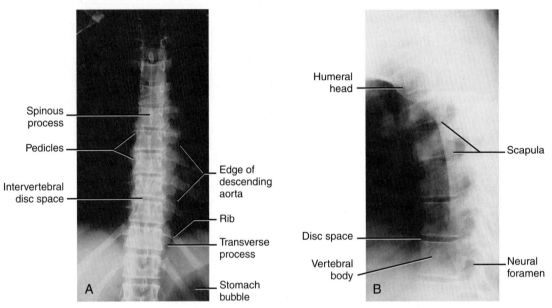

Figure 10-5. Normal anatomy of the thoracic spine. **A,** Anteroposterior, and **B,** lateral views. (From Mettler F. Essentials of Radiology. 2nd ed. Philadelphia: Saunders; 2005.)

9. **What important structures are examined on AP and lateral thoracic radiographs?**
   AP VIEW
   - Soft tissue shadow
   - Spinous process alignment
   - Pedicle: check presence bilaterally
   - Vertebral body, ribs, transverse processes, costotransverse articulations, laminae

   LATERAL VIEW
   - Soft tissue shadow
   - Vertebral body contour and alignment
   - Intervertebral disc space height
   - Pedicles, spinous processes, superior and inferior articular processes, intervertebral foramina

LUMBAR SPINE

10. **What radiographic views are commonly used to assess the lumbar spinal region?**
Standard lumbar spine views include upright (standing) AP and lateral views (Fig. 10-6). Oblique views, lateral flexion-extension views, spot lateral views, and Ferguson views are supplementary views that are valuable in specific situations.

11. **Why should lumbar spine radiographs be obtained with the patient in the standing position whenever possible?**
Lumbar spine pathology (e.g. spondylolisthesis) tends to be exacerbated in the upright position and relieved with recumbency. Most other spinal imaging procedures are performed in the supine position (e.g. CT, magnetic resonance imaging). Standing radiographs provide the opportunity to obtain valuable information about spinal alignment in the erect weight-bearing position.

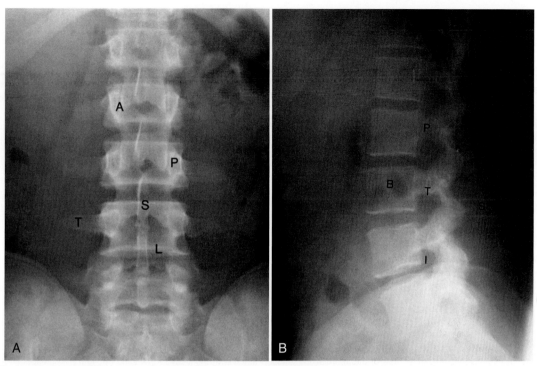

Figure 10-6. Anteroposterior **(A)** and lateral **(B)** view of the lumbar spine. *S,* Spinous process; *P,* pedicle; *T,* transverse process; *L,* lamina; *A,* articular facet joint; *B,* body; *I,* intervertebral foramen. (From Mercier L. Practical Orthopedics. 6th ed. Philadelphia: Mosby; 2008.)

12. What important structures may be assessed on lumbar radiographs?

AP VIEW
- Psoas soft tissue shadow
- Spinous process alignment
- Pedicle; check presence bilaterally
- Vertebral body and disc
- Facet joints
- Sacrum, sacral ala, sacroiliac joints

LATERAL VIEW
- Vertebral body contour and alignment
- Intervertebral disc space height
- Pedicles, spinous processes, superior and inferior articular processes, intervertebral foramina
- Sacrum, sacral promontory

OBLIQUE VIEWS
- Pars interarticularis
- Facet joints
- Neural foramina

13. What is the significance of an absent pedicle shadow?

An absent pedicle shadow on the AP view (Fig. 10-7) is an important radiographic finding because metastatic spinal disease may initially obscure a single pedicle. Pedicle destruction may also result from malignant or primary tumors, histiocytosis, and infection.

14. When are oblique views of the lumbar spine helpful?

- To diagnose spondylolysis
- To assess healing of lumbar posterolateral fusion

15. What anatomic structures comprise the "Scotty dog" on an oblique lumbar radiograph?

On the oblique lumbar radiograph, the vertebra and its processes can be imagined to outline the shape of a dog (Fig. 10-8): ear = superior articular process; head = pedicle; collar/neck = pars interarticularis; front leg/foot = inferior articular process; body = lamina; hind leg/foot = contralateral inferior articular process; tail = spinous process. **Spondylolysis** refers to a defect in the region of the pars interarticularis. It appears as a radiolucent defect in the region of the neck or collar of the *Scotty dog.*

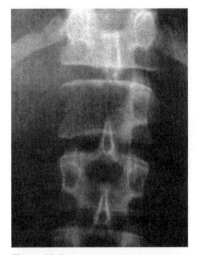

Figure 10-7. Absent pedicle shadow due to vertebral tumor. (From Spine State Art Rev 1998;2(2):178, with permission.)

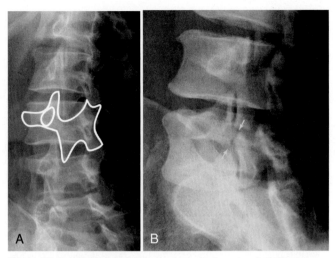

Figure 10-8. Oblique radiographic view of the lumbar spine. **A,** Outline on oblique radiograph resembles a *Scotty dog*. **B,** Spondylolysis is a fracture in the pars interarticularis region, which appears as a radiolucent band in the neck or collar of the dog. (From Pretorious ES, Solomon JA, editors. Radiology Secrets. 2nd ed. Philadelphia: Elsevier; 2006.)

16. What is a Ferguson view and when should it be ordered?

A Ferguson view is an AP view of the lumbosacral junction taken with the x-ray tube angled 30° to 35° cephalad. The x-ray beam goes through the plane of the L5–S1 disc, permitting the anatomy of the lumbosacral junction to be well visualized. This view is ordered when it is difficult to visualize the L5–S1 level in patients with severe spondylolisthesis and to assess an intertransverse fusion at the L5–S1 level (Fig. 10-9).

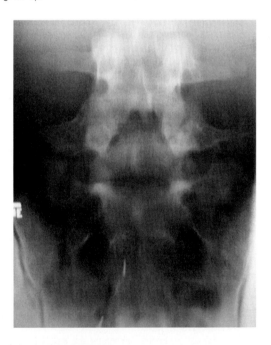

Figure 10-9. Fergusion AP view of the lumbosacral junction. Note the absence of fusion between the transverse processes of L5 and the sacral ala.

17. What are coned-down views? When should they be ordered?

Coned down views or spot views limit scatter of the x-ray beam and are useful to define bone detail for a limited area of the spine. For example, a spot lateral view of the lumbosacral junction is helpful to assess the L5–S1 level in cases of severe spondylolisthesis.

18. Explain the major pitfall involved in interpreting flexion-extension lumbar spine radiographs.

No universally accepted definition of radiographic instability of the lumbar spine exists. In asymptomatic subjects, up to 3 mm of translation and 7° to 14° of angular motion may be present.

19. What is a lumbosacral transitional vertebra?

In the normal spine, the 24th vertebra below the occiput is the last presacral vertebra (L5), and the 25th vertebral segment is the body of S1. In the normal spine, there are five non–rib-bearing lumbar vertebra above the sacrum. People who possess four non–rib-bearing lumbar vertebra are considered to have sacralization of the L5 vertebra. People who possess six non–rib-bearing lumbar vertebra are considered to have lumbarization of the S1 vertebral body. The term lumbosacral transitional vertebra has been adopted because it is difficult to determine whether the transitional vertebra is the 24th or 25th vertebra below the occiput without obtaining additional spinal radiographs. There are a variety of types of lumbosacral transitional vertebra. Vertebral anomalies ranging from hyperplasia of the transverse processes to large transverse processes that articulate with the sacrum or fusion of the transverse process and vertebral body with the sacrum may occur. These abnormalities may be partial or complete, unilateral or bilateral. Proper identification of lumbar spine segments in relation to the sacrum on plain radiographs is essential in planning lumbar spine procedures to ensure that surgery is carried out at the correct spinal level(s).

20. Define the following terms commonly used to describe abnormal vertebral alignment: spondylolisthesis, retrolisthesis, lateral listhesis, and rotatory subluxation.

Spondylolisthesis is defined as the forward displacement of a vertebra in relation to the vertebra below it. The degree of spondylolisthesis is determined by measuring the percentage of vertebral body translation: 0–25% (grade 1); 26%–50% (grade 2); 51%–75% (grade 3); and 76%–100% (grade 4). Other terms used to describe abnormal alignment between adjacent vertebra include **retrolisthesis** (posterior translation of a vertebra in relation to the vertebra below), **lateral listhesis** (lateral subluxation), and **rotatory subluxation** (abnormal rotation between adjacent vertebrae).

SPINAL DEFORMITY ASSESSMENT

21. What standard radiographs are used to evaluate spinal deformities?

Biplanar deformity radiographs (posteroanterior [PA] and lateral 14 × 36-inch radiographs) are the most frequent imaging studies used to assess spinal deformities (Fig. 10-10). The techniques for positioning, shielding, and performing this radiographic examination have been standardized. Radiographs are taken with the patient standing whenever possible. Sitting or supine radiographs may be required for patients who are unable to stand without support, including very young patients, paraplegic patients, and patients with severe neuromuscular disorders.

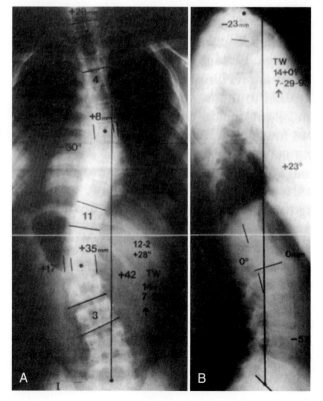

Figure 10-10. A, Posteroanterior (PA) and **B,** lateral spinal deformity radiographs. (From Asher MA. Anterior surgery for thoracolumbar and lumbar idiopathic scoliosis. Spine State Art Rev 1998;12:701–11, with permission.)

22. When should I order a radiograph of a specific spinal region? When should I order a 36-inch radiograph that images the entire spine?

Radiographs of a specific spinal region (cervical, thoracic, lumbar) are obtained for diagnosis and initial assessment of spinal pathology involving a specific vertebral or disc level within a spinal region (e.g. spondylolisthesis, fracture, infection, tumor). Fourteen × thirty-six inch spinal radiographs (long cassette radiographs) are required for assessment of spinal pathology that involves multiple spinal segments (e.g. scoliosis, kyphosis). Fourteen × thirty-six inch spine radiographs are valuable in planning spinal fusion procedures and in the assessment of postoperative spinal alignment.

23. What specialized radiographs are commonly used to assess flexibility of spinal deformities?

- Supine AP side-bending radiographs (Fig. 10-11)
- Supine AP traction radiograph
- Lateral hyperextension radiograph
- Lateral hyperflexion radiograph
- Push-prone PA radiograph

Specialized radiographs are frequently obtained to assist in surgical planning before surgical correction of spinal deformities. *Bending films* are used to aid in selection of spinal levels that should be included in a scoliosis fusion. Supine AP bending films have been shown to be superior to standing bending films for assessing coronal curve flexibility. *Supine AP traction radiographs* are helpful in patients with neuromuscular scoliosis to assess curve flexibility and correction of pelvic obliquity. A *hyperextension lateral radiograph* performed with a bolster placed at the apex of kyphosis may be useful for assessing the flexibility of a kyphotic deformity. A *hyperflexion lateral view* may be helpful to assess the flexibility of a lordotic spinal deformity.

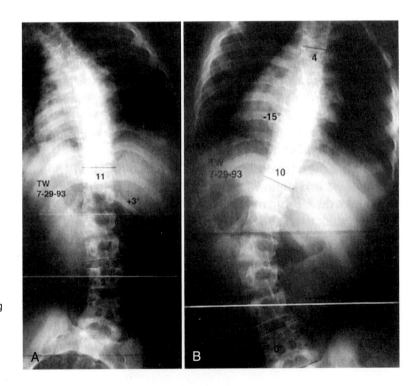

Figure 10-11. Supine 36-inch long cassette side bending radiographs. (From Asher MA. Anterior surgery for thoracolumbar and lumbar idiopathic scoliosis. Spine State Art Rev 1998;12:701–11, with permission.)

24. What is the method used to quantify sagittal and coronal plane curvatures?

The **Cobb method** is most commonly used to quantify curvature in the coronal and sagittal planes (Fig. 10-12). The following steps are involved in this measurement:

1. Identify the end vertebra of the curvature whose measurement is desired.
2. Construct lines along the superior aspect of the upper end vertebra and along the inferior aspect of the lower end vertebra.
3. Next construct lines perpendicular to the lines previously drawn along the end vertebra. Measure the angle between these two lines with a protractor or digital software to determine the Cobb angle.
4. In large curves it is possible to measure the Cobb angle directly from the lines along the end vertebra without the need to construct perpendicular lines.

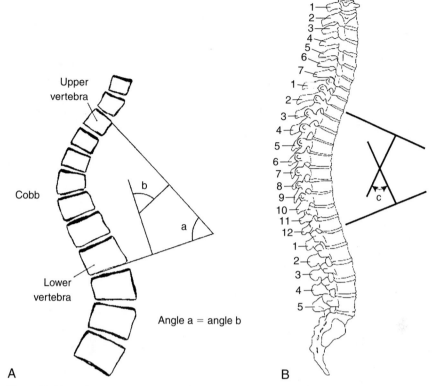

Figure 10-12. **A,** Measurement of scoliosis. **B,** Measurement of kyphosis. (**A** from Katz DS, Math KR, Groskin SA, editors. Radiology Secrets. Philadelphia: Hanley & Belfus; 1998; **B** from Spine State Art Rev 1998;12:1.)

25. What is spinal balance?

Balance has been defined as the ability to maintain the center of gravity of a body within its base of support with minimal postural sway. From the point of view of the spine, it implies that, in both the frontal and sagittal planes, the head is positioned correctly over the sacrum and pelvis in both a translational and angular sense. Normal **coronal plane balance** is present when a plumb line dropped from the center of the C7 vertebral body lies within 1 cm of the middle of the sacrum. Normal **sagittal plane balance** is present when a plumb line dropped from the center of C7 lies within 2.5 cm of the posterior superior corner of S1. Another term for the plumb line measurement is the **sagittal vertical axis (SVA).** By convention, when the SVA falls behind the L5–S1 disc space, the SVA is considered **negative.** When the SVA falls through the L5–S1 disc, the SVA is considered **neutral.** When the SVA fall in front of the L5–S1 disc, the SVA is considered **positive.** In normal patients, the SVA is usually neutral or negative. In the normal patient, the SVA passes anterior to the thoracic spine, through the center of the L1 vertebral body, posterior to the lumbar spine, and through the posterior corner of S1.

26. What are normal values for the sagittal curves of the different spinal regions?

- **Cervical region.** Cervical lordosis (occiput–C7) averages 40°, with the majority of cervical lordosis occurring at the C1–C2 motion segment.
- **Thoracic region.** Normal kyphosis (T1–T12) in young adults ranges from 20° to 50° with a tendency to increase slightly with age. The kyphosis in the thoracic region usually starts at T1–T2 and gradually increases at each level toward the apex (T6–T7 disc). Below the thoracic apex, segmental kyphosis gradually decreases until the thoraco-lumbar junction is reached.
- **Thoracolumbar region.** The thoracolumbar junction (T12–L1) is essentially straight with respect to the sagittal plane. It serves as the transition area between the relatively stiff kyphotic thoracic region and the relatively mobile lordotic lumbar region.
- **Lumbar region.** Normal lumbar lordosis (L1–S1) ranges from 30° to 80° with a mean lordosis of 60°. Lumbar lordosis generally begins at L1–L2 and gradually increases at each distal level toward the sacrum. The apex of lumbar lordosis is normally located at the L3–L4 disc space. (Fig. 10-13)

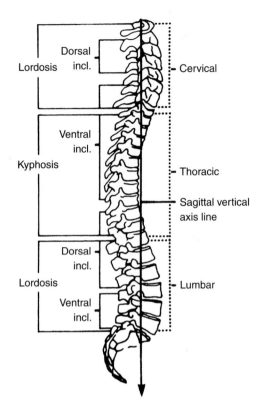

Figure 10-13. The sagittal curves of the spine. (From DeWald RL. Revision surgery for spinal deformity. In: Eilert RE, editor: Instructional Course Lectures. vol. 41, Rosemont, IL: American Academy of Orthopaedic Surgeons; 1992. p. 241, with permission.)

27. Describe the relationship between thoracic kyphosis and lumbar lordosis in normal patients.

The relationship between these two sagittal curves is such that lumbar lordosis generally exceeds thoracic kyphosis by 20° to 30° in a normal patient. This relationship allows the body to maintain normal sagittal balance and maintain the sagittal vertical axis (SVA) in a physiologic position. The body attempts to maintain the SVA in its physiologic position through a variety of compensatory mechanisms. Functionally, the sacrum and pelvis can be considered as one vertebra (pelvic vertebra), which functions as an intercalary bone between the trunk and the lower extremities. Alignment changes in the hip joints and lumbar spine can influence pelvic orientation and, in this manner, alter the sagittal orientation of the base of the spine. The body has an interrelated system of compensatory mechanisms to maintain sagittal balance involving the lumbar spine and pelvis as well as the hip, knee, and ankle joints.

28. What are the sacral parameters that influence sagittal alignment of the spine?

Three sacral parameters (Fig. 10-14) are measured: pelvic incidence (PI), sacral slope (SS), and pelvic tilt (PT). Pelvic incidence (PI) is a fixed anatomic parameter unique to the individual. Sacral slope (SS) and pelvic tilt (PT) are variable parameters. The relationship among the parameters determine the overall alignment of the sacropelvic unit according to the formula **PI = PT + SS**.

* **Pelvic incidence (PI)** is the angle defined by a line perpendicular to the sacral end plate line at its midpoint and a line connecting this point to the femoral rotational axis.
* **Pelvic tilt (PT)** is defined by a vertical reference line and a line from the midpoint of the sacral endplate to the femoral rotational axis.
* **Sacral slope (SS)** is the angle defined by a line along the sacral end plate line and a horizontal reference line.

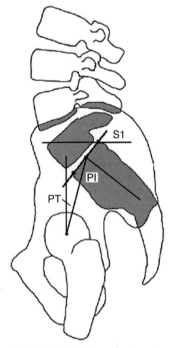

Figure 10-14. Pelvic parameters: pelvic incidence (PI), pelvic tilt (PI), sacral slope (SS, SI). (From Staheli LT, Song KM, editors. Pediatric Orthopaedic Secrets. 3rd ed. Philadelphia: Elsevier; 2007.)

29. What radiographic hallmarks indicate a *flatback syndrome*?

Flatback syndrome is a sagittal malalignment syndrome. Radiographically the hallmarks of flatback syndrome include a markedly positive sagittal vertical axis and decreased lumbar lordosis after a spinal fusion procedure. Classically, it has been reported after use of a straight Harrington distraction rod to correct a lumbar or thoracolumbar curvature. When the thoracic and lumbar spine is fused in a nonphysiologic alignment with loss of lumbar lordosis, the patient cannot assume normal erect posture and assumes instead a stooped forward posture. The patient attempts to compensate for this abnormal posture by hyperextending the hip joints and flexing the knee joints. These compensatory mechanisms are ultimately ineffective in maintaining the SVA in a physiologic position and result in symptoms of back pain, knee pain, and inability to maintain an upright posture. Fixed sagittal malalignment of the spine has many etiologies.

Key Points

1. Systematic review of spine radiographs provides important information regarding spinal alignment, degenerative changes, fractures, and spinal instability.
2. Cervical flexion-extension views should be obtained only in neurologically intact, cooperative, and alert patients and are not advised in the immediate postinjury period.
3. Important radiographic measurements for assessment of spinal deformities include coronal and sagittal plane balance, thoracic kyphosis, lumbar lordosis, and pelvic parameters.

Websites

Standing balance and sagittal plane deformity: analysis of spinopelvic and gravity line parameters: http://www.medscape.com/viewarticle/578313

Three-dimensional terminology of spinal deformity: http://www.srs.org/professionals/glossary/3-d.php

BIBLIOGRAPHY

1. Balderson RA, Auerbach JD. Imaging techniques. Semin Spine Surg 2007;19:57–124.
2. Bernhardt M, Bridwell KH. Segmental analysis of the sagittal plane alignment of the normal thoracic and lumbar spine and lumbosacral junction. Spine 1989;14:717–21.
3. Devlin VJ, Narvaez JC. Imaging strategies for spinal deformities. Spine State Art Rev 1998;12:1.
4. Lonstein JE. Patient evaluation. In: Lonstein JE, Bradford DS, Winter RB, et al., editors. Moe's Textbook of Scoliosis and Other Spinal Deformities. 3rd ed. Philadelphia: Saunders; 1995. p. 45–86.
5. O'Brien MF, Kuklo TR, Blanke KM, et al., editors. Spinal Deformity Study Group Radiographic Measurement Manual. Memphis, TN: Medtronic Sofamor Danek USA, Inc.; 2005.

MAGNETIC RESONANCE IMAGING OF THE SPINE

Vincent J. Devlin, MD

1. How is a magnetic resonance (MR) scan produced?

The hydrogen atoms (protons) in the human body are single charged atoms spinning on random axes such that the body's total magnetic field is zero. During an MR scan, the patient is placed in a magnetic field, which causes the hydrogen nuclei to align parallel with the magnetic field. Application of **radiofrequency (RF) pulses** causes the **hydrogen nuclei** to enter a higher energy state. When the RF pulses are terminated, the excited hydrogen nuclei release energy and return to a lower energy state in a process termed **relaxation.** The energy released during this transition is detected by the MR receiver coil. Signal data are processed in terms of origin within the imaging plane and subsequently displayed on a monitor. The time between RF pulses is termed the **repetition time (TR)**. The time between the application of RF pulses and the recording of the MR signal is termed the **echo time (TE)**. The process of relaxation is described in terms of two independent time constants called **T1** and **T2.**

2. What is signal intensity?

Signal intensity describes the *brightness* of tissues on an MR image. Tissues may be described as high intensity (bright), intermediate intensity (gray), or low intensity (dark). When the tissue intensity of a pathologic process is described relative to the intensity of surrounding normal tissue, it may be described as **hyperintense, isointense,** or **hypointense.** MR signal intensity depends on the T1, T2, and proton density (number of mobile hydrogen ions) of the tissue under evaluation.

3. Explain the differences between T1- and T2-weighted MR images.

T1 (longitudinal plane relaxation time) and T2 (transverse plane relaxation time) are intrinsic physical properties of tissues. Different tissues have different T1 and T2 properties based on how their hydrogen nuclei respond to radiofrequency pulses during the MR scan. Image contrast of a magnetic resonance imaging (MRI) is determined by varying the scanning parameters (TE and TR).

- **T1 images** are produced with a short TR (<1000 msec) and a short TE (<30 msec). T1 images are weighted toward fat. Fat appears bright on T1 images and less bright on T2 images. T1-weighted images are excellent for evaluating structures containing fat, hemorrhage, or proteinaceous fluid, all of which have a short T1 and demonstrate a high signal on T1-weighted images. T1 images demonstrate anatomic structures well because of their high signal-to-noise ratio.
- **T2 images** are produced with a long TR (>1500 msec) and a long TE (>45 msec). T2 images are weighted toward water. Water appears bright on T2 images and dark on T1 images *(mnemonic: water [H₂0] is bright on T2).* Signal intensity on T2 images is related to the state of tissue hydration. Tissue with a high water content (cerebrospinal fluid, cysts, normal intervertebral discs) shows an increased signal on T2 images. T2 images are most useful for contrasting normal and abnormal anatomy. In general, pathologic processes (e.g. neoplasm, infection, acute fractures) are associated with increased water content and appear hyperintense on T2 images and hypointense on T1.

4. Describe the signal intensity of common tissue types on T1- and T2-weighted MR images.

Mineralized tissue (e.g. bone) shows low signal intensity on both T1 and T2 images because it contains few mobile hydrogen ions. Gas contains no mobile hydrogen ions and does not generate an MR signal. The relative signal intensities of different tissue types on T1- and T2-weighted images are summarized (Table 11-1).

5. How do I know whether I am looking at a T1- or T2-weighted image?

One method is to look at the TE (time to echo) and TR (time to repetition) numbers on the scan (Table 11-2).

A simpler method is to recall the signal characteristics of water. Locate a fluid-containing structure (e.g. CSF surrounding the spinal cord). If the fluid is bright, the image is probably a T2-weighted image. If the fluid is dark, the image is probably a T1-weighted image.

The above criteria refer to the most basic pulse sequence, spine echo (SE). In other pulse sequences, contrast phenomenology is more complex.

6. What are pulse sequences?

The term **pulse sequence** refers to a specific method for collecting MR data. The **SE pulse sequence** is commonly used and is obtained by varying the TR and TE as described previously. Additional techniques have been developed to

Table 11-1. Relative Intensity of Different Tissue Types

TISSUE	APPEARANCE ON T1	APPEARANCE ON T2
Normal fluid (e.g. CSF)	Low-intermediate	Bright
Cortical bone	Low	Low
Tendon/ligament	Low	Low
Muscle	Intermediate	Intermediate
Fat	High	Intermediate
Red marrow	Intermediate	Intermediate
Yellow marrow	High	High
Intervertebral disc (central)	Intermediate	Bright
Intervertebral disc (peripheral)	Low	Intermediate

CSF, cerebrospinal fluid.

Table 11-2. T1 vs. T2 Images

IMAGE TYPE	TE	TR
T1	15-30 ms	400-600 ms (<1000)
T2	60-120 ms	1500-3000 ms (>1000)
Proton density	15-30 ms	1500-2000 m

decrease scan time and artifact and to improve visualization of specific pathologic processes. Examples include **fast-spin echo imaging, gradient echo imaging,** and **short tau inversion recovery (STIR) imaging.** As one becomes familiar reading spine MR studies in daily practice, the advantages and disadvantages of specific pulse sequences in relation to various spine pathologies will be appreciated.

7. **What are the contraindications to obtaining an MR scan?**
   MR scans are contraindicated in patients with implanted devices that may be subject to magnetically induced malfunction or potentially harmful movement. Examples include certain cochlear and ocular implants, cardiac pacemakers, certain prosthetic heart valves and stents, implanted pain pumps and neurostimulators, brain aneurysm clips, carotid clips, certain Swan-Ganz catheters, periorbital metal fragments, and certain penile prostheses. When MR imaging (MRI) is performed for intensive care unit (ICU) patients, MRI-compatible ventilators and monitoring devices are required. Pregnancy is considered by some to be a relative contraindication to MRI during the first trimester. Extreme claustrophobia or inability to cooperate with the imaging study (e.g. infants) are relative contraindications and such patients may require sedation.

   Spinal fixation devices are not a contraindication to MRI. However, if these implants are located near the intended site of imaging, significant image artifact may result and render the scan non-diagnostic over the instrumented levels. It is still possible to obtain useful imaging data at spinal segments above and below the instrumented spinal segments. The type of implant metal is also an important consideration. Useful imaging data can be obtained in many cases in the presence of titanium implants. Stainless steel implants generally create excessive artifact, and a computed tomography (CT) or CT-myelogram study is required to evaluate patients with stainless steel spinal implants.

8. **Describe the normal appearance of critical bone and soft tissue structures on MR scans of the cervical spine.**
   See Figure 11-1.

9. **Describe the important anatomic structures of the thoracic spine on MR scans.**
   See Figure 11-2.

10. **What anatomic structures should be routinely assessed on an MR study of the lumbar spine?**
    See Figure 11-3.

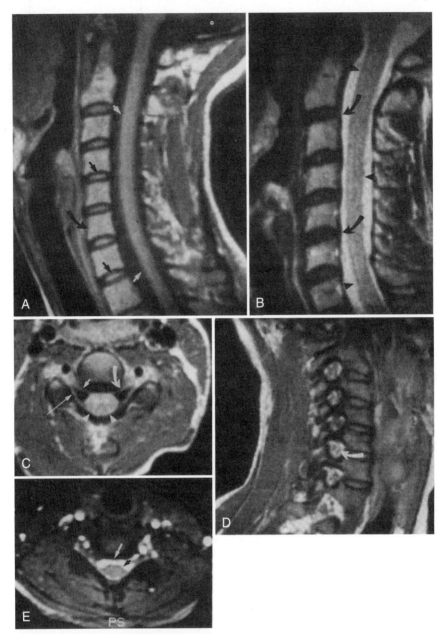

Figure 11-1. Normal cervical spine anatomy. The sagittal T1-weighted image **(A)** provides excellent anatomic delineation of the vertebral bodies (*curved black arrows*), intervertebral discs (*straight black arrows*), and spinal cord (*white arrows*). On the sagittal cardiac gated T2-weighted image **(B)**, a myelographic effect is created by the increased signal intensity in the cerebrospinal fluid (CSF). There is an excellent interface between the posterior margin of the discovertebral joints (*curved black arrows*) and the cerebrospinal fluid, as well as excellent delineation of the spinal cord (black arrowheads). The axial T1-weighted image **(C)** provides excellent delineation of the spinal cord (*white arrowheads*), ventral (*short white arrow*) and dorsal (*long white arrow*) nerve roots, and the intervertebral canals (*curved white arrow*). On the oblique T1-weighted image **(D)**, the fat in the intervertebral canals outlines the neural (*curved arrow*) and vascular structures. On the axial gradient echo image **(E)**, the high signal intensity of the CSF produces excellent contrast for the delineation of the spinal cord (*black arrow*) and the posterior margin of the discovertebral joint (*white arrow*). (From Herzog RJ. State of the art imaging of spinal disorders. Phys Med Rehabil State Art Rev 1990;4:230, with permission.)

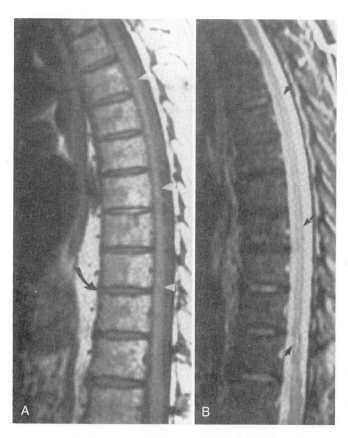

Figure 11-2. Normal thoracic spine anatomy. The sagittal T1-weighted image **(A)** provides excellent anatomic delineation of the vertebral bodies, intervertebral discs (*curved black arrow*), and spinal cord (*white arrowheads*). On the sagittal cardiac-gated T2-weighted image **(B)**, the myelographic effect results in an excellent cerebrospinal fluid (CSF)–extradural interface along with delineation of the thoracic spinal cord (*black arrows*). (From Herzog RJ. State of the art imaging of spinal disorders. Phys Med Rehabil State Art Rev 1990;4:231, with permission).

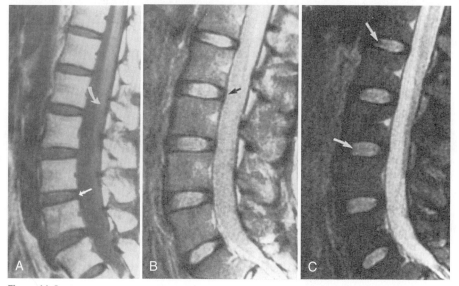

Figure 11-3. Normal lumbar spine anatomy. The sagittal T1-weighted image **(A)** provides excellent delineation of the vertebral bodies, intervertebral discs, thecal sac, lower thoracic cord, and conus medullaris (*curved white arrow*). The high signal intensity of the vertebral bodies is secondary to the fat in the cancellous marrow. The interface between the posterior outer annular fibers (*straight white arrow*) and the CSF is not well defined. On the sagittal proton-density weighted image **(B)**, increased signal intensity in the disc is identified, along with increased signal intensity of the CSF. This results in improved delineation of the posterior annular–posterior longitudinal ligament complex (*arrow*). On the sagittal T2-weighted image **(C)**, increased signal intensity in the disc is identified, along with a linear horizontal area of decreased signal intensity in the center of the disc representing the intranuclear cleft (*arrows*). Increased signal intensity in the CSF creates a myelographic effect and provides an excellent CSF-extradural interface. The sagittal T1-weighted image *continued*

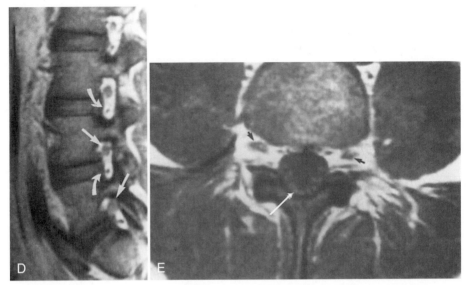

Figure 11-3, cont'd. (D) through the intervertebral canals provides excellent delineation of the dorsal root ganglia (*straight white arrows*) positioned subjacent to the vertebral pedicles. The posterolateral margin of the discs (*curved white arrows*) is well delineated. The axial T1-weighted image **(E)** provides excellent delineation of the individual nerve roots (*long white arrow*) in the thecal sac. The presence of fat in the epidural space and intervertebral canals provides an excellent soft tissue interface to evaluate nerve roots (*short black arrows*), ligaments, and osseous elements. (From Herzog RJ. State of the art imaging of spinal disorders. Phys Med Rehabil State Art Rev 1990;4:232–3, with permission.)

11. When is a screening MRI study indicated for evaluation of the spine?

A screening MRI visualizes the entire spinal cord and vertebral column from foramen magnum to distal sacrum. A screening MRI is indicated to evaluate patients with spinal deformities known to be associated with abnormalities of the neural axis. Examples include left thoracic scoliosis, juvenile scoliosis, congenital scoliosis, and myelodysplasia. Pathologic conditions that may be detected in such patients include syrinx, Arnold-Chiari malformation, diastematomyelia, spinal cord tumor, tethered spinal cord, and congenital spinal stenosis.

A screening MRI is also important in the assessment of patients with metastatic spinal tumor prior to surgical intervention to evaluate for potential multifocal spinal involvement.

12. What are indications for administration of an intravenous contrast agent in conjunction with a spine MR study?

Indications for gadolinium-based intravenous contrast agents include suspected spinal infections, intradural tumors (e.g. *drop metastases*) and evaluation of the spinal canal and its contents following prior laminectomy or discectomy. As gadolinium acts primarily by shortening T1 relaxation times, T1-weighted images are obtained before and after contrast administration. Renal function should be screened prior to contrast administration due to the risk of nephrogenic systemic sclerosis in patients with renal insufficiency and hepatorenal syndrome.

13. Define the terms used to describe abnormal disc morphology on MR studies.

- **Annular tear:** a disruption of the ligament surrounding the periphery of the disc.
- **Bulge:** extension of disc tissue beyond the disc space with a diffuse, circumferential, non focal contour.
- **Protrusion:** displaced disc material extending focally and asymmetrically beyond the disc space. The displaced disc material is in continuity with the disc of origin. The diameter of the base of the displaced portion, where it is continuous with the disc material within the disc space of origin, has a greater diameter than the largest diameter of the disc tissue extending beyond the disc space.
- **Extrusion:** displaced disc material extending focally and asymmetrically beyond the disc space. The displaced disc material has a greater diameter than the disc material maintaining continuity (if any) with the disc of origin.
- **Sequestration:** a fragment of disc that has no continuity with the disc of origin. Another commonly used term is *free disc fragment.* By definition, all sequestered discs are extruded; however, not all extruded discs are sequestered (Fig. 11-4).

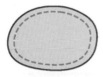

A **Diffuse disc bulge**

B **Broad-based protrusion**
(or focal disc bulge)

C **Focal disc protusion**
AP < mediolateral dimension

D **Disc extrusion**
AP ≥ mediolateral dimension

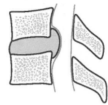

E **Disc extrusion**
Disc migrates above and/or below parent disc, maintaining continuity with it

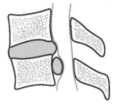

F **Sequestered disc**
Separate from parent disc

Figure 11-4. Abnormalities of disc morphology. **(A) Bulge, (B, C) Protrusion, (D, E) Extrusion, (F) Sequestration.** The *dashed lines* in A and B indicate the vertebral bodies, whereas the *solid lines* represent the discs. AP, anteroposterior. (From Helms CA, Major NM, Anderson, M, et al., editors. Helms: Musculoskeletal MRI. 2nd ed. Philadelphia: Saunders; 2008, with permission.)

14. Match each MR image of a disc abnormality in Figure 11-5A-E with the appropriate description: (1) annular tear, (2) disc bulge, (3) disc protrusion, (4) disc extrusion, and (5) disc sequestration.
Answers: (1) annular tear, B; (2) disc bulge, E; (3) disc protrusion, C; (4) disc extrusion, A; (5) disc sequestration, D.

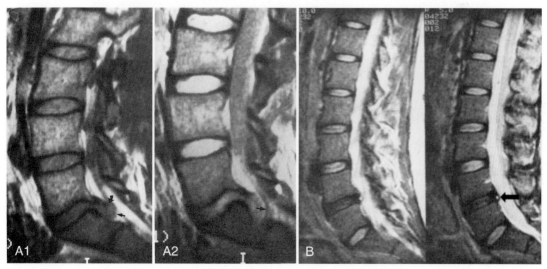

Figure 11-5. Lumbar disc abnormalities **A** from Herzog RJ. State of the art imaging of spinal disorders. Phys Med Rehabil State Art Rev 1990;4:239. **B** from Gundry CR, Heithoff KB, Pollei SR. Lumbar degenerative disk disease. Spine State Art Rev 1995;9:151.

Continued

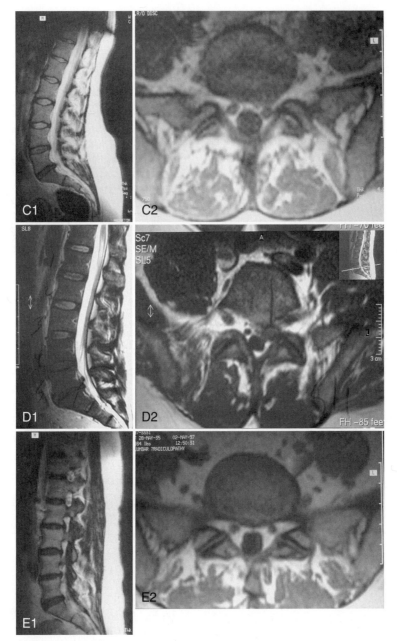

Figure 11-5, cont'd. C, D, and **E** from Russo RB. Diagnosis of low back pain: Role of imaging studies. Phys Med Rehabil State Art Rev 1999;13:437–439, with permission.

15. **Match each cervical MR image in Figure 11-6A-F with the appropriate description. Each image depicts a patient who presents with symptoms consistent with cervical radiculopathy and/or cervical myelopathy.**
   1. Complex cervical spinal deformity. Cervical kyphosis is associated with posterior spinal cord compression at C2 to C4 and anterior spinal cord compression C4 to C6.
   2. Severe multilevel cervical spinal stenosis due to anterior and posterior cord compression.
   3. Single-level cervical disc extrusion associated with severe spinal cord compression.
   4. Multilevel cervical spondylosis superimposed on developmental stenosis. The anteroposterior diameter of the central spinal canal is narrowed on a developmental basis from the C3–C4 level and distally. A cervical disc protrusion is noted at C3–C4, and spondylotic ridges cause mild cord impingement at C4–C5 and C5–C6.
   5. Single-level cervical disc protrusion associated with mild spinal cord compression.
   6. Congenital stenosis of the cervical spinal canal associated with multilevel disc protrusions and severe multilevel spinal cord compression. Congenital fusion of the C6 and C7 vertebral bodies is noted.
      Answers: (1), F; (2), E; (3), C; (4), D; (5), B; (6), A.

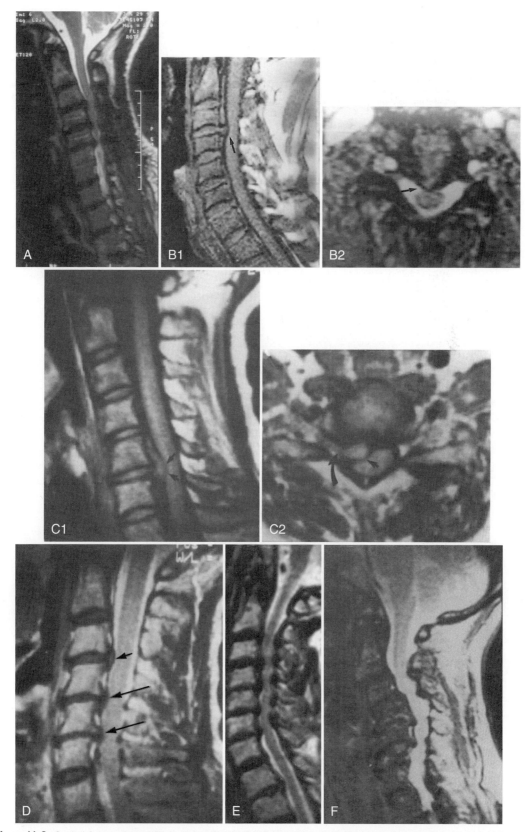

Figure 11-6. Cervical degenerative conditions. (**A** from Oishi M, Onesti ST, Dorfman HD. Pathogenesis of degenerative disc disease of the cervical spine. Spine State Art Rev 2000;14:538. **B** from Schwartz AJ. Imaging of degenerative cervical disease. Spine State Art Rev 2000;14:558. **C** and **D** from Herzog RJ. State of the art imaging of spinal disorders. Phys Med Rehabil State Art Rev 1990;4:236. **E** from Floman Y, Ashkenazi E. Expansive open-door laminoplasty in the management of multilevel cervical myelopathy. Spine State Art Rev 2000;14:639. **F** from Ducker TB. Complex cervical myeloradiculopathy (S-shaped spinal deformity): Case report. Spine State Art Rev 1991;5:317.)

16. Match each lumbar MR image in Figure 11-7A-D with the appropriate description. Each image depicts a patient who presents with symptoms consistent with lumbar spinal stenosis.

1. Ligamentum flavum hypertrophy causing stenosis of the central spinal canal and lateral recess.
2. Hypertrophy of the superior articular process at L5–S1 associated with thickened ligamentum flavum and resulting in front-to-back narrowing of the L5–S1 intervertebral nerve root canal with compression of the L5 ganglion.
3. Synovial cyst arising from the L4–L5 facet joint, resulting in compression of the left side of the thecal sac and left L5 nerve root.
4. Degenerative spondylolisthesis associated with L4–L5 central spinal stenosis.

Answers: (1), D; (2), C; (3), A; (4), B.

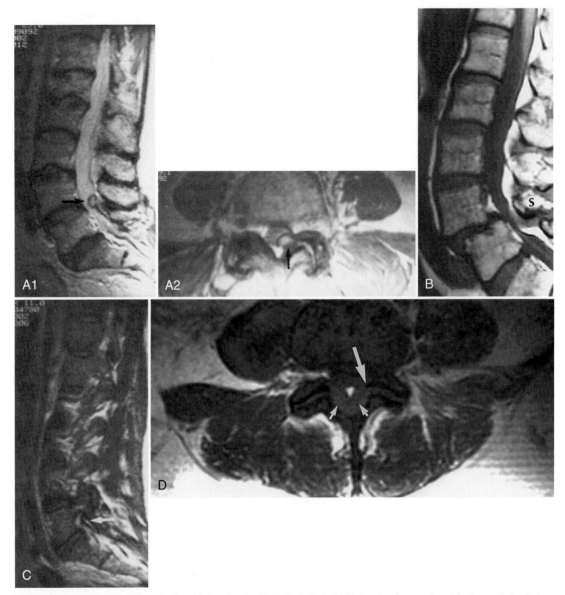

Figure 11-7. Lumbar Spinal Stenosis (**A** and **C** from Gundry CR, Heithoff KB, Pollei SR. Lumbar degenerative disk disease. Spine State Art Rev 1995;9:169. **B** from Barckhausen RR, Math KR. Lumbar spine diseases. In: Katz DS, Math KR, Groskin SA, editors: Radiology Secrets. Philadelphia: Hanley & Belfus; 1998. **D** from Figueroa RE, Stone JA. MR imaging of degenerative spine disease: MR myelography and imaging of the posterior spinal elements. In Castillo M, editor. Spinal Imaging: State of the Art. Philadelphia: Hanley & Belfus; 2001, with permission.

17. A 50-year-old diabetic man presents with a 2-month history of low back pain refractory to bedrest and analgesics. An MRI (Fig. 11-8) is obtained by the patient's primary physician, and the patient is referred for consultation. What is the diagnosis?

The imaging findings are classic for a *disc space infection*. Pyogenic infection typically begins at the vertebral endplates, then involves the disc, and finally spreads to involve the adjacent vertebral bodies. T1-weighted images show decreased signal intensity in the disc and vertebral bodies. T2-weighted images show increased signal intensity in the disc and vertebral bodies. Additional findings may include inflammatory changes in the paravertebral soft tissues and abscess formation in either the epidural space or anterior paravertebral tissues.

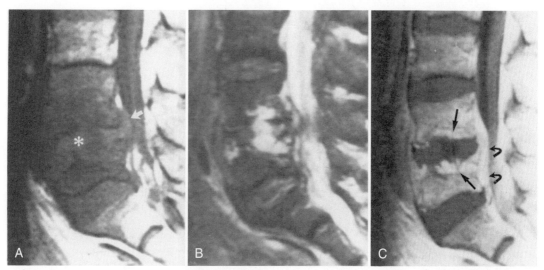

Figure 11-8. Magnetic resonance (MR) of *Streptococcus pneumoniae* discitis/osteomyelitis. **A,** Sagittal T1-weighted conventional spine-echo (CSE) image reveals an extensive hypointensity involving the L4–L5 disc space (*asterisk*) and the adjacent vertebral bodies. An extradural soft tissue mass compresses the thecal sac (*arrow*). **B,** Sagittal T2-weighted CSE image shows mixed hyperintensity and isointensity in the involved L4–L5 intervertebral disc and adjacent vertebrae. **C,** Sagittal T1-weighted CSE image following gadolinium administration reveals peripheral enhancement of the disc (*straight arrows*) and uniform enhancement of the epidural mass (curved arrows), representing discitis and epidural phlegmon. (From Reddy S, Leite CC, Jinkins JRZ. Imaging of infectious disease of the spine. Spine State Art Rev 1995;9:135, with permission.)

18. A 70-year-old woman presents with back pain and a thoracic fracture. She has a history of breast cancer and a documented history of osteoporosis. How can MRI help determine whether the fracture is the result of osteoporosis or metastatic breast cancer?

Findings on MRI that support a diagnosis of *metastatic tumor* include abnormal marrow signal in other vertebrae, a convex posterior margin of the vertebral body (i.e. an expanded appearance), and compression of the entire vertebral body, including its posterior third. Additional features supporting a diagnosis of metastatic disease include involvement of the pedicle, presence of an extraosseous soft tissue mass, and diffuse marrow replacement throughout the vertebral body without focal fat preservation (Fig. 11-9).

Findings on MRI that support a diagnosis of a *benign osteoporotic compression fracture* include normal or mildly abnormal signal in the fractured vertebral body, a wedge-shaped vertebral body without compression of the posterior third, and a horizontally oriented low signal line paralleling the vertebral body endplate (Fig. 11-10).

MRI can be useful in determining the *age of an osteoporotic vertebral fracture.* The presence of marrow edema indicates that the fracture is relatively acute. The STIR pulse sequence is extremely sensitive to marrow edema. Gadolinium contrast will also show enhancement in acute fractures. The absence of marrow edema indicates a more chronic fracture.

The MRI findings in acute osteoporotic compression fractures may overlap the findings in cases of malignant collapse. Fracture edema and hemorrhage can surround a vertebral body and give the appearance of a soft tissue mass. Fracture-related edema in acute osteoporotic fractures may cause diffuse vertebral body enhancement similar to the findings in metastatic disease. However, after osteoporotic fractures heal, signal intensities in the collapsed and adjacent normal vertebral bodies are identical. In equivocal cases, a follow-up MR scan can be performed to reassess the bone marrow for resolution of signal abnormalities and reversion to normal fat signal. A CT-guided biopsy is indicated when questions about the cause of a spine fracture remain after imaging studies have been performed.

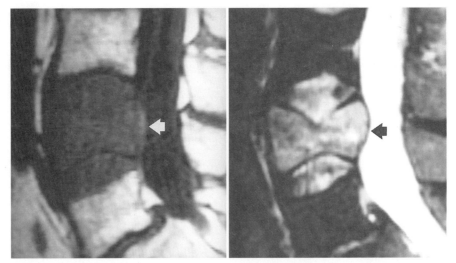

Figure 11-9. Bone metastasis. *Arrows* depict the posterior vertebral cortex, which has a smooth, diffuse bulge and convex contour. (From Palmer WE, Suri R. MR. Differentiation of benign versus malignant collapse. In: Castillo M, editor. Spinal Imaging: State of the Art. Philadelphia: Hanley & Belfus; 2001, with permission.)

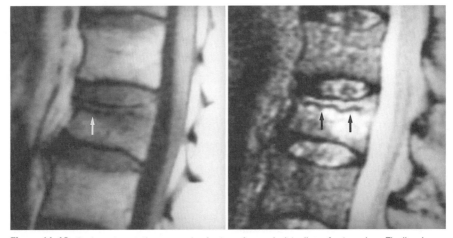

Figure 11-10. Benign osteoporotic compression fracture. *Arrows* depict a linear fracture plane. The line does not extend all the way to the posterior vertebral cortex and posterior cortical height is maintained. (From Palmer WE, Suri R. MR. Differentiation of benign versus malignant collapse. In: Castillo M, editor. Spinal Imaging: State of the Art. Philadelphia: Hanley & Belfus; 2001, with permission.)

Key Points

1. MRI provides excellent visualization of pathologic processes involving the disc, thecal sac, epidural space, neural elements, paraspinal soft tissue, and bone marrow.
2. Gadolinium contrast-enhanced MRI of the spine is valuable for evaluating patients with infection, tumor, or history of prior decompressive surgery.

Website

Radiology web links: http://www.radswiki.net/main/index.php?title=Radiology websites
MRI sequences: http://www.mr-tip.com/serv1.php?type=seq

BIBLIOGRAPHY

1. Castillo M, editor. Spinal Imaging: State of the Art. Philadelphia: Hanley & Belfus; 2001.
2. El-Khoury GY, Bennett L, Stanley M. Essential in Musculoskeletal Imaging. Philadelphia: Saunders; 2003.
3. Helms CA, Major NM, Kaplan PA, et al., editors. Helms: Musculoskeletal MRI. 2nd ed. Philadelphia: Saunders; 2008.
4. Resnick D, Kransdorf MJ, editors. Resnick: Bone and Joint Imaging. 3rd ed. Philadelphia: Saunders; 2005.

COMPUTED TOMOGRAPHY AND CT-MYELOGRAPHY

Vincent J. Devlin, MD

1. What is computed tomography?

Computed tomography (CT) is a noninvasive imaging technology that generates detailed cross-sectional images using a computer and rotating x-ray emitter. The CT scanner is a circular, rotating frame with an x-ray emitter mounted on one side and x-ray detectors mounted on the opposite side. As the patient lies on a mechanical table, which moves through the doughnut-shaped scanner, the scanner rotates and emits an x-ray beam that passes through the body and interacts with a series of rotating detectors. Cross-sectional images are generated based on mathematical reconstruction of tissue beam attenuation. Images are represented on a gray scale in which the shade of gray is determined by the density of the structure. Dense structures such as bone appear white, less dense structures appear as various shades of gray, and the least dense structures (containing gas) appear black. With early-generation CT scanners, termed *sequential CT scanners,* one cross-sectional image was obtained for each complete rotation of the CT frame before the table moved the patient into position for the next image. Contemporary CT scanners, termed *helical* or *spiral CT scanners,* permit the CT scanner to move continuously around the patient as the patient moves through the scanner and utilize multiple rows of x-ray detectors.

2. What are Hounsfield units?

Hounsfield units (HU) measure the relative attenuation or density of a structure imaged on CT. By convention, −1000 is the attenuation for air, 0 for water, and +1000 for dense cortical bone. The operator adjusts the level and width of the displayed range of HU (window) to study different tissues optimally.

3. What is multiplanar reconstruction?

CT data are recorded in the axial plane as image slices composed of small boxes of tissue called *voxels.* These volume elements can be made equivalent in size in three orthogonal axes (isotropic voxels) permitting the axial data to be reconstructed in multiple planes by computer software (e.g. sagittal and coronal reformatted images). Advances in modern software permit reconstruction in nonorthogonal (oblique) planes and curved planes as well. Three-dimensional rendering techniques permit a model of the spine to be created to facilitate understanding of complex three-dimensional anatomy. Contrast agents may be injected into the thecal sac to enhance visualization of the spinal cord and nerve roots or intravenously to permit visualization of vascular structures. (Fig. 12-1)

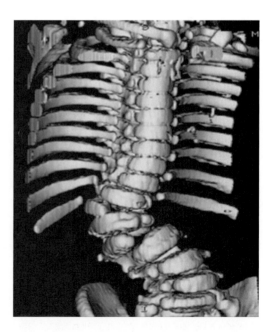

Figure 12-1. Three-dimensional computed tomography (CT) of a patient with scoliosis due to multiple hemivertebra. (From Hedequist DJ. Surgical treatment of scoliosis. Ortho Clin North Am 2007;38:497–509, with permission.)

4. What is the role of CT in assessment of spinal trauma?

Multiplanar CT is the imaging study of choice for evaluation of spine trauma. In many situations, the complex osseous anatomy of the spine is not visualized in sufficient detail on plain radiographs and CT scan is required to accurately diagnose and classify spinal fractures. Magnetic resonance imaging (MRI) plays a complementary role to CT for assessment of ligamentous injury and neurologic compression syndromes in the spine trauma patient (Fig. 12-2).

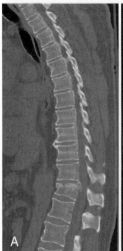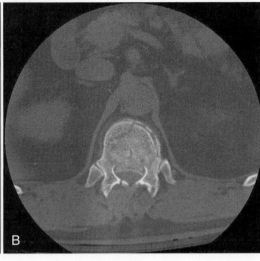

Figure 12-2. T12 burst fracture. **A,** Sagittal image. **B,** Axial image. (From Sethi MK, Schoenfeld AJ, Bono CM, et al. The evolution of thoracolumbar injury classification systems. Spine Journal 2009;9: 780–8, with permission.)

5. Compare the use of CT and MRI for assessment of spinal tumors and spinal infections.

MRI is the optimal test for initial evaluation of spinal tumor and infection after plain radiographs have been obtained. MRI provides information about the spinal canal, disc, bone, and surrounding soft tissues that may not be evident on CT. CT plays a role in determining the extent of bone destruction due to infection or tumor (Fig. 12-3). This determination is important in determining the risk of vertebral fracture and in planning surgical treatment.

6. What questions should be considered before ordering a CT-myelogram study of the spine?

1. Can the pertinent clinical question be answered with noninvasive diagnostic imaging, such as MRI or a combination of MRI and CT?
2. Will the information obtained from the study have an important impact on clinical management of the patient?
3. Does the patient have any history of adverse reaction to iodinated contrast media or any conditions that increase the risk of an adverse reaction to these agents? Some factors considered to increase the risk of a reaction to iodinated contrast include renal insufficiency, diabetic nephropathy, significant cardiac or pulmonary disease, asthma, multiple allergies, and patients at the extremes of age.

7. What types of adverse reactions can occur during a CT-myelogram procedure?

Initially patients may experience discomfort during intrathecal injection of the nonionic water soluble contrast agent. After injection, patients may experience an anaphylactoid (idiosyncratic) reaction (urticaria, facial and laryngeal edema, bronchospasm, hypotension) or a nonidiosyncratic reaction due to the adverse effect of contrast on a specific organ system (nephrotoxicity, cardiac arrhythmia, myocardial ischemia, vasovagal reaction). Specific treatment depends on the exact clinical circumstance.

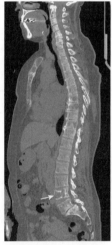

Figure 12-3. Sagittal CT reformation shows multifocal lytic lesions in a patient with multiple myeloma. A pathologic fracture of L4 and lytic lesions in the thoracic spine and sternum are noted. (From Haaga JR, Dogra VS, Forsting M, et al., editors. Haaga: CT and MRI of the Whole Body. 5th ed. St. Louis Mosby; 2008, with permission.)

8. Compare the utility of CT and MRI for assessment of cervical radiculopathy.

Cervical radiculopathy typically results from nerve root impingement in the neural foramen by disc material, bone spurs, or a combination of osseous and disc pathology. MRI is the best test for visualizing disc material, as well as adjacent neural structures, and is generally the first test obtained in the evaluation of cervical radiculopathy. CT is the best test for visualizing osseous pathology responsible for radiculopathy but does not optimally visualize the spinal cord and nerve roots. Use of intrathecal contrast can enhance the ability of CT to visualize adjacent soft tissue and neural structures but requires an invasive procedure and is not required for routine cases.

9. Compare the utility of CT-myelography and MRI for assessment of cervical stenosis presenting with myelopathy.

After plain radiographs are obtained, MRI is usually the next test obtained in the imaging workup for cervical myelopathy. MRI provides a noninvasive means of visualizing the entire cervical spine, including the discs, vertebra, spinal cord, and nerve roots, in multiple planes. CT-myelography plays a role when MRI is contraindicated or when osseous pathology contributes to spinal canal encroachment. In the presence of complex cervical stenosis problems, CT-myelography continues to play a significant role, especially in patients with ossification of the posterior longitudinal ligament (OPLL) where progressive mineralization of this ligament progressively narrows the diameter of the cervical spinal canal (Fig. 12-4A, B). CT images are also valuable in preoperative planning of complex spinal instrumentation procedures for assessment of potential screw fixation sites and their relationship to osseous abnormalities and critical vascular structures (e.g. vertebral artery).

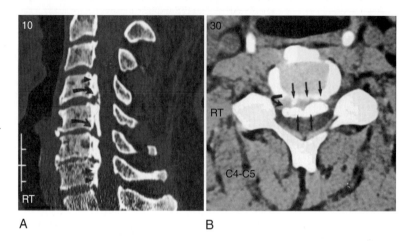

Figure 12-4. Ossification of the posterior longitudinal ligament (OPLL), cervical stenosis, and cervical myelopathy. Sagittal image **(A)** and axial image **(B)** depict continuous OPLL *(straight arrows)*. Double layer sign *(curved arrows)* is pathognomonic for an absent dural plane and risk of cerebrospinal fluid fistula. (From Epstein NE. From the imaging department. Spine Journal 2001;1:77, with permission.)

10. Contrast the utility of CT and MRI for assessment of lumbar disc pathology.

Both CT and MRI are useful techniques for diagnosis of lumbar disc pathology. Both can be used to define disc contour abnormalities (bulge, protrusion, extrusion, sequestration) and guide treatment. The most significant difference between these imaging modalities is the ability of MRI to depict changes in disc pathoanatomy and chemistry (e.g. disc desiccation, annular tears) before changes in disc contour. For this reason, MRI is the imaging modality of first choice for assessment of lumbar disc pathology.

11. How is lumbar spinal stenosis defined and described on CT and MRI?

- *Lumbar spinal stenosis* refers to any type of bone or soft tissue pathology that results in narrowing or constriction of the spinal canal, nerve root canal, or both
- *Central spinal stenosis* refers to compression in the region of the spinal canal occupied by the thecal sac
- *Lateral stenosis* involves the nerve root canal and is described in terms of *three zones*, using the pedicle as a reference point (Fig. 12-5). Spinal stenosis may involve a single spine segment or multiple spinal segments. It may or may not be associated with instability of the spine.

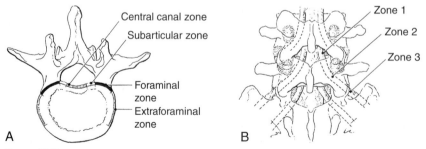

Figure 12-5. Anatomy of spinal stenosis. Axial **(A)** and sagittal **(B)** views demonstrate anatomic relationships of the thecal sac and nerve roots to the surrounding lumbar osseous structures and intervertebral disc. The nerve root may be compressed along its course through the subarticular zone (zone 1), the foraminal zone (zone 2), or the extraforaminal zone (zone 3). In zone 3, the nerve root may be compressed as it exits the nerve root canal or further laterally in the so-called far-lateral region. (From Devlin VJ. Degenerative lumbar spinal stenosis and decompression. Spine State Art Rev 1997;11:107–28, with permission.)

12. A 65-year-old woman presents with symptoms of back pain and neurogenic claudication. Available imaging studies include a lateral myelogram image (Fig. 12-6A) and an axial CT image (Fig. 12-6B). What is the patient's diagnosis? Explain what neural structures are compressed.

The clinical and radiographic findings are classic for L4–L5 degenerative spondylolisthesis (grade 1). The lateral myelogram image shows an intact neural arch at the level of spondylolisthesis, leading to the diagnosis of degenerative spondylolisthesis. Disc degeneration and subluxation with subsequent facet joint and ligamentum flavum hypertrophy result in central spinal stenosis (open arrow and opposing arrows) and zone 1 (subarticular) lateral canal stenosis (*small arrows*). L4–L5 degenerative spondylolisthesis typically results in central spinal stenosis at the L4–L5 level associated with compression of the traversing L5 nerve roots bilaterally. The exiting L4 nerve roots are not typically involved unless there is advanced loss of disc space height, at which time the L4 nerve roots become compressed in the region of the neural foramen. Degenerative spondylolisthesis does not progress beyond a grade 2 (50%) slip unless prior surgery has been performed at the level of listhesis.

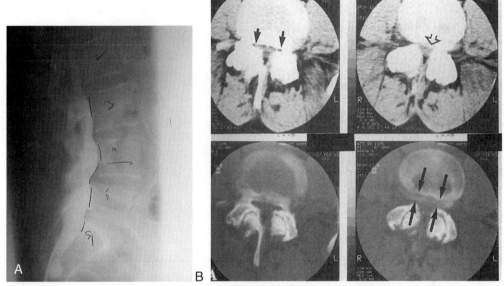

Figure 12-6. A, Lateral myelographic view shows L4-5 spondylolisthesis and spinal stenosis. **B,** Axial computed tomography (CT) scans at the L4–5 level shows central spinal stenosis *(open arrow and opposing arrows)* and zone 1 *(subarticular)* lateral canal stenosis *(small arrows)*. (From Cole AJ, Herring SA. The Low Back Pain Handbook. Philadelphia: Hanley & Belfus; 1997, with permission.)

13. What is the role of CT in evaluation of a patient following spinal decompression and spinal fusion with instrumentation? When should a myelogram be added?

A CT scan can provide critical information following spinal decompression and fusion procedures. A myelogram should be performed in conjunction with the CT scan if it is necessary to assess the spinal canal and nerve root canals at the operative site. Problems that can be diagnosed with CT with or without myelography include:

- Persistent neural compression
- Adjacent level spinal stenosis or instability
- Nonunion following attempted spinal fusion (pseudarthrosis) (Fig. 12-7A, B)
- Incorrect placement of spinal implants including pedicle screws, interbody grafts, or fusion cages (Figure 12-7C).

Although MRI may provide meaningful information in the presence of titanium spinal implants, significant artifact may persist and CT remains the best imaging test. MRI in the presence of stainless steel spinal implants will not provide useful information regarding the instrumented spinal segments due to artifact.

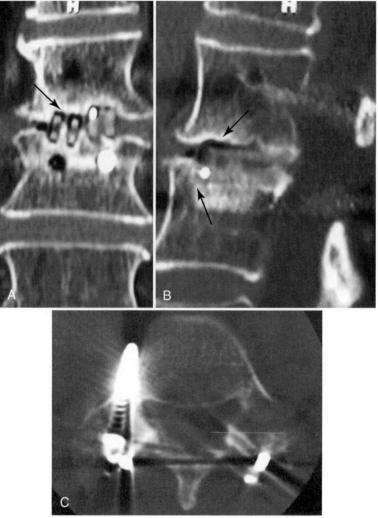

Figure 12-7. A, Coronal computed tomography (CT). **B,** Saggital CT image shows nonunion following attempted L1–L2 posterior interbody fusion. Note the lucencies around the interbody cages *(superior arrows)* and subsidence of cages into the L2 vertebral body *(inferior arrows)*. **C,** Right-sided pedicle screw is improperly placed because it is not contained within bone and impinges on the adjacent nerve root. (A, B, From Fogel GR, Toohey JS, Neidre A, Brantigan JW. The Spine Journal 6: 421-427, 2006. C, From Devlin VJ. Spine Secrets. Philadelphia: Hanley & Belfus; 2003, with permission.)

Key Points

1. Multiplanar CT is the imaging study of choice for evaluating the complex osseous anatomy of the spine.
2. Contrast agents may be injected into the thecal sac or intravenously to enhance CT visualization of the spinal cord, nerve roots, and vascular structures.
3. The radiation dosage associated with CT is an important concern and may be minimized by following appropriate protocols.

Website

Principles of CT and CT Technology: http://tech.snmjournals.org/cgi/content/full/35/3/115

BIBLIOGRAPHY

1. Haaga JR, Dogra VS, Forsting M, et al., editors. Haaga: CT and MRI of the Whole Body. 5th ed. Philadelphia: Mosby; 2008.
2. Resnick D, Kransdorf MJ, editors. Resnick: Bone and Joint Imaging. 3rd ed. Philadelphia: Saunders; 2005.

CHAPTER 13

NUCLEAR IMAGING AND SPINAL DISORDERS

Vincent J. Devlin, MD

1. What nuclear medicine studies are useful in the evaluation of spinal problems?

Technetium-99m bone scan is the most commonly used study for detection of osseous lesions of the spinal column. Additional nuclear imaging studies play a limited role in the diagnosis of spinal infections and include the gallium-67 scan and indium-111 white cell scan. Positron emission tomography (PET) has shown utility in diagnosis of spinal metastatic disease, infection, and bone marrow abnormalities.

2. For which common spinal disorders does a technetium-99m bone scan provide useful diagnostic information?

Technetium-99m bone scanning may provide useful diagnostic information regarding spondylolysis, spine fractures, primary and metastatic spine tumors, and spinal infections.

3. How is a technetium-99m bone scan performed?

A radiopharmaceutical (technetium-99m, typically attached to a diphosphonate derivative) is administered intravenously and rapidly distributed throughout the body. Before excretion through the renal system, the technetium is adsorbed into the hydroxyapatite matrix of bone. A gamma camera is used to record the distribution of radioactivity throughout the body. Areas of increased blood flow and osteoblastic activity are detected by an increased concentration of radionuclide tracer. A decrease or absence of radionuclide tracer reflects either an interruption of blood flow or decreased osteoblastic activity.

4. What is a three-phase bone scan?

A three-phase bone scan is most commonly ordered during a workup for infection. It consists of three parts:
1. **Flow phase study:** assesses vascular spread of the injected radionuclide immediately after radionuclide injection. It detects perfusion abnormalities in suspect tissue.
2. **Blood pool phase study:** detects hyperemia in bone and soft tissue due to abnormal pooling of the radionuclide shortly following contrast injection (5 minutes).
3. **Delayed static phase study:** obtained usually 2 to 4 hours after injection. It can detect abnormal increased uptake in areas of active bone remodeling (Fig. 13-1).

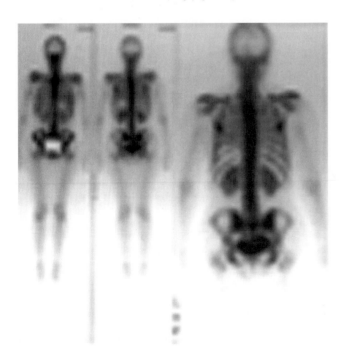

Figure 13-1. Normal technetium bone scan. Uniform activity is present in all bones including the individual vertebra. The bladder and kidneys are visualized. It is common to note increased uptake in the spine or peripheral joints in areas of degenerative disease. (From Pretorius ES, Solomon JA. Radiology Secrets. 2nd ed. St. Louis: Mosby; 2006. p. 409.)

5. **Discuss advantages and disadvantages of a technetium bone scan for diagnosis of spine infections.**

   Advantages of a technetium bone scan include the ability to detect a pyogenic infectious process long before plain radiographs demonstrate any abnormality. A technetium bone scan has a high sensitivity in the diagnosis of spinal osteomyelitis in the absence of prior spine surgery or medical comorbidities.

   Disadvantages of a technetium bone scans is related to its lack of specificity, especially in patients with a history of recent spine surgery, spinal implants, Paget's disease, fracture, or pseudarthrosis. In addition, technetium bone scans are flow-dependent studies and may be falsely negative in situations associated with decreased perfusion to target tissues. A high false-negative rate is associated with their use in the diagnosis of granulomatous infections (e.g. tuberculosis).

6. **What can be done to improve the accuracy of a technetium bone scan for diagnosis of spine infection?**

   A second nuclear imaging modality may be added to increase diagnostic accuracy.
   - A **gallium scan** is the most commonly utilized complementary study for diagnosis of spine infection. Gallium citrate has affinity for iron binding molecules that accumulate at sites of inflammation. False positives may occur in patients with prior surgery or increased bone remodeling (e.g. fracture, pseudarthrosis, recent fusion surgery)
   - **Indium scans** are occasionally used and involve labeling of the patient's leukocytes with indium oxine, which may subsequently accumulate in areas of inflammation following injection. Indium scans have a lower sensitivity but have a higher specificity than gallium scans. Imaging is typically performed at 48 hours following injection for both studies
   - **PET scanning** with 18-F-fluoro-deoxy-D-glucose (FDG) is the newest modality used for diagnosis of spinal infection. FDG is metabolized by activated neutrophils and macrophages involved in inflammation. Advantages include rapid imaging (2 hours following injection) and higher spatial resolution than gallium or indium scans. Disadvantages include limited availability and cost.

7. **What is a SPECT scan?**

   Single-photon emission computed tomography (SPECT) uses a computer-aided gamma camera and the radionuclides of standard nuclear imaging to provide cross-sectional images similar to those of a computed tomography (CT) scan (Fig. 13-2). A SPECT study is more sensitive than planar scintigraphy in detecting lesions in the spine. It allows precise localization of spinal lesions to the vertebral body, disc space, or vertebral arch. SPECT scans are ideal for localizing spondylolysis and identifying small lesions such as an osteoid osteoma.

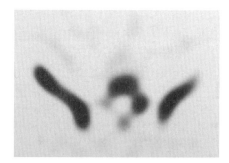

Figure 13-2. Cross-sectional single-photon emission computed tomography (SPECT) image at the L5 level showing increased uptake in the left posterior neural arch consistent with spondylolysis.

8. **What is the role of a technetium bone scan in the evaluation of a pediatric patient with back pain symptoms?**

   A bone scan may be considered for patients with normal spinal radiographs and back pain persisting for longer than 6 weeks. A bone scan can diagnose problems such as spinal osteomyelitis and spinal tumor. A bone scan with SPECT images helps to diagnose a stress reaction (impending spondylolysis) or pars fracture in pediatric patients with back pain.

9. **What information can a bone scan provide about lumbar spondylolysis?**

   A bone scan with SPECT images can provide valuable information about lumbar spondylolysis. It can determine whether a spondylolysis detectable by radiography is acute or chronic. In cases in which radiographs are negative, a bone scan can diagnose an impending spondylolysis (stress reaction). In some cases, the bone scan may be positive on the side opposite a radiographically detectable pars defect and aids in diagnosis of an impending spondylolysis. Bone scans can also be used to assess healing of an acute spondylolysis.

10. **What is the role of a technetium bone scan in the assessment of adults with back pain?**

    The major role of a technetium bone scan in the assessment of adult back pain patients is the diagnosis of serious spine conditions such as infection, tumor, or acute fracture. A technetium bone scan is a good alternative for initial evaluation of a patient with contraindications to spine magnetic resonance imaging (MRI).

11. What is the typical pattern on technetium bone scan in a patient with acute vertebral compression fractures secondary to osteoporosis?

The typical appearance of osteoporotic compression fractures on a technetium bone scan (Fig. 13-3) consists of multiple transverse bands of increased uptake on a posteroanterior image. However, the etiology of the fracture (trauma, tumor, metabolic bone disease) cannot be definitively diagnosed based solely on a bone scan. Increased activity can be noted within 72 hours of fracture, and the average time for a bone scan to revert to normal following an osteoporotic vertebral compression fracture is around 7 months.

12. A 70-year-old woman complains of increasing low back and upper sacral pain. A technetium bone scan was obtained (Fig. 13-4). What is the diagnosis?

The scan shows increased radionuclide activity above the bladder in the sacral area in a H-shaped pattern (Honda sign). Bilateral increased radionuclide uptake in the sacral ala in association with a transverse region of increased radionuclide activity is typical of a sacral insufficiency fracture, most commonly due to osteoporosis.

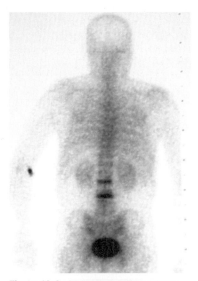

Figure 13-3. Technetium bone scan demonstrates acute two-level osteoporotic compression fractures.

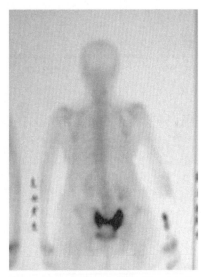

Figure 13-4. Increased radionuclide uptake in an H-shaped pattern (Honda sign) in the sacrum is consistent with an insufficiency fracture.

13. What are the advantages of a technetium bone scan for diagnosis of spinal neoplasms?

A technetium bone scan in association with physical examination and laboratory studies is an effective method for identifying many patients with spinal neoplasms involving the osseous elements of the spinal column. Technetium bone scans can identify occult lesions and multifocal tumor involvement. In addition, if multiple lesions are detected, a bone scan can help identify the most accessible lesion for biopsy.

14. What pitfalls are associated with the use of a technetium bone scan for diagnosis of spinal neoplasms?

Technetium bone scans cannot unequivocally distinguish increased uptake due to tumor from increased uptake due to infection or fracture. In addition, certain tumors (e.g. multiple myeloma, hypernephroma) are not likely to demonstrate increased uptake on technetium bone scans because they do not typically stimulate increased osteoblastic activity. PET scanning using FDG can be useful in symptomatic spinal metastases not identified on radiographs, CT, or technetium bone scan (Fig. 13-5).

15. What is the superscan phenomenon?

The superscan phenomenon occurs when the distribution of disease is so widespread and uniformly distributed that the technetium scan is incorrectly interpreted as negative. Increased radionuclide uptake is noted throughout the skeleton in the presence of diminished or absent uptake in the kidneys and bladder. This phenomenon can occur with metastatic prostate and breast cancer, renal osteodystrophy, and Paget's disease.

16. How is a PET scan performed?

A positron-emitting radionuclide is injected into the body. As the positrons are emitted and travel through tissue they collide with electrons, resulting in production of gamma rays. A PET scanner records and analyzes these data and creates an image. CT or MRI may be combined with PET to maximize diagnostic potential.

FDG is currently the most commonly used radiotracer. It is transported and becomes trapped intracellularly as a result of phosphorylation by hexokinase. FDG accumulates at sites of neoplasia and inflammation as cells in these regions have an increased metabolic rate. Because FDG competes with nonradioactive glucose, recent eating or diabetes with an elevated blood sugar greater than 150 mL/dL will decrease scan sensitivity. 18-F-NaF is a bone-specific tracer that has application in PET imaging of the musculoskeletal system (Fig. 13-6).

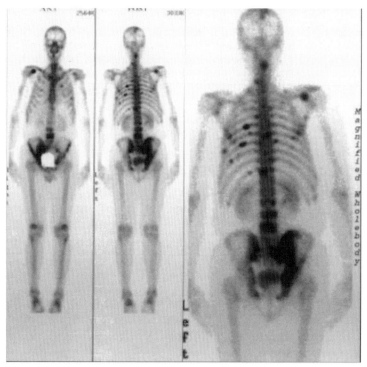

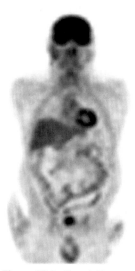

Figure 13-6. Normal 18-F-fluoro-deoxy-D-glucose (FDG) positron emission tomography (PET) scan shows mild diffuse uptake throughout the bowel (a normal variant), mild uptake in the liver, significant uptake in the brain and heart, and marked uptake in the bladder. (From Pretorius ES, Solomon JA. Radiology Secrets. 2nd ed. St. Louis: Mosby; 2006. p. 401.)

Figure 13-5. Anterior and posterior views of a bone scan show a patient with multiple foci of intense activity involving the ribs, spine, skull, right scapula and pelvis due to metastatic cancer. (From Pretorius ES, Solomon JA. Radiology Secrets, 2nd ed. Philadelphia: Mosby, 2006. p. 412)

17. For which common disorders can a PET scan provide useful diagnostic information?
PET scans are most commonly used in the evaluation of cancer for diagnosis, staging, and assessment of treatment effectiveness. Utility in head and neck tumors, colorectal tumors, melanoma, lymphoma, multiple myeloma, lung cancer, and metastatic breast cancer have been reported. The role of PET scans in the diagnosis of spinal infections is evolving.

Key Points

1. A technetium-99m bone scan can detect regions of increased blood flow or osteoblastic activity.
2. A gallium scan or indium-labeled white blood cell scan may be used in conjunction with a technetium bone scan for diagnosis of infection.
3. FGD-PET scans have shown utility in diagnosis of spinal neoplasia and infection.

Websites

Nuclear medicine: http://interactive.snm.org/index.cfm?PageID=972&RPID=924
PET scanning: http://www.petscaninfo.com/zportal/portals/pat/basic

BIBLIOGRAPHY

1. Chen K, Blebea J, Laredo JD, et al. Evaluation of Musculoskeletal Disorders with PET, PET/CT, and PET/MR Imaging. PET Clin 2009;3:451–65.
2. Ell PJ, Gambhir SS. Nuclear Medicine in Clinical Diagnosis and Treatment. 3rd ed. Philadelphia: Churchill Livingstone; 2004.
3. Pretorius ES, Solomon JA. Radiology Secrets. 2nd ed. St. Louis: Mosby; 2006.
4. Ziessman HA, O'Malley JP, Thrall JH. Ziessman: Nuclear Medicine—The Requisites. 3rd ed. St. Louis: Mosby; 2005.

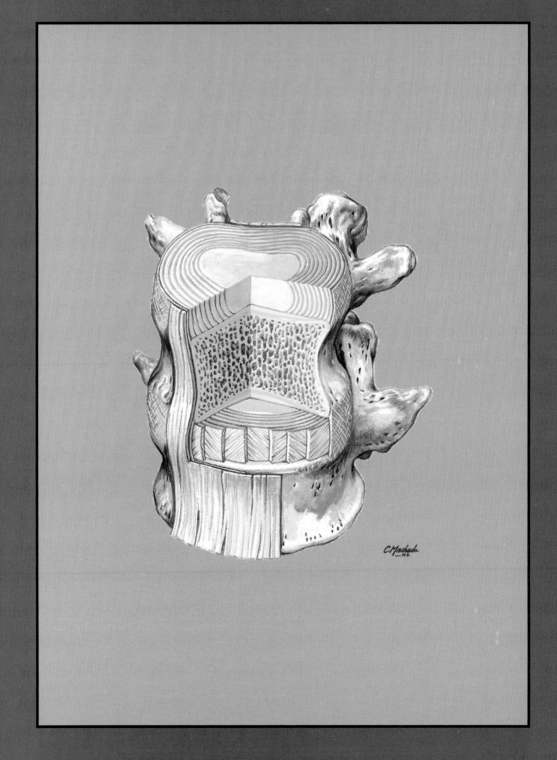

REHABILITATION MEDICINE APPROACHES TO SPINAL DISORDERS

Anna M. Lasak, MD, and Avital Fast, MD

1. What is rehabilitation medicine?

Rehabilitation medicine is a medical specialty focused on the prevention, diagnosis, and treatment of acute and chronic diseases of neuromuscular, musculoskeletal, and cardiopulmonary systems. A holistic and comprehensive approach to medical problems is implemented through a coordinated interdisciplinary team. Multiple simultaneous interventions maximize the patient's physical, psychological, social, vocational, and recreational potential, consistent with physiologic or anatomic impairment and environmental limitations. Rehabilitation medicine addresses both the cause and the secondary effects of injury or illness on a person's life. The scope of rehabilitation medicine is broad and includes spinal disorders, musculoskeletal disorders, stroke, cancer, spinal cord injury, cardiac and pulmonary disorders, chronic pain treatment, geriatric rehabilitation, and vocational rehabilitation.

2. List general goals in rehabilitation of patients with spinal disorders.

- Decrease spinal related pain
- Improve strength, flexibility, balance, motor control, and cardiovascular endurance
- Minimize spine-related disability
- Normalize activities of daily living
- Return to work and vocational activities

3. What are *red flags* in the evaluation of spinal pain?

Red flags are warning signs of potentially serious conditions. They require special attention and further evaluation (lab tests, imaging studies). A careful history and physical examination are mandatory. Findings such as rest pain, pain at night, extremity numbness or weakness, systemic disease, or bowel or bladder dysfunction should prompt detailed assessment. Red flags in evaluation of spinal problems include:

- Fever
- Unexplained weight loss
- Night pain
- Cancer history
- Significant trauma
- Alcohol or drug use
- Age younger than 20 years
- Age older than 50 years
- Osteoporosis
- Failure to improve with treatment

It is also important to recognize patients who are less likely to improve because of psychological or nonmedical problems (i.e. compensation, pending litigation, secondary gain, poor educational level, significant emotional stressors). Such factors increase the risk of developing chronic pain or disability and are termed *yellow flags*.

4. What components are included in a nonoperative spine treatment program?

The initial goal of a nonoperative treatment program is pain control. Bedrest for longer than 2 days is not recommended. Once pain control is achieved, the patient should advance to an exercise program. The ultimate goal of an exercise program is development of adequate dynamic control of the spine to eliminate repetitive injury to pain-sensitive structures (i.e. discs, facet joints). Socioeconomic, psychological, and vocational issues are considered during treatment. It is critical to realize that treatment of acute back pain requires a different approach from the treatment of chronic back pain. Components of a nonoperative treatment program for spinal disorders may include:

- Education (optimize biomechanics involved in the activities of daily living)
- Local modalities: electrotherapeutic modalities (transcutaneous electrical nerve stimulation [TENS], electrical muscle stimulation [EMS], interferential current [IFC]), physical agents (superficial heat [hot packs], cryotherapy [cold packs], ultrasound [US])
- Medication (analgesics, nonsteroidal antiinflammatory drugs [NSAIDs], steroids, anticonvulsants, antidepressants, muscle relaxants, and antispasticity medications)

- Injections (trigger point injections, sacroiliac joint injections, facet joint injections, epidural steroid injections)
- Exercise (reeducation of range of motion and posture, general strengthening and aerobic exercise, specific spinal exercise [flexion, extension, spinal stabilization], pool therapy)
- Orthoses and assistive devices (braces, canes, walkers, wheelchairs, mobility devices)
- Manual therapy (manipulation, mobilization, therapeutic massage)
- Complementary and alternative therapies (acupuncture, yoga)
- Home environment modification (ramps, raised toilet seat, grab bar system for bathroom)
- Ergonomic modifications (chair modification, workstation modification)
- Lifestyle modification (smoking cessation, nutritional counseling, weight reduction)
- Neuroablative procedures (lumbar medial branch neurotomy for facet [zygapophyseal] joint pain)
- Implantable devices (spinal cord stimulator, intrathecal pump)

5. What is the role of therapeutic injections?

Therapeutic injections are used to reduce pain and inflammation and permit initiation of an exercise program.

Local trigger point injections can be done with local anesthetic, with or without steroid, NSAIDs, botulinum toxin, or 5-HT3 receptor antagonists. The analgesic action is explained by inhibition of dorsal horn efferents by nociceptive counter irritant based on gate control theory. Botulinum toxin can be used to decrease painful muscle spasm by blocking acetylcholine release in trigger points (used for treatment of cervical dystonia and piriformis syndrome). Dry needling technique can be used as well to mechanically break the taut muscle fibers in the trigger points.

Prolotherapy involves intraligamentous injection of irritant solution (dextrose, glycerin, phenol) that induces inflammation and proliferation of new cells in incompetent ligament or tendon.

Epidural steroid injections (caudal [CESI], interlaminar [ILESI], transforaminal [TFESI]) are performed under fluoroscopic guidance with contrast enhancement to ensure proper placement of the medication into the epidural space close to the pain generator. Steroids decrease inflammation, stabilize neural membranes, and suppress ectopic neural discharges.

6. What is the role of physical therapy in treatment of spine disorders?

- Instruction in proper exercise technique
- Advancement of the level of therapy based on the patient's symptoms
- Postural correction
- Administration of modalities
- Spinal manipulation
- Assisting the patient with creation of an individual home exercise program
- Providing supervision, motivation, and goal-setting during a therapy program

7. Discuss the role of physical agents in the treatment of spinal pain.

Physical agents utilize physical forces (thermal, acoustic or radiant energy) to promote healing; reduce pain, swelling, and inflammation; or modulate muscle tone. These agents should not be used in isolation but rather as supplements to a therapy program. Heat and cold provide analgesia and muscle tone reduction in superficial structures. Ultrasound increases deep soft tissue extensibility, blood flow, and healing. Hydrotherapy uses agitated water to produce convective heating and massage. Immersion in water reduces spinal loads and can be used as an adjunct to an exercise program.

8. What is TENS?

TENS is the application of small electrical signals to the body via superficial skin electrodes to achieve analgesia (at high frequency 80-100 Hz) or to produce muscle contractions (at low frequency 5-10 Hz). The typical unit consists of a battery, signal generator, and electrode pairs. The exact mechanism of action for TENS is not completely understood. Based on the gate theory of pain, stimulation of large myelinated afferent fibers blocks transmission of pain by small unmyelinated fibers at the level of spinal cord. TENS may also increase endorphin levels in cerebrospinal fluid and enkephalins in the dorsal horn region of the spinal cord. TENS is not a curative modality and should be used as an adjunct tool.

9. How is spinal traction used in the treatment of spinal disorders?

The efficacy of traction in treatment of spinal disorders is controversial. Several techniques are available for applying traction to the spine: manual, mechanical (pulley, free weights), motorized, and autotraction (a device provides lumbar traction when the patient pulls with the arms). Mechanisms proposed for a positive therapeutic effect from traction include distraction of neural foramina and vasa nervorum decompression. Cervical traction can be applied in sitting or supine position with 20 to 30 pounds of traction force. Because approximately 10 pounds are required to counteract the weight of the head, cervical traction tends to be more effective in the supine position. Lumbar traction is generally applied in the supine position with 90 degree of hip and knee flexion. Because of the large forces required to achieve lumbar distraction (50 pounds for posterior vertebral separation, 100 pounds for anterior vertebral separation), lumbar traction is often poorly tolerated by patients.

10. What are the contraindications to use of traction?

Ligamentous instability, previous spine trauma, osteopenia, pregnancy, spine tumor, and spine infection. Advanced age is a relative contraindication to the use of traction.

11. Which spine patients should be referred for assessment by the psychologist or psychiatrist?

Situations in which referral is indicated include alcohol and drug abuse, depression, noncompliance with treatment, behavioral problems, and traumatic stress syndrome.

12. How can a pain clinic assist in the treatment of spinal disorders?

The pain clinic provides an interdisciplinary program for patients with chronic spinal pain syndromes. The Commission on Accreditation of Rehabilitation Facilities (CARF) pain management guidelines require that the team include a physician, nurse, physical therapist, and psychologist or psychiatrist. Interdisciplinary chronic pain treatment uses the strength of specialists working together. The pain clinic is ideal for the following goals:
- Providing medical management, physical therapy, occupational therapy, vocational therapy, and psychotherapy
- Addressing complex issues related to pain behaviors (i.e. patients being paid for remaining disabled behave differently from patients who are not compensated)
- Identification of psychosocial barriers to treatment (i.e. depression, family distress, anxiety, substance abuse)
- Assessment of the patient's psychological strengths and weaknesses and providing individual or group therapy as indicated
- Providing disability management with the goal of returning to employment

13. What are the three levels of nonsurgical care for spinal disorders?

- **Primary care** is applied to patients with acute back and neck pain problems. Symptoms are controlled with medical or surgical management, exercise therapy, medications, modalities, and manual techniques
- **Secondary care** is applied to patients who did not respond to the initial primary care level of treatment. Such patients require more comprehensive management involving the interdisciplinary care of medical specialists, physical therapists, occupational therapists, psychologists, social workers, and disability managers. During this phase restorative exercise and education are applied to prevent deconditioning and chronic disability. Work-conditioning and work-hardening approaches are included in secondary care
- **Tertiary care** is indicated for patients who failed primary and secondary conservative care or surgical treatment. Tertiary care or functional restoration involves interdisciplinary team care with all disciplines on site. Functional restoration programs can be provided by some pain clinics. Functional restoration programs include:
  - Quantification of physical deconditioning (strength, endurance, aerobic capacity)
  - Addressing psychosocial problems (psychopathology, use of narcotics)
  - Identification of socioeconomic factors in disability (compensation, psychogenic pain)
  - Cognitive behavioral training (relaxation techniques, improve self-esteem)
  - Restoration of fitness
  - Work simulation activities
  - Individual, family, and group counseling
  - Disability and vocational management
  - Outcome monitoring

CERVICAL SPINE

14. List the common causes of cervical pain seen in a rehabilitation medicine office practice.

- Myofascial pain
- Cervical spondylosis
- Cervical sprain/strain
- Cervical disc herniation
- Cervical radiculopathy
- Cervical stenosis
- Cervical fractures
- Inflammatory spinal conditions (e.g. rheumatoid arthritis)
- Neoplasm
- Infection

15. Outline a treatment plan for patients with acute neck pain secondary to cervical spondylosis.

Nonoperative options include manual therapy, modalities, isometrics, aerobic conditioning, flexibility exercises, progressive resistance training, disease education, and a home exercise program. Medication (NSAIDs, analgesics, antidepressants, muscle relaxants) also plays a role in treatment.

16. What is the natural history of cervical radiculopathy?

Cervical radiculopathy most commonly results from nerve root compression due to a herniated disc and/or cervical spondylosis. In most cases there is no preceding trauma. Patients commonly present with neck pain, headache, and sharp pain radiating to the upper extremity in a dermatomal distribution. Neck movement, cough, and Valsalva maneuvers tend to exacerbate pain symptoms. Numbness and paresthesias occur most commonly in the distal part of the involved dermatome. Patients may present with weakness of upper extremity muscles, depending on the specific nerve root that is affected. Other patients present with chronic neck pain, limited neck range of motion, and arm weakness. The majority of patients (70%-80%) improve within several weeks. Patients with progressive or persistent neurologic weakness, myelopathy, or intractable pain should be referred for surgical evaluation.

17. Outline a nonsurgical treatment plan for patients with cervical radiculopathy.
- Medication (analgesics, NSAIDs, muscle relaxants, and possibly a short course of oral steroids)
- Cervical traction
- Soft cervical collar
- Cold, heat
- Manual therapy
- Therapeutic injections (cervical epidural injections, trigger point injections)
- Home exercise program
- Ergonomic modifications

18. What is the natural history of cervical spondylotic myelopathy?
Cervical spondylotic myelopathy (CSM) is the most common cause of spinal cord dysfunction in adult patients. Symptoms result from progressive compromise of the spinal cord secondary to degenerative changes in the cervical spine. The first symptoms of CSM are frequently poor balance and lower extremity weakness with resultant gait dysfunction. Patients may also present with gradual weakness and numbness of the hands and fine motor coordination deficits ("clumsy hands"). Some patients may complain of neck pain, although the condition is painless in many patients. Neck flexion may produce a shock-like sensation involving the trunk and upper extremities (Lhermitte's phenomenon). Bowel and bladder function may be affected in later stages of the disease. CSM is a disease with an unpredictable course. Progressive CSM may result in cord ischemia with paralysis due to cervical cord compression. The natural history of CSM has been characterized by long intervals of clinical stability punctuated by short periods of intermittent deterioration in neurologic function.

19. Outline the treatment plan for patients with cervical spondylotic myelopathy.
Nonsurgical management does not alter the natural history of the disease. Surgical intervention is the only treatment that can arrest the progression of CSM and should be considered when feasible. Nonsurgical management may be considered for patients with mild neurologic complaints in the absence of significant disability or patients with advanced CSM whose advanced age and comorbidities significantly increase the risk of surgical intervention. Nonsurgical management may include:
- Immobilization in a cervical collar
- Isometric neck exercises
- Strengthening exercises of upper and lower extremities
- Analgesics, NSAIDs
- Local modalities
- Balance exercises
- Assistive devices (canes, walkers) to minimize risk of falls
- Education. Patients should be instructed to avoid hyperextension of the cervical spine:
  - Adjust headrest in the car
  - Adjust computer screen and TV set height
  - Avoid using high shelves
  - Avoid painting ceilings
  - Avoid certain sports activities with prolonged neck hyperextension, such as breaststroke swimming

  During dental work the dentist should be informed about the neck range-of-motion restrictions; at the hairdresser the patient's face should be positioned toward the sink.

20. What is the treatment of *whiplash injury*?
Whiplash injury is a term used to describe an acute cervical sprain or strain that results from acceleration and deceleration motion without direct application of force to the head or neck. Whiplash commonly affects the cervical facet joints and related musculature (trapezius, levator scapulae, scalene, sternocleidomastoid, and paraspinals). Although the symptoms of nonradicular neck and shoulder pain are often self-limiting (6-12 months), many people continue to experience more chronic symptoms. Treatment options include cervical traction, massage, heat, ice, ultrasound, isometric neck exercises, a soft cervical collar, and NSAIDs and/or short-term analgesic use. Patients with persistent pain may have annular tears, coexisting degenerative joint and disc pathology, nerve root entrapment, spinal stenosis, or myelopathy. Neurologic symptoms or intractable pain symptoms that are not responsive to treatment indicate the need for further evaluation.

THORACIC AND LUMBAR SPINE

21. List common causes of thoracic pain seen in a rehabilitation medicine office practice.
- Thoracic sprain/strain
- Myofascial pain
- Compression fracture (usually due to osteoporosis but occasionally due to tumor)
- Thoracic disc pathology (axial pain, radiculopathy, myelopathy)
- Osteoarthritis

- Scheuermann's disease
- Ankylosing spondylitis
- Forrestier's disease (diffuse idiopathic skeletal hyperostosis [DISH])
- Disc space infection
- Herpes zoster infection and postherpetic neuralgia
- Scoliosis, kyphosis
- Neoplasm
- Extraspinal causes (i.e. pancreatitis, peptic ulcer)

22. Outline a treatment plan for patients with thoracic radiculopathy.

Thoracic radiculopathy may be due to disc herniation or metabolic abnormalities of the nerve root (i.e. diabetes). Patients present with bandlike chest pain. Thoracic radiculopathy is not a common diagnosis, and other possible serious pathology should be excluded (malignancy, compression fracture, infection, angina, aortic aneurysm, peptic ulcer disease). Nonsurgical treatment options for thoracic radiculopathy include medication (NSAIDs, analgesics, oral steroids), modalities, TENS, spinal nerve root blocks, spinal stabilization exercises, strengthening of back and abdominal muscles, orthoses, and postural retraining.

23. List some of the common causes of lumbar pain seen in a rehabilitation medicine office practice.

- Lumbar sprain/strain
- Lumbar disc degeneration
- Myofascial pain
- Fibromyalgia
- Lumbar spondylosis
- Sacroiliac joint dysfunction
- Infection
- Lumbar spondylolysis and spondylolisthesis
- Lumbar spinal stenosis
- DISH
- Spondyloarthropathy (i.e. ankylosing spondylitis)
- Fracture
- Neoplasm
- Extraspinal source (e.g. hip osteoarthritis)

24. How does the probability of recovery change with time after the onset of low back pain symptoms?

The natural history for recovery after an episode of acute back pain is favorable, with recovery noted in most patients by 6 to 12 weeks. From the onset of symptoms, 50% of patients recover by 2 weeks, 70% recover by 1 month, and 90% recover by 4 months. However, despite the high likelihood of recovery after an episode of acute low back pain, over 50% of patients experience another episode within 1 year. Patients who fail to recover by 4 months frequently progress to long-term chronic disability. Patients with chronic back pain are more difficult to treat than those with acute back pain and require different treatment approaches.

25. Describe a treatment plan for patients with acute low back pain.

The natural history of acute low back pain is improvement over time. Patient reassurance; medications (analgesics, NSAIDs, short course of oral steroids, muscle relaxants); and education about back care and exercise are beneficial. Studies suggest that manipulation may decrease pain during the first 3 weeks after onset of symptoms. If pain persists, spinal radiographs should be obtained. Bone scan and/or magnetic resonance imaging (MRI) are indicated if serious underlying pathology is suspected.

26. What is the natural history of a lumbar disc herniation?

The natural history of lumbar disc herniation is quite favorable. Gradual improvement in symptoms over several weeks is noted in the majority of patients. Comparison of nonsurgical and surgical treatment has shown that surgically treated patients recover more quickly from sciatic pain symptoms, report better long-term functional status and higher satisfaction. Both nonsurgical and surgical treatments are associated with clinically significant improvement over time and the differences between treatment groups narrows over time.

27. Outline a nonsurgical treatment plan for lumbar radiculopathy due to lumbar disc herniation.

Treatment goals include pain control, reduction of nerve root inflammation, and rapid return to daily activities. Treatment options for achieving these goals include:

- Medication (NSAIDs, analgesics, muscle relaxants, oral steroids)
- Short-term bedrest
- Modalities (ice, TENS, ultrasound, pool therapy)
- McKenzie exercises
- Lumbosacral stabilization program
- Epidural steroid injection, selective nerve root blocks
- Mobilization techniques
- Ergonomic modification
- Patient education (lifting technique, posture, exercise)
- Surgery

28. What is the natural history of lumbar spinal stenosis?

Lumbar spinal stenosis is a potentially disabling condition, caused by compression of the thecal sac (central stenosis) and nerve roots (lateral stenosis). Patients may present with chronic low back pain, leg pain, and/or neurogenic claudication. Pain is characteristically relieved by sitting or flexion of the trunk. In severe cases, patients may develop bladder dysfunction from compression of sacral roots. The natural history of lumbar spinal stenosis is favorable in only 50% of patients, regardless of initial or subsequent treatment. Significant deterioration in symptoms with nonsurgical treatment is uncommon. Surgery has been shown to be more effective than nonoperative management in patients with lumbar spinal stenosis, as well as degenerative spondylolisthesis associated with spinal stenosis in short- to medium-term follow-up (2–4 years). At long-term follow-up (8–10 years), low back pain relief, predominant symptom improvement, and satisfaction with the current state were similar in patients initially treated surgically or nonsurgically. However, leg pain relief and greater back-related functional status continued to favor those initially receiving surgical care.

29. Outline a treatment plan for a patient with lumbar stenosis.

- Lumbar flexion exercise program (Williams exercises)
- Bicycling
- Uphill treadmill walking
- Modalities (heat, cold, electrotherapy)
- NSAIDs
- Anticonvulsants, antidepressants
- Epidural steroid injections

30. What are flexion exercises (Williams exercises)? When are they appropriate?

Examples of flexion exercises include knee-to-chest exercises (Fig. 14-1), abdominal crunches, and hip flexor stretches. Flexion exercises are commonly prescribed for facet joint pain, lumbar spinal stenosis, spondylolysis, and spondylolisthesis. Flexion exercises increase intradiscal pressure and are contraindicated in the presence of an acute disc herniation. Flexion exercises are also contraindicated in thoracic and lumbar compression fractures and osteoporotic patients.

Flexion exercises have the following goals:
- Open intervertebral foramina and enlarge the spinal canal
- Stretch back extensors
- Strengthen abdominal and gluteal muscles
- Mobilize the lumbosacral junction

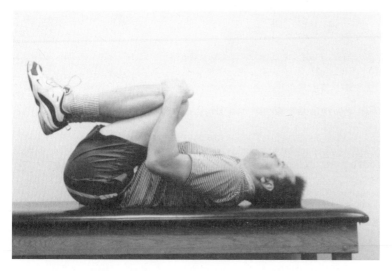

Figure 14-1. Williams exercise: knee to chest.

31. What is the McKenzie exercise approach? How and when is it applied?

McKenzie's method includes both an assessment and intervention component and is commonly referred as a mechanical diagnosis and therapy (MDT). McKenzie's exercise philosophy is based on the finding that certain spinal movements may aggravate pain, whereas other movements relieve pain. McKenzie believed that accumulation of flexion forces caused dysfunction of posterior aspect of the disc. Most of McKenzie's exercises are extension biased. The positions and movement patterns that relieve pain are individually determined for each patient. McKenzie classified lumbar disorders into three syndromes based on posture and response to movement: *postural syndrome, dysfunctional syndrome,* and *derangement syndrome.* Each syndrome has a specific treatment and postural correction. Treatment objectives include identifying the directional preference of lumbosacral movement for an individual patient that induces

centralization of the pain (change in pain location from a distal location in the lower extremity to a proximal or central location). Examples of McKenzie's exercises include:

- Repeat end-range movements while standing: back extension, side gliding (lateral bending with rotation)
- Recumbent end-range movement: passive extension while prone (Fig. 14-2), prone lateral shifting of hips off midline
  McKenzie exercises are most commonly prescribed for disc herniation and lumbar radicular pain.

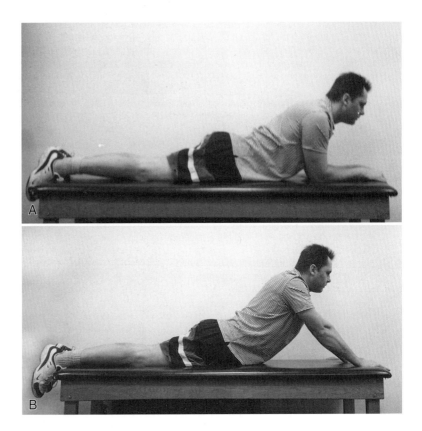

Figure 14-2. McKenzie exercise: passive extension while prone.

32. What are spinal stabilization exercises? When are they used?

Strengthening exercises for a dynamic *corset* of muscle control to maintain a neutral position are known as spinal stabilization exercises. Recently, there has been a special focus on the role of the transversus abdominis and lumbar multifidi muscles in enhancing spinal stability. The goal of stabilization exercises is to reduce mechanical stress on the spine. Spinal stabilization exercises can be prescribed for most causes of low back pain. Key concepts of spinal stabilization exercise program include:

- Determination of the functional range (the most stable and asymptomatic position) for all movements
- Strengthening of transversus abdominis, abdominal obliques (oblique crunches), rectus abdominis (sagittal plane crunches, supine pelvic bracing with alternating arm and leg raises), gluteus maximus (prone gluteal squeezes, supine pelvic bridging, bridging and marching [Fig. 14-3]), and gluteus medius (sidestepping)
- Neuromuscular reeducation, mobility, and endurance exercises
- Progression of therapy from gross and simple movements to smaller, isolated, and complex movements
- Progression to dynamic stabilization exercises (quadriped opposite upper and lower extremity extension [Fig. 14-4], quadriped hip extension and contralateral arm flexion, prone hip extension and contralateral arm flexion, balancing on a gymnastic ball, wall slides, squatting, lifting)

33. What is the role of cardiovascular conditioning in low back pain?

Cardiovascular deconditioning develops secondary to inactivity in patients with chronic low back pain. Aerobic training to improve cardiovascular endurance is an extremely important part of rehabilitation of the low back. Heart-rate limitations for patients with known or suspected cardiac disease are based on stress testing. Aerobic training (i.e. treadmill, bike, stepper, arm and leg ergometer, walking, jogging, swimming) has multiple beneficial effects:

- Increases maximal oxygen consumption (VO_2 max)
- Increases cardiac output
- Increases oxygen extraction

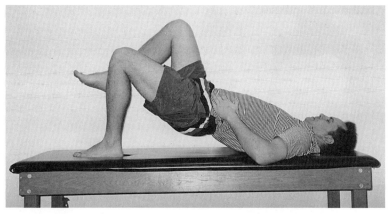

Figure 14-3. Lumbar stabilization exercise: bridging and marching.

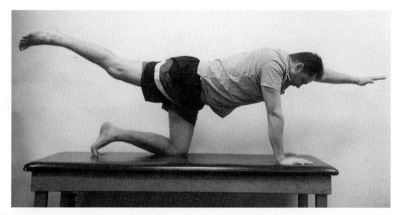

Figure 14-4. Lumbar stabilization exercise: quadruped opposite upper and lower extremity extension.

- Improves oxygen utilization by muscle
- Increases endurance, strength, and coordination of neuromuscular system
- Increases pain threshold (elevates endorphin levels)
- Decreases depression and anxiety
- Promotes healthy lifestyle
- May prevent work-related back injury
- Favorably modifies risk factors for coronary artery disease

34. Define impairment, disability, and handicap.
- **Impairment** is defined as a loss or abnormality of psychological, physical, or anatomic structure or function as determined by medical means. Assessment of impairment is a purely medical determination of deviation from normal health (i.e. weakness of a limb secondary to cervical myelopathy)
- **Disability** is a restriction or inability (resulting from impairment) to perform an activity (i.e. difficulty walking secondary to limb weakness)
- **Handicap** is an inability (resulting from impairment and disability) for a given individual to perform his or her usual interaction with the environment on an appropriate physical, psychological, social, and age level (e.g. inability to climb stairs secondary to limb weakness). A handicap may be overcome by compensating in some way for the impairment (i.e. use of an orthosis or assistive device)

35. How is spinal impairment evaluated?
The practitioner can evaluate spinal impairment by quantifying spinal range of motion, assessing trunk strength and endurance, evaluating balance and motor control, and determining aerobic fitness. Techniques for measuring spinal range of motion include inclinometer, goniometer, modified Schober test, and finger-to-floor distance. There are three basic approaches for testing trunk extensor strength and lifting capacity: isometric (velocity is zero), isokinetic (velocity is constant), and isoinertial (velocity is not constant, but the mass is held constant). Several high-tech machines can be used for testing and training patients (Med X, Cybex, Biodex, Isostation, LIDO, Kin-Com). One can also evaluate the

trunk strength and endurance with standardized tests (i.e. squat endurance test, trunk flexor endurance test, static trunk extensor endurance test) and compare the results with normative databases.

Specific spinal impairment may or may not be related to patient's symptoms or functional abilities. For example, there is weak or nonexisting correlation between spinal range of motion and functional ability. However, decreased trunk extensor endurance correlates with back pain recurrence, chronicity, and first-time episodes of lower back pain symptoms.

36. What is the normal trunk extensor strength?
Approximately 110% to 120% of ideal body weight (IBW) for males and 80% to 95% IBW for females.

37. What deficits in trunk strength are found in patients with chronic low back pain?
The normal average back extensor-to-flexor strength ratio varies from 1.2 to 3.0 (extensors are stronger than flexors). Patients with chronic low back pain have reduced ratio of trunk extensor-to-flexor strength. There is approximately a 50% reduction in isometric extension strength in patients with chronic low back pain compared with asymptomatic individuals.

38. What impairment in trunk strength is noted after lumbar discectomy? After lumbar fusion?
Postfusion patients typically have a greater deficit in trunk extensor strength than postdiscectomy patients. This weakness is secondary to the atrophy and denervation of the multifidi, iliocostalis, and longissimus muscles that result from disuse, as well as injury to the posterior primary rami during posterior fusion surgery. Greater surgical exposure is necessary for fusion compared with discectomy, resulting in greater impairment of trunk extensor strength.

39. What is lifting capacity?
Lifting capacity assesses the spinal functional unit (extensor unit/lumbar paraspinals, gluteals, and hamstrings) and its interaction with the body's other functional units in performance of activities of daily living. Patients with chronic low back pain have a 30% to 50% reduction in lifting capacity. Normal lifting capacity from floor to waist (lumbar lift) is approximately 50% of IBW for men and 35% of IBW for women. Normal lifting capacity from waist to shoulder (cervical lift) is 40% of IBW for men and 25% of IBW for women.

The lifting capacity test is a part of a functional capacity evaluation (FCE). Standardized protocols (i.e. Matheson Functional Capacity Evaluation, EPIC Lift Capacity Test, California Functional Capacity Protocol) are used to evaluate the effect of the spinal impairment for person's ability to perform work tasks.

Key Points

1. The rehabilitation medicine approach to spinal disorders includes a comprehensive assessment of the patient's physical status (strength, flexibility, endurance), psychological status (depression, anxiety), and functional status (ability to perform activities of daily living).
2. Identification and resolution of psychosocial barriers to recovery is critical for successful treatment of chronic spinal pain syndromes.
3. A multidisciplinary team approach (physiatrist, physical therapist, occupational therapist, and psychologist) offers the highest chance for achieving maximum functional improvement in patients with chronic back pain.

Websites

Exercise options for various spine disorders:
http://www.spine-health.com/wellness/exercise
Gateway to Spine Patient Outcomes Research Trial (SPORT) presenting evidence for surgical vs. non-surgical treatment for lumbar disc herniation, spinal stenosis, and degenerative spondylolisthesis: http://www.dartmouth.edu/sport-trial/publications.htm
Rehabilitation: http://www.nlm.nih.gov/medlineplus/rehabilitation.html
Video demonstrations of exercise programs for the spine:
http://www.back.com/articles-exercises.html

BIBLIOGRAPHY

1. Atlas SJ, Keller RB, Wu YA, et al. Long-term outcomes of surgical and nonsurgical management of sciatica secondary to a lumbar disc herniation: 10 year results from the Maine lumbar spine study. Spine 2005;30(8):927–35.
2. DePalma MJ, Slipman CW. Evidence-informed management of chronic low back pain with epidural steroid injections. Spine J 2008;8(1):45–7.
3. Fast A, Thomas MA. Cervical myelopathy. Cervical degenerative disease. In: Frontera WR, Silver JK, editors. Essentials of Physical Medicine and Rehabilitation. Philadelphia: Hanley & Belfus; 2002. p. 3–9, 12–17.
4. Kaelin DL. Thoracic radiculopathy. In: Frontera WR, Silver JK, editors. Essentials of Physical Medicine and Rehabilitation. 1st ed. Philadelphia: Hanley & Belfus; 2002. p. 224–7.
5. Liebenson C, Yeomans S. Quantification of physical performance ability. In: Liebenson C, editor. Rehabilitation of the Spine: A Practitioner's Manual. 2nd ed. Philadelphia, Lippincott, Williams & Wilkins; 2006. p. 226–59.
6. Malanga G, Wolff E. Evidence-informed management of chronic lower back pain with trigger point injections. Spine J 2008;8(1):243–5.
7. Overton EA, Kornbluth ID, Saulino MF, et al. Interventions in chronic pain management. 6. Interventional approaches to chronic pain management. Arch Phys Med Rehabil 2008;89(3 Suppl 1):S61–4.
8. Rinke RC, McCarthy TB. Spinal exercise programs. In: Placzek JD, Boyce DA, editors. Orthopaedic Physical Therapy Secrets. Philadelphia: Hanley & Belfus; 2001. p. 211–15.
9. Standaert CJ, Weinstein SM, Rumpeltes J. Evidence-informed management of chronic low back pain with lumbar stabilization exercises. Spine J 2008;8(1):114–115.
10. Weinstein JN, Lurie JD, Tosteson TD, et al. Surgical compared with nonoperative treatment for lumbar degenerative spondylolisthesis. J Bone Joint Surg Am 2009;91:1295–1304.

15 CHAPTER

PHARMACOLOGIC MANAGEMENT OF CHRONIC SPINAL PAIN

Jerome Schofferman, MD

1. Why is pain management a necessary component in the treatment of spinal disorders?

Despite excellent nonoperative and/or operative care, some patients do not get better. If a surgeon operates on a patient, but the patient does not get better, it remains that surgeon's responsibility to care for the patient or refer the patient for pain management. It is neither responsible nor ethical to abandon the patient. Other patients with spine pain are not candidates for surgery. They too must be treated, and pain management is most likely to help.

2. What are the components of pain management for the patient with a painful spinal disorder?

There is a wide spectrum of treatment options to manage pain, ranging from spinal manipulation to reconstructive surgery. Many patients require a combination of treatments to achieve the best outcome. The preferred treatments will depend on the best medical evidence, clinical expertise of the physician, and the individual patient's values and circumstances. The most common treatments provided include rehabilitation, medications, minimally invasive interventions such as injections or spinal cord stimulation, and surgery. Any or all of these treatments might be accompanied by psychotherapy.

3. What psychological factors are important in the management of chronic pain?

Several psychological systems are potentially at work in the patient with chronic spinal pain. These include the traditional Diagnostic and Statistical Manual of Mental Disorders-IV (DSM-IV) categories, cognitive-behavioral factors, and character traits. In one functional restoration program, 59% of patients with chronic back pain had active psychopathology, which included major depression in 45%, substance abuse disorder in 19%, and anxiety disorder in 17%. Although there were psychological illnesses present before the spinal pain began, most of the disorders developed after the spinal injury. Cognitive-behavioral factors commonly observed include fear, fear-avoidant behavior, and poor coping abilities.

4. What is the definition of pain?

Pain is an unpleasant sensory and emotional experience associated with actual or potential tissue damage or described in terms of such damage. The key points are that pain is unpleasant and always has both sensory (structural) and emotional (psychological) components. In acute pain, the sensory component usually dominates, but there may be anxiety and fear superimposed. In chronic pain, there may be vegetative symptoms and depression in addition to the sensory component.

5. What is acute pain?

Acute pain is pain that has a recent onset. Acute pain usually has a well-defined cause and clear structural etiology. It is expected to follow a familiar natural history and resolve naturally or after appropriate treatment. Acute pain may be accompanied by hyperactivity of the sympathetic nervous system. Acute pain does not imply anything about the level of intensity.

6. What is chronic pain?

Chronic pain is pain that persists well beyond its expected duration. Chronic pain is often associated with significant psychological changes that are usually secondary to the pain and impairment. The hyperactivity of the sympathetic nervous system dissipates and is often replaced by vegetative symptoms such as sleep disturbance, low energy, changes in appetite and weight, decreased libido, and depressed mood.

7. What are some of the types of patients with chronic pain?

There is a spectrum of patients with chronic pain. At the positive end of the spectrum are patients who might be called *adaptive copers* or *persons with chronic pain*. They frequently have identifiable nociceptive or neuropathic stimuli. The psychological changes, when present, are generally consistent with and secondary to the levels of pain and impairment. Patients function at a reasonable level despite their pain. They are compliant with treatment, follow instructions, and tend to respond to medications and other treatments as would be expected.

On the other end of the spectrum are those patients who are dysfunctional and might be called *chronic pain patients.* Their pain seems out of proportion to any identifiable stimulus. They have psychological and behavioral changes that interfere with their lives. They function at a level far lower than would be expected. They may be noncompliant with treatment recommendations, miss appointments, fail to follow directions, and respond poorly to medications and other treatments. They are often a struggle to manage and at times are labeled as *difficult patients.*

8. What are the types of chronic spine pain?

Chronic spine pain can be subdivided into *nociceptive* and *neuropathic types.* **Nociceptive pain** is due to a structural disorder that stimulates small nerve endings (nociceptors). An example is a patient with one or more painful degenerated discs.

Neuropathic pain is due to permanent nerve damage or physiologic change to the peripheral or central nervous system. The nerve is the source of the pain even though it is no longer being stimulated. Neuropathic nerves may have a lowered threshold for firing because they have become sensitized, either peripherally or centrally. As a result, there may be severe pain despite minimal or even no stimulus. Examples include a damaged nerve root due to prolonged neural compression from disc herniation or foraminal stenosis, arachnoiditis, or complex regional pain syndrome (formerly called *reflex sympathetic dystrophy*). Some patients may have both nociceptive and neuropathic pain, a *mixed pain syndrome.*

Neurogenic pain is a confusing term, which is often used to describe pain resulting from direct nerve root compression (e.g. lateral disc herniation or foraminal stenosis). This is considered a variant of nociceptive pain as the nerve root itself contains nociceptive fibers.

9. Why is it important to distinguish nociceptive pain from neuropathic pain?

The distinction is clinically important because some medications are more effective for one type of pain than the other.

10. What are the best drugs for treatment of nociceptive pain?

The best drugs for mild to moderate nociceptive pain are analgesics. These include nonsteroidal antiinflammatory drugs (NSAIDs) and the weak opioids. The best drugs for moderate to severe nociceptive pain are the strong opioids.

11. What are the best drugs for treatment of neuropathic pain?

The drugs of choice for neuropathic pain are anticonvulsants and noradrenergic antidepressants. In addition, some patients will respond to opioids, but higher doses may be needed.

12. What are the classes of analgesics?

These analgesics are sometimes classified as peripherally acting (e.g. NSAIDS) or centrally acting medications (e.g. opioids). Each may have a role in the treatment of chronic spine pain.

13. What are the different types of peripherally acting analgesics?

The peripherally acting analgesics are acetaminophen and the NSAIDs, including aspirin. They are useful for mild to moderate pain and may also act synergistically with centrally acting analgesics. The NSAIDs have two mechanisms to relieve pain, an antiinflammatory effect and a pure analgesic action. Empiric support for this includes the fact that analgesia can begin in less than an hour, long before any antiinflammatory activity could occur, and NSAIDs may relieve pain even when there is no inflammation.

14. What is a good way to select from among the many NSAIDs?

NSAIDs may be classified as nonselective or traditional NSAIDS (e.g. ibuprofen, naproxen) and selective NSAIDS or COX-2 inhibitors (e.g. celecoxib). Traditional NSAIDs act as nonselective inhibitors of the enzyme cyclooxygenase and inhibit both cyclooxygenase-1 (COX-1) and cyclooxygenase-2 (COX-2). Selective NSAIDs were developed in an attempt to provide antiinflammatory action without the gastrointestinal adverse drug reactions attributed to inhibition of COX-1. Additional complications subsequently attributed to these medications include cardiac and renal problems.

Selection of NSAID therapy must take into account patient factors including:
1. Cardiovascular risk
2. Gastrointestinal risk

COX-2 selective inhibitors reduce the risk of NSAID-related ulcers and complications by half when compared with traditional NSAIDs. However, a similar risk profile can be achieved by using a proton pump inhibitor (e.g. Omeprazole 20 mg daily) with a traditional NSAID. The use of aspirin, in combination with an NSAID, is a risk factor for adverse gastrointestinal events. The combination of ibuprofen and aspirin is best avoided.

15. What are some important centrally acting analgesics?

The most important centrally acting analgesics are the opioids. Opioids produce analgesia primarily by binding with opiate receptors in the central nervous system. They work best for nociceptive pain but are somewhat effective for neuropathic pain.

16. What concerns discourage doctors from prescribing opioids?

The major concerns that have discouraged some physicians from using opioids for long-term treatment are:
- Fear of producing addiction and dependence
- Fear of causing organ toxicity
- Fear of disciplinary action by medical licensing boards
- Fear that tolerance will develop requiring progressively increasing doses and eventual lack of effectiveness
- Concerns that opioids are not effective

17. Should physicians who prescribe opioids fear disciplinary action?

No. It is appropriate medical practice to prescribe long-term opioids for chronic pain. Physicians who prescribe opioids for appropriate clinical indications are acting well within the scope of good medical practice. Doctors treating pain and who maintain adequate medical records, perform regular good faith follow-ups, and select patients appropriately are acting well within the scope of practice.

18. What is addiction?

Addiction is a neurobiologic illness with psychological and social components as well. It is the compulsive use of a psychoactive substance resulting in and despite biologic, psychological, or social harm. It is characterized by loss of control. The prevalence of addictive disease in the chronic pain population is about 6% higher than in the general population.

19. What is dependence?

Dependence is a physiological state induced by chronic use of a psychoactive substance (e.g. alcohol or opioids) characterized by an abstinence syndrome upon the abrupt discontinuation of that substance. Dependence must be differentiated from addiction. Virtually all patients on long-term opioids will become dependent, but only a small number will become addicted.

20. What is tolerance?

Tolerance is the progressive lack of efficacy of an analgesic. As a result, it takes more of the analgesic to provide the same response. True tolerance is a biologic phenomenon. However, in some cases of apparent tolerance, the medication is not working as well because the disease has progressed or the activity level has increased, either of which produces relative lack of effectiveness, but not true tolerance. The treatment for this *pseudo-tolerance* is raising the dose or treating the new pathology. In some instances, rotating to another opioid can be helpful.

21. Is tolerance a limiting factor in the long-term use of opioids?

Tolerance is usually not a limiting factor. The experience with the use of long-term opioid analgesics in cancer patients who survive for years has been that tolerance is not a clinical problem. In spine pain, when opioid needs escalate, it is usually because function has increased or there has been progression of the structural disorder, not tolerance.

22. Do opioids produce addiction?

The prevalence of addiction in patients treated with opioids for pain is low. Although opioids may activate an underlying addictive disease, they do not cause it.

23. Are opioids misused by patients?

There are some patients who misuse opioids. Several *patterns of misuse* have emerged. Perhaps the most serious is *drug diversion*, obtaining prescription opioids and subsequently selling them. Another serious problem is the *use of illegal drugs*, such as cocaine or methamphetamine in addition to the opioids. *Unsanctioned dose escalation* is common and can be due to tolerance, poor pain control, or using opioids to treat psychological or other symptoms. Additional *aberrant behaviors* include seeking prescriptions from multiple physicians and forging prescriptions. However, most patients use their medications appropriately.

24. Can opioid misuses be predicted?

Not with any certainty. Although several risk factors have been identified, none have been universally predictive. Factors that should raise a clinician's awareness include past history of illicit drug or alcohol abuse, history of significant psychiatric disorder, and history of legal problems such as driving under the influence.

25. What are some of the warning signs that opioids are being abused?

Certain actions have been identified as being highly suggestive of addictive behavior. They include selling prescription drugs, forging prescriptions, repeatedly borrowing drugs from friends or family, concurrent use of large amounts of alcohol, use of any illicit street drugs, the "loss" of prescriptions or pills, seeking prescriptions from other doctors including emergency department personnel, and frequent missed appointments. Other signs that may raise the suspicion of drug abuse include frequent complaints that the dose is too low, requests for specific drugs, unsanctioned dose escalations, or use of the drug to treat other symptoms. However, some of these behaviors may be due to inadequate pain control, sometimes called *pseudoaddiction*. Despite the best screening, some patients will abuse or misuse opioid analgesics. If abuse or misuse is suspected, the patient should be referred for consultation to a specialist in addiction medicine.

26. Can urine toxicology screening help?

Perhaps, especially in higher risk populations. There is a legitimate argument among pain specialists regarding the role of urine toxicology screening. A so-called *dirty urine* includes the presence of illegal substances such as cocaine and alcohol. A urine sample that does not show the prescribed drug to be present suggests diversion.

27. Are opioids effective for chronic spine pain?

In the past, physicians felt these drugs were ineffective for long-term treatment and the risks were too great, but these opinions were anecdotal and not based on medical evidence. The evidence published over the past decade is quite convincing that long-term opioid therapy can be safe and effective for many well-selected patients with low back pain. Most studies are longitudinal observational studies, but there have now been several randomized placebo-controlled studies in patients with chronic low back pain. In general, opioids seem to reduce pain by at least 50% with acceptable adverse effects. It is necessary to find the best opioid for each patient, and there appears to be a genetic preference. Efficacy has been well maintained, but there are no studies that have reported more than 1-year follow-up.

28. Do opioids cause organ toxicity?

Opioids are not toxic to the liver, kidneys, brain, or other organs. Respiratory depression is rare with oral opioids except in persons with significant pulmonary disease, sleep apnea syndrome, or other serious medical conditions. No evidence of serious organ toxicity has been reported. However, it is not uncommon to see some degree of suppression of testosterone in men and women. This should be watched for and testosterone supplementation administered if levels are suppressed.

29. Which opioid is best for chronic pain?

No single opioid has proven superior to others. About 15% of patients are not able to tolerate long-term opioids due to side effects. Of the patients who can tolerate long-term opioids, about 75% experience meaningful pain relief. Most but not all patients also experience some increase in function. In patients who have been chronically disabled, few return to work. However, in patients who have not been off work at all or have been off for short periods, a meaningful number can return or stay at work.

30. Are side effects common with opioids?

Side effects are common but can usually be managed with adjunctive medications.

31. What are some of the side effects of opioids?

Most patients taking opioids experience side effects. The type and intensity of side effects vary greatly. The most common are somnolence and diminished mental acuity. Interestingly, severe pain can itself cause alteration of cognitive abilities and, when opioids relieve pain, cognitive abilities actually improve. Sedation is common, particularly at initiation of treatment or when medication doses are raised, but it usually improves with time. If the opioid is effective, but there is excess sedation, methylphenidate (Ritalin) or modafinil (Provigil) can be of value.

Nausea is common, especially at initiation of therapy, and usually responds to treatment with antiemetics. Constipation occurs in most patients, and prophylaxis is important, using dioctyl sodium sulfate (DSS) plus Senokot, two to four tablets at night. For more resistant constipation, polyethylene glycol (MiraLax) is often useful. Other side effects include itching (which is not an allergic reaction), sweating, and dry mouth. There may be sexual dysfunction due to opioid-induced lowered testosterone, which is treated by the use of a testosterone patch or gel.

32. What recommendations exist to help with safe and effective use of opioids?

Recommendations for safe and effective use of opioids include:
- A careful evaluation of the patient prior to initiation of therapy
- A written treatment plan stating the goals of therapy
- Informed consent (verbal or written, documented in the medical record)
- Regular follow-up visits with periodic review to evaluate effectiveness of pain control, level of function, side effects, and mood, and to document inquiry regarding aberrant opioid-related behavior
- Consultation with appropriate specialists (e.g. addiction medicine) when necessary
- Maintenance of detailed and appropriate treatment records

33. When is the use of long-term opioids considered appropriate in the management of spinal disorders?

Long-term opioids are appropriate for spine patients with a well-defined structural stimulus that cannot be definitively treated. The pain level should be consistent with the structural disorder present in the spinal column. Aggressive rehabilitation and other appropriate interventions should be pursued, and their failure to relieve pain should be documented. There should be no significant psychological illness or history of addiction or drug abuse. Opioids should not be used to treat nonspecific back or neck pain.

34. What are the two major ways to prescribe opioids?

There are two ways to prescribe analgesics: pain-contingent and time-contingent dosing.
- **Pain-contingent** means taking the analgesic when pain occurs

- **Time-contingent** means taking the analgesic on a regular schedule based on the analgesic half-life of the drug. There is usually better analgesia and fewer side effects with time contingent dosing, which avoids large swings in blood or brain levels. Time-contingent dosing is almost always preferable for chronic pain with rescue doses available for breakthrough pain

35. Are short-acting opioids indicated for long-term use?

The short-acting opioids, such as codeine, hydrocodone (e.g. Vicodin, Norco), or oxycodone (e.g. Roxicodone, Percocet) are not usually used for long-term therapy because there will be wide swings in the blood levels, which leads to poor pain control and more side effects. Toxicity (liver or gastrointestinal) may occur with the use of short-acting opioids formulations containing other pain reducing medications (aspirin, acetaminophen, or ibuprofen). In those rare patients who do better with a short-acting opioid, they should be prescribed in a time-contingent manner. It is best to use a continuous release or long-acting opioid for long-term opioid analgesic therapy, although short-acting opioids should be available for breakthrough pain.

36. Which opioids are available for long-term use?

There are currently six opioids suitable for long-term use: morphine, oxycodone, fentanyl, oxymorphone, methadone, and levorphanol. The synthetic opiate agonist tramadol is an additional therapeutic option. Addiction medicine specialists may also use buprenorphine and butorphanol. There is no best opioid. Patients respond preferentially to some opioids, but not to others, which may make it necessary to try several different ones before finding the best drug for that patient (Table 15-1).

- **Continuous-release morphine** is reasonably easy to use and effective. The opioid is released continuously from the tablet and slowly absorbed from the gut with little accumulation in body tissues. There is effective analgesia for 8 to 12 hours, and the dosing interval is adjusted according to the patient's response. Continuous-release opioids are available in many dose sizes, which makes dose titration convenient. The dose can be titrated upwards once or twice weekly until there is good pain control or significant side effects
- **Oxycontin** is a time-release formula of the analgesic oxycodone and is an alternative to oral morphine
- **Transdermal fentanyl (Duramorph)** is also effective, but there is less dosing flexibility, and some people have difficulty keeping the patches in place
- **Oxymorphone** is available as an extended-release and immediate-release formulation. There are several prospective randomized controlled studies for chronic low back pain that have demonstrated efficacy and tolerable adverse effects
- **Methadone** provides excellent analgesia and is inexpensive, but it is somewhat more difficult to use. This lipophilic drug is well-absorbed from the gut and is then distributed in body fat, taking about 5 to 7 days to reach a steady state. Therefore, the dose should only be adjusted once per week. Once a steady state is reached, there can be 8 to 12 hours of pain relief
- **Levorphanol (Levo-Dromoran)** is a long-acting opioid that is also quite effective, but, several times in the past few years, the manufacturer was not able to produce sufficient quantities. Therefore, it cannot be recommended at this time

37. Is meperidine (Demerol) ever useful for long-term treatment?

Meperidine should rarely, if ever, be used long-term because it is poorly absorbed, provides unreliable analgesia, and may be associated with an unacceptably high level of toxic neurologic side effects.

Table 15-1. Opioid analgesics most useful for chronic pain

CHEMICAL NAME	BRAND NAMES	DURATION OF ANALGESIA (HOURS)	COMMENTS
Morphine	MS-Contin Oramorph Kadian Avinza	8-12 8 12 24	Multiple dose sizes; convenient
Oxycodone	Oxycontin	8-12	Multiple dose sizes; convenient; expensive
Methadone	Dolophine	8-12	Very inexpensive
Fentanyl	Duramorph	48-72	Transdermal
Oxymorphone	Opana-ER	12	Several RCT for LBP*
Levorphanol	Levo-dromoran	6	Only 2-mg dose size; inconvenient
Tramadol	Ultram Ultracet	6 (IR) to 24 (ER)*	Very good data Less potent

ER, extended release; IR, immediate release; RCT, randomized controlled trial.

38. Is there a best dose of an opioid?

The dose and dosing interval is adjusted based on the degree and duration of pain relief and functional improvement balanced against side effects. There is no best or correct dose.

39. When are antidepressants useful for patients with spine problems?

Antidepressants have several potential uses in patients with chronic spinal problems, including the treatment of back pain, neuropathic pain, sleep disturbance, and depression. Only the antidepressants with primarily nonadrenergic activity are useful for pain. The data regarding efficacy of antidepressants for axial pain are equivocal. At best, isolated studies show about 30% reduction in pain in one third of patients. In addition, recent data suggest these drugs are not very effective for radicular pain caused by ongoing neural compression. However, they may be quite effective for neuropathic extremity pain. The sedating antidepressants can be effective for sleep but have not been compared with standard hypnotics. They may have more side effects and greater risk. Most antidepressants can be effective for depression in the patient with chronic spinal pain, but it may take two or three trials before finding the best drug.

40. Are antidepressants useful in patients with pain who are not depressed?

Antidepressants can be effective in patients with no evidence of depression. The analgesic effect, if it occurs, is seen at lower doses than the antidepressant effect. The view that antidepressants improve pain through the treatment of a *masked* depression is no longer held.

41. How do we choose the best antidepressant for patients with spine problems?

The choice of antidepressant depends on the target symptoms: pain, depression, or sleep disturbance.
- Nortriptyline (Pamelor), desipramine (Norpramin), amitriptyline (Elavil), and duloxetine (Cymbalta) are the antidepressants most effective for pain
- Fluoxetine (Prozac), sertraline (Zoloft), paroxetine (Paxil), citalopram (Celexa), and many others are selective serotonin reuptake inhibitors (SSRIs) that may be useful for depression, but not for pain
- Citalopram has fewer drug interactions, and so it may be preferred for patients taking multiple other medications (Table 15-2)

Table 15-2. Antidepressant considerations for patients with chronic pain

GENERIC	BRAND NAME	VALUE FOR PAIN	VALUE FOR DEPRESSION	VALUE FOR SLEEP
Nortriptyline	Pamelor	High	Medium	Medium
Amitriptyline	Elavil	High	Medium	High
Desipramine	Norpramin	High	Medium	Low
Trazodone	Desyrel	Low	Low	High
Fluoxetine	Prozac	Low	High	Poor
Sertraline	Zoloft	Low	High	Poor
Paroxetine	Paxil	Low	High	Low
Citalopram	Celexa	Low	High	Low
Doxepin	Sinequan	Low	Medium	High
Bupropion	Wellbutrin	Low	Medium	Poor
Venlafaxine	Effexor	Low	High	High

42. What are the usual doses for antidepressants?

The initial dose of nortriptyline, desipramine, or amitriptyline is 10 mg at night, which is then increased every 5 days or so in 10-mg increments to 50 mg. After 50 mg, the dose may be increased in 25-mg increments to a target of 75 to 100 mg. Fluoxetine is started at 20 mg each morning, sertraline at 50 mg, paroxetine at 20 mg, and citalopram at 20 mg. Duloxetine is started at 20 mg daily for a week. Dosage is then increased to 30 mg and eventually 60 mg daily. Nausea may limit rapid escalation. Higher doses of all these drugs may best be left to other specialists.

43. What are some of the side effects of the tricyclic antidepressants (TCAs)?

The TCAs are sedating, so they are usually given at night to help sleep. In some patients, there may be excess daytime sedation. Other side effects include dry mouth, urinary retention, constipation, weight gain, blurry vision, and orthostatic hypotension. Usually side effects are mild and decrease with continued use. In contrast, the SSRIs may cause irritability and sexual dysfunction.

44. What other drugs may be useful for neuropathic pain?

Anticonvulsants have become the first line of medications for neuropathic pain. There are occasional reports of effectiveness for axial pain as well, but this is not predictable.

45. Which anticonvulsant is most commonly used for neuropathic pain?

Gabapentin (Neurontin) is currently used most often, although its use for pain is off-label. It may be useful for neuropathic extremity pain due to iatrogenic nerve injury, arachnoiditis, prolonged neural compression, and peripheral neuropathy. It has been shown to be useful in some patients with leg pain due to spinal stenosis. Gabapentin is started at 100 to 300 mg at night and then increased to 300 mg every 8 hours over the days to weeks, and then gradually titrated upward until there is good pain relief or significant side effects. Pain relief may occur at 900 mg per day, but often 1800 mg to 3600 mg per day are necessary. Side effects include dizziness, somnolence, ataxia, and headaches, but these are usually seen at the higher dose levels.

46. What other anticonvulsants have been used for treatment of neuropathic pain?

- Topiramate (Topamax) has been utilized in select patients with radicular pain and axial pain. It is started at 25 mg at night and the dose is increased weekly in 25-mg increments
- Pregabalin (Lyrica) has also been used for neuropathic pain. It is started at 75 mg twice per day
- Clonazepam (Klonopin), a benzodiazepine, is used occasionally for neuropathic pain. It is also effective in reducing myoclonic jerks, a potential side effect of opioids. It is started at 0.5 mg at night and increased in 0.5-mg increments as necessary to a maximum dose of 2 to 4 mg per day in three divided doses

47. What is the role of muscle relaxants in chronic low back pain?

Their role is limited for treatment of chronic back. Muscle relaxants may play a temporary role in the treatment of exacerbations of chronic low back pain. Limited use for 7 to 10 days can be considered. Chronic use should generally be avoided. These medications can be sedating and may cause dependence. There is little evidence that these drugs specifically relax tight muscles. Most of their effects appear to be central rather than peripheral.

48. Which muscle relaxants might be helpful for short-term use?

Cyclobenzaprine (Flexeril) is chemically similar to amitriptyline and may be useful for patients who have a sleep disturbance and decline antidepressants. The dose is 10 mg at night. Baclofen can be effective for the relief of painful spasms, although its effect is in the central nervous system rather than on the muscles. It is started at 10 mg at night and then gradually titrated up to 10 mg every 6 hours. Some other muscle relaxants are orphenadrine (Norflex), carisoprodol (Soma), methocarbamol (Robaxin), metaxalone (Skelaxin), and tizanidine (Zanaflex). There is no good evidence to choose one over another. Diazepam (Valium) is too sedating to use regularly, but lorazepam (Ativan) is occasionally effective for *spasms.*

49. Are sedatives-hypnotics ever indicated in chronic low back pain?

The role of sedative-hypnotics in chronic spine pain is controversial. Adequate restorative sleep is very important for patients with chronic spine pain. Many spine patients have sleep difficulties. The two hypnotics used most often are zolpidem (Ambien) and eszopicine (Lunesta). Limited data suggest zolpidem is somewhat more effective but also has more adverse effects, the most serious of which include sleep walking, talking, and eating, as well as some memory loss. The most serious adverse effects of eszopicine include a very bad taste in the mouth and feelings of anxiety. However, both drugs are generally preferred over the benzodiazepines, such as clonazepam or temazepam (Restoril). Long-acting drugs, such as diazepam or flurazepam (Dalmane), may accumulate with chronic use and produce cognitive impairment and depression, and there may be rebound insomnia when the drugs are discontinued.

50. What is the role of antihistamines for patients with spinal pain?

Antihistamines can help control opioid-induced nausea, vomiting, and itching, but they do not enhance opioid analgesia. Hydroxyzine (Vistaril) and promethazine (Phenergan) are effective for nausea, and both hydroxyzine and cetirizine (Zyrtec) work somewhat for itching. Diphenhydramine (Benadryl) can also be used but is more sedating. Antihistamines should not be used for sleep.

51. What is the role of topical analgesics?

Topical analgesics are applied directly over a painful site. Analgesic activity is limited to the peripheral soft tissues. Common analgesics utilized include:

- **Capsaicin**, the active component of chili peppers, is a topical analgesic cream that depletes substance P in small nociceptors. It may provide pain relief in patients with peripheral neuropathy, arthritis of small joints, and occasionally complex regional pain syndrome
- **Lidoderm 5% patch** is another topical treatment. The patch is applied over small areas of neuropathic pain. Anecdotally, some patients with focal nociceptive pain also respond. The patches are worn for 12 hours and then taken off for 12 hours, but the analgesia is sustained. It is FDA approved for the treatment of postherpetic neuralgia

Key Points

1 It is important to differentiate nociceptive pain from neuropathic pain because certain medications are more effective for one type of pain than another.
2 Analgesics are the most effective medications for nociceptive pain and include peripherally acting analgesics (e.g. acetaminophen, aspirin, NSAIDs) or centrally acting analgesics (e.g. opioids).
3 The drugs of choice for neuropathic pain are anticonvulsants and noradrenergic antidepressants.
4 Muscle relaxants are a class of medications that do not specifically relax tight muscles but instead exert a therapeutic effect through sedation and central depression of neuronal transmission.
5 NSAIDs are extensively prescribed for spinal pain but have serious potential side effects related to the gastrointestinal tract, renal, and cardiovascular system.

Websites

1. American Pain Society Clinical Practical Guidelines: http://www.ampainsoc.org/pub/cp_guidelines.htm
2. Online educational resources: http://www.stoppain.org/for_professionals/default.asp
3. Pain evaluation and management: http://www.nlm.nih.gov/medlineplus/pain.html
4. Pain management topics: http://www.pain.com/
5. United States Regulations for Controlled Substances: http://www.justice.gov/dea/pubs/abuse/index.htm

BIBLIOGRAPHY

1. Chang V, Gonzalez P, Akuthota V. Evidence-informed management of chronic low back pain with adjunctive analgesics. Spine J 2008;8:21–7.
2. Gallagher R, Welz-Bosna M, Gammaitoni A. Assessment of dosing frequency of sustained release opioid preparations in patients with chronic nonmalignant pain. Pain Medicine 2007;8:71–4.
3. Katz N, Adams E, Benneyan J, et al. Foundations of opioid risk management. Clin J Pain 2007;23:103–18.
4. Malanga G, Wolff E. Evidence-informed management of chronic low back pain with nonsteroidal anti-inflammatory drugs, muscle relaxants and simple analgesics. Spine J 2008;8:173–84.
5. McNicol E, Horowicz-Mehler N, Fisk RA, et al. Management of opioid side effects in cancer-related and chronic non-cancer pain: A systematic review. J Pain 2003;4:231–56.
6. Schofferman J, Mazanec D. Evidence-informed management of chronic low back pain with opioid analgesics. Spine J 2008;8:185–94.
7. Urquhart D, Hoving J, Assendelft W, et al. Antidepressants for non-specific low back pain. Cochrane Database Syst Rev 2008;23:CD001703.
8. Yaksi A, Ozgonenel L, Ozgonenel B. The efficiency of gabapentin therapy in patients with lumbar spinal stenosis. Spine 2007;32:939–42.

DIAGNOSTIC AND THERAPEUTIC SPINAL INJECTIONS

Vincent J. Devlin, MD

1. What specialists perform diagnostic and therapeutic spinal injections?
A diverse community of physicians from many specialties perform spinal injections including anesthesiologists, physiatrists, interventional radiologists, neurologists, and spine surgeons.

2. What is the preferred setting for performing spinal injections?
The preferred setting for both diagnostic and therapeutic spinal injections is the sterile environment of an outpatient/ambulatory surgery suite or hospital operating room. Fluoroscopy is used to improve accuracy, safety, and efficacy of injections. Monitoring, including pulse oximetry, blood pressure, and pulse, should be recorded during the procedure and during the recovery period in case of an adverse reaction to the injected local anesthetic or intravenous sedation. Emergency resuscitating equipment, including crash carts, should be available.

3. What instructions should be given to patients prior to a spine injection procedure?
Patients are instructed to continue with their usual medications except those that affect bleeding. The risk-benefit of discontinuing anticoagulation should be discussed with the patient and prescribing physician. Many practitioners advise that nonspecific nonsteroidal antiinflammatory agents be discontinued 5 to 7 days before the procedure. Aspirin-based products and platelet inhibitors (e.g. Plavix) are discontinued 7 to 10 days prior to injection. Warfarin should be discontinued 5 to 7 days before injection and the international normalized ratio (INR) checked at least 1 day prior to the procedure. When low-molecular-weight heparin is used as an anticoagulant, it should be stopped at least 18 hours prior to the injection. If the injection is to occur in the afternoon, a light breakfast in the morning is recommended. A driver is needed to transport the patient to and from the surgery center, especially if conscious sedation is used during the procedure.

4. What are the pain generators of the spine?
Symptoms of axial and radicular pain may be attributed to pathology involving bone, spinal soft tissues (muscles, ligaments, tendons), intervertebral discs, facet joints, sacroiliac joints, and neurologic structures (spinal cord and nerve roots). The interventional pain physician uses injection techniques in an attempt to identify a specific pain generator responsible for a patient's symptoms and guide subsequent treatment. It may be challenging or impossible to identify a specific pain generator in the setting of diffuse age-related degenerative spinal pathology. Consensus regarding the scientific basis for a single pain generator to explain the morbidity of chronic axial pain does not exist.

Soft tissue sprain or **strain** (muscle, tendon, ligament) is the most common disorder responsible for low back and neck pain. This diagnosis is generally based on clinical assessment without the need for interventional procedures. Frequently, the diagnosis of soft tissue sprain or strain is made by exclusion of more serious pathology and may alternately be described as *nonspecific back pain syndrome*.

Intervertebral disc displacement may impinge on a nerve root, resulting in radicular pain that involves the arm or leg. Evidence also suggests that the disc itself can cause pain in the absence of neural compression. **Discogenic pain** is the term used to describe such pain. Histologic studies demonstrate the presence of nerve endings throughout the outer third of the annulus fibrosus. These nerve endings are branches of the sinuvertebral nerves, the gray rami communicantes, and the lumbar ventral rami. Annular tears may result from injury or degeneration. These fissures in the outer margins of the annulus may lead to pain due to mechanical or chemical irritation.

Facet joints (zygapophyseal joints or *z-joints*) are paired synovial joints in the posterior column of the spine, which are innervated by medial branches of primary dorsal rami. Lumbar facet pathology may result in referred pain involving the buttock, groin, hip, or thigh. Cervical facet joint pathology can manifest as neck pain, referred pain involving the scapular area or headaches.

Sacroiliac joints are a potential pain generator due to the presence of nociceptors in and around these joints. However, clinical diagnosis and appropriate treatment remains controversial.

5. List the basic interventional spine procedures.
Epidural injections, medial branch blocks, facet injections, discography, and sacroiliac joint injections.

6. Is fluoroscopy necessary to perform spinal injections?
For many years, epidural injections were performed without the use of radiographic guidance. Success depended on the operator's experience and the ability of the operator to palpate the landmarks of the spine. Even in the hands of an experienced practitioner, needle placement without radiographic guidance during epidural injection is incorrect in more

than 25% of cases. The use of fluoroscopy to guide the needle into the epidural space has greatly enhanced the accuracy of injections. In addition, injection of a small amount of contrast dye can help avoid inadvertent epidural venous injection or intrathecal injection. The use of fluoroscopy is mandatory to perform procedures such as facet injections, medial branch blocks, and transforaminal epidural injections.

7. What are the different approaches for injections into the epidural space?

Epidural steroid injections have been used to treat low back and radicular pain since the early 1900s. The epidural space is a potential space within the spinal canal and outside the dura mater. A mixture of local anesthetic and corticosteroid is injected into the epidural space via various approaches: interlaminar, transforaminal, or caudal.

The **interlaminar approach** is the most commonly used approach for cervical, thoracic, and lumbar epidural injections (Fig. 16-1). Epidural needles (Crawford or Tuohy type) are directed between the lamina via a midline or paramedian approach. As the needle penetrates the ligamentum flavum, the epidural space is identified by the loss-of-resistance method. Typically 5 to 10 mL of corticosteroid and local anesthetic solution is injected in the lumbar and thoracic spine. In the cervical spine, 3 to 5 mL is injected. The injectate is delivered to the posterior epidural space, and indirect spread to the anterior epidural space is anticipated.

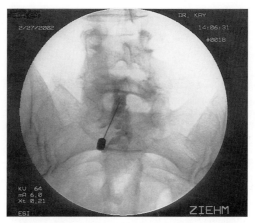

Figure 16-1. Lumbar epidural-interlaminar approach.

The **transforaminal approach** is used to inject the medication directly into the neuroforamen. The injectate is delivered to the anterior epidural space in the region of the targeted pathology (Fig. 16-2). Transforaminal injection should be performed only under fluoroscopic guidance for accuracy and safety. The needle is directed obliquely to a specific target area in the neuroforamen. Because the needle is placed directly at the target nerve root, less volume is required to achieve pain relief. In the lumbar spine, 3 to 5 mL of corticosteroid and local anesthetic solution is injected. In the cervical spine, 1 to 1.5 mL is required to adequately block the target nerve root.

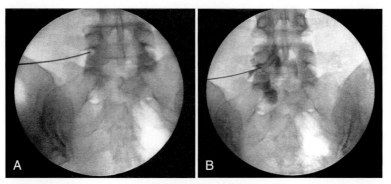

Figure 16-2. A, Lumbar epidural-transforaminal approach. The needle is placed in the left L5 neuroforamen. **B,** Injection of contrast shows epidural dye flow.

The **caudal approach** is the safest approach for injection into the lumbar epidural space and has the least risk of dural puncture. The needle is inserted between the sacral cornu into the sacral hiatus, which leads to the caudal epidural space. The drawback of this approach is the large volume of the injection required to reach the target area in the lumbar spine. Frequently, 10 to 15 mL of corticosteroid and local anesthetic solution is needed to achieve pain relief.

Use of an epidural catheter to deliver the medication to the lumbar spine is helpful in patients with prior history of spine surgery (Fig. 16-3). Various manufacturers offer epidural catheters specifically designed for pain procedures. An introducer needle is placed caudally, and the flexible epidural catheter is advanced cephalad to the target. These catheters can also be steered to the left or right to reach the target area. With the use of a catheter, less volume is necessary to achieve pain relief if the catheter tip is in close proximity to the target area.

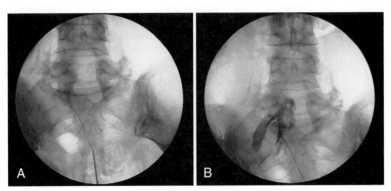

Figure 16-3. A, Lumbar epidural-caudal approach using epidural catheter. Note that the patient had previous decompression and fusion. The catheter tip is in the vicinity of the left L5 neuroforamen. **B,** Injection of contrast showing epidural dye flow and left L5 and S1 radiculogram.

8. What are the indications for epidural injections?

Epidural steroid injections have been shown to be effective in treatment of radicular symptoms due to disc herniation, central spinal stenosis, and neuroforaminal stenosis. Limited evidence supports the role of epidural injections for axial pain. Axial pain subgroups, such as those with annular tears or disc end-plate inflammatory changes, are considered more likely to benefit from epidural steroids than patients with nonspecific axial pain. Limited evidence supports efficacy of injections for ongoing radicular and/or axial pain following prior spine surgery.

Injections are indicated when pain is refractory to less invasive treatments, such as physical therapy and medication. Repeat injections are indicated in patients with partial relief of symptoms after the initial injection. Many practitioners limit the number of epidural injections to three per year to minimize the side effects from repeated corticosteroid injections. Each practitioner is advised to weigh the risks and the benefits before proceeding with each injection.

9. What are the contraindications to epidural steroid injections?

Contraindications for epidural steroid injections include local infection at the injection site, systemic infection, bleeding diathesis, uncontrolled diabetes mellitus, and uncontrolled cardiovascular disease. Injections in the presence of local or systemic infection may spread the infection to other areas of the body, including the epidural space. There is a risk of epidural hematoma in patients with bleeding diathesis. Blood glucose may be even more difficult to control after epidural steroid injections in patients with uncontrolled diabetes mellitus. Patients with congestive heart failure, hypertension, or cardiac disease may experience worsening of their condition after corticosteroid injection because of its effects on fluid and electrolyte balance.

10. What are some possible complications associated with epidural injections?

- **Vasovagal reaction**
- **Allergic reaction** to injected medications or topical antiseptic
- **Infection:** Superficial infection or deep infection (epidural abscess) may occur. Adrenal suppression by corticosteroids may unmask systemic infection
- **Bleeding:** Hematoma may develop in superficial tissue sites or in the epidural space
- **Dural puncture and subarachnoid injection:** Spinal headache may occur due to spinal fluid leak secondary to inadvertent dural puncture. Frequently, the dural puncture site seals by itself with bedrest. Epidural blood patch is the treatment for persistent spinal headache. Injection of medication intended for the epidural space into the subarachnoid space may lead to respiratory depression, arachnoiditis, and pain
- **Intravascular injection:** May lead to spinal cord infarction or anesthetic toxicity (seizures, cardiac arrest, death). The advantage of the transforaminal approach due to its delivery of the injectate to the anterior epidural space must be weighed against the potential risk of spinal cord or brain infarction due to unrecognized intravascular injection, which is less likely to occur with the caudal or translaminar approaches

- **Neurologic complications:** May occur as a result of direct penetrating trauma to spinal nerves or the spinal cord, infarction due to intravascular injection into a radicular artery, ischemia resulting from neural compression by hematoma, or neurotoxicity secondary to injected medication
- **Miscellaneous complications:** Pneumothorax (following lung injury during thoracic or lower cervical injections) or bladder dysfunction (due to blockade or sacral nerve roots)

11. Discuss the side effects of corticosteroids.

Adverse effects may be associated with spinal corticosteroid injections. Fortunately, the amount of steroid used and the frequency of injection are limited. For this reason, fewer complications occur following spinal injections compared with chronic steroid use. Dose-dependent side effects of corticosteroids include nausea, facial flushing, insomnia, low-grade fever (usually < 100° F), and nonpositional headache. Corticosteroid-related immune suppression can mask an existing infection or unmask a new one. Peptic ulcer disease can be exacerbated by injection of corticosteroid. A large dose of corticosteroid can result in changes in fluid balance, electrolyte levels, and blood pressure. It is not uncommon to see elevation in blood glucose after a steroid injection. With repeat injections, the risk of osteoporosis is increased. Avascular necrosis is also a concern with use of corticosteroids. Adrenal suppression may occur following repeat injections.

12. How long do typical epidural injections last?

The length of time that the effects of epidural injection last varies widely depending on the type of spinal pathology. Typically, epidural injections using combination of corticosteroid and local anesthetic last between 3 weeks and 3 months. The therapeutic effect of corticosteroids is attributed to their antiinflammatory properties.

13. Explain the difference between a facet joint injection and a medial branch block.

A painful facet joint can be blocked by injecting into the joint itself or by blocking the nerves that supply the painful joint. The medial branch of the posterior primary ramus of the spinal nerve innervates the facet joint. The medial branch of the adjacent dorsal rami carries the nociceptive fibers supplying the facet joint. Because each facet joint is dually innervated by the medial branch above and below the joint, it can be blocked by injecting the medial branch above and below the joint. For example, the L4–L5 facet is innervated at its upper aspect by branches from L3 and at its lower aspect by branches from L4. Therefore, two injections are necessary to block the innervation of this single facet joint. To block the medial branch, particular attention should be paid to needle placement to avoid inadvertent injection into the neuroforamen (Fig. 16-4).

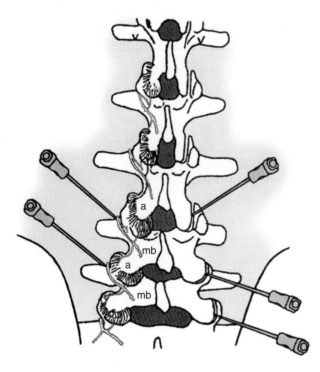

Figure 16-4. Posterior view of lumbar spine showing location of medial branches (**mb**) of dorsal rami, which innervate lumbar facet joints (**a**). Needle position for L3 and L4 medial branch blocks shown on left half of diagram would be used to anesthetize L4–L5 facet joint. Right half of diagram shows L3–L4, L4–L5, and L5–S1 intraarticular facet joint injection positions. (From Canale S, Beaty J. Campbell's Operative Orthopaedics. 11th ed. Philadelphia: Mosby; 2007. Redrawn from Boduk N. Back pain: zygapophyseal blocks and epidural steroids. In: Cousins MJ, Bridenbaugh PO, editors. Neural Blockade in Clinical Anesthesia and Management of Pain. 2nd ed. Philadelphia: Lippincott; 1988.)

14. How long does a facet joint injection last?

Facet joint injections can be performed purely as a diagnostic block by injecting only local anesthetic or for therapeutic purposes by adding corticosteroid to the local anesthetic. A local anesthetic block lasts only for a few hours. An injection using a corticosteroid and local anesthetic combination may last up to 2 weeks (see Figs. 16-5 and 16-6).

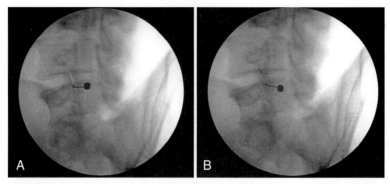

Figure 16-5. **A,** Lumbar facet injection. The needle is placed in the left L4–L5 facet joint. **B,** Injection of contrast shows dye flow into joint space, confirming the needle placement.

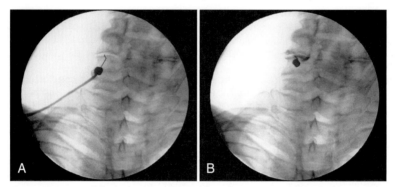

Figure 16-6. **A,** Cervical facet injection. The needle is placed in the cervical facet joint. **B,** Injection of contrast confirms needle placement.

15. Explain radiofrequency neurotomy.

Radiofrequency neurotomy is used to denervate a painful facet joint by thermocoagulating the medial branch that supplies its sensation. Each facet joint is innervated by the medial branch above and below the joint. To denervate a particular joint, the medial branch above and below the joint needs to be treated. The insulated probe is inserted percutaneously to the target nerve tissue and connected to the generator, which supplies a radiofrequency current. This current generates heat in the surrounding tissues, creating a lesion that destroys the nerve tissue. Pain relief may last for 6 to 9 months following a single treatment (Fig. 16-7).

16. Describe pathophysiologic changes associated with discogenic pain.

Disc degeneration refers to abnormal disc morphology secondary to aging or injury. Discs that exhibit decreased signal intensity in their central region on a T2-weighted magnetic resonance imaging (MRI) are frequently termed *degenerative.*

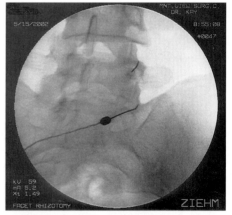

Figure 16-7. Radiofrequency probe in position for lumbar medial branch neurotomy.

Not all degenerative discs are painful. In certain patients, it is thought that the disc becomes sensitized and generates pain as a result of chemical or mechanical irritation. Histologic studies have demonstrated the presence of nerve endings throughout the outer third of the annulus fibrosus. These nerve endings are branches of the sinuvertebral nerves, the gray rami communicantes, and the lumbar ventral rami. Phospholipase A_2, a known inflammatory mediator, is found in high levels in the intervertebral disc. Chemical irritation is most likely due to leaking of inflammatory mediators, such as phospholipase A_2 from the nucleus with subsequent irritation of nerve endings in the annulus.

17. What is provocative discography?

Provocative discography is a test used to identify a painful intervertebral disc. A needle is placed percutaneously into the center of the disc in the awake patient. Once the needle placement is confirmed, a small amount of fluid (usually contrast dye) is injected. As the contrast is injected, the lateral fluoroscopic projection is used to monitor the contrast pattern. In theory, if the particular disc is a source of pain, the patient will experience the familiar type of back or leg pain as the pressure builds up within the disc on injection of fluid. The volume of fluid injected is recorded for each disc level. The resistance of each disc to injection and the quality of the endpoint with injection are recorded. A disc with an intact annulus will have a high resistance to injection and a firm endpoint. A severely degenerated disc is likely to have reduced resistance to injection and almost no endpoint as the contrast leaks out of the disc without pressurizing the disc. Many practitioners use manometry to monitor pressure as dye is injected and record the opening pressure and pressure at which pain is reproduced. In addition to the suspected disc(s), at least one adjacent disc is tested as a control. Injection of normal discs is not generally associated with pain. Communication must occur between the discographer and patient during the procedure. The patient must report whether the pain experienced during injection is the typical pain for which he or she is seeking relief. The patient should rate the degree of pain on an analog scale for each injected level.

Postdiscography images are recorded as plain x-rays (Fig. 16-8) or as a computed tomography (CT) scan to document the contrast dye pattern (nucleogram). Nucleograms can be described as cotton ball, lobular, irregular, fissured, or ruptured (Fig. 16-9). Cotton ball and lobular nucleogram patterns are considered normal. As the disc degenerates, nucleograms deteriorate from irregular to fissured and finally to a ruptured pattern.

Figure 16-8. **A,** Lumbar discography, anteroposterior view. **B,** Lateral view showing normal lobular nucleogram of the top disc and abnormal posterior fissures in the lower two discs.

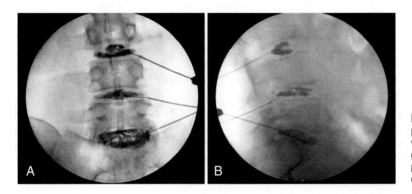

Discogram type		Degeneration
1. Cottonball	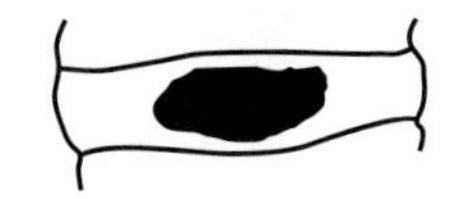	No signs of degeneration. Soft white amorphous nucleus
2. Lobular	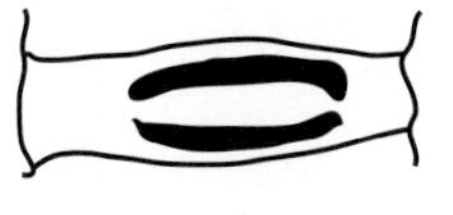	Mature disc with nucleus starting to coalesce into fibrous lumps
3. Irregular	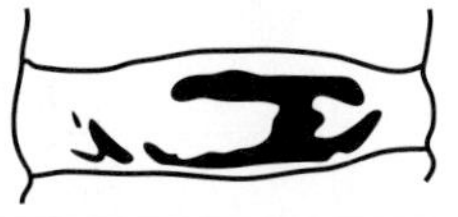	Degenerated disc with fissures and clefts in the nucleus and inner annulus
4. Fissured	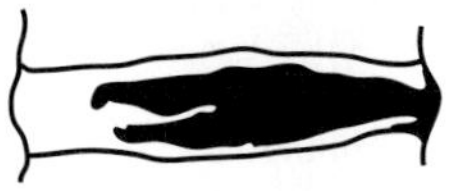	Degenerated disc with radial fissure leading to the outer edge of the annulus
5. Ruptured	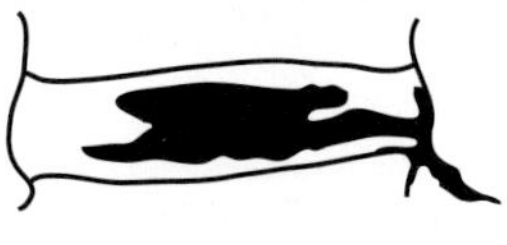	Disc has a complete radial fissure that allows injected fluid to escape. Can be in any state of degeneration.

Figure 16-9. The five types of discogram and the stages of disc degeneration that they represent. (From Adams M, Dolan P, Hutton W. The stages of disc degeneration as revealed by discograms. J Bone Joint Surg 1986;68B:36–41, with permission.)

18. What criteria are used to make the diagnosis of discogenic pain based on provocative discography?

To diagnose discogenic pain, one must document evidence of disc degeneration on a nucleogram and concordant pain during injection of the target disc. Injection of adjacent normal control discs should not elicit pain. The sole purpose of discography is to identify painful intervertebral discs. At least one normal-appearing adjacent disc is tested as a control. A valid test requires the absence of pain in the control disc. It has been observed that some discs can be made painful if sufficient pressure is applied. False-positive results can be reduced by using manometry to record pressure during discography. The following criteria for diagnosis of lumbar discogenic pain using manometry are recommended:

1. Stimulation of the suspected disc reproduces concordant or familiar pain
2. The pain that is reproduced is registered as at least 7 on a 10-point visual analog scale
3. The pain that is reproduced occurs at a pressure less than 50 psi or less than 15 psi above the opening pressure. (Opening pressure is defined as the amount of pressure that must be exerted to start the flow into the disc.)
4. Stimulation of adjacent discs provides controls such that when only one adjacent disc can be stimulated, that disc is painless or pain from that disc is not concordant and is produced at a pressure greater than 15 psi above opening pressure

19. Discuss the controversy surrounding provocative discography.

Discography remains a controversial test. Proponents of discography opine that disc morphology on MRI cannot be used to distinguish a painful disc from asymptomatic age-appropriate degenerative changes as justification for this test. Opponents of discography cite a high percentage of false-positive results in patients with psychological distress, chronic pain syndromes, increased somatic awareness, anular disruption, and individuals involved in litigation or workers' compensation cases. In addition, provocative discography has not been shown to improve treatment outcomes for patients with axial pain syndromes and may lead to unnecessary and ineffective spinal surgery. Use of discography to identify candidates for surgical treatment, such as a lumbar fusion, remains controversial.

20. What are the possible complications of discography?

Nausea, headache, and increased pain may occur but are typically limited and readily treatable. Discitis is the most serious common complication with an incidence of 0.7% to 2.7%. Other complications relate to misplacement of the needle, including nerve injury, dural puncture, and bowel perforation. Accelerated progression of disc degeneration following discography is also a concern.

21. What are the treatment options for discogenic pain?

There is no consensus concerning the optimal treatment of discogenic pain. Nonsurgical treatment options include therapeutic exercise, medication, injections, and use of a lumbar support. Surgical treatment options include spinal fusion and disc replacement surgery.

22. When are sacroiliac (SI) joint injections indicated?

Patient history and physical examination have been shown to be unreliable in the diagnosis of SI joint pain. An analgesic response to a properly performed diagnostic SI joint block is considered the most reliable test to diagnose SI joint-mediated pain. Patients with low back, buttock, or groin pain not attributed to other causes can be considered for SI joint injection. The patient is positioned in the prone oblique position to facilitate visualization of the inferior portion of the joint. A 22-gauge spinal needle is placed in the inferior aspect of the joint, and a small amount of contrast is injected to confirm needle position. Then a small amount of corticosteroid, combined with a local anesthetic, is injected (Fig. 16-10).

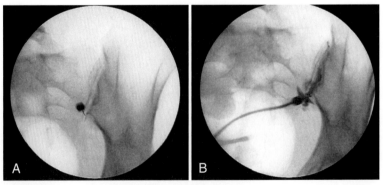

Figure 16-10. **A,** Sacroiliac joint injection. The needle is placed in the joint space. **B,** Injection of contrast shows dye flow in the joint space, confirming needle placement.

23. What injection techniques can help differentiate other pain generators that mimic cervical and lumbar pathology?

Shoulder pain can frequently mimic cervical disorders. Careful examination of the shoulder joint should always be performed in a patient presenting with neck pain. Diagnostic injection into the subacromial space and the acromioclavicular joint can differentiate pain originating from the shoulder region from pain originating in the cervical spine.

Degenerative arthritis of the hip joint may present with symptoms that mimic an upper lumbar disc herniation or spinal stenosis. Injection of the hip joint with a local anesthetic under fluoroscopic guidance can help differentiate hip and spine pathology.

Key Points

1. Options for epidural injections include translaminar, transforaminal, and caudal approaches.
2. Facet-mediated pain may be blocked with an intraarticular facet injection or medial branch block.
3. Use of provocative discography in the management of axial pain syndromes remains controversial.
4. An analgesic response to a properly performed diagnostic SI joint block is considered the most reliable test to diagnose SI joint-mediated pain.

Discography: http://emedicine.medscape.com/article/1143705-overview
Epidural steroid injections: http://emedicine.medscape.com/article/325733-overview
Injection, sacroiliac: treatment and medication:
http://emedicine.medscape.com/article/103399-treatment
Paraspinal injections – facet joint and nerve root blocks: http://emedicine.medscape.com/article/345382-overview

BIBLIOGRAPHY

1. Abbasi A, Malhotra G, Malanga G, et al. Complications of interlaminar cervical epidural steroid injections. Spine 2007;32:2144–51.
2. Adams MA, Dolan P, Hutton W. The stages of disc degeneration as revealed by discograms. J Bone Joint Surg 1986;68B:36–41.
3. Carragee EJ, Cohen S. Diagnostic injections in the spine. In: Herkowitz HN, Garfin SR, Eismont FJ, et al., editors. The Spine. 5th ed. Philadelphia: Saunders; 2006.
4. Carragee EJ, Hurwitz EL, Cheng I, et al. Treatment of neck pain: injections and surgical interventions: Results of the Bone and Joint Decade 2000-2010 Task Force on neck pain and its associated disorders. Spine 2008;33:S153–S169.
5. Chou R, Loeser JD, Owens DK, et al. Interventional therapies, surgery and interdisciplinary rehabilitation for low back pain: An evidence-based clinical practice guideline from the American Pain Society. Spine 2009;34:1066–77.
6. Dreyer SJ, Dreyfuss P, Cole AJ, et al. Injection procedures. In: Cole AJ, Herring SA, editors. Low Back Pain Handbook. 2nd ed. Philadelphia: Hanley & Belfus; 2003. p. 277–96.
7. Dreyfuss P, Lagattuta FP, Kaplansky B, et al. Zygaphophyseal joint injection techniques in the spinal axis. In: Physiatric Procedures in Clinical Practice. Philadelphia: Hanley & Belfus; 1995. p. 206–26.
8. Malhotra G, Abbasi A, Rhee M. Complications of transforaminal cervical epidural steroid injections. Spine 2009;34:731–9.
9. Young IA, Hyman G, Packia-Raj L, et al. The use of lumbar epidural/transforaminal steroids for managing spinal disease. J Am Acad Orthop Surg 2007;15:228–38.

ELECTRODIAGNOSIS IN SPINAL DISORDERS

Mark A. Thomas, MD, and Emal Wahezi, MD

1. List the common reasons for requesting electrodiagnostic tests (EDX) in the evaluation of patients with spinal disorders.

- *To establish and/or confirm a clinical diagnosis.* EDX may help differentiate whether neck, low back, or extremity symptoms are due to radiculopathy, peripheral entrapment neuropathy, or polyneuropathy
- *To localize nerve lesions.* EDX can assist in differentiation between root lesions (radiculopathy), brachial or lumbosacral plexus lesions (plexopathy), and peripheral nerve lesions (entrapment neuropathy). EDX can help distinguish central lesions (e.g. motor neuron disease) from peripheral neuropathy and spinal stenosis
- *To determine the severity and extent of nerve injury.* EDX can differentiate a neuropraxic injury (conduction block) from active axonal degeneration or compromise of the entire peripheral nerve (neurotomesis). EDX can help to determine whether a lesion is acute or chronic, progressive or improving, or preganglionic versus postganglionic
- *To correlate findings noted on spinal imaging studies.* EDX can determine whether an abnormality noted on spinal magnetic resonance imaging (MRI) is the cause of nerve root pathology
- *To provide documentation in medical-legal settings*

2. When should EDX be avoided in the assessment of patients with spinal disorders?

- *During the first 2 to 4 weeks after symptom onset.* During this time many EDX findings are difficult to detect, and testing is not recommended
- *When the diagnosis of radiculopathy is unequivocal.* EDX adds nothing of value to the plan for treatment and is not required in this setting
- *When findings will not change medical or surgical management* (e.g. patients with extreme illness, patients who refuse treatment)
- *Patients with potential contraindications to EDX testing* (e.g. anticoagulated patients, patients with open skin lesions, patients with transmissible diseases, patients with pacemakers and defibrillators)

3. What are the basic components of an electrodiagnostic examination?

EDX is an extension of the history and physical examination. Its goal is to help in distinguishing among the variety of causes for numbness, weakness, and pain. The standard EDX examination consists of two parts: *electromyography* (EMG) and *nerve conduction studies* (NCS).

EMG (needle electrode examination) uses a needle "antenna" to detect and record electrical activity directly from a muscle. The four standard components of the examination assess:

1. Insertional activity
2. Spontaneous activity
3. Motor-unit potentials
4. Recruitment

The distribution of abnormalities identifies the site of nerve or muscle pathology. **EMG is the most useful electrodiagnostic test for the evaluation of radiculopathy.**

NCS record and analyze electric waveforms of biologic origin elicited in response to an electric stimulus. NCS assess the ability of a specific nerve to transmit an impulse between two sites along the course of an axon. When NCS are abnormal, they give information that a specific nerve is not conducting impulses in the measured area. Both sensory and motor nerve conduction studies can be performed. Sensory, motor, and mixed nerves can be assessed. **NCS are useful for diagnosis of peripheral entrapment neuropathy and peripheral neuropathy.** They are generally expected to be normal in radiculopathy because the lesion is usually preganglionic. Specialized NCS—H-reflex, F-wave, and somatosensory evoked potentials (SEP)—may play a limited role in diagnosis of radiculopathy.

4. What is the anatomic basis for EDX as it relates to the assessment of spinal disorders?

The purpose of the EDX is to assess the motor and sensory function related to the spinal nerves. Each spinal nerve contains both motor and sensory fibers and contributes to the formation of the peripheral nerve. The cell bodies for the motor axons are situated within the anterior horn of the spinal cord. The cell bodies for the sensory axons are located within the dorsal root ganglion near its junction with the ventral root. There it forms the mixed spinal nerve in the region of the intervertebral foramina. After exiting the neural foramen, the spinal nerve root divides into anterior and posterior rami. The anterior rami supply the anterior trunk muscles and, after entering the brachial or lumbosacral plexus, the muscles of the extremities. The posterior rami supply the paraspinal muscles and skin over the neck and trunk (Fig. 17-1).

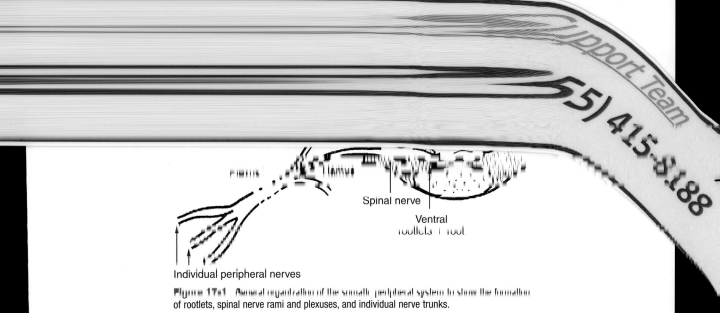

Spinal nerve

Ventral
rootlets + root

Plexus

Ramus

Individual peripheral nerves

Figure 17-1 General organization of the somatic peripheral system to show the formation of rootlets, spinal nerve rami and plexuses, and individual nerve trunks.

Lesions can be classified as either preganglionic (localized to spinal cord or nerve root) or postganglionic (localized to plexus or distal mixed peripheral nerve). Lesions within the spinal canal (myelopathy, radiculopathy) compromise sensory fibers proximal to their cell bodies in the dorsal root ganglion. Such lesions do not affect the sensory NCS studies because the injured sensory fibers degenerate centrally between the cell body in the dorsal root ganglion and the nerve root. Cells in the dorsal root ganglion continue to supply nutrition to the peripheral sensory fibers, thereby preserving sensory nerve conduction in this region. With more peripheral lesions (e.g. within and distal to the plexuses), sensory fibers degenerate distally, resulting in abnormal sensory NCS. In contrast, nerve root compression distal to the motor cell bodies in the anterior horn cell results in distal degeneration of motor fibers that can be detected on motor NCS and EMG studies.

It is possible for the dorsal root ganglion to be situated slightly more proximal in the foramina and be affected by direct compression or indirectly by vascular insult and edema formation. The dorsal root ganglion can also be damaged in diseases such as diabetes mellitus, herpes zoster, and malignancy. In these conditions, the sensory NCS may be abnormal. However, abnormal sensory NCS rarely occur with discogenic radiculopathies.

5. Explain how EMG is used to assess patients with spinal disorders for the presence of a radiculopathy.

Specific muscles are selected for EMG assessment. Six upper limb muscles, including paraspinal muscles, consistently identify more than 98% of cervical radiculopathies that are confirmable by electrodiagnosis. For upper-limb EMG evaluation, a suggested screen includes deltoid, triceps, pronator teres, abductor pollicis brevis, extensor digitorum communis, and cervical paraspinal muscles. Six lower limb muscles, including paraspinal muscles, consistently identify more than 98% of electrodiagnostically confirmable lumbosacral radiculopathies. A suggested lower-limb EMG screen for optimal identification includes the vastus medialis, anterior tibialis, posterior tibialis, short head of biceps femoris, medial gastrocnemius, and lumbar paraspinal muscles. For both lumbosacral and cervical disorders, when paraspinal muscles are not reliable to study, eight distal muscles are needed to achieve optimal identification.

Localization of a nerve injury to a specific root level is achieved by testing a variety of muscles in a multisegmental distribution that are innervated by different peripheral nerves. If the abnormalities are confined to a single myotome but cannot be localized to the distribution of a single peripheral nerve, the diagnosis is consistent with radiculopathy. The paraspinous musculature is generally affected in radiculopathies. However, on occasion, especially in cervical radiculopathies and long-standing radiculopathies, the paraspinous muscles may be normal.

There are four distinct steps in the needle EMG examination of each muscle:
1. Assessment of insertional activity
2. Assessment of spontaneous activity
3. Examination of motor unit potentials
4. Assessment of recruitment

Abnormal resting potentials include fibrillations, positive sharp waves, fasciculations, and high-frequency repetitive discharges. Electrodiagnostic findings must be interpreted in view of the time interval between the onset of the lesion and the performance of the electrical study. Table 17-1 further identifies the pathophysiology and diseases associated with EMG abnormalities.

Table 17-1. Needle electromyographic findings

EMG FINDING	PATHOPHYSIOLOGY	ASSOCIATED DISEASES
Increased insertional activity	Insertion injury of muscle fibers	Acute inflammatory myopathy, acute neuropathy, lower motor neuron disease such as radiculopathy
Fibrillation potentials	Denervation of muscle fibers Membrane instability	Myopathy, neuropathy, anterior horn cell disease, neuromuscular transmission disorders, radiculopathy
Positive sharp waves	Denervation of muscle fibers Membrane instability	Myopathy, neuropathy, anterior horn cell disease, neuromuscular transmission disorders, radiculopathy (may be present in normal foot and paraspinal muscles)
Fasciculation	Motor unit irritation	Neuropathy (can be a normal variant)
Increase in duration, amplitude, and phase number (polyphasics)	Reduced motor unit number Collateral sprouting Muscle fiber reinnervation	Neurogenic lesion Late-stage muscle disease
Decrease in duration, amplitude, and phase number	Necrotic muscle fibers Reinnervation	Early myopathy Late-stage neuropathy
Increase in firing rate	Reduced motor unit number Increased temporal recruitment	Neuropathy, anterior horn cell disease (early) Botulism
Decrease in firing rate	Reduced activation from the CNS	Upper motor neuron disease, pain, poor patient effort

CNS, central nervous system; EMG, electromyography.

6. What is the earliest EMG finding in acute radiculopathy?

The earliest EMG finding in acute radiculopathy is a decrease in the number of motor unit potentials (MUPs) seen on recruitment. The recruitment frequency (the rate of firing of the first motor unit recruited at the moment when the second motor unit appears) is increased early in radiculopathy. In other words, the initial motor unit recruited must fire faster before being able to recruit a second unit because there are fewer MUPs to recruit.

7. Describe the temporal sequence of electrophysiologic abnormalities seen in a radiculopathy.

Table 17-2.

Table 17-2. Temporal sequence of electrophysiologic abnormalities seen in a radiculopathy

DAYS AFTER ONSET	ELECTROPHYSIOLOGIC ABNORMALITIES
0+	Reduced number of motor unit potentials Reduced recruitment interval Increased firing rates of motor potentials Fasciculations may appear H-reflex latency prolonged Reduced number of F waves
4+	Compound motor action potentials amplitude is reduced
7+	Positive sharp waves appear in paraspsinal muscles
12+	Positive sharp waves appear in proximal limb muscles Fibrillations in paraspinal muscles
15+	Positive sharp waves appear in distal limb muscles Fibrillations occur in proximal limb
18+	Fibrillations potentials seen in most affected muscles

8. What are fibrillation potentials? Why are they important in assessing radiculopathy?

Fibrillation potentials are spontaneous and regularly firing action potentials of individual denervated muscle fibers. Fibrillation potentials are a sensitive indicator of motor axon loss. They can be observed in neuropathy, direct nerve and muscle trauma, myopathy, and some neuromuscular junction

10. What are the limitations of needle EMG in the diagnosis of radiculopathy?
1. Needle EMG detects recent motor axon loss but does not detect sensory axon loss, demyelination, or conduction block
2. False-negative studies can occur in instances of focal demyelination secondary to root compression, when axon loss involves only sensory root fibers, when only a few motor fibers are injured by root compression, during the early postinjury period before denervation potentials appear, or several months after the onset of a radiculopathy (late postinjury period) when significant reinnervation is present
3. False-positive studies are possible when reinnervation is the sole evidence of radiculopathy
4. A normal EMG of the paraspinal muscles does not rule out the presence of root lesions
5. Positive sharp waveforms can be found in normal people without low back pain and are not significant

11. How are NCS obtained? For what diagnoses are NCS most likely to be helpful?
NCS are obtained by application of an electrical impulse at one point, resulting in an action potential (motor or sensory) that is recorded at a second point at a predetermined distance along the course of the nerve. The NCS measures the time (latency) required to travel between the stimulating and recording site as well as the velocity (nerve conduction velocity [NCV]) and amount of potential conducted (amplitude). Sensory responses (sensory nerve action potential [SNAP]) are picked up over a sensory nerve, whereas motor responses are picked up by recording over a muscle (compound motor action potential [CMAP]). The compound SNAP represents the sum of the action potentials of the sensory fibers of individual sensory or mixed nerves. The CMAP is the sum of the action potentials of individual muscle fibers. It is also called the M-wave. The CMAP amplitude reflects the number of muscle fibers activated by nerve stimulation. Special types of nerve conduction studies include F wave, H reflex, SEPs, and motor-evoked potentials (MEPs).

NCS are most likely to yield positive findings in conditions that may mimic the symptoms of radiculopathy, such as compression neuropathy or peripheral neuropathy. Sensory NCS are expected to be normal in radiculopathy because the pathologic lesion is almost always preganglionic. Motor NCS can be abnormal in severe radiculopathy (i.e. reduced CMAP amplitude).

12. What are H reflexes and F waves?
H reflexes and F waves are special types of conduction studies that give information about nerve conduction in proximal sections of nerves that are difficult to assess by standard NCS techniques. These studies are of limited value in diagnosing radiculopathy, although they are excellent screening tests for polyneuropathy.

13. How is the F wave elicited? What is its value in the assessment of radiculopathy?
The F wave is a compound action potential evoked from a muscle by a supramaximal electric stimulus to its related peripheral nerve. This procedure results in an antidromic activation of the motor neuron. The F wave has variable configuration, latency, and amplitudes. Amplitudes generally range between 1% and 5% of the M wave. F waves are abnormal immediately after nerve root injury, even when the needle EMG is normal. However, an F-wave study has low utility for diagnosing a radiculopathy because a muscle is innervated by multiple roots and any lesion along these multiple neural pathways can render it abnormal. Abnormal F waves are observed only in multiple and severe motor root compromise. Clinically, F waves have been shown to be useful in the diagnosis of multiple root lesions such as Guillain-Barré syndrome and extensive proximal neuropathies such as plexopathies.

14. Describe the H wave and its clinical use.
The H reflex is a monosynaptic spinal reflex first described by Hoffmann in 1918. It is the electrical equivalent of the triceps surae reflex when recorded from the gastrocnemius/soleus muscle. An abnormal H reflex localizes the lesion to the S1 root or any points along this neural pathway. Prolonged latency and reduced amplitude may indicate an S1 radiculopathy. However, H-reflex studies are neither highly sensitive nor specific. H reflexes demonstrate approximately a 50% sensitivity for S1 root involvement and may be used to distinguish S1 from L5 radiculopathies. Once abnormal, the H reflex remains so indefinitely, independent of the patient's clinical status. The H reflex is frequently absent bilaterally after lumbar laminectomy and in patients over 60 years of age.

15. What is SEP testing? What is its value in the investigation of radiculopathy?

SEPs are waveforms recorded over the scalp or spine following electrical stimulation of a mixed or sensory nerve in the periphery. SEPs are conducted in the posterior columns of the spinal cord, which represent nerve fibers carrying joint position and vibratory sensation. These nerve fibers usually remain unaffected in radiculopathy. SEPs are used successfully in monitoring spinal cord function during spinal surgery, and prolonged SEP latency can be the earliest sign in extensive multiroot lesions. However, this modality is of limited value for the diagnosis of cervical or lumbar radiculopathy. The range of normal SEP values is broad, and the test has poor sensitivity and specificity for assessing nerve root function.

16. What are the EDX findings in a single-level radiculopathy?

- Abnormal EMG findings in a myotomal distribution
- Normal sensory NCS
- Normal motor NCS or reduced CMAP amplitude with normal conduction velocity when motor root compromise is severe
- Normal F waves
- Abnormal H reflex in most S1 radiculopathies

17. What is the most common root level of cervical radiculopathy?

The C7 root is most commonly involved in cervical radiculopathy (31%–81%), followed by C6 (19%–25%), C8 (4%–10%), and C5 (2%–10%). Nerve roots C1 to C4 have no extremity representation, and lesions affecting these roots cannot be diagnosed on EDX testing.

18. What are the significant EDX findings in a C5 radiculopathy?

Abnormalities are noted on EMG testing of the rhomboids, supraspinatus, infraspinatus, levator scapulae, and deltoid muscles. EMG abnormalities may also be seen in the biceps and brachialis, although more distally innervated muscles should be normal.

19. What are the significant EDX findings in a C6 radiculopathy?

EMG abnormalities are commonly seen in the biceps, pronator teres, extensor carpi radialis, and occasionally in the flexor carpi radialis. Rarely are EMG abnormalities detected in the deltoid, supraspinatus, or infraspinatus muscles with C6 radiculopathy. Conditions that may mimic C6 radiculopathy include carpal tunnel syndrome, median nerve entrapment at the elbow, and radial sensory nerve entrapment. These conditions may be differentiated on the basis of abnormal NCS.

20. What are the key muscles to assess for EMG diagnosis of C7 radiculopathy?

The most specific muscles include the anconeus, pronator teres, flexor carpi radialis, triceps, and extensor digitorum communis muscles. NCS may show unilateral abnormalities of the flexor carpi radialis H reflex. Carpal tunnel syndrome may be confused with C7 radiculopathy but can be distinguished with median nerve motor and sensory nerve testing.

21. What are the key muscles to assess for the diagnosis of C8 and T1 radiculopathies?

It is difficult to differentiate C8 from T1 root lesions. The key muscles for the diagnosis of C8–T1 compromise are the flexor digitorum profundus, abductor digiti minimi, first dorsal interosseous, pronator quadratus, abductor pollicis brevis, and opponens pollicis. If abnormalities are found in the extensor indicis proprius and cervical paraspinal muscles but not the pronator teres or extensor carpi radialis muscles, a C8 root lesion may be present because the radial nerve contains very few T1 fibers. The diagnosis of T1 radiculopathy is rare. NCS should be performed to rule out ulnar neuropathy at the elbow or wrist, as well as brachial plexopathy and thoracic outlet syndrome.

22. What are the significant EDX findings in L4 radiculopathies?

EMG abnormalities may be seen in the quadriceps, adductors, and occasionally in the tibialis anterior muscle. EMG abnormalities are noted in the paraspinal muscles in radiculopathy and are absent in lumbar plexopathy and femoral neuropathy.

23. What are the significant EDX findings in L5 radiculopathy?

EMG abnormalities are most commonly seen in the peroneal innervated musculature. To differentiate L5 radiculopathy from a peroneal neuropathy, EMG abnormalities should be sought in the flexor digitorum longus and tibialis posterior, as well as in the proximal muscles with L5 innervation (tensor fascia lata, gluteus medius and minimus, and lumbar paraspinal muscles).

24. What are the significant EDX findings in S1 radiculopathy?

EMG abnormalities are most frequently seen in the gastrocnemius and soleus muscles, as well as the lateral hamstring, gluteus maximus, and lumbar paraspinal muscles. EMG abnormalities may also be noted in the intrinsic foot muscles. If EMG abnormalities are limited to the intrinsic foot muscles, the diagnosis of tarsal tunnel syndrome should be confirmed or excluded by NCS.

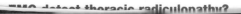

abnormally prolonged SEPs may be helpful in the ... needle examination.

27. Why is the EDX evaluation of limited value after a laminectomy?

Postoperative EDX studies are of limited value. Abnormalities in the paraspinal muscles are difficult to interpret because denervation potentials can originate from traumatic muscle injury secondary to surgery. Within the first 10 to 14 postoperative days, the EDX study reveals only preexisting abnormalities. Between 3 weeks and 4 months after surgery, EDX results can reliably investigate a previously unsuspected lesion or be used to assess postoperative weakness. When the EDX examination is performed 4 to 6 months after cervical laminectomy or 6 to 12 months after lumbar laminectomy, it is difficult to interpret the significance of findings. Abundant fibrillation potentials found in proximal and distal muscles of the myotome may suggest a recurrent or ongoing radiculopathy.

Key Points

1. Electrodiagnostic evaluation is useful to establish and/or confirm a clinical diagnosis of radiculopathy.
2. EMG has limited usefulness in the evaluation of spinal stenosis.
3. Electrodiagnostic testing should be deferred during the first 2 to 4 weeks following clinical onset of radiculopathy because false-negative studies are common during this time period.

Websites

1. Electrodiagnostic Testing, North American Spine Society: http://www.spine.org/Documents/EMG_2006.pdf
2. Electrodiagnostic Testing, American Academy of Orthopaedic Surgeons: http://orthoinfo.aaos.org/topic.cfm?topic=A00270
3. Practice Guidelines, American Association of Neuromuscular & Electrodiagnostic Medicine: http://www.aanem.org/Practice/Practice-Guidelines.aspx

BIBLIOGRAPHY

1. Chiodo A, Haig AJ, Yamakawa KS, et al. Magnetic resonance imaging vs. electrodiagnostic root compromise in lumbar spinal stenosis: A masked controlled study. Am J Phys Med Rehabil 2008;87(10):789–97.
2. Dumitru D, editor. Textbook of Electrodiagnostic Medicine. 2nd ed. Philadelphia: Hanley & Belfus; 2001.
3. Lomen-Hoerth C, Aminoff MJ. Clinical neurophysiologic studies: Which test is useful and when? Neurol Clin North Am 1999;17:65–74.
4. Nadin RA, Patel MR, Gudas TF, et al. Electromyography and magnetic resonance imaging in the evaluation of radiculopathy. Muscle Nerve 1999;22:151–55.
5. Pezzin LE, Dillingham TR, Lauder TD, et al. Cervical radiculopathies: Relationship between symptom duration and spontaneous EMG activity. Muscle Nerve 1999;22:1412–18.
6. Robinson LR. Role of neurophysiologic evaluation in diagnosis. J Am Acad Orthop Surg 2000;8:190–99.
7. Spindler HA, Felsenthal G. Electrodiagnostics and spinal disorders. Spine State Art Rev 1995;9:597–610.
8. Streib EW, Sun SF, Paustian FF, et al. Diabetic thoracic radiculopathy: Electrodiagnostic study. Muscle Nerve 1986;9:548–53.
9. Tsao B. The electrodiagnosis of cervical and lumbosacral radiculopathy. Neurol Clin 2007;25(2):473–94.

SPINAL ORTHOSES

Vincent J. Devlin, MD

1. What is a spinal orthosis?

A spinal orthosis is a device that provides support or restricts motion of the spine. Spinal orthoses may also be prescribed to treat spinal deformities such as scoliosis. All orthoses are force systems that act on body segments. The forces that an orthosis generates are limited by the tolerance of the skin and subcutaneous tissue.

2. List some common indications for prescribing a spinal orthosis.

- To prevent or correct a spinal deformity (e.g. scoliosis, kyphosis)
- To immobilize a painful or unstable spinal segment (e.g. spinal fracture)
- To protect spinal instrumentation from potentially dangerous externally applied mechanical loads

3. How are spinal orthoses classified?

Orthoses have been described according to location of origin (e.g. Milwaukee brace, Charleston brace), inventor (e.g. Knight, Williams), or appearance (e.g. halo). The most universally accepted classification system describes spinal orthoses according to the region of the spine immobilized by the orthosis:

- Cervical orthosis (CO): e.g. Philadelphia collar
- Cervicothoracic orthosis (CTO): e.g. SOMI brace
- Cervicothoracolumbosacral orthosis (CTLSO): e.g. Milwaukee brace
- Thoracolumbosacral orthosis (TLSO) e.g. Jewett brace
- Lumbosacral orthosis (LSO): e.g. Chairback brace
- Sacroiliac orthosis (SIO): e.g. Sacroiliac belt

4. What factors require consideration in order to prescribe the most appropriate orthosis for a specific spinal problem?

- The patient's body habitus
- Likelihood of patient compliance
- The intended purpose of the orthosis (motion control, deformity correction, pain relief, protection of spinal implants)
- The location of the spinal segment(s) that require immobilization
- The degree of motion control required

5. What orthoses are available for treating cervical disorders?

- Cervical orthoses (CO)
- Cervicothoracic orthoses (CTO)
- Halo skeletal fixator

6. When are COs prescribed? How do they work? What are the commonly used types of COs?

COs are commonly prescribed for pain associated with cervical spondylosis, for stabilization following cervical spinal surgery, and for protection and immobilization of the cervical spine following trauma. COs are cylindrical in design and encircle the neck region. They may be anchored to the mandible and/or the occiput to increase stiffness and motion control.

COs may be soft or rigid. Soft collars provide no meaningful motion control. Rigid COs (e.g. Philadelphia, Miami-J) restrict flexion-extension in the middle and lower cervical region. However, restriction of rotation and lateral bending is less effective, and control of flexion-extension in the occiput to C2 region is limited. COs are inadequate for immobilization of unstable spine fractures. Common types of COs include:

SOFT COLLAR (Fig. 18-1)

Design: Nonrigid; made of firm foam covered by cotton and fastened posteriorly with Velcro. Provides minimal restriction of cervical movement

Indications: Cervical spondylosis, cervical strains. Allows soft tissues to rest, provides warmth to muscles, and reminds the patient to avoid extremes of

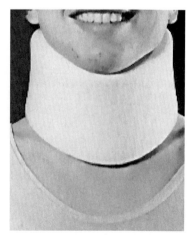

Figure 18-1. Soft collar.

...Philadelphia collar. More appropriate for use in patients with altered mental status because collar-skin contact pressures generated by this brace are below maximal capillary skin pressure

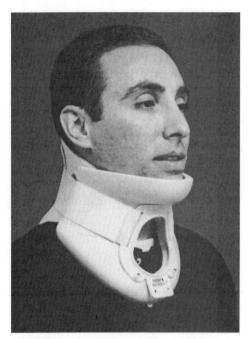

Figure 18-2. Philadelphia collar. (From Fisher TJ, Williams SL, Levine AM. Spinal orthoses. In: Browner BD, Jupiter JB, Levine AM, et al, editors. Skeletal Trauma. 4th ed. Philadelphia: Saunders; 2008.)

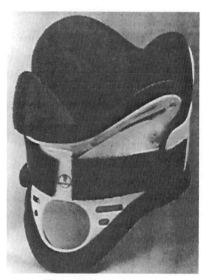

Figure 18-3. Miami-J collar.

7. When are CTOs prescribed? How do they work? What are the commonly used types of CTOs?

CTOs are prescribed when greater motion restriction is desired in the middle and lower cervical spine compared with the restriction achieved with COs. CTOs use chin and occiput fixation attached to the trunk via straps or rigid circumferential supports. Two to four rigid uprights are used to increase stiffness and improve motion control. These designs are generally reported to be more uncomfortable by patients. Common types of CTOs include:

TWO-POSTER CTO (Fig. 18-4)

Design: A metal orthosis consisting of single anterior and posterior uprights. Occipital, mandibular, sternal, and thoracic pads are attached. Difficult to use if the patient cannot sit erect

Indications: Provision of support following cervical fusion procedures

FOUR-POSTER CTO (Fig. 18-5)

Design: Similar to two-poster but with two anterior and two posterior uprights

Indications: Provision of support following cervical fusion procedures

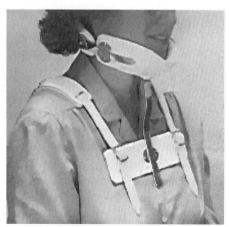

Figure 18-4. Two-poster orthosis.

SOMI CTO (Fig. 18-6)

Design: The sternal occipital mandibular immobilizer (SOMI) derives its name from its points of attachment. It consists of a sternal plate with shoulder components, a waist belt, and occipital and mandibular pads connected by uprights to create a three-post design. A head band may be added and is useful if the chin piece must be temporarily removed due to skin irritation. This orthosis can be more easily fitted to the supine patient than poster type CTOs because the uprights that maintain position of the occipital pad are attached anteriorly to the sternal plate. This brace is not compatible with magnetic resonance imaging (MRI)

Indications: Provision of additional support after cervical fusion procedures, immobilization of stable cervical fractures, and as a transition brace after treatment with a halo orthosis

ASPEN CTO SYSTEM (Fig. 18-7)

Design: Consists of a CO attached to a thoracic vest via two or four posts

Indications: For maximum possible stabilization of the lower cervical and upper thoracic spinal regions. Indicated for minimally unstable fractures

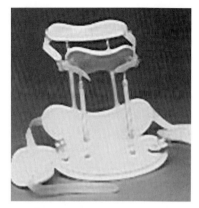

Figure 18-5. Four-poster orthosis.

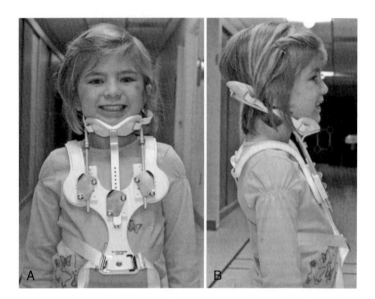

Figure 18-6. Sternal occipital mandibular immobilizer cervicothoracic orthosis. (From Kim DH, Ludwig SC, Vaccaro AR, et al, editors. Atlas of Spine Trauma. Philadelphia: Saunders; 2008. p. 523.)

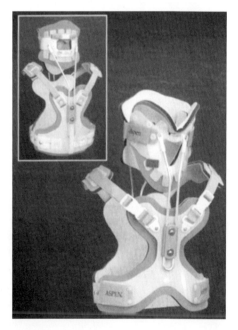

Figure 18-7. Aspen cervicothoracic orthosis. (From Kim DH, Ludwig SC, Vaccaro AR, et al, editors. Atlas of Spine Trauma. Philadelphia: Saunders; 2008. p. 95.)

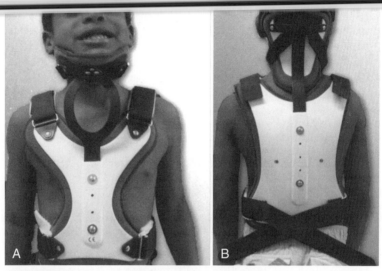

Figure 18-8. Minerva cervicothoracic orthosis. (From Kim DH, Ludwig SC, Vaccaro AR, et al, editors. Atlas of Spine Trauma. Philadelphia: Saunders; 2008. p. 96.)

8. Describe the components of a halo vest orthosis.

The halo vest orthosis (Fig. 18-9) stabilizes the cervical spine by fixing the skull in reference to the chest through an external mechanical apparatus. A rigid ring is fixed about the periphery of the skull. A snug-fitting fleece-lined plastic vest immobilizes the chest. Adjustable rods and bars stabilize the ring and vest with respect to each other. This orthosis provides the most effective restriction of cervical motion, especially for the upper cervical region. Traction may be applied to the cervical spine by use of turnbuckles.

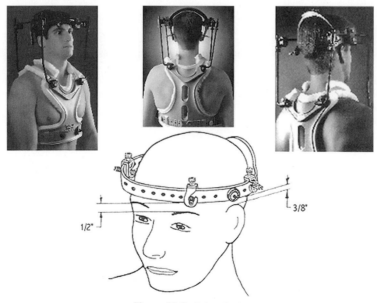

Figure 18-9. Halo orthosis.

9. When should a halo orthosis be prescribed?

Indications for use of a halo skeletal fixator include:

1. Treatment of select cervical fractures (especially C1 and C2 fractures)
2. Postoperative immobilization (e.g. to supplement and protect nonrigid spinal fixation such as C1–C2 wiring)
3. Maintenance of cervical spinal alignment when spinal stability is compromised by tumor or infection and surgical stabilization has not yet been performed or is contraindicated

10. How is the halo skeletal fixator applied?

The patient is placed supine with the head position controlled by the physician in charge (Fig. 18-10). The correct ring size (permits 1–2 cm of circumferential clearance around the skull) and vest size are determined. Critical measurement to determine correct vest size include:

1. Waist circumference
2. Chest circumference at level of xiphoid
3. Distance from shoulder to iliac crest

Pin sites are identified. The skin is cleaned with Betadine, and pin sites are injected with 1% lidocaine. The patient is instructed to keep the eyes closed during placement of the anterior pins to prevent skin tension in the eyebrow area, which could cause difficulty with eyelid closure. Anterior pins are placed 1 cm above the orbital rim, below the equator (greatest circumference) of the skull, and above the lateral two thirds of the orbit. This pattern avoids the temporalis muscle laterally and the supraorbital and supratrochlear nerves and frontal sinus medially. Posterior pins are placed opposite the anterior pins at the 4 o'clock and 8 o'clock positions. The pins are tightened to 8 in-lb (0.9 Nm) in adults. The vest is applied, and the upright posts are used to connect the ring to the vest. Cervical radiographs are obtained to check spinal alignment. The pins are retightened with a torque wrench once at 24 to 48 hours after initial application. The pin sites are cleaned daily with hydrogen peroxide.

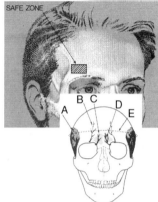

Figure 18-10. Halo pin placement. **A,** Temporalis muscle. **B,** Supraorbital nerve. **C,** Supratrochlear nerve. **D,** Frontal sinus. **E,** Equator. (From Garfin SR, Bottle MJ, Waters RL, et al. Complications in the use of the halo fixation device. J Bone Joint Surg 1986;68A:320–25.)

11. What problems have been associated with the use of halo orthosis?

Complications associated with use of a halo orthosis include pin-loosening, pin-site infection, discomfort secondary to pins, scars after pin removal, nerve injury, dysphagia, pin-site bleeding, dural puncture (following trauma to the halo ring), pressure sores secondary to vest irritation, reduced vital capacity, brain abscess, and psychological trauma.

Although the halo is the most restrictive of the various CTOs, significant motion may occur due in part to difficulty in fitting the brace securely to the chest. Both supine and upright radiographs should be assessed to ensure that cervical alignment and restriction of cervical motion are maintained with changes in posture. A phenomenon termed *snaking* may occur, in which there is movement between individual cervical vertebra without significant motion between the head and the spine. Use of the halo orthosis is not well tolerated in senior citizen patients, patients with severe rheumatoid arthritis and coexistent hip and knee arthritis, or patients with severe kyphotic deformities (e.g. ankylosing spondylitis). Such patients experience difficulties with ambulation, balance, feeding, and self-care. In such patients rigid internal fixation of the spine to avoid halo use is the preferred treatment option when feasible.

12. What special techniques are required to apply a halo vest orthosis in pediatric patients?

General anesthesia is frequently required. Various ring and vest sizes are required. A computed tomography (CT) scan of the skull is obtained to guide pin placement in very small children. This permits assessment of skull thickness and aids in avoiding suture lines and skull anomalies associated with congenital malformations. There is risk of perforation of the inner table of skull during pin placement in pediatric patients. In patients younger than 3 years, use of multiple pins (10–12 pins) inserted with a maximum torque of 2 in-lb is recommended. In children 4 to 7 years of age, 8 pins are used, and the pins are tightened with 4 in-lb of torque. In children 8 to 11 years of age, 6 to 8 pins are used, and the pins are tightened with 6 in-lb of torque. For children 12 years or older, the adult guidelines for halo placement are used (4 pins, 8 in-lb of torque).

13. What is a noninvasive halo system? (Fig. 18-11)

A noninvasive halo system attempts to provide immobilization of the cervical spine approaching that of a conventional halo in a less invasive fashion. This orthosis avoids the use of skull pins, which eliminates many of the complications associated with the conventional halo system. It consists of a total contact orthosis made of Kydex. Anterior and posterior bars connect the vest to an attachment, which encompasses the occiput, mandible, and forehead. This orthosis provides immobilization from C1 to T1, with similar intersegmental immobilization of the cervical spine as a halo except at the C1–C2 segment. It provides a less invasive alternative to the halo orthosis or an alternative for post-halo immobilization.

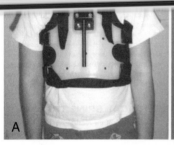 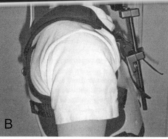

Figure 18-11. Noninvasive halo system. (From Kim DH, Ludwig SC, Vaccaro AR, et al, editors. Atlas of Spine Trauma. Philadelphia: Saunders; 2008. p. 527.)

14. Describe three methods for classifying TLSOs.

TLSOs are prescribed for disorders involving the thoracic and lumbar regions. TLSOs may be classified according to:
1. **Method of fabrication**: TLSOs may be *prefabricated* (e.g. cruciform anterior spinal hyperextension [CASH] brace, Jewett brace), *custom-molded* to the body contours of the individual patient (custom TLSO, body cast), or *hybrid* (prefabricated module customized to a specific patient)
2. **Intended function**: TLSOs may be further differentiated on the basis of intended function:
   - *Static support and immobilization* (e.g. treatment of stable thoracic and lumbar fractures, postoperative bracing after spine fusion)
   - *Deformity correction* (spinal deformities such as idiopathic scoliosis, Scheuermann's kyphosis)
   - *Postural support* (e.g. to relieve axial pain)
3. **Degree of soft tissue contact**: TLSOs can be distinguished by the degree of contact with skin and soft tissues. *Limited contact orthoses* (e.g. Jewett, CASH, Knight-Taylor) utilize discrete pads or straps to restrict motion. *Full-contact orthoses* (TLSO, body cast) distribute orthotic pressure over a wide surface area

15. What motions do TLSOs attempt to restrict?

The thoracic region is the most stable and least mobile portion of the spinal column. The thorax provides inherent stability with its connecting ribs and sternum. The coronal orientation of the thoracic facet joints is such that rotation is the major motion requiring restriction. This motion is difficult to control and requires a custom-molded orthosis if maximal motion control is required. The thoracolumbar junction is a transition region between the stable upper and middle thoracic regions and the mobile lumbar region. Facet joint orientation transitions from a coronal to a sagittal orientation in this region. The lumbar region is more mobile than the thoracic region with flexion-extension motion predominating due to the sagittal orientation of the lumbar facet joints. Experimental studies have shown that full-contact TLSOs can effectively restrict motion between T8 and L4. If motion control is required above T8, a cervical extension should be added to the TLSO. Experimental studies have also shown that a TLSO paradoxically increases motion at the L4–L5 and L5–S1 levels. As a result, a thigh cuff must be added to the TLSO if motion control is desired at the L4–L5 and L5–S1 levels. Because limited contact braces function by applying forces via sternal and pubic pads, these orthoses provide only mild restriction of sagittal plane motion (flexion-extension) and do not effectively limit coronal or transverse plane motion.

16. What are the most commonly used types of limited contact TLSOs?

JEWETT (Fig. 18-12)

Design: Consists of a three-point fixation system with anterior pads located over the sternum and pubic symphysis and a posterior pad located over the thoracolumbar region. This orthosis restricts flexion but permits free extension. It is reported to be uncomfortable due to force concentration over a small area as a result of its three-point design

Indication: For pain relief associated with minor stable thoracic and upper lumbar fractures (e.g. fractures secondary to osteoporosis)

CASH (Fig. 18-13)

Design: The CASH orthosis is shaped like a cross with bars and pads anteriorly that are opposed by a posterior thoracolumbar strap

Indication: Similar to Jewett

KNIGHT-TAYLOR (Fig. 18-14)

Design: Pelvic and thoracic bands are connected by a pair of posterior and lateral metal uprights. An interscapular band stabilizes the uprights and serves as an attachment for axillary straps. Over the shoulder straps attempt to limit lateral bending and flexion-extension. A cervical extension may be added. Poor rotational control is provided by this orthosis

Indications: Minor stable fractures and stable soft tissue injuries

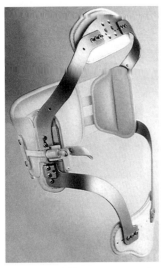

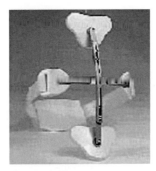

Figure 18-13. Cruciform anterior spinal hyperextension orthosis.

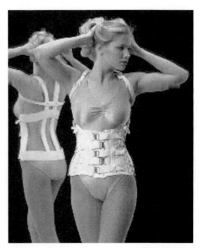

Figure 18-14. Knight-Taylor thoracolumbosacral orthosis.

Figure 18-12. Jewett orthosis.

17. What are the most commonly used types of full-contact TLSOs?

CUSTOM-MOLDED TLSO (Fig. 18-15)

Design: Plastic jacket provides total body contact except over bony prominences. Available in one- or two-piece construction with anterior, posterior, or side-opening styles

Indications: Immobilization of the spine between T8 and L4. Provides adequate rotational control for treatment of stable spine fractures in this region

CUSTOM-MOLDED TLSO WITH CERVICAL EXTENSION (Fig. 18-16)

Design: Custom-molded TLSO with attached chin and occiput support

Indications: Immobilization of the spine between T1 and T7. Provides adequate rotational control for treating stable spine fractures in this region

CUSTOM-MOLDED TLSO WITH THIGH CUFF (Fig. 18-17)

Design: Custom-molded TLSO with attached thigh cuff. Thigh cuff may be fixed or may be attached via hinges with a drop lock

Indications: Immobilization of the spine between L4 and S1

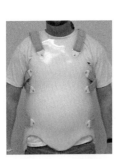

Figure 18-15. Custom-molded thoracolumbosacral orthosis.

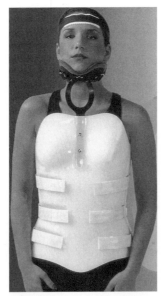

Figure 18-16. Custom-molded thoracolumbosacral orthosis with cervical extension.

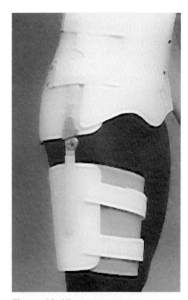

Figure 18-17. Custom-molded thoracolumbosacral orthosis with thigh cuff.

18. **When an orthosis is indicated for immobilization of a stable thoracic or lumbar fracture, what are the most important factors to consider in selection of the appropriate type of orthosis?**

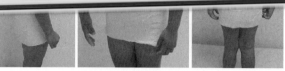

Figure 18-18. Hyperextension cast.

The *level of injury* is a critical factor to consider in orthotic selection for a thoracic or lumbar fracture. For an orthosis to limit motion in a specific region of the spine, the orthosis must extend proximal and distal to the level of injury and immobilize the adjacent spinal segments. A TLSO is generally recommended if rigid immobilization is required from the T8 to L4 level. If the fracture involves L5, a thigh cuff should be added. If control is required proximal to T8 level, a cervical extension should be added. A halo or Minerva orthosis can effectively immobilize from the T1 level cephalad. The *type of spine fracture*, *associated injuries* (e.g. pulmonary, abdominal), and the patient's *body habitus* are additional important factors to consider in decision making.

19. **What are some contraindications to orthotic treatment for thoracic and lumbar spine fractures?**
    - Unstable fracture types (fracture-dislocation, significant ligamentous injury, e.g. Chance fracture, flexion-distraction injury)
    - Incomplete neurologic deficit (surgery for decompression and stabilization indicated)
    - Morbid obesity
    - Polytrauma or associated injuries that prohibit brace wear (e.g. pulmonary or abdominal injury)
    - Impaired mental status
    - Impaired skin sensation
    - Noncompliant patient

20. **What are reasons to consider use of an orthosis following a spinal fusion procedure?**
    At present, spinal fusion procedures are most commonly performed in conjunction with the placement of segmental spinal instrumentation. If the patient is reliable, possesses good bone quality, and multiple fixation points are used, postoperative bracing is not mandatory after a spinal instrumentation and fusion procedure. Reasons to consider use of a spinal orthosis following a spinal fusion procedure:
    - To provide a splinting effect to relieve pain and limit trunk motion. Use of an orthosis can increase intraabdominal pressure, which has the potential to provide a splinting effect that may help relieve pain during the initial recovery period. An orthosis can also provide a postural reminder to limit extreme body motions
    - To protect spinal implants from excessive forces. Young children tend to become active prematurely and may disrupt spinal fixation. Adults with osteopenia may also benefit from bracing to protect the implant-bone interface
    - To provide immobilization after a lumbar fusion performed without use of spinal implants

21. **What are the most commonly prescribed orthoses for treatment of lumbar and lumbosacral disorders?**
    Various types of LSOs exist ranging from custom-molded LSOs to elastic binders. LSOs stabilize the lumbar and sacral regions by encircling the upper abdomen, rib cage, and pelvis. Motion restriction provided by molded LSO does not approach the restriction provided by a molded TLSO. In contrast to a TLSO, an LSO does not extend over the thorax and cannot limit motion by a three-point bending mechanism. Instead, LSOs function by fluid compression of the abdominal cavity and restriction of gross body motion. They provide only mild restriction of flexion and extension and minimal restriction of side bending and rotation. LSOs are not sufficiently restrictive for immobilization of lumbar spine fractures. Nonrigid LSOs such as corsets, sports supports, and binders do not provide meaningful restriction of spinal motion but exert an effect providing a reminder to maintain proper posture, supporting weak abdominal musculature and reducing pain by limiting gross trunk motion.

    CUSTOM-MOLDED LSO (Fig. 18-19)
    Design: Custom made from patient mold
    Indications: Chronic low back pain of musculoskeletal origin, postsurgical immobilization

CHAIRBACK LSO (Fig 18-20)

Design: Composed of a posterior frame of Kydex with a fabric abdominal panel. Adjustable laces provide side closure and front straps provide front tightening

Indications: Low back pain exacerbated by lumbar extension

CORSET (Fig 18-21)

Design: Canvas garment with side-pull tightening straps and paraspinal steel stays

Indications: Mechanical low back pain

ELASTIC BINDER (Fig. 18-22)

Design: Broad elastic straps are fastened with Velcro closure

Indications: For postural support with minimal discomfort. Good choice for a patient with a pendulous abdomen or weak abdominal musculature

SPORTS SUPPORT (Fig. 18-23)

Design: Consists of a heavy-duty elastic binder with a posterior neoprene pocket. The pocket holds a thermoplastic panel that is heated and contoured to the patient's lumbosacral region

Indications: For patients whose shape or activity level precludes use of a more restrictive orthosis

SACROILIAC ORTHOSIS (Fig. 18-24)

Design: Belts that wrap around the pelvis between the trochanters and the iliac crests

Indications: During pregnancy when laxity of the sacroiliac or anterior pelvic joints may cause pain or for other conditions affecting the sacroiliac joints

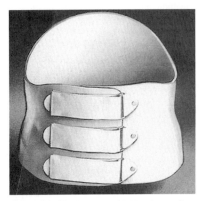

Figure 18-19. Custom molded lumbosacral orthosis.

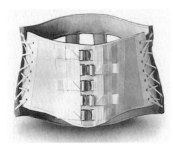

Figure 18-20. Chairback lumbosacral orthosis.

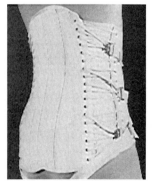

Figure 18-21. Corset.

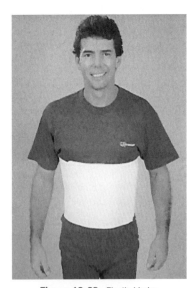

Figure 18-22. Elastic binder.

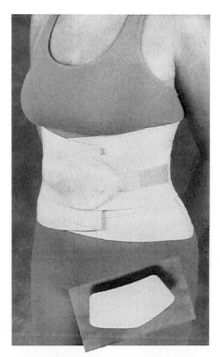

Figure 18-23. Sports support.

Figure 18-24. Sacroiliac orthosis.

22. What orthoses have been shown to be effective for treatment of adolescent idiopathic scoliosis?

Orthoses are recommended for adolescent idiopathic scoliosis patients who have curves of 20° to 40° and who are likely to have significant growth remaining. Patients with curves less than 20° are usually observed for progression, whereas those with curves approaching 50° are generally considered for surgical treatment. There is a lower likelihood of successful orthotic treatment in male patients with scoliosis and for patients with significant curves detected prior to age 10. Options for orthotic treatment include:

- **Milwaukee brace** (Fig. 18-25): Basic components include a custom molded pelvic girdle, one anterior and two posterior uprights extending from the pelvic girdle to a plastic neck ring, corrective pads, straps, and accessories. This brace can be used for all curve types and is the most effective orthosis for curves with an apex above T8. The cosmetic appearance of this brace is a concern to patients and limits compliance

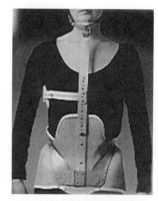

Figure 18-25. Milwaukee brace.

- **TLSO** (Fig. 18-26): The TLSO encompasses the pelvis and thorax. Curve correction is obtained through placement of corrective pads within the orthosis. This orthosis is effective for treatment of thoracic curves with an apex located below T8, as well as thoracolumbar and lumbar scoliosis. The best known orthosis in this category is the Boston brace

- **Charleston brace** (Fig. 18-27): The Charleston brace is designed to be worn only at night while the patient is lying down. This permits fabrication of a brace that overcorrects the curve and creates a mirror image of the curve. For example, a left lumbar curve is treated by designing a brace that creates a right lumbar curve. The relative success of this brace depends on the flexibility of the spine. It is most effective for single curves in the lumbar or thoracolumbar region. It provides a treatment option for patients who are noncompliant with daytime brace use

- **SpineCor brace** (Fig. 18-28): This novel design is a flexible brace that utilizes fabric pelvic and thoracic harnesses connected by elastic straps. The elastic straps are tightened to provide lateral and rotational corrective forces

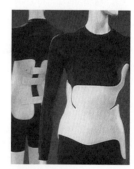

Figure 18-26. Thoracolumbosacral orthosis (Boston).

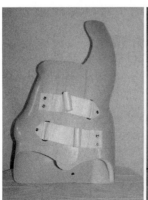 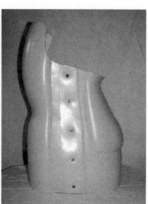

Figure 18-27. Charleston brace.

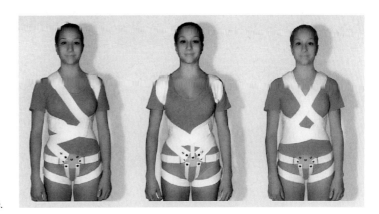

Figure 18-28. SpineCor brace.

23. What are the orthosis options for treatment of an adolescent with Scheuermann's kyphosis?

The CTLSO (Milwaukee brace) is the traditional method for orthotic management of sagittal plane (kyphotic) deformities of the spine in adolescents, but its appearance limits patient acceptance. A TLSO with an anterior sternal extension or padded anterior shoulder outriggers may be considered as an alternative. A TLSO is most effective for treatment of low thoracic kyphotic deformities (apex below T9) or thoracolumbar-lumbar Scheuermann's disease. In very severe deformities, cast treatment can be considered prior to use of an orthosis to gain greater deformity correction.

24. What are the orthosis options for treatment of an adolescent with low back pain and spondylolysis?

Adolescent athletes may sustain injuries to the lumbar region that result in spondylolysis or stress fracture in the pars interarticularis. Various types of braces have been advised for treatment of this condition. Improvement in symptoms following bracing has been reported whether or not healing of the stress fracture occurs. Orthotic options for an adolescent with spondylolysis include a corset, Boston-type LSO, or custom TLSO.

Key Points

1. A spinal orthosis may be prescribed to provide support to the spine, restrict spinal motion, or correct a spinal deformity.
2. Spinal orthoses are classified according to the region of the spine immobilized by the orthosis: cervical orthosis (CO), cervicothoracic orthosis (CTO), or thoracolumbar sacral orthosis (TLSO).
3. The halo vest orthosis is associated with a higher rate of complications than other cervical orthoses and is not well tolerated in the elderly population.
4. The TLSO provides effective motion restriction between T8 and L4 but paradoxically increases motion at the L4–L5 and L5–S1 levels.

Websites

Scoliosis Research Society Brace Manual: http://www.srs.org/professionals/bracing_manuals/
Spinal Orthoses:
http://www.spine-health.com/conditions/scoliosis/bracing-treatment-idiopathic-scoliosis
Spinal Orthotics: http://emedicine.medscape.com/article/314921-overview

BIBLIOGRAPHY

1. Agabegi SS, Asghar SS, Herkowitz HN. Spinal orthoses. J Am Acad Orthop Surg 2010; 18:657-67.
2. Bible JE, Biswas D, Whang PG, et al. Postoperative bracing after spine surgery for degenerative conditions: A questionnaire study. Spine J 2009;9:309–16.
3. Botte MJ, Byrne TP, Abrams RA, et al. Halo skeletal fixation: Techniques of application and prevention of complications. J Am Acad Orth Surg 1996;4:44–53.
4. Carter KD, Roberto RF, Kim KD. Nonoperative treatment of cervical fractures: Cervical orthoses and cranioskeletal traction in patients with cervical spine fractures. In: Kim DH, Ludwig SC, Vaccaro AR, et al, editors. Atlas of Spine Trauma. Philadelphia: Saunders; 2008. p. 88–103.
5. Howard A, Wright JG, Hedden D. A comparative study of TLSO, Charleston and Milwaukee braces for idiopathic scoliosis. Spine 1998;23:2404–11.

CHAPTER 19

COMPLEMENTARY AND ALTERNATIVE MEDICINE TREATMENTS FOR BACK PAIN

Mark A. Thomas, MD, and Sayed E. Wahezi, MD

1. List common treatment approaches to back pain that are considered to be part of complementary and alternative medicine (CAM).
- Manipulation
- Swedish massage
- Acupuncture
- Herbal therapy
- Aromatherapy
- Shiatsu
- Reflexology
- Acupressure
- T'ai chi
- Mind-body treatments
- Magnetic therapy
- Homeopathy
- Prolotherapy
- Nutritional therapy

2. Define chiropractic medicine and chiropractic manipulation.
Chiropractic medicine is a holistic approach to patient care that focuses on the normal relationships among the spinal column, nervous system, and soft tissues. Imbalance or misalignment of the spinal column is considered to be responsible for impaired or abnormal nerve function, resulting in subsequent disease and pain.

Chiropractic manipulation is a realignment or balancing of the spine or extremities to restore normal relationships and health. This goal is achieved by movement of body parts to increase range of motion and to relax muscles.

3. Define somatic dysfunction.
Somatic dysfunction is defined as impaired or altered function of related components of the somatic (body framework) system: skeletal, arthrodial, and myofascial structures and related vascular, lymphatic, and neural elements. Physical findings associated with somatic dysfunction are summarized by the acronym TART:

T = **T**enderness
A = **A**symmetry of bony structures
R = **R**ange-of-motion alterations
T = **T**issue texture changes

4. When is manipulation or manual medicine indicated for treatment of low back pain (LBP)?
Manual medicine utilizes techniques to attempt to restore full range of motion (ROM) to joints that have restrictive barriers. Manipulation is useful for patients with acute LBP (<4 weeks of symptoms) and a related somatic dysfunction who have no progressive neurologic deficit. Limited supporting data help to define when or how to use manual medicine for the treatment of chronic LBP.

5. What are the goals of manual medicine in the treatment of LBP?
- Restore maximal, painless movement of the musculoskeletal system
- Restore spinal postural balance
- Decrease pain
- Improve global health

6. How does manual medicine achieve a positive effect in the treatment of LBP?
Manipulation is thought to work by:
- Restoring normal and symmetric disc or facet alignment
- Restoring spinal range of motion and optimal muscle function
- Reducing afferent-nociceptor signal transmission to the spinal cord through a gate effect
- Stimulating endorphin release, which increases the pain threshold or reduces pain severity
- Providing a strong placebo effect

7. What are the main manual medicine techniques used to treat LBP?
Manual medicine techniques may be classified as thrusting manipulation and nonthrusting manipulation.

10. Who performs thrusting and nonthrusting manipulation and when are these techniques prescribed?
Osteopathic physicians and chiropractors are trained in HVLA and commonly perform these techniques. Nonthrusting techniques are typically performed by physical therapists. Both therapies are prescribed in cases of acute musculoskeletal back pain.

11. How is muscle energy manipulation performed? When is it useful?
Muscle energy manipulation requires that the patient perform a voluntary contraction of muscle in a specific direction, at increasing levels of intensity, against a counterforce applied by the practitioner. For a specific segmental dysfunction, the patient is passively moved to the pathologic barrier to motion and then asked to move away from the barrier with gentle muscle contractions of a 3- to 5-second duration. This action is thought to relax the muscle involved in moving the joint toward the barrier. After 1 to 2 seconds of relaxation, the practitioner moves the affected joint directly through the previous pathologic barrier toward the normal physiologic barrier. This technique is commonly applied to segmental dysfunction affecting the lumbar spine segments, as well as dysfunction of the pelvis and sacrum.

12. What does muscle energy manipulation accomplish in the treatment of LBP?
Muscle energy techniques lengthen shortened or contracted paraspinal muscles, relax muscle spasm, and strengthen weak muscle groups. Theoretically, muscle energy therapy also reduces local myoedema, relieves passive congestion, and mobilizes spinal articulations with restricted segmental mobility.

13. What is strain-counterstrain? How is it applied in the treatment of back pain?
Strain-counterstrain is a passive, indirect adjustment technique in which a spinal segment is placed into its position of greatest comfort or *ease* to decrease pain and restore normal segmental motion. Strain-counterstrain might correct abnormal neuromuscular reflexes that generate small, but significant, anatomic changes in lumbar spine musculature that cause pain. After identifying a tender point, the patient is moved into a position of pain relief and maintained in this position for 90 to 120 seconds with subsequent slow and gradual return to the neutral position. This treatment is time consuming and passive. Therefore, it must be combined with an active exercise program to achieve a lasting, meaningful outcome.

14. Describe myofascial release.
Myofascial release is a manual therapy that applies tension to tight or painful soft tissues through a combination of manual traction and torsion. The goal of myofascial release is to decrease tightness and restore normal tissue mobility. Direct and indirect release techniques are used. In the direct technique the resistance to tissue motion (the pathologic barrier) is engaged with a constant force from the practitioner's hand until release occurs. In the indirect technique the practitioner moves the tissue along the path of least resistance until free motion is obtained. Because of its passive nature, however, myofascial release needs to be performed in the context of active treatment such as exercise. Myofascial release is commonly used to treat myofascial LBP.

15. What can manual medicine offer the patient with back pain?
Evidence indicates that manual medicine treatment may result in early, albeit temporary relief of LBP. This relief may help the patient to begin an active treatment program with more lasting effect. When patients are appropriately selected (again, the somatic dysfunction must be identified), good outcomes can be obtained. The use of manual medicine techniques remains controversial, especially for persons with known disc herniation. Limited evidence demonstrates long-term efficacy in LBP treatment. It is recommended that treatment be discontinued if the patient experiences no measurable benefit after 6 to 8 visits over a 2-week period.

16. What physiologic effects of massage are useful in the treatment of back pain?
- Tissue relaxation
- Increased local or regional blood flow
- Disruption or loosening of adhesions
- Reduction of edema by stimulating venous and lymphatic drainage
- Activation of a gate mechanism in the dorsal horn of the spinal core resulting in pain reduction

- Stimulation of sensory fibers to produce a state of reduced adrenocortical stress reactivity
- Centrally mediated effects (reflexology)

17. What are the different types of massage therapy?

The most useful and frequently used massage schools for treatment of LBP include Swedish massage, acupressure (ischemic compression), shiatsu, reflexology, and structural integration (Rolfing).

18. Describe shiatsu massage.

Shiatsu is a type of massage that synthesizes Western principles of anatomy and physiology with the Oriental principle of energy flow (chi). Stretching and digital manual pressure are applied over acupuncture meridians to smooth and balance energy flow.

19. What are the major contraindications to massage?

- Malignancy
- Cellulitis
- Lymphangitis
- Recent trauma or bleeding
- Deep venous thrombosis
- Recent scuba diving with rapid ascent (nitrogen bubble release)

20. What is acupressure? When is it useful in treating LBP?

Acupressure is the application of thumb or finger pressure to traditional acupuncture points. When applied to a myofascial trigger point, it is called ischemic compression. Acupressure techniques are reported to achieve a therapeutic effect by producing ischemia, muscle relaxation, and reactive hyperemia. When trigger points are identified in back musculature, acupressure techniques may produce rapid muscle relaxation and pain relief. One advantage of acupressure is the ease of application. The patient can use a tennis ball, cane, or other object to provide appropriate pressure independently. Alternatively, a family member or friend can be trained to provide acupressure treatment.

21. How does reflexology work?

Reflexology is based on the tenet that a homuncular map of the body is present on the earlobe, palm, and sole of the foot. Circular deep friction or longitudinal pressure is applied to the specific area on the homunculus that corresponds to an identified area of somatic dysfunction. The goal of this type of treatment is to stimulate and restore a balance of energy in the abnormal tissue.

22. What is mind-body therapy?

The theory of mind-body techniques is based on a belief that the mind and body are inseparable. Most mind-body interventions are movement techniques that seek to enhance awareness of posture and movement. Mind-body therapies include relaxation techniques, cognitive-behavioral interventions, biofeedback, hypnosis, and meditation.

23. Provide a brief description of the types of mind-body therapy that have been used to treat patients with LBP.

1. **Cognitive-behavioral programs** are a component of many established pain treatment centers. These programs focus on educating patients and teaching coping skills in a highly structured group setting under the guidance of a clinical psychologist. They frequently incorporate hypnosis, meditation, and biofeedback techniques
2. The **Alexander technique** is a method of modifying chronic patterns of back and neck muscle tension through an instructor's verbal direction and awareness exercises. Patients are encouraged to experience a state of proper alignment and functional movement by improving their sense of proprioception
3. The **Feldenkrais method** uses multiple repetitions of a particular movement to establish new *engrams*. It emphasizes consideration of whole-body effects from even simple motions. The method relies on the capacity to learn new movement patterns and bypass the *thinking mind*
4. **Pilates-based methods** condition the entire musculoskeletal system and assist the patient in recovering from an injury that produces a weak link in the kinetic chain. Pilates emphasizes eccentric muscle contractions with little or no resistance and then reintroduces more aggressive strengthening and function by providing gradually incremental tasks
5. **T'ai chi** consists of a series of linked, slow, and constant movements. Its origin dates back to seventeenth-century China. Special postures and graceful motion are assumed to achieve a balanced energy flow (chi) throughout the body. T'ai chi develops strength, flexibility, and conscious muscle relaxation
6. **Yoga** is a lifestyle that provides direction in philosophy, ethics, social responsibility, and nutrition. The patient with back pain most commonly practices yoga to improve strength, flexibility, and relaxation. The aims of therapeutic yoga are to increase range of motion and flexibility in the spine and to decrease tightness in the lower extremities
7. **Therapeutic touch** or energy therapy is based on modulating and balancing the flow of *chi*. The therapist's hands move over the patient's body (physical touch or noncontact *touch*), redirecting and rebalancing the *energy field* of the patient with back pain. The goal of energy therapy is to reduce pain and stress-related symptoms

25. How has acupuncture been used for treatment of LBP?

Use of acupuncture has been reported in the treatment of acute LBP, chronic LBP, myofascial pain syndrome, muscle strain and ligament sprain, and vertebral fractures.

26. Describe aromatherapy.

Aromatherapy is based on the concept that exposure to specific odors, in the form of essential oils, can have a therapeutic effect through physiologic and emotional changes. Its efficacy is controversial. Oils are extracted from jasmine flowers, almonds, and lavender. Aromatherapy for LBP is commonly provided by the addition of essential oils to therapeutic massage.

27. Describe herbal therapy.

Herbal medicine is most often associated with traditional Chinese medicine, Indian traditional medicine (Ayurveda), or Western herbalism. It is a form of botanical medicine that uses plant extracts to treat various diseases. Patients should be aware that herbal therapies are not without potential for adverse interactions with other medications. In addition, herbal remedies are not regulated by the Food and Drug administration (FDA).

Two herbs commonly used to treat LBP are arnica and St. John's wort. Arnica, which is derived from a flowering plant, is used for musculoskeletal injuries such as acute lumbar strain. St. John's wort (*Hypericum performatum*) is utilized for the treatment of depression, fibromyalgia, arthritic pain, LBP, and neuropathic pain. St. John's wort **should not** be used with psychotropic medications, including other antidepressants.

28. What is magnet therapy?

Magnet therapy attempts to balance the patient's energy field in order to decrease pain. It has become a popular treatment for various musculoskeletal conditions, including LBP. Magnets are available in small pads and discs for local or circumscribed application and as mattress pads and seat cushions for total body coverage. The strength of the therapeutic magnetic field ranges from 300 to 5000 gauss.

29. How does magnet therapy work?

In theory, the application of a magnetic field increases blood flow by acting on calcium channels located in vascular muscle. Increased circulation improves tissue oxygenation with subsequent elimination of inflammatory byproducts that elicit pain. Magnets also may influence the metabolism and energy flow in both positive and negative ways. The positive magnetic pole is thought to decrease the metabolic rate (negative effect), whereas the negative pole normalizes the body's metabolic and energy function (beneficial effect). In addition, a membrane-stabilizing effect on nociceptive fibers may occur, rendering these fibers less excitable and reducing the firing frequency of unmyelinated C fibers. Research findings do not support claims regarding efficacy of magnetic therapy.

30. What are the contraindications for magnetic therapy?

Magnetic therapy is contraindicated in the presence of implanted electrical devices (pacemakers, defibrillators, neurostimulators), active bleeding, or pregnancy.

31. How does homeopathic therapy work?

Homeopathy is based on the theory that disease results from an imbalance in the innate human homeostasis. Homeopathic therapy uses minute or diluted doses of natural substances (homeopathic remedies) that would produce illness in larger or more concentrated doses. These remedies restore health by stimulating the body to restore homeostasis through normal healing and immune mechanisms.

32. Describe prolotherapy and its use in LBP.

Prolotherapy treats back pain that is related to motion and due to weakened or incompetent ligaments and tendons. The injury-repair sequence is initiated by scraping the tissue or adjacent periosteum with a needle and then injecting a dextrose solution to induce fibroblast proliferation and scarring/repair of tissue. Prolotherapy can increase tendon size and strength. Success (less pain, less tenderness) in patients with chronic LBP who have not responded to conventional treatment is reported.

33. What kinds of nutritional therapy have been used in the treatment of back pain?

Appropriate and healthy diet may reduce pain by decreasing weight, improving mobility, increasing functional activity level, and contributing to a positive sense of well-being. Low-fat, low-cholesterol diets are thought to aid healing of joints involved in back pain through improvement of vascular flow. Diets rich in antiinflammatory components have also been recommended based on the principle that pain has an underlying inflammatory component. Such antiinflammatory diets are high in omega-3 and omega-6 fatty acids and linoleic acid and low in saturated fats, processed meats, and sugar. A wide variety of vitamins and minerals has been advocated for treatment of back pain including vitamin A; B vitamins (B_1, B_6, B_{12}); vitamins C, D, E; glucosamine; methylsulfonylmethane (MSM); S-adenosylmethionine (SAM-e); and D-L phenylalanine (DLPA).

34. What CAM treatments work best for the treatment of back pain?

Popularity or personal testimonials do not prove or disprove treatment efficacy. CAM therapies are most frequently administered in combination with traditional therapeutic interventions for back pain using nonstandardized protocols. The medical evidence to support specific CAM treatments for back pain may be unavailable, insufficient, or conflicting depending on the specific intervention that is evaluated. Nevertheless, standardized reviews and randomized controlled trials have been published supporting CAM treatments, such as spinal manipulation and mobilization, acupuncture, prolotherapy, cognitive-behavioral therapy, and nutritional supplementation. Treatments should be pursued on an individual basis, taking into account the patient's total health picture.

Key Points

1. Complementary and alternative medicine (CAM) therapies are most frequently administered in combination with traditional therapeutic interventions for back pain.
2. The medical evidence to support specific complementary and alternative medicine (CAM) treatments for back pain may be unavailable, insufficient, or conflicting depending on the specific intervention that is evaluated.

Websites

National Institute for Health, National Center for Complementary Medicine: http://nccam.nih.gov/
Review of traditional and complementary non-surgical treatments for back pain: http://www.dartmouth.edu/sport-trial/NonSurgGuideFinal_wcvr.pdf

BIBLIOGRAPHY

1. Ammendolia C, Furlan AD, Imamura M, et al. Evidence-informed management of chronic low back pain with needle acupuncture. Spine J 2008;8(1):160–72.
2. Atchison JW, Taub NS, Cotter AC, et al. Complementary and alternative medicine treatments for low back pain. In: Lox DM, editor. Physical Medicine and Rehabilitation: Low Back Pain. Philadelphia: Hanley & Belfus; 1999. p. 561–86.
3. Bronfort G, Haas M, Evans R. Evidence-informed management of chronic low back pain with spinal manipulation and mobilization. Spine J 2008;8(1):213–25.
4. Collacott EA, Zimmerman JT, White DW, et al. Bipolar permanent magnets for the treatment of chronic low back pain: A pilot study. JAMA 2000;283:1322–25.
5. Dagenais S, Mayer J, Haldeman S. Evidence-informed management of chronic low back pain with prolotherapy. Spine J 2008;8(1):203–12.
6. Gagnier JJ. Evidence-informed management of chronic low back pain with herbal, vitamin, mineral, and homeopathic supplements. Spine J 2008;8(1):70–9.
7. Gatchel RJ, Rollings KH. Evidence-informed management of chronic low back pain with cognitive behavioral therapy. Spine J 2008;8(1):40–4.
8. Haldeman S, Dagenais S. What have we learned about the evidence-informed management of chronic low back pain? Spine J 2008;8(1):266–77.
9. Imamura M, Furlan AD, Dryden T, et al. Evidence-informed management of chronic low back pain with massage. Spine J 2008;8(1):121–33.
10. Kalauokalani D, Cherkin DC, Sherman KJ, et al. Lessons from a trial of acupuncture and massage for low back pain: Patient expectations and treatment effects. Spine 2001;26:1418–24.
11. Rakel D. Integrative Medicine. 2nd ed. Philadelphia: Saunders; 2007.
12. Wai EK, Rodriguez S, Dagenais S, et al. Evidence-informed management of chronic low back pain with physical activity, smoking cessation, and weight loss. Spine J 2008;8(1):195–202.

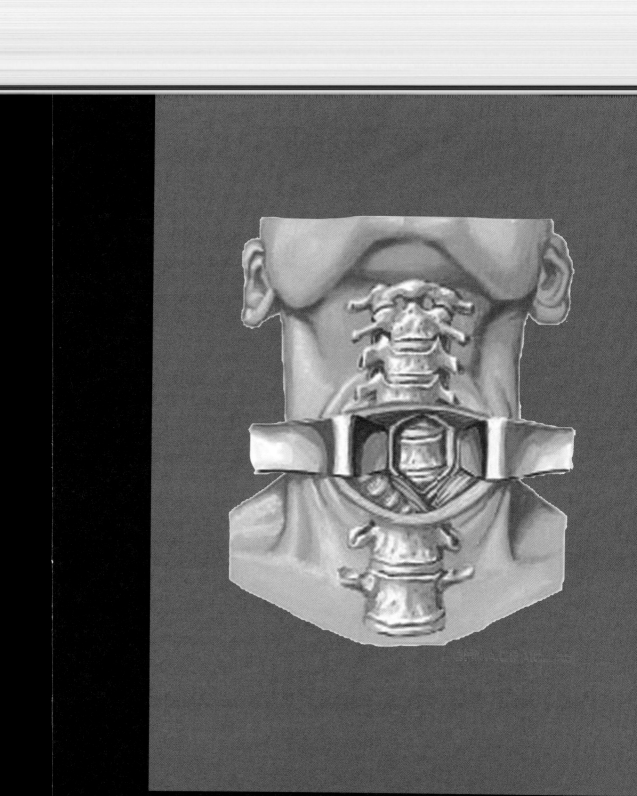

INDICATIONS FOR SURGICAL INTERVENTION IN SPINAL DISORDERS

Vincent J. Devlin, MD, and Paul Enker, MD, FRCS, FAAOS

1. Why are the indications for a spine procedure of such critical importance?

Poor patient selection guarantees a poor surgical result despite how expertly a surgical procedure is performed.

2. What factors determine success after a spinal procedure?

The critical factors that determine success after spinal surgery are the:
- Surgical indication (I)
- Surgical technique (T)
- Patient psychosocial factors (PS)
- Biologic unknowns (BU)

It is critical to perform surgery for the appropriate indication with technical proficiency. However, patient psychosocial factors (workers' compensation, litigation, depression) or biologic unknowns (the multitude of factors that affect healing of a spinal fusion or neural recovery after decompression) can negatively influence the outcome of appropriate and well-executed surgery in powerful ways. Furthermore, these factors are often beyond the control of the surgeon. The relationship among these factors has been summarized in a formula by Enker:

$$\text{Surgical success} = \frac{I \times T}{PS^4 \times BU}$$

3. What are the three major indications for spinal procedures?
- Decompression
- Stabilization
- Realignment

4. Name common indications for spinal decompression procedures.

Spinal decompression is indicated for symptomatic spinal cord or nerve root impingement. Common indications for decompression procedures include disc herniation, spinal stenosis, and cord and/or nerve root impingement secondary to fracture, tumor or infection.

5. Name common indications for spinal stabilization procedures.

Spinal stabilization is performed when the structural integrity of the spinal column is compromised to prevent initial or additional neurologic deficit, spinal deformity, or intractable pain. Common indications for spinal stabilization procedures include fractures, tumors, spondylolisthesis, and spinal instability after laminectomy.

6. Name common indications for spinal realignment procedures.

Spinal realignment procedures are performed to correct spinal deformities. Spinal deformities may result from single-level spinal pathology (e.g. spondylolisthesis, fracture, tumor) or pathology involving multiple spinal levels (kyphosis, scoliosis).

7. How are indications for spinal surgery prioritized?

Indications for spinal surgery are prioritized based on the physician's responsibility to prevent irreversible harm to the patient as a result of spinal pathology and the window of time within which surgical intervention is effective. Although there is no universally accepted classification, surgical indications can be separated into three broad categories:

1. **Emergent indications.** Patients in this category are likely to experience a negative outcome if surgery is not performed emergently. Examples include patients with cauda equina syndrome (most commonly due to a massive lumbar disc herniation) and patients with progressive loss of motor function (e.g. secondary to fracture or spinal tumor)

2. **Urgent indications.** Patients in this category have a serious spinal condition and require surgical intervention to prevent development of a significant permanent neurologic deficit or spinal deformity. Absence of a severe initial neurologic deficit or progressive neurologic deficit permits the opportunity for additional spinal imaging studies,

Only in limited specific circumstances. Back pain is a symptom, not a diagnosis. The lifetime prevalence of back pain exceeds 70%. Surgery is not indicated for nonspecific low back pain. However, back pain may be a prominent symptom in patients with neural impingement, spinal instability, or certain spinal deformities. In such situations, appropriate spinal decompression, stabilization, and realignment may improve back pain symptoms related to serious underlying spinal pathology. In select degenerative disorders, spinal fusion is a reasonable option following adequate nonsurgical treatment if a definite nociceptive focus is identified in a patient without negative psychosocial factors. Caution is crucial when the indication for surgery is pain because this complaint is often subjective and personal and surgical results are uniformly poor when issues of secondary gain exist.

9. When is surgery indicated for a lumbar disc herniation?

Cauda equina syndrome is the only emergent indication for surgical treatment of a lumbar disc herniation. If a patient is developing a progressive motor deficit, it is reasonable to intervene promptly. Indications for elective lumbar disc excision include:
- Functionally incapacitating leg pain in a specific nerve root distribution
- Nerve root tensions signs with or without neurologic signs
- Failure of nonoperative treatment for at least 4 to 8 weeks

It is critical to confirm that magnetic resonance imaging (MRI) findings correlate with the patient's symptoms before considering surgical treatment.

10. When is surgical treatment indicated for lumbar spinal stenosis?

Patients with spinal stenosis generally present with varying combinations of low back and buttock pain, neurogenic claudication, and lower extremity radicular symptoms. Severe progressive neurologic deficits are not typically present, although they can occur. Surgery is considered for patients who have failed nonsurgical management; patients with persistent functional incapacity; patients with neurologic deficits; and patients with persistent buttock, thigh, and/or leg pain. The patient's general medical condition requires consideration in the decision whether or not to pursue surgical treatment. Patient education regarding realistic expectations and goals following surgical treatment is important. Surgical goals may include improved function, decreased pain, and improvement or halted progression of neurologic deficits.

11. What are the indications for surgical treatment of cervical radiculopathy due to cervical disc herniation?

- Persistent or recurrent arm pain unresponsive to nonoperative treatment
- Progressive functional neurologic deficit
- Static neurologic deficit associated with significant radicular pain
  The patient must have positive imaging studies that correlate with clinical findings.

12. What are the indications for surgical treatment of cervical spinal stenosis?

Patients with cervical stenosis may present with radiculopathy, myelopathy, or a combination of radiculopathy and myelopathy. Surgical indications for cervical spondylotic radiculopathy are similar to those for a cervical disc herniation. Surgical treatment of cervical myelopathy is recommended for patients with pain refractory to nonsurgical measures, progressive neurologic deficit or progressive impairment of function (e.g. ambulation, balance, upper extremity coordination).

13. When is surgical intervention indicated for spinal infection?

- To perform open biopsy to obtain tissue for culture when closed biopsy has failed or is considered dangerous
- Failure of medical management in a patient with persistent pain and elevated erythrocyte sedimentation rate and/or C-reactive protein levels
- Drainage of an abscess
- Decompression for spinal cord and/or nerve root compression with impending or associated neurologic deficit
- Correction of progressive or unacceptable spinal deformity
- For progressive or unacceptable spinal instability

14. When is surgical intervention indicated for primary spinal tumors?

- Open biopsy to obtain tissue for definitive diagnosis
- Failure of medical therapy (e.g. chemotherapy, radiation)

- For treatment of tumors known to be resistant to medical therapy
- Decompression for spinal cord and/or nerve root compression with impending or associated neurologic deficit
- Correction of progressive or unacceptable spinal deformity
- For progressive or unacceptable spinal instability

15. What are the indications for surgical intervention for metastatic spinal tumors?
- Open biopsy to obtain tissue for definitive diagnosis
- Treatment for tumors resistant to radiotherapy and/or chemotherapy
- Decompression for spinal cord and/or nerve root compression with impending or associated neurologic deficit
- Correction of progressive or unacceptable spinal deformity
- For progressive or unacceptable spinal instability
- Intractable pain and/or neurologic deterioration during radiation therapy despite steroids
- Impending pathologic fracture/instability

16. When is surgical treatment indicated for spinal fractures?
Surgical treatment is indicated for unstable spine fractures. Clinical stability has been defined by White and Panjabi as the ability of the spine under physiologic loads to limit the patterns of displacement so as not to damage or irritate the spinal cord or nerve roots and, in addition, to prevent incapacitating deformity or pain due to structural changes. Classification systems for fractures involving specific levels of the spine are used to guide treatment.

17. What factors are considered in deciding whether surgical treatment is indicated for adolescent idiopathic scoliosis?
Indications for surgical treatment are based on curve magnitude, clinical deformity, risk of curve progression, skeletal maturity, and curve pattern. Curves greater than 50° should undergo surgical treatment because of the risk for continued curve progression in adulthood. Curves in the 40° to 50° range are analyzed on an individual basis. Curves greater than 40° with documented progression are indicated for surgery. Curves greater than 40° in skeletally immature patients (e.g. premenarchal female) should be treated surgically because of the natural history of continued curve progression with growth. Clinical deformity plays a role in decision making for select lumbar curves (35–40°). Some curves cause marked waistline asymmetry and may be considered for surgery on this basis. Sagittal plane alignment is also an important consideration. In a small subgroup of patients with severe thoracic hypokyphosis or actual thoracic lordosis, surgical treatment should be considered even if the coronal plane curve is less than 40°.

18. What are some common indications for surgical treatment of adult scoliosis?
Unlike adolescent patients with scoliosis, adult patients commonly present for evaluation of back pain symptoms. Indications for surgical treatment of adult patients with scoliosis include pain, progressive deformity, cardiopulmonary symptoms, neurologic symptoms, and cosmesis.

19. When a patient reports that an initial spinal procedure has failed to improve their condition, when is revision spine surgery indicated?
A comprehensive clinical and imaging assessment is required to address this complex question. Pain severity or disability, in and of itself, is not an indication for additional spinal surgery. It is also important to recognize that a patient with unrealistic expectations and goals will not benefit from additional surgical intervention. Surgery may potentially be indicated if surgically correctable pathology is present and the patient's symptoms can be explained on the basis of this pathology. Factors to sort out during a patient's work-up include whether the persistent symptoms are related to a prior spinal decompression (e.g. incomplete decompression, undecompressed adjacent level stenosis, recurrent disc herniation) or spinal fusion (e.g. pseudarthrosis, instrumentation-related issues, suboptimal spinal alignment). Previously undetected spinal infection must always be ruled out. Timing of symptom onset in relation to the initial procedure is an important clue in sorting out the diagnosis. Commonly encountered problems for which revision spinal surgery may provide benefit in the appropriately selected patient include:
- Recurrent or persistent disc herniation
- Recurrent or persistent spinal stenosis
- Postlaminectomy instability
- Infection
- Symptomatic pseudarthrosis
- Sagittal imbalance syndrome (flatback deformity)
- Adjacent-level degenerative changes or stenosis (transition syndrome)

20. Describe common indications for posterior spinal instrumentation and fusion procedures.
- **Posterior spinal decompression and stabilization.** Symptomatic spinal stenosis is most commonly decompressed from a posterior approach. Concomitant posterior fusion and spinal instrumentation can restore posterior spinal column integrity and prevent future spinal deformities. A wide range of pathology (e.g. fractures, tumors, spondylolisthesis) requiring decompression and fusion may be treated from a posterior approach

intervertebral disc and/or vertebral body. Debridement, decompression, arthrodesis, and stabilization are most directly achieved from an anterior approach
- **Anterior correction of spinal deformity.** Anterior fusion combined with use of anterior spinal instrumentation is an effective method for treatment of select cases of scoliosis and other spinal deformities
- **To enhance arthrodesis.** The anterior spinal column provides a highly vascularized fusion bed, which promotes successful arthrodesis. The addition of an anterior fusion increases the rate of successful arthrodesis when a posterior spinal instrumentation and fusion are performed for challenging cases
- **Anterior release or destabilization to enhance posterior spinal deformity correction.** Improved correction of rigid spinal deformities using posterior spinal instrumentation can be achieved by resection of disc or bone from the anterior spinal column
- **To restore anterior spinal column lead sharing.** Normally 80% of axial load is transmitted through the anterior spinal column and 20% through the posterior spinal column. Restoration of anterior spinal load sharing is required to restore stability to mechanically compromised spinal segments

22. **What are common indications for surgically addressing the anterior spinal column in conjunction with posterior spinal fusion and instrumentation?**
- Spinal pathology that compromises anterior spinal column load sharing, as well as the posterior spinal tension band (e.g. isthmic spondylolisthesis, vertebral destruction of major proportions due to tumor, infection, trauma)
- To enhance arthrodesis (e.g. pseudarthrosis repair, treatment of postlaminectomy instability)
- Treatment of severe spinal deformities (e.g. adult scoliosis, rigid spinal deformities)
- To prevent *crankshaft phenomenon* (spinal deformity progression occurring after a healed posterior fusion due to continued anterior spinal growth) in pediatric patients with congenital scoliosis, neuromuscular scoliosis and early-onset idiopathic scoliosis

An anterior column fusion can be performed through either a posterior approach or a separate anterior surgical approach depending on clinical circumstances (Fig. 20-1).

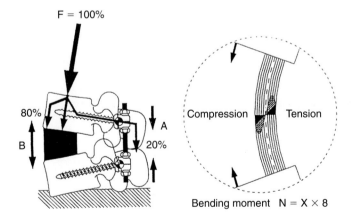

Figure 20-1. Anterior column load sharing and the posterior tension band principle. The normal biomechanics of the lumbar spine is such that 80% of axial load passes through the anterior spinal column and 20% of load passes through the posterior spinal column **(A)**. The posterior spinal column is controlled by the erector muscles of the trunk, which apply dorsal compression forces against an intact anterior spinal column (tension band principle). The efficacy of the tension band principle directly depends on the intactness of the anterior spinal column **(B)**. (From Harms J. Screw-threaded rod system in spinal fusion surgery. Spine State Art Rev 1992;6:541–75, with permission.)

23. **Describe factors that may influence decision making regarding spinal surgery in clinical scenarios where multiple treatment options exist or evidence to support the best treatment is unclear. How can patients and physicians work together in this situation?**
Decision making regarding treatment options for spinal disorders, such as symptomatic degenerative disc problems, is challenging as the best available evidence regarding treatment is conflicting. Factors that have been reported to influence surgeon decision making include surgeon training, anecdotal experience, value judgments regarding patients,

and local standards, as well as external and/or market forces. In these scenarios where several choices for treatment exist, the use of *shared decision making* is advocated. The surgeon's role is to:

1. Describe the patient's condition accurately
2. Present the best available medical evidence regarding risks, benefits, and realistic outcomes of various treatment options
3. Assist the patient in clarifying his or her preferences and values regarding treatment alternatives
4. Guide the patient through this process while maintaining neutrality. Use of *decision aids* is an option to facilitate this process. However, patient desire to be involved in the decision-making process varies from person to person. Although all patients want to be well informed, some prefer to delegate basic decisions and technical details to their surgeons.

Key Points

1. General indications for surgical intervention for spinal disorders include decompression, stabilization, and deformity correction.
2. By providing evidence-based information on surgical options and outcomes, surgeons can partner with patients through *shared decision making* to determine the preferred treatment course for spine pathologies having multiple potential treatment options.

Websites

1. Dartmouth-Hitchcock Center for Shared Decision Making: http://www.dhmc.org/shared_decision_making.cfm
2. Specific Indications for Spine Surgery (video): http://www.uwtv.org/programs/displayevent.aspx?rID=4166
3. Spine Surgery: What you need to know. http://www.spineuniverse.com/displayarticle.php/article3502.html

BIBLIOGRAPHY

1. Bridwell KH, DeWald RL. The Textbook of Spinal Surgery. 2nd ed. Philadelphia: Lippincott-Raven; 1997.
2. Enker P. Formula for a successful surgical outcome. Presented at the Fourth Annual International Spine Workshop, Cleveland Spine and Arthritis Center at Lutheran Hospital, Cleveland, OH, February, 1992.
3. Frymoyer JW, Wiesel SW. The Adult and Pediatric Spine. 3rd ed. Philadelphia: Lippincott; 2004.
4. Herkowitz HN, Garfin SR, Eismont FJ, et al. Rothman and Simeone The Spine. 5th ed. Philadelphia: Saunders; 2006.
5. Patchell RA, Tibbs PA, Regine WF, et al. Direct decompressive surgical resection in the treatment of spinal cord compression caused by metastatic cancer: A randomized trial. Lancet 2005;366:643–8.
6. Weiner BK, Essis FM. Patient preferences regarding spine surgical decision making. Spine 2006;31:2857–60.
7. Weinstein JN. The missing piece: Embracing shared decision making to reform health care. Spine 2000;25:1–4.
8. White AA, Panjabi MM. Clinical Biomechanics of the Spine. 2nd ed. Philadelphia: Lippincott; 1990.

1. **In what situations is it unrealistic to perform surgery for a patient with a spinal disorder?**

   Decisions can only be made on a case-by-case basis after a complete physical examination, imaging workup, and medical risk assessment have been completed. Some situations in which spinal surgery would not be advised include:

   - When the general medical condition of the patient is a contraindication to an appropriate surgical procedure
   - In the presence of global spinal pathology not amenable to focal surgical treatment (e.g. axial pain secondary to diffuse degenerative disc changes involving the cervical, thoracic, and lumbar spine may be beyond surgical remedy)
   - Poor soft tissue coverage over the posterior aspect of the spine, which is not reconstructible with plastic surgery techniques
   - Severe infection that cannot be eradicated
   - Lack of correlation between imaging studies and the patient's symptoms
   - Patients with unrealistic expectations and goals with respect to surgical outcome
   - Patients with profound psychological disorders

2. **How is surgical decision making for degenerative spinal disorders different from decision making for spinal disorders secondary to trauma, tumor, or infection?**

   Spinal disorders secondary to tumor, trauma, and infection frequently require surgical intervention on an emergent or urgent basis. These disorders are structural problems in which surgical decision making involves determination of the need for spinal decompression and the optimal surgical procedure to restore spinal biomechanics. Degenerative spinal problems usually require surgery on an elective basis. The patient has the opportunity to maximize available nonsurgical treatment options before considering surgery. Decision making for degenerative disorders not only involves restoration of spinal biomechanics but also encompasses a multitude of psychologic and socioeconomic issues. It is important that patients undergoing elective spine surgery for degenerative disorders be educated about realistic expectations and goals regarding pain and physical function in relation to surgery.

3. **What surgeon factors negatively influence the decision to proceed with a spinal operation?**

   Spinal surgery has a significant risk of serious complications, including problems such as permanent neurologic deficit. This type of surgery should be performed by surgeons with prerequisite training and experience. There is little role in modern spinal surgery for the surgeon who performs only occasional spine surgery. The current trend is for spinal surgery to be performed by orthopedic surgeons or neurosurgeons who devote the majority of their practice to the diagnosis and treatment of spinal disorders in facilities with adequate equipment and support staff.

4. **What patient factors can be modified before a spinal fusion procedure to improve surgical outcome?**

   - *Nutritional status:* Poor nutritional status increases the risk of infection and wound-healing problems
   - *Smoking:* Nicotine use decreases fusion success and increases risk of postoperative pulmonary complications
   - *Use of nonsteroidal antiinflammatory medication:* Nonspecific NSAIDs inhibit platelet aggregation, whereas COX-2 specific agents lack this effect. Although a controversial area, there is some evidence to suggest an association between decreased fusion rates and use of NSAIDs
   - *Assessment and treatment of osteoporosis:* Osteoporosis compromises spinal fixation and is associated with adjacent-level fractures following spinal fusion with posterior instrumentation

5. **What patient psychosocial factors may negatively influence the decision to proceed with a spinal operation?**

   Substance abuse (alcoholism, drug dependence), severe depression or other psychologic disturbance (e.g. borderline personality), secondary gain (litigation, financial, social), chronic pain, as well as childhood developmental risk factors (physical abuse, sexual abuse, abandonment, neglect, chemically dependent parents).

6. **What is the role of Waddell signs in deciding whether or not to proceed with a lumbar spine operation?**

A brief screening for nonorganic signs as described by Waddell is valuable. These signs include:
- *Tenderness* (superficial and/or nonanatomic)
- *Simulation* (low back pain with axial loading of the skull or rotation of shoulders and pelvis)
- *Distraction* (marked improvement of pain on straight leg raising with distraction)
- *Regional disturbance* (nonanatomic findings on sensory or motor examination)
- *Overreaction* (disproportionate pain behaviors during examination)

The presence of three of more of these signs suggests that the patient does not have a straightforward physical problem and that psychologic factors also need to be considered. Certain patients require both operative management of their spinal pathology and careful management of the psychosocial and behavioral aspects of their illness. Assessment of behavioral signs is not a complete psychological assessment and should not be used to deny appropriately indicated treatment.

7. **Why is the presence of degenerative disc changes, disc herniation, or spinal stenosis on magnetic resonance imaging (MRI) an insufficient basis for determining the need for surgical intervention?**

MRI of the spine is a highly sensitive but not highly specific. Many findings reported on spinal imaging studies are common in asymptomatic individuals. Decisions about the need for surgical intervention must rely on correlation of symptomatology and imaging studies.

8. **A 50-year-old male executive presents to the office of a surgeon after a lumbar MRI scan ordered by his primary care physician. The patient has experienced symptoms of intermittent mechanical low back pain without radiculopathy over the past 3 months. According to the radiologist's report, the patient has severe degenerative disc disease. The patient is extremely worried and is interested in having the disease corrected with an operation. Is surgical treatment indicated?**

No. Degeneration of the lumbar intervertebral disc is part of the normal aging process and is not properly termed a disease. In a study of lumbar MRI scans in asymptomatic subjects, degenerative disc changes were seen in 34% of patients between 20 and 39 years, 59% of patients between 40 and 50 years, and in 93% of patients between 60 and 80 years. This patient should be evaluated with standing radiographs of the lumbar spine and undergo a detailed history and physical examination. If evaluation reveals no serious underlying problem, the patient can be reassured and nonsurgical treatment can be initiated.

9. **A 15-year-old football player is evaluated on a preseason examination and reports a history of intermittent low back pain. Presently he is not experiencing low back pain symptoms. Radiographs show an L5 spondylolysis. Is surgical treatment indicated?**

No. The patient is asymptomatic, and prophylactic surgery is not indicated. Children and adolescents with spondylolysis and low-grade spondylolisthesis usually respond to nonoperative treatment measures and often can avoid surgery.

10. **A 40-year-old man is referred for consultation after a lumbar MRI showed a large extruded disc fragment at L5–S1 level. The patient noted the onset of severe back and radicular pain 1 month ago. Since that time, the patient reports greater than 50% reduction in back and leg pain. The patient reported initial mild weakness of ankle plantarflexion, which has improved. The patient has no difficulty with gait and has no symptoms to suggest cauda equina syndrome. The patient is presently working at an office job. Should surgery be recommended at this time?**

No. This patient is likely to experience a good outcome with nonsurgical treatment. Prognostic factors that suggest a positive outcome with nonoperative care include:
- A large disc extrusion or sequestration
- Progressive return of neurologic function within the first 12 weeks
- Relief or greater than 50% reduction in leg pain within the first 6 weeks of onset
- Absence of spinal stenosis
- Absence of pain with crossed straight leg raising
- Positive response to corticosteroid injection
- Limited psychosocial issues

11. **When is revision lumbar spinal surgery contraindicated?**

Revision spinal surgery is contraindicated in the absence of surgically correctable pathology. Severity of pain or disability, in and of itself, is not an indication for additional surgery. Symptomatic patients with problems such as recurrent herniated discs, spinal instability, pseudarthrosis, or spinal stenosis are potential candidates for additional surgery. Patients with symptoms due to problems such as scar tissue (arachnoiditis, perineural fibrosis), systemic medical disease, or psychosocial instability are unlikely to have positive outcomes if surgery is undertaken.

13. When can pyogenic spinal infections be treated without surgery?
The majority of spinal infections can be managed effectively with appropriate antibiotic therapy and brace treatment. Biopsy and blood cultures are mandatory to select appropriate antibiotic therapy. Parenteral antibiotics should be administered for a minimum period of 6 weeks. Effectiveness of antibiotic therapy can be assessed with serial erythrocyte sedimentation rates and C-reactive protein levels. The indications for surgical intervention are limited and well defined.

14. What types of spinal fractures can be treated without surgery?
CERVICAL SPINE
- Select atlas (C1) fractures
- Select type 1 and type 3 odontoid (C2) fractures
- Most hangman's fractures (C2) except type 3 injuries
- Subaxial cervical compression fractures without posterior ligamentous injury
- Isolated undisplaced fractures of the posterior elements

THORACIC AND LUMBAR SPINE
- Many compression fractures
- Select neurologically intact patients with stable thoracolumbar burst fractures without disruption of the posterior osteoligamentous complex. Fracture patterns with less than 25° kyphosis and less than 50% canal compromise in patients without associated closed-head injury or multitrauma are most appropriate.

Key Points

1. Inappropriate patient selection guarantees a poor surgical result despite how expertly a surgical procedure is performed.
2. Surgical decision making for neck and low back pain without symptomatic neurologic compression remains controversial.

Websites

1. Back pain often ends without surgery: http://www.webmd.com/back-pain/news/20070530/back-pain-often-ends-without-surgery
2. Fair and balanced view of spine fusion surgery: http://www.spine.org/Pages/ConsumerHealth/NewsAndPublicRelations/NewsReleases/2004/AFairandBalancedViewofSpineFusionSurgery.aspx
3. Patient selection for spine surgery: http://www.spineuniverse.com/displayarticle.php/article3072.html

BIBLIOGRAPHY

1. Akbarnia B, Ogilvie JW, Hammerberg KW. Debate: degenerative scoliosis: To operate or not operate. Spine 2006;31:S195–S201, 2006.
2. Boden SD, Davis DO, Dina T, et al. Abnormal magnetic resonance scans of the lumbar spine in asymptomatic subjects. J Bone Joint Surg 1990;72A:403–8.
3. Currier BL, Kim CW, Eismont FJ. Infections of the spine. In: Herkowitz HN, Garfin SR, Eismont FJ, et al, editors. Rothman and Simeone The Spine. 5th ed. Philadelphia: Saunders; 2006. p. 1265–1316.
4. Maguire JK. Nonsurgical management of acute injuries to the spine. In: Fardon DF, Garfin SR, editors. Orthopaedic Knowledge Update–Spine 2. Rosemont, IL: American Academy of Orthopaedic Surgeons; 2002. p. 167–76.
5. Main CJ, Waddell G. Spine update: Behavioral response to examination. A reappraisal of the interpretation of "nonorganic signs." Spine 1998;23:2367–71.
6. Mirza S, Deyo R. Systematic review of randomized trials comparing lumbar fusion surgery to nonoperative care for treatment of chronic back pain. Spine 2007;32:81–23.
7. Weinstein JN, Lurie JD, Tosteson TD, et al. Surgical vs. nonsurgical treatment for lumbar degenerative spondylolisthesis. N Engl J Med 2007;356:2257–70.
8. Weinstein JN, Tosteson TD, Lurie JD, et al. Surgical vs. nonoperative treatment for lumbar disc herniation: The Spine Patient Outcomes Research Trial (SPORT): a randomized trial JAMA 2006;296:2451–2459.
9. Weinstein JN, Tosteson TD, Lurie JD, et al. Surgical vs. nonsurgical therapy for lumbar spinal stenosis. N Engl J Med 2008;358:794–810.

PREOPERATIVE ASSESSMENT AND PLANNING FOR PATIENTS UNDERGOING SPINE SURGERY

Vincent J. Devlin, MD, and William O. Shaffer, MD

1. Name five factors that influence complication rates associated with spine procedures.
- Type of procedure
- Whether elective or emergency
- Chronologic age of the patient
- General health status of the patient
- Facility where surgery is performed (e.g. experience of surgeons, anesthesiologists, hospitalists, intensivists; availability of state-of-the-art imaging and spinal monitoring)

2. What types of elective spinal procedures are associated with the lowest risk of complications and perioperative morbidity?
When performed in patients without significant medical comorbidities, the following elective spinal procedures have the lowest risk profiles:
- Lumbar microdiscectomy
- Lumbar laminectomy
- Anterior cervical discectomy and fusion
- Single-level lumbar spinal instrumentation and fusion (anterior or posterior)
- Posterior instrumentation and fusion for adolescent idiopathic scoliosis

3. What types of spinal procedures are associated with a high risk of complications and perioperative morbidity?
- Revision spinal deformity procedures
- Same-day multilevel anterior-posterior spinal procedures
- Emergent spinal procedures for tumor, infection, and trauma
- Instrumentation and fusion for spinal deformities in patient with neuromuscular scoliosis

4. What types of patients are at increased risk of complications after spinal surgery?
- Pediatric patients with spinal deformities secondary to neuromuscular disease
- Patients older than 60 years requiring extensive fusion procedures, especially anterior fusions or anterior/posterior fusions
- Patients with major preoperative neurologic deficits
- Patients requiring surgery for tumor or infection
- Patients with a history of chronic steroid use
- Patients with multiple medical comorbidities

5. Once a patient has decided to pursue elective spine surgery, what three general issues require attention before the day of surgery?
1) Appropriate interdisciplinary medical evaluation to confirm that the patient is a reasonable medical candidate for anesthesia and proposed surgery
2) Coordination of equipment and personnel required for the surgical procedure
3) Patient education regarding diagnosis, treatment, and eventual recovery, including discharge planning
Exact details vary with patient factors:
- Pediatric vs. adult patients
- Associated medical comorbidities
- Procedure type (decompression vs. fusion)
- Magnitude of surgery (number of levels fused, anterior vs. posterior vs. combined procedures)
- Surgical setting (outpatient vs. inpatient)

medical problems). Medical subspecialty consultation (e.g. cardiology, pulmonology) as indicated.

7. **List key points to assess during the preoperative medical evaluation of a patient undergoing major spinal reconstructive surgery.**
   - **Cardiovascular:** Cardiac risk factors, presence of carotid disease, history of transient ischemic attacks, presence of peripheral vascular disease and/or vascular claudication, history of thromboembolic disease, presence and types of stents or pacemaker, use of antiplatelet therapy or anticoagulants. Consider option of inferior vena cava filter in select patients
   - **Pulmonary:** Specific problems noted with neuromuscular disorders, severe thoracic scoliosis, chronic obstructive pulmonary disease (COPD), sleep apnea, emphysema, and smokers
   - **Neurologic:** Document preoperative neurologic status and baseline cognitive status. Check antiseizure medication levels when appropriate
   - **Hematologic:** History of abnormal bruising or bleeding or conditions associated with coagulopathy including renal and hepatic disorders. Assess issues regarding blood donation and blood transfusion. Determine plan for antiplatelet and anticoagulation medication management in perioperative period
   - **Endocrine:** Assess risk factors for osteoporosis, optimize control of blood glucose in diabetic patients, determine need for perioperative steroids in chronic steroid users or adrenal insufficiency
   - **Renal:** Special precautions and preoperative consultation for patients with chronic renal insufficiency to assess for dialysis preoperatively
   - **Hepatic:** Increased perioperative morbidity in presence of chronic or active liver disease
   - **Rheumatologic:** Assess for cervical instability in rheumatoid arthritis patients. Consultation for perioperative management of disease modifying antirheumatic drugs, especially tumor necrosis factor (TNF)-alpha inhibitors
   - **Immune status:** Caution is required if surgery planned for immune compromised patients (e.g. oncology, human immunodeficiency virus [HIV], rheumatology patients)
   - **Nutritional status:** Assess nutritional status as deficits result in impaired wound healing and increased risk of infection
   - **Orthopaedic:** Assess for extremity contractures, presence of total joint replacements, cervical instability, or previously undiagnosed cervical myelopathy, which will influence safety of patient positioning prior to and during spine surgery
   - **Medications:** Obtain list of all medications and nutritional supplements, evaluate potential impact on spine surgery, and determine plan for perioperative medication management
   - **Patient habits:** History of smoking, alcohol use, analgesic use, drug abuse
   - **Psychological and social factors:** Assess barriers to recovery including depression and lack of home/family support

8. **What is the leading cause of death after noncardiac surgery?**
   Cardiac events in the perioperative period are the leading cause of death after noncardiac surgery.

9. **What tests are useful to assess patients at risk of a cardiac event before spinal surgery?**
   Tests for assessment of cardiac status include 12-lead ECG, treadmill exercise stress testing, pharmacologic stress testing (e.g. adenosine, dipyridamole, dobutamine), nuclear imaging, echocardiography, and cardiac catheterization. Indications for testing are based on cardiac risk factors and the patient's functional status according to American College of Cardiology/American Heart Association (ACC/AHA) guidelines.

10. **How is cardiac risk stratified before surgery?**
    Guidelines for cardiac risk stratification developed by the American College of Cardiology and American Heart Association include assessment of:
    A. *CLINICAL RISK FACTORS*
    - Major: Unstable coronary syndromes, decompensated congestive heart failure (CHF), significant arrhythmia, severe valvular disease
    - Intermediate: Mild angina pectoris, prior myocardial infarction, compensated CHF, diabetes mellitus, renal insufficiency
    - Minor: Advanced age, abnormal ECG, rhythm other than sinus, low functional capacity, history of stroke, uncontrolled hypertension

B. *PROCEDURAL RISK FACTORS*
- High risk: Major emergency surgery, vascular surgery, any procedure that is prolonged with large fluid shifts, blood loss, or both
- Intermediate risk: General orthopedic procedures, carotid endarterectomies, peritoneal and thoracic procedures
- Low risk: Endoscopic procedure, superficial procedure, cataract surgery, breast surgery

C. PATIENT'S FUNCTIONAL STATUS. RATED AS EXCELLENT, MODERATE, OR POOR
Application of an algorithm based on these guidelines leads to a decision to proceed with surgery, to cancel surgery pending coronary artery intervention, or to delay surgery for additional noninvasive cardiac testing. The most recent guidelines (2007) determine the need for additional cardiac evaluation prior to elective surgery based on a **Revised Cardiac Risk Index** and the patient's **functional status** quantified in metabolic equivalents (METS).

11. What are the risk factors for perioperative stroke?
Major risk factors include advanced age, history of transient ischemic attacks, hypertension, cardiac abnormalities (e.g. atrial fibrillation), diabetes, and prior stroke. Patients with a history of transient ischemic attacks should be referred for a duplex ultrasonography before undergoing an elective spine procedure. Carotid bruits in the absence of symptoms do not necessarily warrant additional workup.

12. When is a pulmonary consultation advisable before spinal surgery?
- Thoracic spinal deformities
- Neuromuscular spinal deformities
- Patients with known pulmonary problems (asthma, COPD, sleep apnea, emphysema) or smoking history

13. What results on preoperative arterial blood gas testing suggest the presence of significant pulmonary disease?
A baseline arterial carbon dioxide pressure ($PaCO_2$) of greater than 50 mm Hg or chronic hypoxemia should raise concern about the possibility of pulmonary hypertension or cor pulmonale. Such patients have an increased risk of postoperative respiratory failure.

14. Which patients are likely to require ventilatory support after spinal surgery?
Patients are extubated following spine surgery according to accepted anesthesia protocols. Specific situations where extubation may be delayed include:
- Patients with significant preoperative impairment of pulmonary function
- Patients undergoing same-day multilevel anterior and posterior thoracolumbar fusion procedures involving extensive blood loss and fluid shifts
- Patients undergoing extensive anterior or circumferential cervical surgery due to risk of postoperative neck edema and resultant airway obstruction

15. Why are smokers at increased risk of complications following spinal procedures compared with nonsmokers?
Smoking increases the risk of cardiopulmonary problems after surgery (e.g. atelectasis, pneumonia). Cessation of smoking 2 months before surgery reduces the risk of pulmonary complications fourfold. Smoking also decreases the rate of successful spinal fusion.

16. List key points relating to neurologic assessment before spinal procedures.
- Document the presence of any preoperative neurologic deficits
- Determine the patient's ability to cooperate with a wake-up test (rarely required)
- Consider a neurology consultation if a history of seizure disorder is present
- Obtain neurosurgery consultation if spinal deformity correction is planned in a patient with a central nervous system (CNS) shunt

17. Why is nutritional assessment important? How is a patient's nutritional status quantified?
Malnutrition increases the chance of postoperative infection and wound healing complications. Serum albumin less than 3.5 mg/dL, total lymphocyte count less than 1500 to 2000 cells/mm, transferrin less than 200 mg/dL, and prealbumin less than 20 mg/dL are considered to represent clinical malnutrition.

18. What are the options for blood transfusion if significant blood loss is anticipated during a spinal procedure?
- **Autologous blood (use of the patient's own blood).** Candidates for this option typically require a hematocrit of at least 34%, weigh at least 100 pounds, are 12 to 75 years old, and do not have significant medical comorbidities. The patient's own blood may also be salvaged during surgery through use of a cell saver
- **Directed donor blood.** The patient may specify family members or selected individuals to donate blood before surgery. In general, a safety margin is not provided to the patient by selecting his or her blood donors

before surgery in select patients. An autologous blood donation program also ensures increased marrow production of blood. Hematology consultation is valuable for complex patients.

20. Does the presence of diabetes increase the risk of complications associated with spine surgery?

Yes. The presence of diabetes increases the risk of impaired wound healing and wound infection in patients undergoing spine surgery. In addition, insulin-dependent diabetic patients who undergo decompression for radiculopathy have less favorable outcomes, especially if peripheral neuropathy is present. Optimization of blood glucose levels preoperatively can result in improved wound healing and decreased infection rates.

21. What laboratory tests can be used as a screen for alcoholism in the preoperative period?

Increased red-cell mean corpuscular volume (MCV) and increases in the hepatic enzyme gamma glutamyltransferase have been described as confirmatory markers for alcoholism.

22. What problems may occur in alcoholic patients who undergo spine surgery?

- Alcohol withdrawal symptoms (autonomic dysfunction, seizures, hallucinations, delirium)
- Altered metabolism of medications including anesthetic agents
- Abnormal hemostasis due to decrease in vitamin K-dependent clotting factors and platelet abnormalities
- Metabolic abnormalities: hypoglycemia, ketoacidosis, malnutrition, nutrient deficiencies (thiamine, folate and magnesium)

23. What problems are encountered following spinal procedures in patients who abuse opioids or benzodiazepines?

Postoperative problems include difficulty with pain control due to drug tolerance and patient anxiety.

24. List basic equipment/facility requirements for undertaking complex spinal surgical procedures.

- Range of spinal implants and ancillary instrumentation
- Power equipment (e.g. surgical drills and burrs)
- Imaging capability (radiographs, fluoroscopy)
- Radiolucent spine table
- Anesthesiologists familiar with anesthetic requirements for intraoperative neurophysiologic monitoring
- Spinal monitoring capability
- Surgical microscope
- Blood recovery system (cell saver)
- Bone bank access
- Appropriate perioperative medical and surgical support services including intensive care facilities when indicated

25. What is the best way to ensure that a patient has been adequately educated about diagnosis, treatment, and recovery before an elective spinal procedure?

Arrange a conference with the patient and his or her significant others before surgery. Important points to cover during this meeting include:

- Review patient's specific spinal problem and treatment alternatives
- Review pertinent diagnostic studies
- Explain specific surgical procedures using spine models (incisions, bone graft, implants, Food and Drug Administration [FDA] status of spinal devices)
- Discuss realistic expectations and goals of surgical treatment (pain relief, deformity correction, neurologic improvement, likely outcome of procedure)
- Discuss possible surgical complications, obtain informed consent, and document this process in the medical record
- Confirm arrangements for blood donation, cessation of aspirin and antiinflammatory medication, cessation of smoking, spinal monitoring, review of wake-up test (if needed), and orthosis (if needed).
- Order any additional imaging studies required for preoperative planning
- Review final recommendations and evaluations by consultants (anesthesiologist, internist, cardiologist, pulmonologist)

- Outline events on the day of surgery for the patient and family: check-in procedures and waiting area, duration of surgery, and patient's postoperative location and status (ICU vs. step down vs. standard floor vs. outpatient; discuss need for postoperative ventilatory support (when appropriate). Arrange for hospital tour (if appropriate)
- Review anticipated hospital course/discharge arrangements: length of stay, discharge planning concerns, work-related issues, psychologic support during recovery period, and chemical dependency issues related to use of narcotic medication

26. What common complications should be explained to the patient before performing a procedure for decompression of the spinal cord and/or nerve roots?

- Neurologic injury
- Dural tear
- Spinal instability
- Persistent or increased back and/or extremity pain
- Blood loss
- Wound infection
- Complications related to the surgical approach
- Potential need for subsequent spinal surgery including stabilization procedures
- Medical complications—urinary tract infection, myocardial infarction, deep vein thrombosis
- Anesthetic complication
- Arachnoiditis
- Death

27. What common complications should be explained to the patient before surgical procedures that involve spinal instrumentation and fusion?

- Implant/bone graft failure, misplacement, or dislodgement
- Neurologic injury, including paralysis and loss of bowel and bladder control
- Pseudarthrosis (failure of fusion)
- Bone graft donor site pain
- Infection
- Blood loss
- Diseases transmitted by blood transfusion or allograft bone
- Dural tear
- Persistent or increased back and/or extremity pain
- Need for subsequent spinal surgery
- Medical complications: urinary tract infection, myocardial infarction, pneumonia, deep vein thrombosis, pulmonary embolism, stroke
- Allergic reaction (to drugs, metallic devices)
- Surgical approach-related complications (e.g. hernia, retrograde ejaculation in men, vascular injury, visceral injury, dysphagia)
- Visual difficulty or blindness
- Pressure sores on chest, facial areas, pelvis, and lower extremities
- Anesthetic complication
- Death

Key Points

1. Comprehensive preoperative evaluation and planning decreases perioperative complications and optimizes patient outcomes following spine surgery.
2. Patient education regarding diagnosis, treatment alternatives, complications, and anticipated recovery is an integral component of the preoperative planning process.

Websites

1. 2007 ACC/AHA practice guideline on perioperative cardiovascular evaluation for noncardiac surgery: http://circ.ahajournals.org/cgi/reprint/CIRCULATIONAHA.107.185700
2. 2002 ACC/AHA practice guideline on perioperative cardiovascular evaluation for noncardiac surgery: http://americanheart.org/downloadable/heart/1013454973885perio_update.pdf
3. Perioperative pocket manual: http://enotes.tripod.com/periop-0.htm
4. Medical consultation guidelines: http://medicine.ucsf.edu/education/resed/handbook/HospH2002_C14.htm

BIBLIOGRAPHY

1. Baldus C, Blanke K. Preoperative nursing care. In: Bridwell KH, DeWald RL, editors. The Textbook of Spinal Surgery. ed. 2. Philadelphia: Lippincott-Raven; 1997. p. 3–10.
2. Devlin VJ, Williams DA. Decision making and perioperative care of the patient. In: Margulies JY, Aebi M, Farcy JP, editors. Revision Spine Surgery. St. Louis: Mosby; 1999. p. 297–319.
3. Eagle KA, Berger PB, Calkins H, et al. ACC/AHA guidelines update for perioperative cardiovascular evaluation for noncardiac surgery-executive summary. J Am Coll Cardiol 2002;39:542–53.
4. Faciszewski T, Jensen R, Rokey R, et al. Cardiac risk stratification of patients with symptomatic spinal stenosis. Clin Orthop Rel Res 2001;384:110–15.
5. Fleisher LA, Beckman JA, Brown KA, et al. ACC/AHA 2007 guidelines on perioperative cardiovascular evaluation and care for noncardiac surgery: Executive summary. Circulation 2007;116:1971–96.
6. Hu SS, Berven SH. Preparing the adult deformity patient for spine surgery. Spine 2006;31:S126–S131.
7. Reeg SE. A review of comorbidities and spinal surgery. Clin Orthop Rel Res 2001;384:101–9.

1. **What steps can spinal surgeons follow to maximize the likelihood of a successful outcome after spinal decompression procedures?**
   - Rely on high-quality imaging studies (computed tomography [CT], magnetic resonance imaging [MRI], CT-myelography) for preoperative planning
   - Operate only when the clinical history and physical examination correlate with spinal imaging studies
   - Use prophylactic intravenous antibiotics immediately prior to surgery
   - Minimize exposure-related damage to spinal structures (muscles, ligaments, facet joints, bone, nerve tissue)
   - Operate with adequate lighting, exposure, and use of loupe magnification or a microscope
   - Confirm that the proper surgical level(s) have been exposed by taking an intraoperative radiograph or fluoroscopic image
   - Assess spinal stability before wound closure. Perform a spinal fusion if spinal instability has been created as a result of the decompression procedure or if spinal instability was present before surgery

2. **Distinguish among laminotomy, laminectomy, and laminoplasty.**
   All three procedures are performed through a posterior approach and are intended to provide posterior decompression of neural structures.
   A **laminotomy** consists of partial lamina or facet joint removal to expose and decompress the nerve root and/or dural sac (see Fig. 23-1B).
   A **laminectomy** consists of removal of the spinous process and the entire lamina to achieve decompression (see Fig. 23-1C).

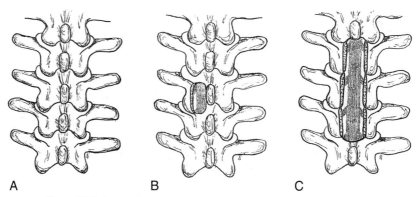

Figure 23-1. Lumbar decompression. **A,** Preoperative. **B,** Laminotomy. **C,** Laminectomy.

A **laminoplasty** provides decompression of the neural elements by enlarging the spinal canal with a surgical technique (Fig. 23-2) that avoids removal of the posterior spinal elements. Various laminoplasty techniques permit preservation and reconstruction of the posterior osseous and ligamentous structures of the spinal column without the need for fusion. Laminoplasty techniques are most commonly utilized in the cervical spine.

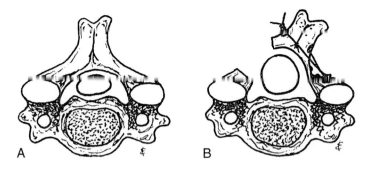

Figure 23-2. Cervical laminoplasty: **A,** Preoperative. **B,** Postoperative.

A

B

3. Distinguish among anterior discectomy, corpectomy, and vertebrectomy.

- An **anterior discectomy** procedure is indicated to relieve anterior neural compression localized to the level of the disc space. It involves removal of the intervertebral disc and any osteophytes that compress the neural elements. The space formerly occupied by the disc is filled with bone graft or a fusion cage (Fig. 23-3)
- A **corpectomy** (*corpus,* another word for vertebral body) entails removal of the vertebral body combined with removal of the superior and inferior adjoining discs (Fig. 23-4). The resultant anterior spinal column defect is reconstructed with an anterior bone graft or fusion cage and usually stabilized with anterior and/or posterior spinal instrumentation. A corpectomy is indicated to relieve anterior neural compression that extends behind a vertebral body or to remove a vertebral body whose structural integrity is compromised (e.g. tumor, infection, fracture)
- A **vertebrectomy** is a more radical procedure consisting of removal of the posterior spinal elements (spinous process, lamina, pedicles) in addition to removal of the vertebral body. This procedure creates severe spinal instability and is performed in conjunction with anterior and posterior spinal instrumentation and fusion

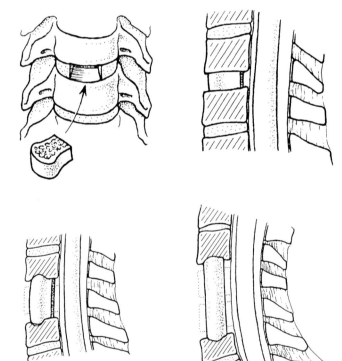

Figure 23-3. Anterior cervical decompression: discectomy. (From Miller, EJ, Aebi M. Anterior fusion of the cervical spine. Spine State Art Rev 1992;6: 459–74.)

Figure 23-4. Anterior cervical decompression: single level and multilevel corpectomy. (From Miller, EJ, Aebi M. Anterior fusion of the cervical spine. Spine State Art Rev 1992;6:459–74.)

exposure of the axillary process, a thin rim... junction is required for treatment of tumors (e.g. chordoma in the region of the clivus) and for resection of the odontoid process in rheumatoid arthritis patients with irreducible C1–C2 subluxations.

6. What are the options for surgical decompression of a C5–C6 disc herniation?
- An **anterior approach** is most commonly used to remove a cervical disc herniation, especially when it is large and centrally located. Anterior surgical options include anterior discectomy and fusion or artificial disc replacement. Anterior **discectomy and fusion** are initiated by removing the majority of the disc and leaving the lateral annulus on either side intact. The posterior annulus and posterior longitudinal ligament are removed, and any loose disc fragments are removed from the epidural space. After the disc is removed, a bone graft is placed in the disc space. Typically, an anterior cervical plate is applied as well. Alternatively, an **artificial disc replacement** may be placed into the defect, which provides for stabilization but preserves segmental spinal motion
- An alternative surgical option is to perform a **posterior laminoforaminotomy.** A posterior laminoforaminotomy approach is appropriate for removal of disc fragments located posterolaterally but does not provide sufficient exposure for safe removal of central disc herniations

7. Discuss the indications for a cervical laminotomy.
A cervical *laminotomy* is performed for treatment of a posterolateral disc herniation or foraminal stenosis. The lamina and facets are partially removed to provide posterior exposure of the nerve root and adjacent disc. Direct decompression of the nerve root is termed a *foraminotomy.*

8. When is the posterior surgical approach considered for decompression of cervical spinal stenosis?
Posterior surgical approaches for cervical spinal stenosis are most commonly recommended when three or more levels require decompression. An important prerequisite to successful decompression from a posterior approach is the presence of a neutral to lordotic sagittal alignment, which permits dorsal migration of the spinal cord away from anterior compressive pathology.

9. When is the anterior surgical approach considered for decompression of cervical spinal stenosis?
Anterior surgical approaches for treatment of cervical spinal stenosis are widely used for treatment of cervical spinal stenosis in patients with three or fewer levels of involvement. Successful decompression can be achieved regardless of whether the patients has lordotic, neutral, or kyphotic sagittal plane alignment. Multilevel discectomy and interbody fusion are appropriate when neural compression is localized to the level of the disc space. Anterior corpectomy and strut grafting are appropriate when cord compression extends beyond the disc level or when a significant kyphotic deformity is present.

10. When is a combined anterior and posterior approach considered for treatment of cervical spinal stenosis?
- Multilevel cervical stenosis requiring three or more levels of anterior decompression
- Multilevel cervical stenosis requiring two or more levels of corpectomy
- Multilevel cervical stenosis associated with cervical kyphotic deformity
- Rigid post-traumatic or postlaminectomy kyphotic deformities

11. Compare the advantages and disadvantages of cervical laminectomy, cervical laminoplasty, and cervical laminectomy with fusion for treatment of multilevel cervical spinal stenosis.
- **Cervical laminectomy** has been widely used for decompression of cervical stenosis with satisfactory results in a high percentage of patients. Its advantage is its simplicity. Disadvantages include the tendency to produce segmental instability, postoperative kyphotic deformity, and late neurologic deterioration in certain patients
- **Cervical laminoplasty** has been popularized to address some of the problems associated with cervical laminectomy. Retention of the posterior spinal elements decreases the likelihood of postoperative spinal instability and extensive postoperative epidural scar formation. Because the procedure is performed without fusion, cervical motion is preserved. However, postoperative neck pain may be problematic after laminoplasty procedures
- **Cervical laminectomy combined with lateral mass fusion and screw-rod fixation** continues to play a role in the treatment of multilevel cervical spinal stenosis. It is an effective means of decompressing the spinal canal in

patients with neutral or lordotic cervical alignment. Fusion prevents the development of postoperative kyphosis and can improve neck pain symptoms. Disadvantages include loss of cervical motion and the complexity of the procedure

12. What nerve root injury is most common after cervical laminectomy or laminoplasty?

C5 nerve root dysfunction is the most common nerve root problem after cervical laminectomy or laminoplasty. Nerve root dysfunction may be noted immediately after surgery, or it may develop 1 to 5 days after surgery. The exact cause of C5 dysfunction is not entirely clear, but it has been attributed to the following factors: (1) the C5 root is the shortest cervical root, (2) C5 is usually located at the midpoint of the decompression—the segment that undergoes the greatest dorsal shift after decompression, and (3) C5 root deficits are easily detectable on clinical examination because the C5 root provides sole innervation to the deltoid muscle.

13. Give three examples of clinical situations in which a cervical corpectomy is indicated.

A corpectomy is indicated for anterior spinal cord compression due to:
1. Vertebral body tumor extending into the spinal canal
2. Vertebral body fracture with retropulsion of bony fragments into the spinal canal
3. Ossification of the posterior longitudinal ligament in a patient with kyphotic deformity

14. What factors are involved in determining the appropriate surgical approach for treatment of a thoracic disc herniation?

Factors to consider in determining the appropriate surgical approach (anterior vs. posterior) include:
- Location of the disc herniation relative to the spinal cord (central, centrolateral, lateral)
- Level of the disc herniation (upper thoracic, midthoracic, thoracolumbar junction)
- Nature of the herniated disc material (calcified vs. noncalcified)
- Surgeon's familiarity with different surgical approaches

15. Is laminectomy a reasonable approach for treatment of a thoracic disc herniation?

No! Midline laminectomy approaches should be avoided because of their poor historical results. This approach is associated with a high rate of complications, including paraplegia. Laminectomy provides poor access to the centrolateral aspect of the disc space, and retraction of the spinal cord is not advised because of the risk of paraplegia.

16. What anterior surgical approaches are used for treatment of a thoracic disc herniation?

- **Open thoracotomy approach:** Best for disc herniations between T4 and T12
- **Thoracoscopic approach:** Easiest for midthoracic disc herniations but requires specialized equipment and training
- **Transsternal or medial clavisectomy approach:** Anterior access from T2 to T4 is difficult with the first two approaches and may require one of these more complex approaches. Both are associated with significant exposure-related morbidity

17. What posterior surgical approaches are used for treatment of a thoracic disc herniation?

- **Costotransversectomy approach:** The transverse process–rib articulation is disrupted, and the portion of the rib overlying the disc is removed. This approach provides posterolateral access to the vertebral body and the disc
- **Lateral extracavitary approach:** This approach is similar to but more extensive than the costotransversectomy approach. Portions of the transverse process, rib head, pedicle, and facet are resected to provide more extensive access to the disc space
- **Transpedicular approach:** This midline approach involves removal of the facet joint and medial portion of the pedicle to achieve access to the portion of the disc space lateral to the spinal cord without the need to retract this structure

18. Describe the three basic steps involved in performing a thoracic or lumbar corpectomy after the exposure has been performed, including ligation of the segmental vessels.

1. The discs above and below the target vertebral body are removed. This procedure facilitates removal of the vertebral body by providing reference landmarks for the depth and position of the spinal canal.
2. The vertebral body is then removed. The anterior two thirds of the vertebral body is rapidly removed with a rongeur, osteotome, or burr. The remaining posterior wall of the vertebral body is thinned with a burr. This procedure facilitates the more delicate removal of the posterior vertebral cortex with a curette or Kerrison rongeur to expose the spinal canal, posterior longitudinal ligament, and dural sac.
3. The space created after corpectomy is filled with a structural bone graft or a cage to restore anterior column support. Anterior and/or posterior spinal implants are used to provide additional stability.

An anterior approach is most commonly utilized for treatment of infections involving the disc and vertebral bodies and for drainage of paravertebral abscesses. The disc space is the most common location for pyogenic infection. As the disc space becomes infected and purulent material enters the anterior epidural space, anterior neural compression develops. An anterior epidural abscess may occur. A paravertebral abscess may develop as infection spreads along the anterior or anterolateral aspect of the spinal column.

21. In treatment of spinal infections, when is a posterior surgical approach indicated?
A posterior approach is used when an epidural abscess develops posterior to the dural sac in the absence of anterior disc space infection. In this case, a laminectomy or bilateral laminotomies is performed.

22. Describe three techniques for decompression of a thoracolumbar burst fracture associated with a retropulsed bone fragment that causes neurologic deficit.
1. Indirect decompression achieved by use of posterior spinal instrumentation, fusion, *ligamentotaxis,* and realignment of the spinal deformity
2. Direct posterolateral decompression via a laminectomy or transpedicular approach, combined with use of posterior spinal instrumentation and fusion
3. Direct anterior decompression with corpectomy and reconstruction, combined with anterior and/or posterior spinal instrumentation

23. What structures typically compress the spinal cord and nerve roots in patients with congenital scoliosis or kyphosis?
Spinal cord compression in congenital scoliosis and kyphosis is frequently caused by the posterior part of a hemivertebra. When scoliosis is present, a pedicle at the apex of the curvature may compress the spinal cord and nerve roots.

24. Describe two ways that decompression can be performed to treat a patient with congenital kyphosis and symptomatic spinal cord compression.
1. Perform a first-stage transthoracic or transabdominal anterior approach and then perform a corpectomy including removal of the pedicle. Subsequent posterior decompression and spinal stabilization are also required
2. Remove the pedicle, transverse process, rib, and portion of the body compressing the spinal cord via a posterolateral approach. Posterior spinal stabilization is performed as part of the procedure

25. What determines the approach for decompression of a lumbar disc herniation?
In contrast to the cervical and thoracic spinal regions, posterior approaches are typically utilized for lumbar discectomy. The neural elements in the lumbar region include the cauda equina and individual nerve roots, which may be retracted without fear of iatrogenic injury. The primary factor guiding selection of the operative approach is the **location of the disc fragment**. Disc herniations located in the central or posterolateral region of the spinal canal are easily removed through a **laminotomy approach.** Disc herniations located in the foraminal and extraforaminal zone are most directly decompressed through a **paraspinal or intertransverse approach.**

26. Describe a lumbar laminotomy procedure for removal of a disc herniation.
A laminotomy is performed on the side of the disc herniation. An intraoperative radiograph or fluoroscopic image is taken to confirm the proper level of exposure. Sufficient bone and ligamentum flavum are removed to permit visualization of the lateral edge of the nerve root. Retraction of the nerve root and removal of the disc fragment are performed under magnification (loupes or microscope).

27. Describe a paraspinal approach for removal of a foraminal lumbar disc herniation.
The muscles attached to the midline bony structures are left intact. An incision is made in the fascia lateral to the midline. Blunt dissection is carried down to the transverse processes. The transverse processes are identified, and the intertransverse membrane is exposed. A radiograph is obtained to confirm that the correct spinal level has been exposed. The intertransverse membrane is then released, the nerve root is identified and retracted medially, and the disc herniation is removed.

28. What are the surgical options for decompression of lumbar spinal stenosis?
- **Single or multilevel laminotomy.** This technique can be used for single-level or multilevel stenosis when the neural compression is localized to the level of the disc space. This technique has the advantage of preserving the stability

provided by midline bony and ligamentous structures. It is somewhat more difficult and more time-consuming than a laminectomy when performed for multilevel stenosis (Fig. 23-1B).

- **Single-level or multilevel laminectomy.** This technique may be used for any type of spinal stenosis problem and is required for treatment of congenital lumbar spinal stenosis. The disadvantage of this technique is its tendency to destabilize the spinal column (Fig. 23-1C).

29. **When should the surgeon perform a spinal arthrodesis after decompression for lumbar spinal stenosis?**
   - Following intraoperative destabilization (removal of more than 50% of both facet joints, complete removal of a single facet joint, disruption of the pars interarticularis)
   - For patients with significant lumbar scoliosis
   - For patients with spondylolisthesis or lateral listhesis at the level of decompression

Key Points

1. The selection of the appropriate procedure for spinal decompression depends on a variety of factors including clinical symptoms, spinal level, location of compression, number of involved levels, and the presence/absence of spinal instability or spinal deformity.
2. Spinal arthrodesis and spinal instrumentation are indicated in conjunction with decompression in the presence of spinal deformity or spinal instability or when decompression results in destabilization at the surgical site.

Websites

Spine surgical procedures: http://www.orthospine.com/index.php/surgical-procedures-mainmenu-27
Laminotomy versus laminectomy: http://www.spineuniverse.com/treatments/surgery/laminotomy-versus-laminectomy

BIBLIOGRAPHY

1. Bilsky MH, Boland P, Lis E, et al. Single-stage posterolateral transpedicle approach for spondylectomy, epidural decompression and circumferential fusion of spinal metastases. Spine 2000;25:2240–50.
2. Edwards CC, Heller JG, Hideki M. Corpectomy versus laminoplasty for multilevel cervical myelopathy: An independent matched-cohort analysis. Spine 2002;27:1168–75.
3. Kim DH, Henn JS, Vaccaro AR, et al. Surgical Anatomy and Techniques to the Spine. Philadelphia: Saunders; 2006.
4. McCulloch JA, Young PH. Essentials of Spinal Microsurgery. Philadelphia: Lippincott-Raven; 1998.
5. Osterman H, Seitsalo S, Karppinen J, et al. Effectiveness of microdiscectomy for lumbar disc herniation: A randomized controlled trial with 2 years of follow-up. Spine 2006;31:2409–14.
6. Vaccaro AR, Baron EM. Spine Surgery: Operative Techniques. Philadelphia: Saunders; 2006.

1. Define spinal arthrodesis.

Spinal arthrodesis is defined as the elimination of motion across an intervertebral segment as a result of bony union (fusion). During surgery adjacent bone surfaces are decorticated, bone graft material is applied, and spinal instrumentation or subsequent external immobilization is used to decrease motion at the surgical site and facilitate fusion.

2. What are the three main categories of spinal arthrodesis procedures?

Anterior column fusion, posterior column fusion, and circumferential fusion (also called 360° fusion, global fusion, or combined anterior and posterior column fusion).

3. What is the role of spinal instrumentation in spinal arthrodesis procedures?

Spinal instrumentation may be used to correct a spinal deformity or to stabilize a spinal segment whose structural integrity has been compromised by spinal pathology such as a fracture, tumor, or infection. Spinal instrumentation may be used to limit intersegmental motion and to create a favorable mechanical environment that increases the likelihood of successful fusion.

4. Name common indications for performing a spinal arthrodesis and provide at least one clinical example for each indication.

- *Trauma:* burst fractures, fracture-dislocations, flexion-distraction injuries
- *Tumor:* pathologic spine fracture secondary to metastatic or primary tumor
- *Infection:* spinal instability due to disc space infection or vertebral osteomyelitis
- *Rheumatologic disorders:* C1–C2 instability due to rheumatoid arthritis
- *Spinal deformities:* scoliosis, kyphosis, congenital deformities
- *Degenerative spinal disorders:* degenerative spondylolisthesis with spinal stenosis

5. What factors influence successful healing of a spinal fusion?

1. **Type of bone graft used** (autograft, allograft, synthetic biomaterials)
2. **Local factors:**
- Quality of the soft tissue bed into which bone graft is placed
- Method of preparation of the graft recipient site
- Mechanical stability of the spine segment(s) to be fused
- Graft location (anterior vs. posterior spinal column)
- Spinal region (the cervical region is considered a more favorable environment for fusion than the thoracic or lumbar regions)
3. **Systemic host factors:**
- Metabolic bone disease (e.g. osteoporosis)
- Nutrition
- Perioperative medication
- Smoking

6. How does tobacco use interfere with spinal fusion?

The rate of successful spinal arthrodesis in smokers is lower than in nonsmokers. Cigarette smoking has been shown to interfere with bone metabolism and inhibit bone formation. Nicotine is considered the agent responsible for these adverse effects. The precise mechanisms responsible remain under investigation and include inhibition of graft revascularization and neovascularization, as well as osteoblast suppression. These effects are mediated by inhibition of cytokines.

7. What common medications may potentially interfere with healing of a spinal fusion?

Certain medications have potential to impair fusion if used in the perioperative period because they inhibit or delay bone formation. Examples include nonsteroidal antiinflammatory drugs (e.g. ibuprofen, Toradol), cytotoxic drugs (e.g. methotrexate, doxorubicin), certain antibiotics (e.g. ciprofloxacin), and anticoagulants (e.g. Coumadin). Recent evidence has shown that the adverse effects of nonsteroidal antiinflammatory medications on spinal fusion are related to dose and duration of administration. Low-dose ketorolac tromethamineToradol (30 mg intravenous every 6 hours for 48 hours) has been shown to lack an adverse effect on lumbar fusion rates.

8. **What are the common sources for bone graft material used in spinal arthrodesis procedures?**

Graft options for spinal fusion include autograft, allograft, and synthetics. Sources for autograft bone include the patient's fibula, ribs, and ilium. Autograft may be procured as a structural or nonstructural graft. The ratio of cancellous to cortical bone varies depending on the bone graft site and technique of graft procurement. Allograft bone is human cadaveric bone that can be stored as either a fresh-frozen or freeze-dried preparation. It is available in a variety of shapes and composition similar to autograft bone. Allograft bone may also undergo processing by acid extraction to remove bone mineral while retaining collagen and noncollagenous proteins. The end product is demineralized bone matrix (DBM), an allograft form with osteoinductive activity. Additional graft materials available for use in fusion procedures include ceramics, polymers, composite materials, and bone morphogenetic proteins (BMPs). Bone marrow aspirate (BMA) may be combined with graft material to improve its osteogenic potential.

9. **Discuss fundamental differences between cortical and cancellous bone graft in spinal applications.**

Cortical bone can be used to provide immediate structural stability. Cortical bone is incorporated by creeping substitution, which occurs slowly over years. Cancellous bone provides a porous matrix essential for osteogenesis in areas not requiring immediate structural support. Cancellous bone is incorporated much more rapidly than cortical bone because of direct bone apposition onto the scaffold provided by bony trabeculae.

10. **Compare and contrast the healing potential of the anterior spinal column and posterior spinal column with respect to spinal fusion.**

Biomechanical factors are different in the anterior and posterior spinal columns. In the lumbar region it is estimated that 80% of the body's load passes through the anterior spinal column, and 20% passes through the posterior spinal column. Thus, bone graft placed in the anterior column is subjected to compressive loading, which promotes fusion. In the anterior spinal column, the wide bony surface area combined with the excellent vascularity of the fusion bed creates a superior biologic milieu for fusion. In contrast, bone graft placed in the posterior column is subjected to tensile forces, which provide a less favorable healing environment. In the posterior spinal column, fusion is more dependent on biologic factors such as the presence of osteogenic cells, osteoinductive factors, and the quality of the soft tissue bed into which the graft material is placed. Thus, the posterior spinal column is a more challenging environment in which to achieve a spinal fusion.

11. **What anatomic structures provide potential sites for posterior spinal arthrodesis?**

In the *cervical region*, posterior spinal fusions are achieved by applying bone graft to the lamina, facet joints, and spinous process. In the *thoracic and lumbar regions*, the lamina, facet joints, spinous processes, and transverse processes are available sites for arthrodesis. These bone surfaces require meticulous preparation including removal of all overlying soft tissue prior to graft application. In addition, it is critical to remove the outer cortical bone surface (decortication) in order to expose underlying cancellous bone and provide access to the pluripotent stem cells within the patient's bone marrow in order to achieve a consistent and high likelihood of successful fusion. See Figure 24-1.

Figure 24-1. Posterior spinal arthrodesis technique. **A,** Posterior fusion. Posterior osseous structures (lamina, facet joints, transverse processes) are cleaned of soft tissue, and the outer cortical bone is removed (decortication) to expose underlying cancellous bone. **B,** Facet joint fusion. The facet joint cartilage is excised, and the joint surfaces are prepared for bone graft application. (From Laurin CA, Riley LH Jr, Roy-Camille R. Atlas of Orthopaedic Surgery. vol. 1. General principles. Spine. Chicago: Year Book Medical Publishers, inc., and Paris: Masson; 1989.)

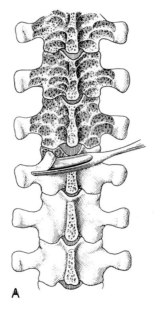

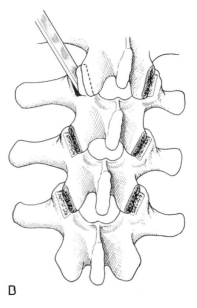

A   B

patient undergoing posterior fusion, an alternative form of autogenous bone graft (e.g. rib) or a mixture of autogenous local bone graft from the surgical site in combination with a graft extender or enhancer (morselized allograft, DBM, BMA) is recommended to increase the likelihood of successful posterior fusion. Recent studies have provided evidence to support the use of bone morphogenetic protein (rhBMP-2) in combination with synthetic carriers or combined with local autograft in posterior fusion applications. However, at the current time posterior use of rhBMP-2 remains an off-label use. Additional graft materials include ceramics, polymers, and composite materials, which may be combined with BMA or synthetic osteoinductive factors.

13. **What bone graft alternatives are available for use in anterior spinal fusion procedures?**
Both autograft and allograft bone graft have been reported to provide reasonable fusion rates in the anterior spinal column. The high rate of fusion obtained with autograft must be weighed against the morbidity of harvesting large sections of autogenous bone graft from the pelvis. Use of anterior and/or posterior spinal instrumentation can improve fusion rates when structural allograft bone grafts are used. Additional graft options include synthetic cages used in combination with BMPs, nonstructural allograft, or synthetic osteoconductive materials.

14. **Explain the difference between nonstructural and structural bone grafts.**
Bone grafts placed in the anterior spinal column may be classified as:
- **Nonstructural grafts** (also termed *morselized* grafts) typically consist of particles of cancellous bone (e.g. from the iliac crest) placed into a defect in the anterior spinal column (e.g. after discectomy). This type of graft is intended to promote arthrodesis between adjacent vertebral bodies. The graft itself does not restore structural stability to the anterior spinal column. Use of adjunctive spinal instrumentation is generally required to facilitate bony union
- **Structural grafts** contain a cortical bone surface that can provide mechanical support during the process of fusion consolidation. Anterior bone graft constructs may be classified according to location as *strut grafts*, *interbody grafts*, or *transvertebral grafts*
See Figure 24-2.

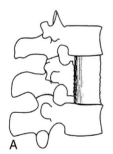 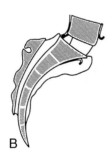 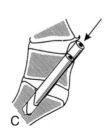

A　　　　　B　　　　　C

Figure 24-2. **A,** Anterior graft constructs may be described as strut grafts; **B,** interbody grafts or **C,** transvertebral grafts. (From Devlin VJ, Pitt DD. The evolution of surgery of the anterior spinal column. Spine State Art Rev 1998;12:493–528.)

15. **What graft options are available for interbody fusion in the cervical, thoracic, and lumbar spinal regions?**
- In the **cervical region,** the most frequently used interbody graft material is allograft bone graft. Iliac autograft bone graft remains an excellent option but has become less popular due to associated donor site morbidity and the widespread availability of allograft. The most common interbody graft configurations are a tricortical horseshoe-shaped graft or a cylindrical cortical graft. Fusion cages are an additional option for use in cervical interbody fusion
- In the **thoracic region,** graft options include rib graft, autogenous iliac graft, structural and nonstructural allograft, and fusion cages combined with autograft and/or allograft
- In the **lumbar spine,** both nonstructural and structural grafts are used depending on a variety of factors. Structural graft options for interbody fusion include autograft (iliac crest); allograft (femur, ilium, tibia); and a variety of interbody fusion cage devices that are generally used in combination with nonstructural bone graft, BMPs, or synthetic osteoconductive materials
See Figure 24-3.

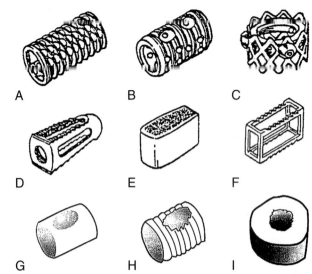

Figure 24-3. Options for lumbar interbody fusion. **A,** Ray cylindrical threaded fusion cage. **B,** BAK cylindrical threaded fusion cage. **C,** Surgical titanium mesh. **D,** Tapered (lordotic) fusion cage. **E,** Iliac crest autograft or allograft bone. **F,** Carbon fiber fusion cage. **G,** Nonthreaded femoral cortical bone dowel. **H,** Threaded femoral cortical bone dowel. **I,** Femoral ring allograft. (From Devlin VJ, Pitt DD. The evolution of surgery of the anterior spinal column. Spine State Art Rev 1998;12:493–528.)

16. What are fusion cages?

Fusion cages are devices intended to provide structural support to the anterior spinal column following removal of an intervertebral disc or vertebral body. These devices are generally used in conjunction with bone graft and supplemental fixation. The cage is intended to restore immediate mechanical stability to the anterior spinal column and provide a favorable environment for bone graft healing. Cages are available in a variety of shapes and materials (titanium, carbon fiber, PEEK, cortical bone). Cages may be implanted from a variety of surgical approaches (e.g. anterior, lateral, posterolateral, transforaminal) depending on the specific spinal region and type of pathology requiring surgical treatment.

17. What graft options are available after corpectomy in the cervical, thoracic, and lumbar spinal regions?

- In the **cervical region,** one- or two-level corpectomies are most commonly reconstructed using tricortical iliac autograft or fibula allograft combined with spinal instrumentation. For reconstruction of two or more vertebral levels, a fibular allograft graft or fusion cage is most commonly used in combination with spinal instrumentation
- In the **thoracic and lumbar regions,** a wide variety of structural graft options are available including autograft, allograft, fusion cages, and bone cement. Adjunctive spinal instrumentation is used in combination with strut grafts
    See Table 24-1.

18. What is the most common indication for placement of a transvertebral graft?

A transvertebral graft is most commonly used in the surgical treatment of high-grade lumbar spondylolisthesis when a reduction or resection procedure is undesirable. Typically a fibular autograft or allograft is placed from either a posterior or anterior approach to bridge L5 and the sacrum. The graft is typically combined with posterolateral spinal fusion and instrumentation.

19. When does a surgeon use the anterior iliac crest or the posterior iliac crest for harvesting bone grafts?

Factors to consider in selecting the graft site include the volume of bone graft required and the patient's position during surgery. The posterior iliac crest can supply a greater volume of bone than the anterior iliac crest. Patient position during surgery is also a factor. When the patient is in the prone position, the posterior third of the ilium is more easily accessible, whereas in the supine position the anterior third of the ilium is easier to access.
    See Figure 24-4.

20. List complications associated with harvesting autograft from the ilium.

- Infection
- Donor site pain
- Superior gluteal artery injury
- Pelvic fracture
- Sacroiliac joint violation
- Damage to the sciatic nerve
- Meralgia paresthetica (lateral femoral cutaneous nerve injury)
- Lumbar hernia
- Cluneal nerve transection

21. Define nonunion following a spinal fusion procedure.

Nonunion or pseudarthrosis is defined as the failure of an attempted fusion to heal within 1 year after surgery.

Autograft—rib	Can be harvested during surgical exposure	Low initial strength precludes use as a structural graft
Allograft—structural (e.g. femur, tibia)	High initial strength No donor site morbidity Versatile Can be filled with autograft	Slow osseous incorporation Low risk of disease transmission
Vascular graft—rib	Relative ease of harvest Rapid healing even in compromised fusion bed	Low initial strength Use of adjunctive structural support required
Vascular graft—fibula	High initial strength Straight geometry Rapid healing even in compromised fusion bed	Technical procedure Time-consuming Donor site morbidity
Bone cement (PMMA)	No donor morbidity Adequate resistance to compressive loading	Biologically inert Finite lifespan Late loosening and failure
Synthetic fusion cage	High strength No donor site morbidity Can be customized to fill any bony defect Serrations provide resistance to shear forces	Subsidence in osteopenic bone may be problematic Osseous integration uncertain Long-term follow-up indeterminate

PMMA, polymethylmethacrylate. From Devlin VJ, Pitt DD. The evolution of surgery of the anterior spinal column. Spine State Art Rev 1998;12:493–528.

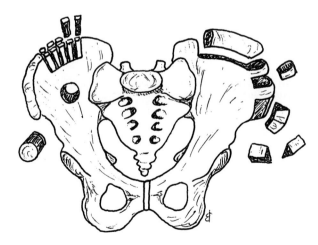

Figure 24-4. Types of anterior and posterior iliac grafts.

22. **What are the major risk factors for nonunion following a spinal fusion procedure?**
    • **Biologic factors:** Tobacco use, medication (steroids, nonsteroidal antiinflammatory medication), deep wound infection, metabolic disorders
    • **Mechanical factors:** Inadequate spinal fixation
    • **Inadequate surgical technique:** Inadequate preparation of the fusion site
    • **Graft-related factors:** Inadequate volume of bone graft, inappropriate selection of graft material (e.g. use of allograft as the sole graft material in an adult posterior fusion)

23. How is a failed spine fusion diagnosed?

Clinical symptoms such as localized pain over the fusion site should prompt suspicion of a nonunion. Confirmatory tests include plain radiographs (include flexion-extension radiographs) and computed tomography with multiplanar reconstructions. Radiographic findings that suggest pseudarthrosis include broken or loose spinal implants, progressive spinal deformity after surgery, and discontinuity in the fusion mass on radiography. Surgical exploration is the most reliable method of determining whether a fusion has successfully healed.

24. Does the presence of a nonunion after an attempted spinal fusion always cause symptoms?

No. Although many patients who develop a nonunion report pain symptoms, this is not always the case. Fusion success does not always correlate with patient outcome. However, many studies support a strong positive correlation between successful arthrodesis and positive patient outcomes.

Key Points

1. Graft options for spinal arthrodesis include autograft bone, allograft bone, synthetics, and bone morphogenetic protein (BMPs).
2. Successful posterior fusion is dependent on meticulous preparation of the graft bed, decortication of the osseous elements, and application of sufficient and appropriate graft material.
3. Fusion cages are devices intended to provide structural support to the anterior spinal column following removal of an intervertebral disc or vertebral body.

Websites

Bone graft alternatives: http://www.knowyourback.org/Documents/bone_grafts.pdf
Bone graft substitutes: http://aatb.kma.net/aatb/files/ccLibraryFiles/Filename/000000000101/AAOSbonegraftsubstitutes.pdf
Lumbar pseudarthrosis: http://www.medscape.com/viewarticle/462180

BIBLIOGRAPHY

1. Boden SD. Overview of the biology of lumbar spine fusion and principles for selecting a bone graft substitute. Spine 2002;27:S26–S31.
2. Buchowski JM, Liu G, Bunmaprasert T, et al. Anterior cervical fusion assessment: Surgical exploration versus radiographic evaluation. Spine 2008;33:1185–91.
3. Buttermann GR, Glazer PA, Hu SS, et al. Revision of failed lumbar fusions: Comparison of anterior autograft and allograft. Spine 1997;22:2748–55.
4. Fischgrund JS, Mackay M, Herkowitz HN, et al. Degenerative lumbar spondylolisthesis with spinal stenosis: A prospective, randomized study comparing decompressive laminectomy and arthrodesis with and without spinal instrumentation. Spine 1997;22:2807–12.
5. Glassman SD, Carreon LY, Djurasovic M, et al. RhBMP versus iliac crest bone graft for lumbar spine fusion: A randomized, controlled trial in patients over sixty years of age. Spine 2008;33:2843–49.
6. Pradhan BP, Tatsumi RL, Gallina J, et al. Ketorolac and spinal fusion: Does the perioperative use of ketorolac really inhibit spine fusion? Spine 2008; 33:2079–82.
7. Sandhu HS, Grewal HS, Parvataneni H. Bone grafting for spinal fusion. Orthop Clin North Am 1999;30:685–98.
8. Yazici M, Asher MA. Freeze-dried allograft for posterior spinal fusion in patients with neuromuscular spinal deformities. Spine 1997;22:1467–71.
FDA Disclosure: The U.S. Food and Drug Administration (FDA) has approved the clinical use of rhBMP-2, marketed as InFUSE™ Bone Graft, in anterior lumbar interbody fusion with rhBMP-2 on an absorbable collagen sponge carrier within specific titanium cages. Use of this product for an indication not in the approved or cleared labeling is considered "off-label use."

1. **What are the various surgical approaches to the anterior and posterior cervical spine?**

   A. Anterior
   - Transoral approach
   - Extra/lateral/retropharyngeal approaches
   - Anterolateral (Smith-Robinson) approach

   B. Posterior
   - Midline approach

POSTERIOR APPROACH TO THE CERVICAL SPINE

2. **What are the major palpable posterior anatomic landmarks and their corresponding anatomic levels?**
   - *Posterior occipital prominence:* Inion (external occipital protuberance)
   - *First palpable spinous process:* C2 spinous process
   - *Most prominent spinous process at cervicothoracic junction:* Vertebra prominens (C7)

3. **Describe the posterior exposure of the upper cervical spine.**
   The patient is placed into a reverse Trendelenburg position with a midline incision made from the external occipital protuberance to the spinous process of C2. The C2 vertebra (axis) has a large lamina and bifid spinous process that provides attachments for the rectus major and inferior oblique muscles. The bony topography between the lamina and the lateral mass of the axis is indistinct. Surgical dissection on the occiput and the ring of the atlas should be done in a careful manner. It is advisable to use gentle muscle retraction and Bovie (monopolar and bipolar) cauterization rather than any forceful subperiosteal stripping.

4. **What is the significance of the ligamentum nuchae?**
   The ligamentum nuchae (Fig. 25-1) represents the midline fascial confluence. Dissection should be carried through this ligament to decrease blood loss and to maintain a stout tissue layer for closure.

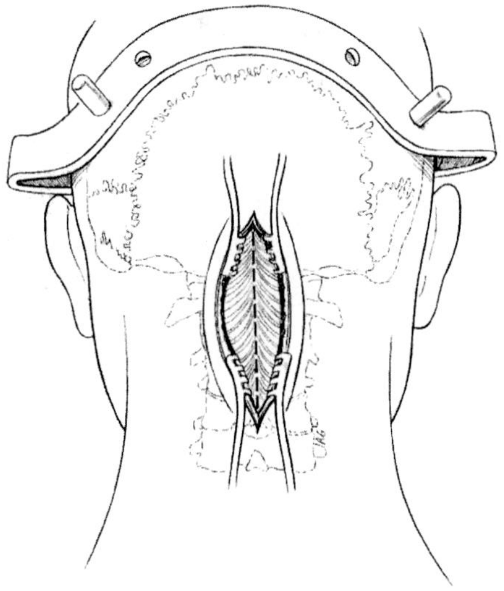

5. **What structure is at risk with lateral dissection of the atlas?**
   The vertebral artery lies lateral to the ring of the atlas (Fig. 25-2); therefore, the dissection should not be carried more than 1.5 cm lateral to the posterior midline and 8 to 10 mm laterally along the superior C1 border to avoid injury to the vertebral artery. Once the greater occipital nerve is encountered and the fragile venae comitantes of the paravertebral venous plexus are exposed, further lateral dissection endangers the vertebral artery.
   If bleeding is encountered from disruption of the venous plexus between C1 and C2, packing and hemostatic agents are usually adequate to control bleeding. If vertebral artery injury occurs, direct repair, manual pressure, and ligation are options for control of hemorrhage.

Figure 25-1. Ligamentum nuchae. (From Winter R, Lonstein J, Denis F, et al. Posterior upper cervical procedures: Atlas of Spinal Surgery. Philadelphia: Saunders; 1995. p. 21.)

6. **Describe the course of the vertebral artery in the cervical spine.**
   The vertebral artery arises from the subclavian artery. It enters the transverse foramen at C6 in 95% of people and courses upward through the foramina above. At C1, the vertebral artery exits from the foramen, courses medially on the superior groove of the posterior ring of the atlas, and enters the foramen magnum to unite with the opposite vertebral artery to form the basilar artery.

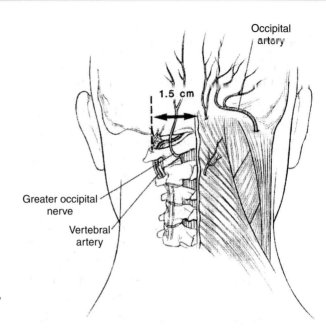

Occipital artery

1.5 cm

Greater occipital nerve

Vertebral artery

Figure 25-2. Vertebral artery. (From Winter R, Lonstein J, Denis F, et al. Posterior upper cervical procedures: Atlas of Spinal Surgery. Philadelphia: Saunders; 1995. p. 23.)

7. **Where is the vertebral artery injured most frequently in upper cervical spine exposures?**
   The vertebral artery is injured most frequently just lateral to the C1–C2 facet articulation and at the superior lateral aspect of the arch of C1.

8. **Why is the patient placed in a reverse Trendelenburg position?**
   The reverse Trendelenburg position allows venous drainage away from the surgical field and toward the heart, which decreases bleeding during the procedure.

9. **Describe the posterior exposure of the lower cervical spine.**
   The midline posterior exposure is the most common approach used in the cervical spine. Care is taken to carry dissection through the ligamentum nuchae to minimize blood loss. Once the tips of the spinous processes are identified at the appropriate levels through radiographic confirmation, subperiosteal dissection of the posterior elements is then carried out. The posterior approach is extensile and is easily extended proximally to the occiput and distally to the thoracic spinal region.

10. **What functional consequences may arise from lateral dissection of the paraspinal muscles?**
    Lateral dissection carries the potential risk of denervation of the paraspinal musculature. Inadequate approximation of the posterior cervical musculature may lead to a fish gill appearance of the posterior paraspinal muscles and possible loss of the normal cervical lordosis.

11. **Why is it important to expose only the levels to be fused, especially in children?**
    A process termed *creeping fusion extension* may occur when unwanted spinal levels are exposed during the fusion procedure. This is especially common in children and may lead to unintended fusion at these spinal levels.

12. **What complications are associated with the posterior approach to the cervical spine?**
    Complications include postlaminectomy kyphosis due to muscular denervation or following decompression, radiculopathy, epidural hematoma, and loss of neck range of motion. Postoperative paralysis and paresis, particularly of the C5 nerve root, are also associated with a posterior cervical laminectomy or laminoplasty.

ANTERIOR APPROACHES TO THE CERVICAL SPINE

13. **What are the indications for a transoral approach to the upper cervical spine?**
    Pathology at the craniocervical junction (CCJ) with an anterior midline component (e.g. tumor), which is not amenable to decompression by a posterior approach. A transoral approach allows direct access to CCJ from mid-clivus to the superior aspect of C3.

the pharyngeal mucosa and muscle. The anterior longitudinal ligament and tubercle of the atlas are exposed subperiosteally, and the longus colli muscles are mobilized laterally. A high-speed burr may be used to remove the anterior arch of the atlas to expose the odontoid process (Fig. 25-4).

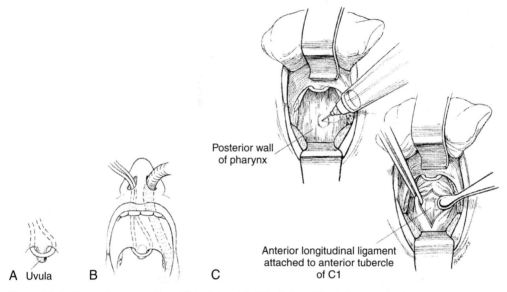

Posterior wall
of pharynx

Anterior longitudinal ligament
attached to anterior tubercle
A Uvula   B   C   of C1

Figure 25-3. Transoral exposure. (From Winter R, Lonstein J, Denis F, et al. Posterior upper cervical procedures: Atlas of Spinal Surgery. Philadelphia: Saunders; 1995. p. 3.)

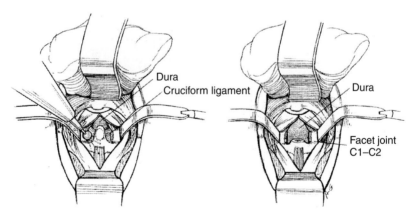

Dura
Cruciform ligament   Dura

Facet joint
C1–C2

Figure 25-4. Removal of C1 arch. (From Winter R, Lonstein J, Denis F, et al. Posterior upper cervical procedures: Atlas of Spinal Surgery. Philadelphia: Saunders; 1995. p. 5.)

16. What preoperative patient care factors must be addressed before undergoing a transoral decompression?

All oropharyngeal or dental infections must be treated before elective surgery because wound infection rates are high with this approach. The oral cavity is cleansed with chlorhexidine before surgery, and after surgery perioperative antibiotics are given for 48 to 72 hours (often a cephalosporin and metronidazole).

17. Describe the incision and superficial dissection for the retropharyngeal approach to the upper cervical spine.

A skin incision is made along the anterior aspect of the sternocleidomastoid muscle and is curved toward the mastoid process. The platysma and the superficial layer of the deep cervical fascia are divided in the line of the incision to expose the anterior border of the sternocleidomastoid. The submandibular gland and digastric muscle are identified (Figs. 25-5 and 25-6).

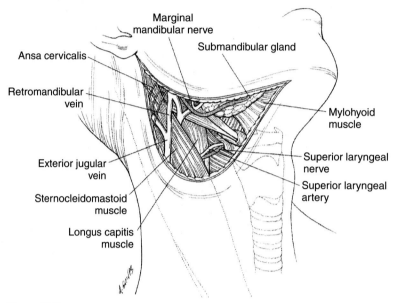

Figure 25-5. Anterior retropharyngeal approach. (From Winter R, Lonstein J, Denis F, et al. Posterior upper cervical procedures: Atlas of Spinal Surgery. Philadelphia: Saunders; 1995. p. 10.)

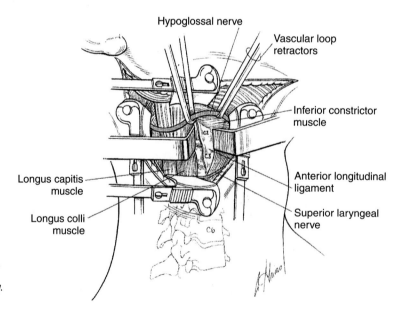

Figure 25-6. Anterior retropharyngeal approach–deep dissection. (From Winter R, Lonstein J, Denis F, et al. Posterior upper cervical procedures: Atlas of Spinal Surgery. Philadelphia: Saunders; 1995. p. 11.)

18. What two vessels are ligated once the sternocleidomastoid is retracted?

The superior thyroid artery and the lingual vessels.

19. What nerve may be potentially injured in this approach, resulting in a painful neuroma?

The marginal branch of the facial nerve.

23. Name the palpable anatomic landmarks used to identify the level of exposure of the lower cervical spine.

The angle of the mandible (C2–C3), the hyoid bone (C3), upper aspect of thyroid cartilage (C4–C5), cricoid membrane (C5–C6), carotid tubercle (C6), and the cricoid cartilage (C6).

24. Describe the anterior lateral or Smith-Robinson approach to the lower or subaxial cervical spine.

A transverse incision is made over the interspace of interest in Langer's lines to improve the cosmetic appearance of the surgical scar. The incision is carried slightly laterally beyond the anterior border of the sternocleidomastoid muscle and almost to the midline of the neck. The subcutaneous tissue is divided in line with the skin incision. The platysma may be divided along the line of the incision, or its fibers may be bluntly dissected and its medial-lateral divisions retracted (Fig. 25-7). The anterior border of the sternocleidomastoid is identified, and the fascia anterior to this muscle is incised. The sternocleidomastoid is retracted laterally and the strap muscles are retracted medially to permit incision of the pretracheal fascia medial to the carotid sheath. The sternocleidomastoid and carotid sheath are retracted laterally, and the strap muscles and visceral structures (trachea, larynx, esophagus, thyroid) are retracted medially. The anterior aspect of the spine, including the paired longus colli muscles, are now visualized.

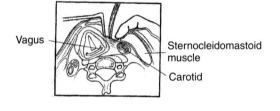

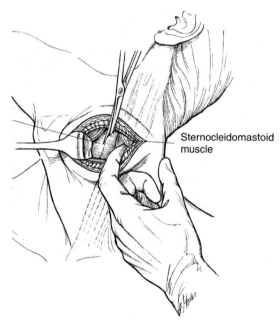

Figure 25-7. Exposure of the lower anterior cervical spine. (From Winter R, Lonstein J, Denis F, et al. Posterior upper cervical procedures: Atlas of Spinal Surgery. Philadelphia: Saunders; 1995. p. 53.)

25. What is the function of the platysma muscle and its corresponding innervation?

The platysma is an embryologic remnant serving no functional importance. It receives its innervation from the seventh cranial nerve.

26. Once the platysma and the superficial cervical fascia are divided, what neurovascular structure is at risk for injury?

The carotid sheath. It contains three neurovascular structures: internal jugular vein, carotid artery, and vagus nerve.

27. What structures are at risk when dissecting through the pretracheal fascia of the neck?

The superior and inferior thyroid arteries may be injured during dissection through the pretracheal fascial layer. Dissection is normally done in a longitudinal manner, using digital dissection.

28. What fascial layer is encountered after dissection through the pretracheal fascia?

After dissection through the pretracheal fascia, the prevertebral fascia or retropharyngeal space is encountered. The prevertebral fascia is split longitudinally, exposing the anterior longitudinal ligament. The longus colli muscle is elevated bilaterally and retracted laterally until the anterior surface of the vertebral body is exposed.

29. What structures are at risk when the dissection is carried too far laterally on the vertebral body in the subaxial spine?

Dissection carried too far laterally may risk injury to the vertebral artery traversing through the foramen transversarium or damage the sympathetic plexus.

30. What are the advantages and disadvantages of approaching the cervical spine anteriorly from the right or left side?

Smith and Robinson advocated using the left-sided approach to decrease the risk of damaging the recurrent laryngeal nerve. On the right side, this nerve loops beneath the right subclavian artery and then travels in a relatively horizontal course in the neck, increasing its chances of damage with exposure in this region. However, most right-handed surgeons find the right-sided approach more facile because the mandible is not an obstruction. A right-sided exposure avoids damage to the thoracic duct. Also, the cervical esophagus is retracted less due to its normal anterior position on the left side of the neck. Overall, either side can be used for the anterior approach because evidence does not suggest one side to be safer than the other.

31. Name the potential causes of dysphagia after anterior cervical surgery.

Dysphagia may be secondary to postoperative edema, hemorrhage, denervation (recurrent laryngeal nerve), or infection. If persistent dysphagia is present, a barium swallow or endoscopy should be considered.

32. Damage to the sympathetic chain may result in what clinical condition?

Horner's syndrome, which is manifested by a lack of sympathetic response resulting in anhydrosis, ptosis, miosis, and enophthalmos. The cervical sympathetic chain lies on the anterior surface of the longus colli muscles posterior to the carotid sheath. Subperiosteal dissection is important to prevent damage to these nerves. Horner's syndrome is usually temporary; permanent sequelae occur in less than 1% of cases.

33. Describe the rare but serious complication of esophageal perforation.

Patients usually manifest symptoms in the postoperative period related to development of an abscess, tracheoesophageal fistula, or mediastinitis. The usual treatment consists of intravenous antibiotics, nasogastric feeding, drainage, debridement, and repair.

Key Points

1. The transoral approach to the craniocervical junction is indicated for fixed deformity causing anterior midline neural compression.
2. The posterior midline approach is extensile and provides access from the occiput to the thoracic region.
3. A key to the anterior approach to the cervical spine is understanding the anatomy of the fascial layers of the neck.

Websites

Approaches to the spinal column: http://medind.nic.in/jae/t02/i1/jaet02i1p76.pdf
Anterior transoral resection: http://www.beverlyhillsspinesurgery.com/webdocuments/siddique-a2.pdf

BIBLIOGRAPHY

1. An H. Surgical exposures and fusion techniques of the spine. In: An H, editor. Principles and Techniques of Spine Surgery. Baltimore: Williams & Wilkins; 1998. p. 31–62.
2. Liu J, Apfelbaum R, Schmidt M. Anterior surgical anatomy and approaches to the cervical spine. In: Kim D, Vaccaro A, Fessler R, editors. Spinal Instrumentation: Surgical Techniques. New York: Thieme; 2005. p. 59–69.
3. McAfee PC, Bohlman HH, Riley LH Jr, et al. The anterior retropharyngeal approach to the upper part of the cervical spine. J Bone Joint Surg 1987;69A:1371–83.
4. Misra S. Posterior cervical anatomy and surgical approaches. In: Kim D, Vaccaro A, Fessler R, editors. Spinal Instrumentation: Surgical Techniques. New York: Thieme; 2005. p. 267–74.
5. Winter R, Lonstein J, Denis F, et al. Atlas of Spinal Surgery. Philadelphia: Saunders; 1995. p. 1–104.

1. **What are the indications for an anterior surgical approach to the thoracic and lumbar spine?**
   - Anterior spinal decompression and stabilization (e.g. tumor, infection, fracture)
   - Anterior correction of spinal deformity (e.g. scoliosis)
   - To enhance arthrodesis (e.g. for treatment of posterior pseudarthrosis)
   - Anterior release or destabilization to enhance posterior spinal deformity correction (e.g. for treatment of severe, rigid spinal deformities)
   - To improve biomechanics of posterior implant constructs (e.g. to restore anterior column load sharing when anterior spinal column integrity has been compromised)
   - To enhance restoration of sagittal alignment
   - To eliminate asymmetric growth potential (e.g. congenital scoliosis)

2. **List situations in which an anterior thoracic or lumbar surgical approach may not be advised.**
   - Patients who have undergone prior anterior surgery to the same spinal region. Dissection will be difficult because of adhesions and will increase the risk of visceral or vascular injury
   - Patients with poor pulmonary function may have an unacceptable risk of complications after an anterior thoracic approach
   - Patients with extensive calcification of the aorta are not ideal candidates for anterior lumbar approaches. Extensive mobilization of the great vessels is required and is associated with an increased risk of vascular complications

3. **What anterior surgical approaches may be used to expose the upper thoracic spine (T1–T4)?**
   Access to the T1 vertebral body is generally possible through a standard anterior cervical approach medial to the sternocleidomastoid muscle. Anterior exposure between T1 and T3 is challenging. Options for exposure include a modified sternoclavicular approach, a third-rib thoracotomy, or a median sternotomy. Each approach has advantages and disadvantages, depending on patient anatomy, type of spinal pathology, number of levels requiring exposure, and type of surgery required.

4. **What standard surgical approach is used to expose the anterior aspect of the spine between T2 and T12?**
   The anterior aspect of the thoracic spine between T2 and T12 is approached by a thoracotomy.

5. **What is the preferred method of positioning a patient for an approach to the anterior thoracic spine?**
   The lateral decubitus position with an axillary roll under the down-side axilla (Fig. 26-1). Many surgeons prefer approaching the thoracic spine from the left side because it is easier to work with the aorta than the vena cava.

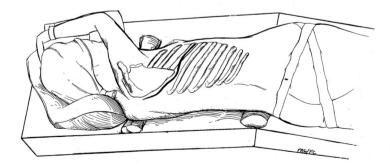

Figure 26-1. Positioning of the patient for an anterior approach to the thoracic spine. (From Majd ME, et al. Anterior approach to the spine. In: Margulies JY, Aebi M, Farcy JP, editors. Revision Spine Surgery. St. Louis: Mosby; 1999. p. 139.)

However, the type of spinal pathology may dictate the side of approach. For example, in the anterior treatment of scoliosis, the surgical approach should be on the convex side of the curve.

6. What factors determine the level of rib excision when the thoracic spine is exposed through a thoracotomy approach?

If the procedure requires exposure of a long segment of the thoracic spine (e.g. for treatment of scoliosis or kyphosis), a rib at the proximal end of the region requiring fusion is removed. For example, removal of the fifth rib allows exposure from T5 to T12.

If the patient requires treatment of a single vertebral body lesion, the rib two levels proximal to the involved vertebral body is removed. Alternatively, the rib directly horizontal to the target vertebral level at the mid-axillary line on the anteroposterior (AP) thoracic spine x-ray is removed.

If the surgeon requires only a limited exposure (e.g. to excise a thoracic disc herniation), the rib that leads to the disc should be removed (e.g. the eighth rib is removed for a T7–T8 disc herniation).

7. What are some tips for counting ribs after the chest cavity has been entered during a thoracotomy?

The first cephalad palpable rib is the second rib. The first rib is generally located within the space occupied by the second rib and cannot be easily palpated. The distance between the second and third rib is wider than the distance between the other ribs. Application of a marker on a rib with subsequent radiographic verification is important to identify the level of exposure.

8. During an anterior exposure of the thoracic spine, the parietal pleura is divided longitudinally over the length of the spine. What landmarks may be used for identification of critical anatomic structures?

The vertebral bodies are located in the depressions, and the discs are located over the prominences (Fig. 26-2). The segmental vessels are identified as they cross the vertebral bodies (depressions). This has been referred to as the *hills-and-valleys concept* (i.e. discs are the hills and vertebral bodies are the valleys).

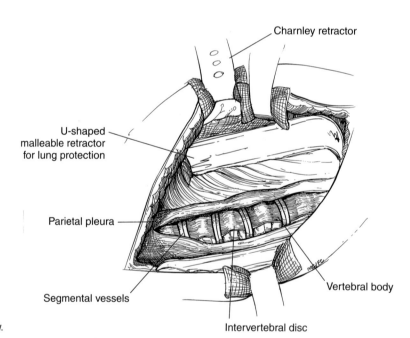

Figure 26-2. Intraoperative view of the anterior exposure of the thoracic spine. (From Majd ME, Harkess JW, Holt RT, et al. Anterior approach to the spine. In Margulies JY, Aebi M, Farcy JP, editors. Revision Spine Surgery. St. Louis: Mosby; 1999. p. 142.)

9. After the initial surgical exposure, what study should be obtained by the surgeon before proceeding with an anterior discectomy or corpectomy?

A radiograph or fluoroscopic view should be obtained to confirm that the correct spinal level has been exposed. Even if one knows anatomy very well, mistakes can be made. This strategy is very important because wrong-level surgery is not an uncommon claim in malpractice lawsuits against spine surgeons.

10. Are there any risks associated with ligation of the segmental artery and vein as they cross the vertebral bodies?

Ligation of the segmental vessels is required to obtain comprehensive exposure of the vertebral body. Unilateral vessel ligation is safe. However, ligation too close to the neural foramina may damage the segmental feeder vessels to the spinal cord. Temporary and reversible occlusion of segmental vessels may be used when the risk of paraplegia is high (congenital kyphoscoliosis, severe kyphosis, patients who have undergone prior anterior spinal surgery with vessel ligation). If there is no change in spinal potential monitoring after temporary vessel occlusion, permanent ligation may be carried out safely.

11. After thoracotomy, placement of a chest tube is necessary. What are the proper placement criteria?

The chest tube should be placed at the anterior mid-axillary line at least two interspaces from the incision. Placement of the chest tube too posteriorly has potential for kinking and can cause subsequent blockage of drainage in the supine position. In addition, posterior placement is uncomfortable and painful when the patient lies supine.

12. During a thoracic spinal exposure via thoracotomy, a creamy discharge is noted in the operative field. What anatomic structure has been violated?

The thoracic duct. Thoracic duct injuries are uncommon. Most injuries heal without intervention. Repair or ligation of the area of leakage can be attempted. Leaving the chest tube in place for several additional days can be considered. This strategy may help to avoid a chylothorax by allowing the thoracic duct to heal. If a chylothorax should develop postoperatively, treatment options include chest tube drainage, a low-fat diet, or hyperalimentation.

13. What is the standard surgical approach for exposure of the anterior aspect of the spine between T10 and L2 (thoracolumbar junction)?

Exposure in this region is achieved through a transdiaphragmatic thoracolumbar approach, also termed a *thoracophrenolumbotomy* (Fig. 26-3). The patient is positioned as for a thoracotomy. The incision typically begins over the tenth rib and extends distally to the costochondral junction, which is transected. The incision extends distally into the abdominal region as required. Dissection through the layers of the abdominal wall is carried out, and the peritoneum is mobilized from the undersurface of the diaphragm. The diaphragm is then transected from its peripheral insertion. The peritoneal sac and its contents are mobilized off the anterolateral aspect of the lumbar spine. This strategy provides the surgeon with wide continuous exposure of the spine across the two major body cavities (thoracic cavity and abdominal cavity).

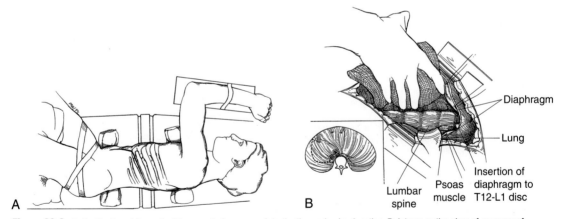

Diaphragm

Lung

Insertion of diaphragm to T12-L1 disc

Psoas muscle

Lumbar spine

A

B

Figure 26-3. **A,** Positioning of the patient for an anterior approach to the thoracolumbar junction. **B,** Intraoperative view of exposure of the thoracolumbar region. Note how the diaphragm requires detachment from its insertion along the lateral chest wall. (From Majd ME, et al. Anterior approach to the spine. In Margulies JY, Aebi M, Farcy JP, editors. Revision Spine Surgery. St. Louis: Mosby; 1999. p. 146, 147.)

14. A patient with an L1 lesion underwent an uneventful left-sided thoracoabdominal approach and corpectomy of L1. After surgery the patient complained of weakness of left hip flexion and difficulty in climbing stairs. What is the most probable cause of this problem?

In this case, the most probable cause is retraction and mobilization of the psoas muscle causing trauma to the muscle during surgery. The patient's symptoms should gradually improve without further treatment. The psoas major muscle attaches on both sides to the last thoracic and all five lumbar vertebral bodies. The psoas major is innervated by the anterior rami of the upper lumbar nerves. Its principal actions are flexion and medial rotation of hip joint. In addition, the muscle flexes the lumbar spine both anteriorly and laterally. In the sitting position, the psoas muscle is relaxed and permits kyphosis of the lumbar spine. In the standing position, the psoas muscle is taut and thus induces physiologic lumbar lordosis.

15. What are the surgical approach options for exposure of the lumbar spine and lumbosacral junction?

The most commonly used open surgical approaches to the lumbar spine and lumbosacral junction are the retroperitoneal flank approach and the medial incision retroperitoneal approach. A minimal incision direct lateral approach has recently been popularized and is applicable to all lumbar levels except L5-S1. Less commonly used approaches include the transperitoneal approach and the laparoscopic approach.

16. Describe a medial incision retroperitoneal approach to the lumbar spine.

In a medial incision retroperitoneal approach (Fig. 26-4), the patient is positioned supine. A vertical left paramedian or midline incision is commonly used. Transverse or oblique incisions are also options. The rectus sheath is incised, and the muscle is retracted to expose the transversalis fascia. The fascia is incised to enter the retroperitoneal space. Alternatively, if exposure of only L5–S1 is required, the retroperitoneal space can be entered below the arcuate line, thus avoiding the need for incising any fascia. The peritoneal sac is swept off the abdominal wall and anterior aspect of the spine to complete initial exposure.

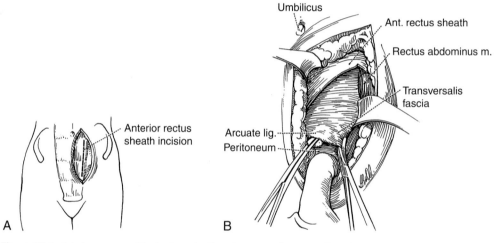

Figure 26-4. Anterior exposure of the lumbar spine through a paramedian retroperitoneal approach. **A,** A longitudinal incision is made through the fascia overlying the rectus muscle to expose the muscle belly. **B,** The arcuate ligament marks the point of entry into the retroperitoneal space. Using a sponge stick caudad to the ligament in a gentle sweeping motion, the surgeon pushes down and toward the midline to free the peritoneal sac from the fascia and displace it toward the midline, thereby exposing the spine. (From Majd ME, et al. Anterior approach to the spine. In Margulies JY, Aebi M, Farcy JP, editors. Revision Spine Surgery. St. Louis: Mosby; 1999. p. 151.)

17. What are the advantages and disadvantages of a medial incision retroperitoneal approach?

ADVANTAGES
- Provides excellent exposure from L2 through S1
- This muscle-sparing approach is less painful than a muscle-incising approach
- The direct anterior exposure facilitates graft placement and anterior decompression

DISADVANTAGES
- It cannot easily provide exposure above L2
- The anterior peritoneum is thin and easily perforated in this area
- Use of this approach is best limited to cases with moderate spinal deformity (scoliosis <40° or kyphosis <25°)

18. Describe a retroperitoneal flank approach.

In the retroperitoneal flank approach (Fig. 26-5), the patient is typically positioned in the lateral decubitus position with the left side upward. After an oblique skin incision, the layers of the abdominal wall are transected (external oblique, internal oblique, and transversus abdominis). The transversalis fascia is incised, and the peritoneum is mobilized medially to permit exposure of the psoas muscle, which overlies the anterolateral aspect of the spine.

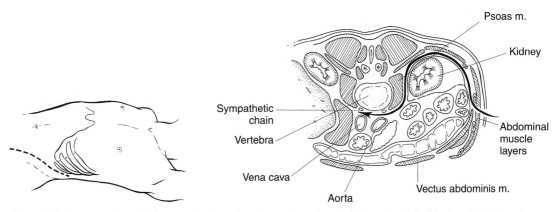

Figure 26-5. The retroperitoneal flank approach to the lumbar spine may be performed with the patient in the lateral position or the supine position. Dissection passes anterior to the psoas muscle to expose the spine. (From An HS. Surgical exposure and fusion techniques of the spine. In An HS, editor. Principles and Practice of Spine Surgery. Baltimore: Williams & Wilkins; 1985. p. 56.)

19. What are the advantages and disadvantages of the retroperitoneal flank approach?

ADVANTAGES
- Allows exposure of the entire lumbar spine and lumbosacral junction
- The extensile nature of this approach allows exposure above L2
- Useful for cases of severe spinal deformity (scoliosis >40° or kyphosis >25°)

DISADVANTAGES
- This muscle-incising approach is more painful than a muscle-splitting approach
- Muscle hernias can occur
- Exposure of the L5–S1 disc can be more difficult than with the medial incision approach

20. What are the disadvantages of a transperitoneal approach?
Extensive mobilization of the abdominal organs and packing of the intestinal contents out of the operative field increases operative time and complications. Manipulation of the abdominal contents increases the risk of postoperative ileus and intestinal adhesions. There is also a higher risk of retrograde ejaculation in male patients compared with the retroperitoneal approach.

21. What are some of the potential complications of an anterior approach to the lower lumbar and lumbosacral spine?
- Surgical sympathectomy
- Vascular injury
- Ureteral injury
- Deep vein thrombosis
- Incisional hernia
- Retrograde ejaculation

22. During the retroperitoneal exposure of the lumbosacral spine, approximately what percentage of cases is complicated by vascular injuries?
Vascular injury rates during anterior lumbar spine surgery range from 1% to 15%. These intraoperative injuries are usually recognized during surgery and repaired with simple suture techniques. The rates of postoperative morbidity and major complications from deep venous thrombosis or arterial embolization are low.

23. What is the most important factor in avoiding vascular injury during anterior lumbar spine surgery?
Knowledge of the relationship of vascular structures to the anterior lumbosacral spine is the key to avoiding vascular complications during anterior exposure of the spine (Fig. 26-6).

First, the surgeon should plan exactly how many anterior disc spaces require exposure. If exposure of only the L5–S1 disc is required, the necessary dissection is limited. However, if exposure of the L4–L5 level or multiple anterior disc levels is required, extensive vascular mobilization is necessary and the exposure will be complex.

Next, the surgeon should assess the level of the bifurcation of the aorta and vena cava. Most commonly the great vessels bifurcate at the L4–L5 disc space or at the upper part of the L5 vertebral body. However, the location of the bifurcation may vary from L4 to S1.

For exposure of the L5–S1 disc, it is necessary to ligate the middle sacral artery and vein, which lie directly over the L5-S1 disc. Exposure of the L5–S1 disc is usually achieved by working in the bifurcation of the aorta and vena cava.

For exposure of the L4–L5 disc it is generally necessary to mobilize branches originating from the distal aorta and vena cava as well as from the external iliac artery and vein. These branches tether the great vessels to the anterior aspect of the spine and limit safe left-to-right retraction of the vascular structures overlying the L4–L5 disc space.

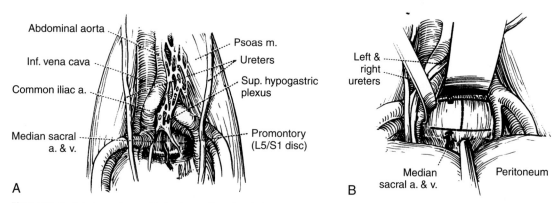

Figure 26-6. Anterior anatomy at the lumbosacral junction. **A,** Anatomic structures related to the anterior L4 to S1 region—ureter, sympathetic plexus, aorta, vena cava, and bifurcation of these vessels. **B,** Exposure of the L5–S1 disc following ligation of the middle sacral vessels. Note that both the left and right ureters are retracted toward the right side. (From Majd ME, et al. Anterior approach to the spine. In Margulies JY, Aebi M, Farcy JP, editors. Revision Spine Surgery. St. Louis: Mosby; 1999. p. 152.)

It is especially critical to identify and securely ligate the iliolumbar vein and various ascending lumbar veins. Failure to control the vessels before attempting to retract the great vessels off the L4–L5 disc can result in uncontrolled hemorrhage and even death. The segmental vessels overlying the L4 vertebral body and proximal vertebral levels may also require ligation, depending on how many levels require exposure.

24. What is the transpsoas approach to the lumbar spine?

A surgical approach has been developed for lumbar interbody graft placement from a direct lateral approach passing through the posterior retroperitoneum and the anterior portion of the psoas muscle. Tubular retractors and electrophysiologic monitoring are integral to this approach. The technique is feasible for all lumbar levels except the L5–S1 interspace.

25. A 46-year-old man underwent implantation of two cylindrical fusion cages in the L5–S1 disc space through an anterior surgical approach. One year later, the surgeon decided to revise the cages through an anterior retroperitoneal approach because the fusion did not heal and the cages were migrating out of the disc space. During the procedure scar tissue made exposure difficult, and the surgeon was concerned that an injury to the ureter had occurred. What is the best way to evaluate for this problem? What treatment is indicated if a ureteral injury exists?

Intravenous injection of 5 mL of methylene blue can appear within 5 to 10 minutes in the surgical field and confirm the ureteral injury. Urologic consultation and repair or stenting of the ureter are required. Placement of a ureteral stent before surgery helps to identify the ureter during revision anterior surgical procedures and may help to prevent this complication.

26. A 40-year-old man underwent a L5–S1 anterior lumbar interbody fusion with implantation of an anterior fusion cage. He complains of erectile dysfunction after the procedure. What should the surgeon advise the patient?

The patient should be advised that prognosis for recovery is good because erection is not controlled by any of the neural structures that course over the anterior aspect of the L5–S1 disc. The patient's difficulty is not related to the anterior approach and other underlying causes should be evaluated.

Erection is predominantly a parasympathetic function through control of the vasculature of the penis. The parasympathetic fibers responsible for erection originate from the L1–L4 nerve roots and arrive at their target area via the pelvic splanchnic nerves. Somatic function from the S1–S4 levels is carried through the pudendal nerve.

Anterior spine surgery at the L5–S1 level has the potential to disrupt the superior hypogastric plexus. This sympathetic plexus crosses the anterior aspect of the L5–S1 disc and distal aorta. The superior hypogastric plexus controls bladder neck closure during ejaculation. Failure of closure of the bladder neck during ejaculation causes ejaculate to travel in a retrograde direction into the bladder and can result in sterility.

27. During an anterior approach to the lumbosacral junction, the Bovie is used to coagulate the middle sacral artery and vein. This technique, as opposed to bipolar electrocoagulation or a suture ligation of the middle sacral artery and vessel, increases the risk for what complication?

Retrograde ejaculation. This complication has been reported more commonly with the endoscopic approach to the lumbosacral junction than with an open surgical approach. This finding has been attributed to use of a Bovie with subsequent damage to the sympathetic plexus. Male patients undergoing an anterior L5–S1 exposure should always be forewarned of this possible complication. Many surgeons do not offer an anterior exposure to men in their reproductive years for fear of this complication and its medical/legal ramifications.

28. **After the left-sided retroperitoneal approach to the lumbar spine, the patient wakes up complaining of coolness in the right lower extremity compared with the left. Palpation of pulses demonstrates good dorsalis pedis and posterior tibia pulses bilaterally, and the right leg does appear to be cooler than the left leg. How are these clinical findings explained?**
The sympathetic chain lies on the lateral border of the vertebral bodies and is often disrupted during an anterior surgical exposure. A sympathectomy effect occurs and allows increased blood flow to the left leg compared with the right. This process explains the temperature increase and occasional swelling noted in the lower extremity on the side of the surgical exposure. Patients should be forewarned of this possible result of an anterior spine procedure and told that it will not impair the ultimate outcome surgery.

29. **After a left-sided retroperitoneal exposure of the lumbosacral junction, the patient awakens in the recovery room complaining of increased pain in the left lower extremity. The left leg is noted to be cooler than the right leg. What test should be ordered immediately?**
An arteriogram should be ordered on an emergent basis. This clinical scenario cannot be explained on the basis of a sympathectomy effect by which the ipsilateral leg on the side of the exposure becomes warmer. When the distal extremity on the side of the exposure becomes cooler, it is usually due to dislodgement of an arteriosclerotic plaque. Thus, assessment of the vasculature with an arteriogram is the study of choice to determine whether the plaque has lodged in the trifurcation in the popliteal fossa. Immediate consultation with an experienced vascular surgeon is appropriate.

30. **The technique for implantation of an artificial disc requires the surgeon to place the implant as far posteriorly as possible along the vertebral endplates. During the procedure for one type of artificial disc, sequential dilators are placed in the L5–S1 interspace until a loud pop is heard or felt. This noise represents the disruption of the posterior longitudinal ligament. Aside from fainting, what should the surgeon do if a large return of blood is noted in the wound after this popping noise?**
In the case of rapid bleeding after distraction and disruption of the posterior longitudinal ligament, the presumptive diagnosis is disruption of the epidural venous plexus. The most appropriate technique at this point is to place gel foam soaked with thrombin into the posterior aspect of the interspace and then remove the distraction from the interspace. After several minutes the bleeding will stop, and the procedure may continue.

Key Point

1. Knowledge of the relationship of the visceral, vascular, and neurologic structures to the anterior and lateral aspect of the spine is the key to avoiding complications during surgical exposure.

Websites

Anterior exposure of the thoracic and lumbar spine: http://archsurg.ama-assn.org/cgi/content/full/141/10/1025
Thoracotomy for exposure of the spine: http://www.ctsnet.org/sections/clinicalresources/thoracic/expert_tech-37.html

BIBLIOGRAPHY

1. DeWald RL. Anterior exposures of the thoracolumbar spine. In: Bridwell KH, DeWald RL, editors. The Textbook of Spinal Surgery. 2nd ed. Philadelphia: Lippincott-Raven; 1997. p. 253–60.
2. Kim DH, Henn JS, Vaccaro AR, et al. Surgical Anatomy and Techniques to the Spine. Philadelphia: Saunders; 2006.
3. Majd ME, Harkess JW, Holt RT, et al. Anterior approach to the spine. In: Margulies JY, Aebi M, Farcy JP, editors. Revision Spine Surgery. St. Louis: Mosby; 1999. p. 138–55.

POSTERIOR SURGICAL APPROACHES TO THE THORACIC AND LUMBAR SPINE

Vincent J. Devlin, MD

1. **Describe the options for patient positioning for posterior surgical approaches to the thoracic and lumbar spinal regions.**
Typically patients are positioned prone on a radiolucent operative frame for posterior approaches to the thoracic and lumbar spine. An exception is the use of a lateral decubitus position during simultaneous anterior and posterior surgical procedures.

2. **What are the basic types of positioning frames for posterior spinal procedures?**
   - **Four-post frame:** Proximal pads are placed beneath the pectoral region and distal pads are placed in the region of the anterior superior iliac spines. The hip joints and lower extremities are positioned parallel with the trunk. Spine-specific operating room tables are available, which incorporate this design (e.g. Jackson spinal table)
   - **Wilson frame:** Longitudinal curved pads are attached to a frame, which can be raised or lowered to alter lumbar lordosis
   - **Knee-chest frame:** The patient's hips and knees are positioned at 90° and the patient's abdominal and lower extremity mass is supported by the patient's knees

3. **Discuss major considerations for selecting the appropriate positioning frame for a specific spinal procedure.**
A four-post frame design is preferred for multilevel fusion procedures. This type of frame permits extension of the hips and thighs, which preserves or enhances lumbar lordosis. Use of a frame that decreases lumbar lordosis (Wilson frame, knee-chest frame) is preferred for lumbar discectomy procedures. Decreasing lumbar lordosis facilitates access to the lumbar spinal canal as the distance between the spinous processes and lamina is increased. Care is necessary when positioning a patient for spinal stenosis decompressions. Spinal stenosis patients are symptomatic in extension. Positioning such patients on a frame that decreases lumbar lordosis and flexes the spine may result in failure to fully appreciate the extent of neural decompression required to relieve symptoms.

4. **Outline the steps involved in a midline posterior exposure of the thoracic and lumbar spine.**
   - Incise the skin and subcutaneous tissues with a scalpel
   - Place Weitlander and cerebellar retractors to tamponade superficial bleeding by exerting tension on surrounding tissues
   - Electrocautery dissection is carried out down to the level of the spinous processes
   - Cobb elevators and electrocautery are used to elevate the paraspinous muscles from the lamina at the level(s) requiring exposure. This provides sufficient exposure for discectomy and laminectomy procedures
   - If a fusion is planned, Cobb elevators and electrocautery are used to elevate the paraspinous muscles laterally to the tips of the transverse processes on each side. Subsequently the facet joints are excised and prepared for fusion. Care is taken to preserve the soft tissue structures (interspinous ligaments, supraspinous ligaments and facet capsules) at the transition between fused and nonfused levels
   - Hemostasis is maintained by coagulating bleeding points with electrocautery and packing with surgical sponges

5. **Where are blood vessels encountered during posterior spinal exposures?**
The arterial blood supply of the posterior thoracic and lumbar spine is consistent at each spinal level (Fig. 27-1). Arteries are encountered at the lateral border of the pars interarticularis, the upper medial border of the transverse process, and the intertransverse region. Sacral arteries exit from the dorsal sacral foramen. The superior gluteal artery enters the gluteal musculature and may be encountered during iliac crest bone grafting.

6. **What methods are used to guide the surgeon in exposing the correct anatomic levels during a posterior approach to the thoracic or lumbar spine?**
A combination of methods is used to guide exposure of correct anatomic levels:
   - **Preoperative radiographs** are reviewed to determine bony landmarks and presence of anatomic variants that may affect numbering of spinal levels (i.e. altered number of rib-bearing thoracic vertebra, lumbarized or sacralized vertebra)

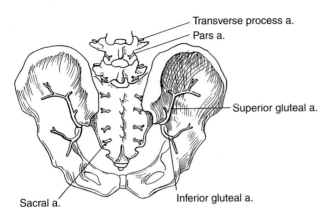

Transverse process a.

Pars a.

Superior gluteal a.

Sacral a.

Inferior gluteal a.

Figure 27-1. Blood vessels encountered during posterior midline approach. (From Wiesel SW, Weinstein JN, Herkowitz H, et al, editors. The Lumbar Spine. 2nd ed. Philadelphia: Saunders; 1996.)

- **Intraoperative osseous landmarks** are referenced: C7 (vertebra prominens), T8 (inferomedial angle of the scapula), T12 (most distal palpable rib), L4–L5 (superior lateral edge of ilium)
- An **intraoperative radiograph** with a metallic marker at the level of exposure is obtained. A permanent copy should be made to document the correct level of exposure for every procedure

7. **How is the location of the thoracic pedicle identified from the posterior midline approach?**
   The thoracic pedicle is located at the intersection of the pars interarticularis and the proximal third of the transverse process just lateral to the midpoint of the superior articular process. The exact location of the pedicle at each thoracic level varies slightly. A rongeur or power burr is used to remove the outer bony cortex and expose the entry site to the pedicle.

8. **How is the location of the lumbar pedicle identified from the posterior midline approach?**
   The lumbar pedicle is located at the intersection of two lines. The vertical line passes along the lateral aspect of the superior articular process and passes lateral to the pars interarticularis. The horizontal line passes through the middle of the transverse process, where it joins the superior articular process.

9. **What is a thoracic transpedicular approach?**
   After the spine is exposed by a posterior midline approach, the thoracic pedicle can be used as a pathway to access anterior spinal column pathology. This approach is most commonly used for non-calcified disc herniations located lateral to the spinal cord. The facet joint at the level and side of the disc herniation is resected. The superior aspect of the pedicle below the herniation is removed with a motorized burr. Sufficient working room is created for removal of disc material. This approach is also useful for vertebral biopsy.

10. **What is a costotransversectomy approach?**
    A costotransversectomy approach is a posterolateral approach to the thoracic spine (Fig. 27-2). It provides unilateral access to the posterior spinal elements, lateral aspect of the vertebral body, and anterior aspect of the spinal canal without the need to enter the thoracic cavity. Exposure includes resection of the posteromedial portion of the rib and transverse process. This approach was initially developed for drainage of tuberculous abscesses. It remains useful for

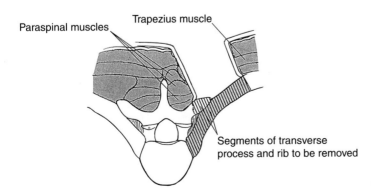

Paraspinal muscles

Trapezius muscle

Segments of transverse process and rib to be removed

Figure 27-2. Costotransversectomy approach. (From Winter RB, Lonstein JE, Dennis F, Smith MD, editors. Atlas of Spine Surgery. Philadelphia: Saunders; 1995.)

biopsies and disc excision (lateral and paracentral disc herniations) in patients who cannot tolerate a formal thoracotomy. It does not provide sufficient exposure of the ventral spinal canal to permit removal of central disc herniations or placement of an anterior strut graft/cage.

11. What is a lateral extracavitary approach?

A lateral extracavitary approach is a posterolateral extrapleural approach to the thoracic spine and thoracolumbar junction (Fig. 27-3). It provides greater exposure of the anterior spinal column and anterior aspect of the spinal canal than is achieved with a costotransversectomy. This approach requires removal of portions of the rib, costotransverse joint, facet, and pedicle. The exposure achieved is sufficient to permit removal of central disc herniations, corpectomy, and placement of an anterior strut graft or cage. This approach is usually combined with posterior segmental spinal instrumentation and fusion as this approach results in significant spinal instability.

12. Describe the paraspinal approach to the lumbar spine.

The paraspinal (Wiltse) approach is a posterolateral approach to the lumbar region (Fig. 27-4). It utilizes the plane between the multifidus and longissimus muscles. It permits direct access to disc herniations and spinal stenosis located in the extraforaminal zone without the need to resect the pars interarticularis or facet complex. It is also a useful approach for lumbar intertransverse fusion and instrumentation procedures.

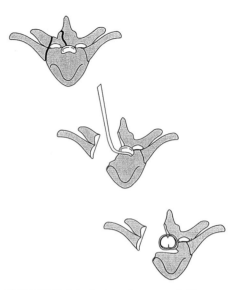

Figure 27-3. Lateral extracavitary approach. (From Amundson GM, Garfin SR. Posterior spinal instrumentation for thoracolumbar tumor and trauma reconstruction. Semin Spine Surg 1997;9:262.)

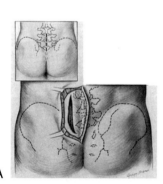

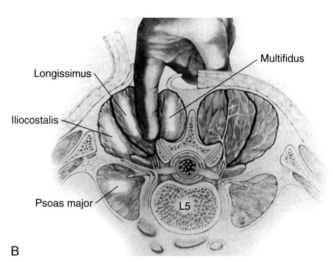

Figure 27-4. Lumbar paraspinal approach. (From Zindrick MR, Selby D. Lumbar spine fusion: different types and indications. In Wiesel SW, Weinstein JN, Herkowitz H, et al, editors. The Lumbar Spine. 2nd ed, vol. 1. Philadelphia: Saunders; 1996. p. 609.)

13. What is a PLIF approach?

Posterior lumbar interbody fusion (PLIF) refers to placement of intracolumnar implant(s) into a lumbar disc space from a posterior approach (Fig. 27-5). The disc space must be prepared to receive the interbody devices. Steps involved in this process include laminectomy, discectomy, restoration of disc space height, and decortication of the vertebral endplates. One interbody device is generally placed on each side of the disc space, and posterior pedicle instrumentation is used to stabilize the spinal segment.

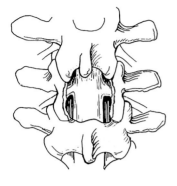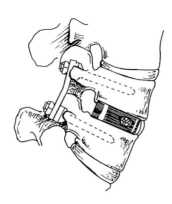

Figure 27-5. Posterior lumbar interbody fusion (PLIF). (From Zindrick MR, Wiltse LL, Rauschning W. Disc herniations lateral to the intervertebral foramen. In White AH, Rothman RH, Ray CD, editors. Lumbar Spine Surgery: Techniques and Complications. St. Louis: Mosby; 1987. p. 204.)

14. What is a TLIF approach?

Transforaminal lumbar interbody fusion (TLIF) refers to placement of intracolumnar implant(s) into a lumbar disc space through a unilateral posterior approach (Fig. 27-6). Unilateral removal of the pars interarticularis and facet complex provides posterolateral access to the disc space. This technique minimizes the need for significant retraction of neural elements and preserves the contralateral facet complex. The working space is sufficient to permit placement of two interbody fusion devices or a single large device through a unilateral approach. Posterior pedicle instrumentation is used to stabilize the spine segment.

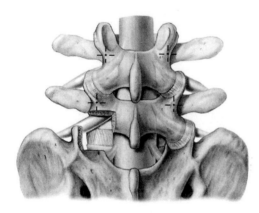

Figure 27-6. Transforaminal lumbar interbody fusion (TLIF). (Courtesy of DePuy AcroMed, Raynham, MA.)

15. What is a vertebral column resection?

A vertebral column resection (VCR) is a procedure to treat severe rigid spinal deformity. Using modern techniques, VCR can be performed entirely from a posterior approach in appropriate cases. The procedure involves removal of one or more spinal segments including the spinous process, lamina, transverse processes, pedicles, cephalad and caudad intervertebral discs, and vertebral body. When the resection is performed at a thoracic spinal level, rib resection is also required. Placement of temporary screw-rod fixation prior to osseous resection is critical to prevent neurologic injury during the procedure. Following the resection, the deformity is corrected by shortening the spinal column. An intervertebral cage is often placed into the anterior column defect to serve as a fulcrum for deformity correction and to prevent excessive spinal column shortening. The procedure is associated with significant neurologic risk and intraoperative neurophysiologic monitoring is mandatory.

Key Points

1. Posterior approaches to the thoracic and lumbar spine are extremely versatile and permit posterior decompression, fusion, and instrumentation from T1 to the sacrum.
2. Modern surgical techniques permit circumferential decompression and fusion of the thoracic and lumbar spine utilizing a single-stage posterior approach.

Website

Posterior lumbar fusion approaches: http://ukpmc.ac.uk/articlerender.cgi?accid=PMC2697340&tool=pmcentrez
Vertebral column resection:
http://www.spinal-deformity-surgeon.com/vcr-paper.html

BIBLIOGRAPHY

1. Harms J, Tabasso G, editors. Instrumented Spinal Surgery: Principles and Technique. New York: Thieme Verlag; 1999.
2. Steffee AD, Sitkowski DJ. Posterior Lumbar Interbody Fusion and Plates. Clin Orthop 1988;227:99–102.
3. Vaccaro AR, Baron EM, editors. Operative Techniques: Spine Surgery. Philadelphia: Saunders; 2008.

CERVICAL SPINE INSTRUMENTATION

Kern Singh, MD, Vincent J. Devlin, MD, Justin Munns, MD, Alexander R. Vaccaro, MD, PhD

CHAPTER 28

1. What are the indications for use of cervical spinal instrumentation?
- To immobilize an unstable segment
- To promote bony union
- To improve soft tissue healing
- To correct spinal deformity
- To decrease the need for external immobilization

2. How are the various types of cervical spinal implants classified?
No universal classification exists. Cervical spinal implants may be classified descriptively by:
- *Location of implant:* Anterior spinal column versus posterior spinal column
- *Spinal region stabilized:* Occipitocervical (O–C1); odontoid (C2); atlantoaxial (C1–C2); subaxial (C3–C7); cervicothoracic (C7–T2)
- *Method of osseous attachment:* Screw, hook, wire, cable
- *Type of longitudinal member:* Rod, plate, other (e.g. rib graft)

3. What types of cervical spinal implants are most commonly utilized today?
Posterior cervical instrumentation most commonly involves use of rod-screw systems. Screws may be placed in the occiput, C1 (lateral mass), and C2 (pedicle vs. pars vs. translaminar screws). In the subaxial cervical region, lateral mass screws are most commonly used at the C3 to C6 levels, whereas pedicle screws are typically used at C7 and distally in the thoracic region. Anterior cervical plates are the most commonly used implants in the C3 to C7 region. Reconstruction of the anterior spinal column following discectomy or corpectomy may be performed with bone graft or fusion cages (Fig. 28-1A and B).

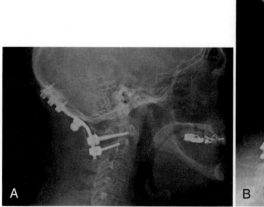
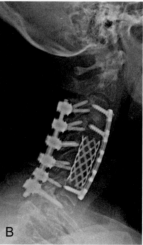

Figure 28-1. A, Posterior occiput to C2 spinal instrumentation, **B,** Posterior spinal instrumentation C3 to T1 and anterior reconstruction with C3–C4 allograft bone graft and titanium mesh cage from C4-C7.

4. What are the indications for use of spinal instrumentation in the occipitocervical region?
- Trauma
- Ligamentous instability
- Select odontoid fractures
- Rheumatoid arthritis (basilar invagination)
- Infection
- Neoplasm
- Select skeletal dysplasias
- Arnold-Chiari malformations
- Select metabolic bone diseases

5. What implant options are available for use at the occipitocervical junction?

- **Anterior options:** Implants are infrequently placed in this region because it is challenging to achieve surgical exposure here. Bone graft or cages are used to reconstruct osseous defects. Occasionally specialized plates (e.g. C2 to clivus plate) or C1-occipital condyle screws are used
- **Posterior options:** Rod-screw systems are the most commonly used implant. A hybrid rod-plate combination is an additional option. Contoured rods with wire or cable fixation are an option for special circumstances. Bone grafts and wires may be used in conjunction with other implants but are rarely used in isolation because they are not sufficiently stable to permit patient mobilization without extensive external immobilization, such as a halo device

6. Where can a surgeon safely place screws in the occiput when performing posterior occipitocervical instrumentation?

Occipital bone is thickest and most dense in the midline below the external occipital protuberance (inion). This region provides an excellent surface for screw purchase. Occipital bone thickness decreases laterally and inferiorly from the inion. Screws should be placed below the superior nuchal line that overlies the transverse sinuses, which can be injured during drilling or screw placement (Fig. 28-2).

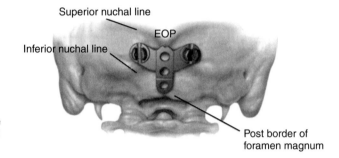

Figure 28-2. Safe placement of occipital screws is in the region adjacent to the external occipital protuberance and below the superior nuchal line. (DePuy Spine, Inc. All rights reserved.)

7. How are occipital screws connected to a rod system?

The surgeon has several options including:

- *Modular midline screw-plates:* A midline plate permits screw purchase in the thick midline bone and permits minor adjustments to facilitate linkage to an independent dual rod construct (Fig. 28-3A)
- *Hybrid rod-plate fixation:* Plates attach laterally to the midline of the occiput and connect with rods for fixation in the cervical spine distally. Specialized implants consisting of a single rod that transitions to a plate are available (Fig. 28-3B)
- *Rod with specialized connectors:* Occipital screws are linked to rods via offset screw-rod connectors (Fig. 28-3C)

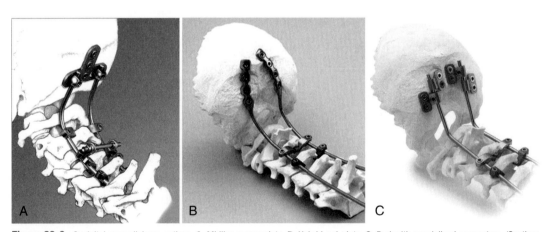

Figure 28-3. Occipital screw linkage options. **A,** Midline screw-plate. **B,** Hybrid rod-plate. **C,** Rod with specialized connectors. (Synthes Spine. All rights reserved.)

8. How is posterior screw fixation performed at C1?

Two basic techniques are utilized:

- In the first technique, the screw is placed directly in the lateral mass of C1. The entry point is at the junction of the C1 lateral mass with the undersurface of the C1 posterior arch (Fig. 28-4A). The extensive venous plexus in this region makes dissection challenging. In addition, the C2 nerve root is in proximity to the screw entry point and must be retracted distally. A modified technique involves creation of a notch on the undersurface of the C1 arch to facilitate drill/screw placement to minimize dissection in the region of this venous plexus. Screws are directed with 5 to 10 degrees of convergence and parallel to the C1 arch (Fig. 28-4B)

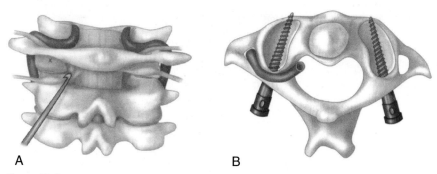

Figure 28-4. **A,** Posterior landmark for C1 screw placement. **B,** C1 screw trajectory in the axial plane. (From Vaccaro AR, Baron EM. Spine Surgery: Operative Techniques. Philadelphia: Saunders; 2008, with permission.)

- The second technique uses an entry point on the C1 arch and places a screw through the pedicle analog of C1 and into the C1 lateral mass. The vertebral artery is at greater risk with this technique and one must not mistake a common anomaly in which a bony bridge, the arcuate foramen, overlies the vertebral artery or the screw will injure the vertebral artery. This osseous anomaly has been termed the *ponticulus posticus*. With either technique, excessive superior C1 screw angulation will violate the occiput-C1 joint. An excessively long C1 screw may potentially compromise the internal carotid artery or hypoglossal nerve.

9. What are the options for achieving screw fixation in C2?
Three options exist: C2 pars screws, C2 pedicle screws, and C2 translaminar screws.

10. How is a C2 pars screw placed?
The *pars interarticularis* is defined as the portion of the C2 vertebra between the superior and inferior articular processes. The screw entry point is 3 to 4 mm superior and 3 to 4 mm lateral to the inferior medial aspect of the C2–C3 facet joint. Screw trajectory is parallel to the C2 pars interarticularis with approximately 10 degrees of medial angulation (Fig. 28-5).

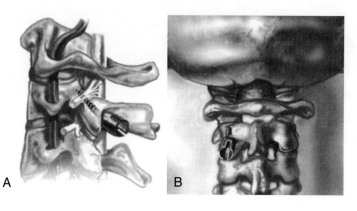

Figure 28-5. C2 pars screw placement. **A,** Lateral view. **B,** Anteroposterior view. (From McLaughlin MR, Haid RW, Rodts GE. Atlas of Cervical Spine Surgery. Philadelphia: Saunders; 2005, with permission.)

11. How is a C2 pedicle screw placed?
The *C2 pedicle* is defined as the portion of the C2 vertebra connecting the posterior osseous elements with the vertebral body and consists of the narrow area between the pars interarticularis and the vertebral body. The entry point is approximated by the intersection of a vertical line through the center of the C2 pars interarticularis and a horizontal line through the center of the C2 lamina. The screw entry point is in the cranial and medial quadrant defined by these landmarks. The screw is placed with 15 to 30 degrees of medial angulation and parallel to the superior surface of the C2 pars interarticularis. The medial wall of the C2 pars can be palpated as an additional guide to placement (Fig. 28-6).

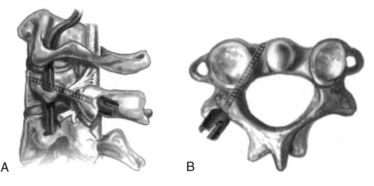

Figure 28-6. C2 pedicle screw placement. **A,** Lateral view. **B,** Anteroposterior view. (From McLaughlin MR, Haid RW, Rodts GE. Atlas of Cervical Spine Surgery. Philadelphia: Saunders; 2005, with permission.)

12. Compare and contrast a C2 pedicle screw with a C2 pars screw.

The C2 pedicle screw trajectory is more superior and medial than the pars screw and has less risk of injury to a high-riding vertebral artery. A longer screw length may be achieved using a C2 pedicle screw than a C2 pars screw. A C2 pedicle screw can be safely placed with bicortical screw purchase. A C2 pars screw is typically a unicortical screw that stops short of the transverse foramen to prevent potential injury to the vertebral artery.

13. When might a C2 translaminar screw be preferred over alternative C2 screw fixation methods?

A *translaminar screw* is preferred when the trajectory for placement of a C2 pars or pedicle screw is compromised by an aberrantly coursing vertebral artery or aberrant osseous anatomy. The technique is straightforward and consists of creating a small entry window at the junction of the C2 spinous process and lamina. A blunt probe or hand drill is used to create a pathway for screw placement in the cancellous bone of the contralateral lamina. The process is repeated on the opposite side for placement of a second screw that crosses above or below the initial screw. An additional *window* can be created at the facet-laminar junction to visualize *screw-exit* to ensure that the screw has not inadvertently violated the inner cortical surface of the lamina (Fig. 28-7).

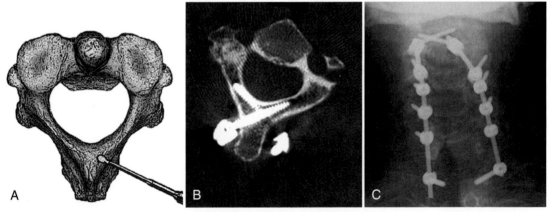

Figure 28-7. C2 translaminar screw placement technique. **A,** Creation of screw tract, **B,** Axial CT view after screw placement, **C,** Anteroposterior radiograph after screw placement. (A from Jea A, Sheth R, Vanni S, et al. Modification of Wright's technique for placement of C2 translaminar screws: technical note. Spine J 2008;8:656–60, with permission.)

14. What are the indications for spinal implant placement in the atlantoaxial (C1–C2) region?

Atlantoaxial instability due to traumatic etiologies (e.g. unstable odontoid fractures), midtransverse ligament disruption, odontoid nonunion, an unstable os odontoideum, or nontraumatic disorders, such as rheumatoid arthritis, congenital malformations, and metabolic disorders.

15. What are the types of implants most commonly used to stabilize the atlantoaxial (C1–C2) joint?

C1–C2 stabilization is most commonly performed from a posterior approach using C1–C2 transarticular screws or C1–C2 screw-rod constructs. Posterior wire/cable techniques or rod-clamps are less frequently utilized. Anterior placement of transarticular screws is a specialized technique, which is occasionally used to salvage failed posterior C1–C2 fusions and for unique cases.

16. Describe the technique for posterior C1–C2 transarticular facet screw fixation.
The starting point for a *transarticular screw* is 3 to 5 mm above the C2–C3 facet joint and as medial as possible without breaking through the medial aspect of the C2 isthmus. Screw insertion can be guided by exposing the posterior C1–C2 facet complex and the isthmus of C2. The transarticular screws traverse the inferior articular process of C2, the isthmus of C2, the superior endplate of C2, the C1–C2 facet joint, and the lateral mass of C1 (Fig. 28-8).

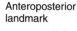

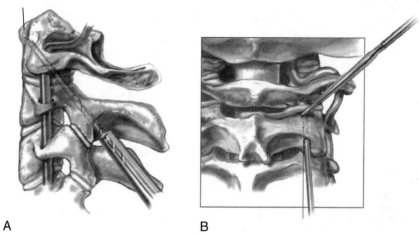

A   B

Figure 28-8. C1-C2 transarticular screw placement. **A,** Lateral view, **B,** Anteroposterior view. (From McLaughlin MR, Haid RW, Rodts GE. Atlas of Cervical Spine Surgery. Philadelphia: Saunders; 2005, with permission.)

17. What are some complications and challenges associated with transarticular screw placement?
The technique carries a risk of vertebral artery injury. It cannot be performed in up to 20% of patients due to vertebral artery anomalies. A preoperative computed tomography (CT) scan is required to look for a high-riding vertebral artery whose aberrant path is along the planned screw trajectory. Proper screw placement requires anatomic reduction of the C1–C2 joints prior to screw placement. Excessively long screws may injure the internal carotid artery or hypoglossal nerve. In addition, screw placement in patients with increased thoracic kyphosis is challenging because it is difficult to achieve the required screw trajectory in this setting.

18. Describe advantages of C1–C2 screw rod systems versus transarticular screws.
C1–C2 screw-rod systems have several advantages over transarticular screws for stabilization of the C1–C2 region. C1–C2 screw-rod systems are more versatile. Preoperative reduction of the C1–C2 joints is not required prior to instrumentation. In fact, the independent placement of screws in C1 and C2 can be used as a tool to facilitate reduction, which can be checked with fluoroscopy and modified without the need to replace screws. In addition, C1–C2 screw rod systems can be used in cases where transarticular screws are contraindicated (e.g. vertebral artery anomalies, severe kyphosis).

19. Why are transarticular screws or screw-rod constructs preferred over posterior wire or cable procedures?
Transarticular screws and screw rod techniques provide much greater stability than wire/cable techniques and avoid the need for postoperative external mobilization with a halo vest. In addition, these techniques are associated with higher rates of successful fusion than wire/cable techniques. Screw-based techniques avoid the risk of wire passage adjacent to the spinal cord. Screw-based techniques can be used in the presence of fractured or absent lamina, whereas wire/cable techniques rely on intact posterior elements to provide fixation.

20. Describe two common techniques used to achieve C1–C2 stabilization using wires or cables?
- The *Gallie technique* begins with sublaminar wire (double-looped) passage from caudal to cranial under the posterior arch of C1. Following wire passage, a structural corticocancellous iliac graft is harvested and shaped to conform to the posterior processes of C1 and C2. The two free ends of the wire are then passed through the leading wire loop and then passed over the graft and around or through the spinous process of the axis. The free ends of the wire are then twisted in the midline, thereby securing the graft position between C1 and C2 (Fig. 28-9A)

- The *Brooks technique* involves the passage of dual or doubled sublaminar wires (cables/tape) from caudal to cranial under the arch of C2 and then C1. Following the passage of the wire, two separate triangular or rectangular cortico-cancellous iliac grafts are harvested and placed over the posterior elements of C1 and C2. The ends of the wires on each side are then tightened together, thereby securing the position of the grafts (Fig. 28-9B)

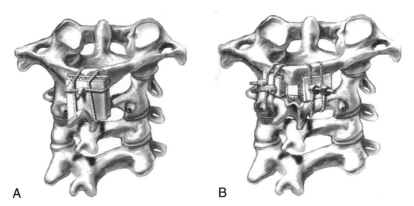

Figure 28-9. C1–C2 wire techniques. **A,** Gallie technique, **B,** Brooks technique. (From McLaughlin MR, Haid RW, Rodts GE. Atlas of Cervical Spine Surgery. Philadelphia: Saunders; 2005, with permission.)

21. Describe the fixation of choice for select odontoid fractures treated through an anterior approach.

One or two screws may be used to stabilize a type 2 odontoid fracture. The critical transverse outer diameter for the placement of two 3.5-mm cortical screws is 9 mm. Cadaveric biomechanical studies have demonstrated that one central screw, which engages the cortical tip of the dens, is just as effective as two screws. Two screws more effectively counter the rotational forces created by the alar ligaments. Single-screw options include the use of a single 4.5-mm cannulated Herbert screw or a single 3.5/4.0-mm standard lag screw (Fig. 28-10).

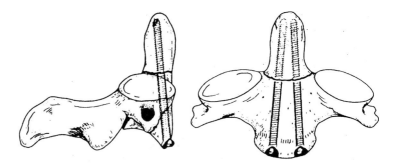

Figure 28-10. Odontoid screw fixation. **Left,** Lateral view. **Right,** Anteroposterior view.

22. What are some contraindications for the use of odontoid screw fixation?

- Patients who possess anatomic obstructions to appropriate screw placement (e.g. short neck, excessive thoracic kyphosis, barrel chest deformity)
- Unfavorable fracture patterns (e.g. fracture obliquity in the same direction as screw placement—i.e., a sagittal plane fracture that courses posterior superiorly to anterior inferiorly, low type 3 odontoid fractures, fractures requiring a flexed neck position to maintain reduction)
- Poor bone quality (a pathologic fracture with compromised bone quality, significant osteoporosis)

23. What are the indications for posterior subaxial cervical instrumentation?

Fracture fusion and stabilization, posterior stabilization following an anterior nonunion, adjunctive stabilization following a long segment anterior fusion, or fusion and stabilization following a posterior decompression for cervical myelopathy.

24. Describe three techniques for placement of lateral mass screws.

Three commonly employed techniques for lateral mass screw placement (C3-C6) have been described by Roy-Camille, Magerl, and An and are summarized in Table 28-1. Laterally directed screws are not utilized at C2 due to concerns regarding vertebral artery proximity.

Table 28-1. Recommended landmarks for lateral mass screw placement

TECHNIQUE	ROY-CAMILLE	MAGERL	AN
Starting position (lateral mass)	Center	1 mm medial and 1–2 mm cephalad to the center	1 mm medial to the center
Cephalad tilt	0	30	15
Lateral tilt	10	25	30

At C7, the lateral mass is frequently quite small, and a lateral mass screw risks causing C8 nerve root irritation. For this reason, pedicle screws are more commonly utilized at this level, although C7 lateral mass fixation remains a valid technique depending on individual patient anatomy (Fig. 28-11).

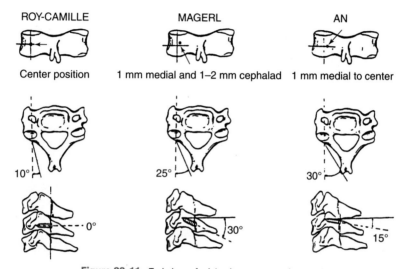

ROY-CAMILLE   MAGERL   AN

Center position   1 mm medial and 1–2 mm cephalad   1 mm medial to center

Figure 28-11. Techniques for lateral mass screw placement.

25. What is the role of pedicle screws in the cervical spine?
Pedicle screws are useful and relatively safe at the C2 and C7 levels. In the majority of patients, the vertebral artery enters the foramen transversarium of C6 and is not at risk with C7 pedicle screw placement. Pedicle screw placement at the C3 through C6 levels is not widely practiced in North America due to concern relating to the risk of vertebral artery injury.

26. Describe the most common technique used for C7 pedicle screw placement.
Most commonly, a laminoforaminotomy is created at C6–C7 to palpate and visualize the medial border of the C7 pedicle. Next, a small drill or pedicle probe can be used to cannulate the C7 pedicle while visualizing for a medial pedicle breech. This is followed by screw placement.

27. What are some advantages of lateral mass and pedicle screw fixation versus posterior wire or cable fixation?
Cervical lateral mass and pedicle screw fixation affords significantly increased stability in rotation and extension, compared with posterior wiring or cable fixation. Spinal implant fixation to the lateral mass and pedicles obviates the need for intact laminae or spinous processes, which are necessary for most wire/cable techniques. Rigid postoperative cervical immobilization is not required with screw fixation techniques. Loss of wire fixation, due to wire failure or bony pullout, is the most common complication associated with wire/cable techniques but is rarely seen with screw-based techniques.

28. What techniques have been described for use of wires and cables in the subaxial cervical region?
Wires or cables may be placed beneath the lamina (sublaminar), between adjacent spinous processes (interspinous or *Rogers wiring*), through the facet joints, or between the facet joint and the spinous process. The *Bohlman triple-wire technique* combines midline interspinous wiring with passage of separate wires through adjacent spinous processes, which are used to secure a corticocancellous bone graft to the decorticated posterior elements on each side of the spinous processes.

29. What are the indications for anterior cervical plating?

To decrease the incidence of graft or cage subsidence and dislodgement, to minimize kyphotic collapse of the fused interface, to improve fusion rates, and to minimize the need for postoperative external immobilization.

30. Describe the design features of the first anterior cervical plates.

The original Caspar (Aesculap Instrument Company) and Orozco (Synthes Spine) systems were non-constrained, load-sharing plates that required bicortical screw purchase. Due to the non-constrained nature of the screw plate interface, excessive motion at the screw plate junction occasionally led to screw loosening or pullout. Engagement of the posterior vertebral cortex was required to minimize screw loosening. This is technically challenging and an increased risk of neurologic injury is associated with this technique.

31. What solution was developed to address the difficulties associated with anterior cervical plates requiring bicortical screw purchase?

Because of the technical difficulty associated with bicortical screw purchase, constrained systems that firmly lock the screws to the plate were developed. The first solution was a plate system (cervical spine locking plate [CSLP]) that used a screw with an expandable cross-split head that locks into the plate after insertion of a small central bolt (Synthes Spine). Securing the screws to the plates allows a more direct transfer of the applied forces from the spine to the plate and improved construct stiffness without the need for bicortical screw purchase. Alternative methods were developed to secure the screw to the plate to prevent screw back-out and included a variety of screw head coverage mechanisms (ring locks, blocking heads, screw covers) (Fig. 28-12).

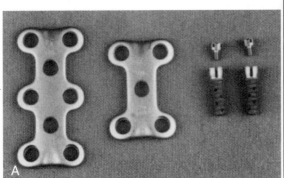
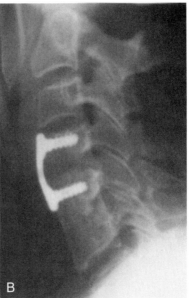

Figure 28-12. Anterior cervical locking plate (Synthes Spine). **A,** The screw head is locked to the plate by insertion of a conical bolt, thereby ensuring angular stability between the plate and the screws. **B,** Anterior cervical locking plate application after interbody fusion. Note that penetration of the posterior vertebral body cortex is not required to achieve a stable implant construct.

32. How are current anterior cervical plating systems classified?

Anterior cervical plate systems can be broadly classified as either static (constrained) plates or dynamic (semi-constrained) plates.

- **Static plates** rely on screws, which are rigidly locked to the plate. A direct transfer of applied forces from spine to plate is assured, but the theoretical possibility of stress shielding of the anterior spinal column is present
- **Dynamic plates** utilize screws that are restricted from backing out from the plate but attempt to allow some degree of load sharing between the plate and the anterior spinal column. This load sharing is achieved through three mechanisms, which may be used singularly or in combination: *screw rotation, screw translation,* or *plate shortening. Semiconstrained rotational plates* permit rotation at the plate-screw interface as graft subsidence occurs. *Semiconstrained translational plates* permit screws to slide longitudinally (fixed screws) within slotted holes in the plate. Some designs permit only longitudinal translation (fixed screws), whereas others permit both longitudinal screw translation and screw rotation (variable screws). The last type of plate permits translation by means of plate shortening. The ends of the plate are rigidly fixed to adjacent vertebra, but the plate itself shortens under physiologic loading (Fig. 28-13)

Rotational vs. Translational

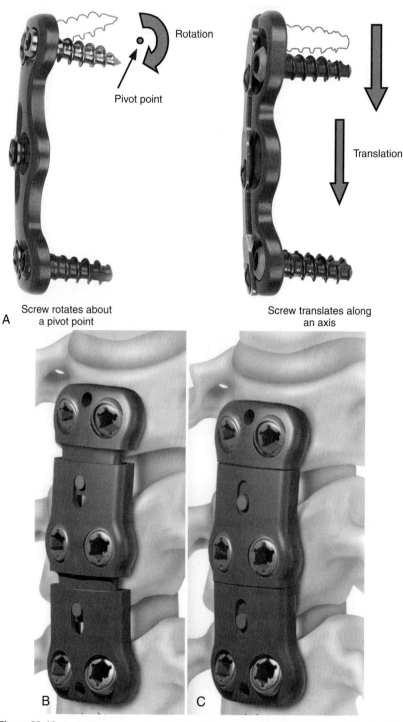

Figure 28-13. **A,** Rotational versus translational anterior cervical plate. **B,** Cervical translation through plate shortening. **C,** Note plate length intraoperatively compared with postoperatively, (A, from Medtronic Sofamor Danek, 2005. All rights reserved. B and C, from DePuy Spine, Inc. All rights reserved.)

33. Which type of anterior cervical plate is superior—a static plate or a dynamic plate?

This is a controversial area. In the setting of trauma, a *static plate* is indicated because it provides greater immediate stability. In the treatment of degenerative disorders, no studies have established superiority of one particular type of plate. With use of *dynamic plates*, graft settling may lead to segmental kyphosis, foraminal stenosis, and plate impingement on the superior adjacent disc space. However, when multilevel corpectomies are stabilized with anterior plates, graft subsidence may be accommodated by translational plates and potentially decrease the rate of anterior plate fixation failure.

34. What is a buttress plate?

A *buttress or junctional plate* is an alternative to long segment anterior cervical plates that are subject to large cantilever forces, particularly at the caudal plate-screw-bone junction. The buttress plate spans only the caudal or cephalad graft-host junction, thereby theoretically preventing graft extrusion. The plate is most commonly used at the caudal end of the graft where the cantilever forces are the greatest. A surgeon should use supplemental posterior segmental fixation in the setting of a long anterior strut graft fusion and junctional plate stabilization to prevent dislodgement of the buttress plate with potentially catastrophic consequences (Fig. 28-14).

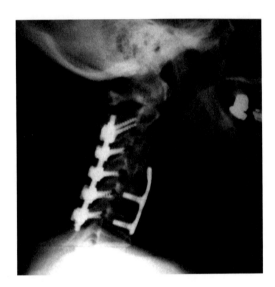

Figure 28-14. The buttress plate prevents anterior graft dislodgement in combination with posterior cervical instrumentation. (From Vaccaro AR, Baron EM: Spine Surgery: Operative Techniques. Philadelphia: Saunders; 2008, with permission.)

Key Points

1. Posterior cervical instrumentation typically involves use of rod-screw systems. Screws may be placed in the occiput, C1 (lateral mass), and C2 (pedicle vs. pars vs. translaminar screws). In the subaxial cervical region, lateral mass screws are most commonly used at the C3 to C6 levels, whereas pedicle screws are typically used at C7 and distally in the thoracic region.
2. Anterior cervical plates are the most commonly used implants in the C3 to C7 region and may be classified as static or dynamic plates.
3. The anterior spinal column may be reconstructed with autogenous bone graft (iliac or fibula), allograft bone graft, or synthetic materials (e.g. titanium mesh cages, carbon fiber cages, polyetheretherketone [PEEK] cages).

Websites

Anterior cervical plate nomenclature of cervical spine study group: http://cme.medscape.com/viewarticle/424941_1
Posterior occipital cervical fixation: http://www.spineuniverse.com/displayarticle.php/article288.html
Trends in surgical management for type II odontoid fracture: 20 years of experience at a regional spinal cord injury center: http://www.orthosupersite.com/view.asp?rID=28891

BIBLIOGRAPHY

1. Harms J, Melcher RP. Posterior C1-C2 fusion with polyaxial screw and rod fixation. Spine 2001;26:2467–71.
2. Jea A, Sheth R, Vanni S, et al. Modification of Wright's technique for placement of C2 translaminar screws: technical note. Spine J 2008;8:656–60.
3. Jeanneret B, Magerl F. Primary posterior fusion C1-2 in odontoid fractures: indications, technique and results of transarticular screw fixation. J Spinal Disord Tech 1992;5:464–75.
4. McLaughlin MR, Haid RW, Rodts GE. Atlas of Cervical Spine Surgery. Philadelphia: Saunders; 2005.
5. Reilly TM, Sasso RC. Anterior odontoid screw techniques. Tech Ortho 2002;17(3):306–15.
6. Rhee JM, Riew KD. Dynamic anterior cervical plates. J Am Acad Orthop Surg 2007;15(11):640–6.
7. Sekhon LH. Posterior cervical lateral mass screw fixation: analysis of 1026 consecutive screws in 143 patients. J Spinal Disord Tech 2005;18(4):297–303.
8. Stock GH, Vaccaro AR, Brown AK, et al. Contemporary posterior occipital fixation. J Bone Joint Surg 2006;88A:1642–9.
9. Vaccaro AR, Baron EM. Spine Surgery: Operative Techniques. Philadelphia: Saunders; 2008.
FDA Disclosure: The use of screw-based fixation in lateral mass or pedicle in the posterior cervical spine is not FDA cleared or approved.

THORACIC AND LUMBAR SPINE INSTRUMENTATION

Edward A. Smirnov, MD, D. Greg Anderson, MD, and Vincent J. Devlin, MD

GENERAL CONSIDERATIONS

1. **Summarize the functions of spinal instrumentation in thoracic and lumbar fusion procedures.**
   - **Enhance fusion.** Spinal implants immobilize spinal segments during the fusion process and increase the rate of successful arthrodesis
   - **Restore spinal stability.** When pathologic processes (e.g. tumor, infection, fracture) compromise spinal stability, spinal implants can restore stability
   - **Correct spinal deformities.** Spinal instrumentation can provide correction of spinal deformities (e.g. scoliosis, kyphosis, spondylolisthesis)
   - **Permit extensive decompression of the neural elements.** Complex spinal stenosis problems requiring extensive decompression create spinal instability. Spinal instrumentation and fusion prevent development of postsurgical spinal deformities and recurrent spinal stenosis

2. **Why is surgical stabilization of the spine considered a two-stage process?**
   In the short term, stabilization of the spine is provided by spinal implants. However, long-term stabilization of the spine occurs only if fusion is successful. If the fusion does not heal, spinal implant failure will ultimately occur. The surgeon influences this process through meticulous fusion technique, selection of the appropriate location for fusion (anterior, posterior, or combined anterior and posterior column fusion), and use of appropriate spinal implants to adequately support the spine during this process.

3. **What is meant by the terms *tension band principle* and *load-sharing concept*?**
   - A tension band is a portion of a construct that is subjected to tensile stresses during loading. In the normal spine, the posterior spinal musculature maintains normal sagittal spinal alignment through application of dorsal tension forces against the intact anterior spinal column. This is termed the **tension band principle.** The posterior spinal musculature can function as a tension band only if the anterior spinal column is structurally intact
   - Biomechanical studies have shown that in the normal lumbar spine approximately 80% of axial load is carried by the anterior spinal column and the remaining 20% is transmitted through the posterior spinal column. This relationship is termed the **load-sharing concept** (Fig. 29-1)

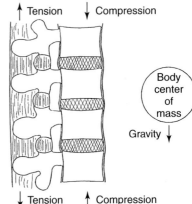

Figure 29-1. Anterior column load-sharing and posterior tension band principle.

4. **What is the relevance of the load-sharing concept to the selection of appropriate spinal implants?**
   Load sharing between an instrumentation construct and the vertebral column is a function of the ratio of the axial stiffness of the spinal instrumentation and the axial stiffness of the vertebral column. If the anterior spinal column is incompetent, the entire axial load must pass through the posterior spinal implant. In the absence of adequate anterior column support, normal physiologic loads exceed the strength of posterior spinal implant systems. In this situation, posterior spinal implants will fail by fatigue, permanent deformation, or implant migration through bone. Thus, it is critical to reconstruct an incompetent anterior spinal column when using posterior spinal implant systems.

POSTERIOR SPINAL INSTRUMENTATION

5. **Name three posterior spinal instrumentation systems that are considered to be the precursors of contemporary posterior spinal instrumentation systems.**
   Harrington instrumentation, Luque instrumentation, and Cotrel-Dubousset instrumentation.

6. What is Harrington instrumentation?

The initial instrumentation developed by Paul Harrington consisted of a single rod with ratchets on one end in combination with a single hook at each end of the rod. Distraction forces were applied to obtain and maintain correction of spinal deformities. This system was introduced 1960 in Texas and was utilized to treat various spinal problems, especially scoliosis, for more than 25 years. Shortcomings of this system included the need for postoperative immobilization to prevent hook dislodgement and the inability to correct and maintain sagittal plane alignment. Various modifications were introduced to address these problems, including square-ended hooks, use of compression hooks along a convex rod, and use of supplemental wire fixation (Fig. 29-2).

7. What is Luque instrumentation?

In the 1980s, Edwardo Luque from Mexico introduced a system that provided segmental fixation consisting of wires placed beneath the lamina at multiple spinal levels. Wires were tightened around rods placed along both sides of the lamina. Corrective forces were distributed over multiple levels, thereby decreasing the risk of fixation failure. The increased stability provided by this construct eliminated the need for postoperative braces or casts. The ability to translate the spine to a precontoured rod provided better control of sagittal plane alignment than Harrington instrumentation (Fig. 29-3).

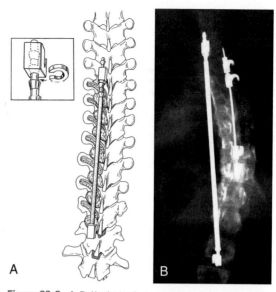

Figure 29-2. A, B, Harrington instrumentation. (**A** from Winter RB, Lonstein JE, Denis F, et al. Atlas of Spine Surgery. Philadelphia: Saunders; 1995. **B** from Errico TJ, Lonner BS, Moulton AW. Surgical Management of Spinal Deformities. Philadelphia: Saunders; 2009.)

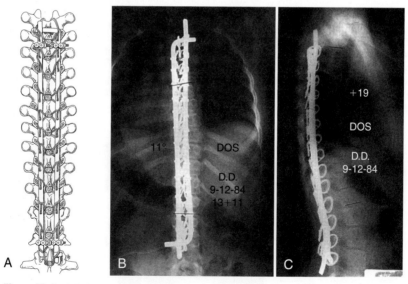

Figure 29-3. A, B, C, Luque instrumentation. (From Winter RB, Lonstein JE, Denis F, et al. Atlas of Spine Surgery. Philadelphia: Saunders; 1995.)

8. What is Cotrel-Dubousset instrumentation?

In 1984, Cotrel and Dubousset from France introduced their segmental fixation system, which became known as the CD system. It consisted of multiple hooks and screws placed along a knurled rod. The use of multiple fixation points permitted selective application of compression and distraction forces along the same rod by altering hook direction. A rod rotation maneuver was introduced in an attempt to provide improved three-dimensional correction of scoliosis. Rod contouring permitted improved correction of the sagittal contour of the spine. The stable segmental fixation provided by this system obviated the need for postoperative immobilization (Fig. 29-4).

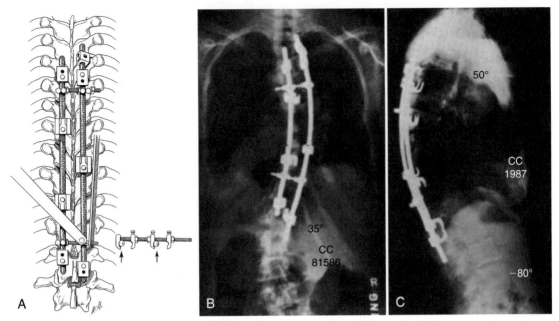

Figure 29-4. A, B, C, Cotrel-Dubousset instrumentation. (A from Winter RB, Lonstein JE, Denis F, et al. Atlas of Spine Surgery. Philadelphia: Saunders; 1995. B, C, from Lonstein JE, Bradford DS, Winter RB, et al. Moe's Textbook of Scoliosis and Other Spinal Deformities. 3rd ed. Philadelphia: Saunders; 1995.)

9. What is meant by the term *posterior segmental spinal fixation*?

Posterior segmental spinal fixation is a general term used to describe a variety of contemporary posterior spinal instrumentation systems that attach to the spine at multiple points throughout the instrumented spinal segments. A complete implant assembly is termed a **spinal construct.** Typically, spinal instrumentation constructs consist of a **longitudinal member** (rod or plate) on each side of the spine connected by **transverse connectors** (cross-linking devices) to increase construct stability. **Segmental fixation** is defined as the connection of the longitudinal member to multiple vertebrae within the construct. Options for achieving segmental fixation include the use of hook, wire, and pedicle screw **anchors.** Various corrective forces can be applied to the spine by means of segmental anchors including compression, distraction, rotation, cantilever bending, and translation. The Isola system, developed by Marc Asher and colleagues, popularized the integration of hook, wire, and screw fixation within a single implant construct. Such implant constructs are referred to as **hybrid constructs** (Fig. 29-5).

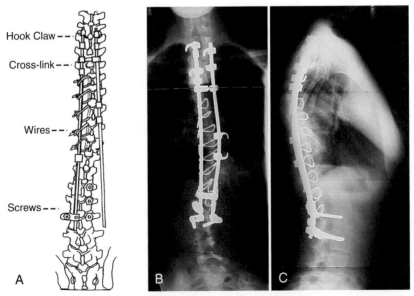

Figure 29-5. A, B, C, Contemporary hybrid posterior segmental spinal instrumentation.

10. Describe the use of hook anchors in posterior segmental spinal constructs.

Hook anchors may be placed above or below the T1 to T10 transverse processes, under the thoracic facet joints, and above or below the thoracic and lumbar lamina. When blades of adjacent hooks face each other, this is termed a **claw configuration.** Compression forces can be applied to adjacent opposing hooks, thereby securing the hooks to the posterior elements. A claw may be composed of hooks at a single spinal level (intrasegmental claw) or hooks at adjacent levels (intersegmental claw). Hooks placed in a claw configuration provide more secure fixation than a single hook anchor. For this reason, claw fixation is typically used at the proximal and distal ends of spinal constructs.

11. Describe the use of wire anchors in posterior segmental spinal contructs.

Wire anchors (and more recently cables) can be placed at every level of the spine. Possible attachment points for wire anchors include the base of the spinous process, underneath the lamina (sublaminar position), or underneath the transverse process. Spinous process wires are placed through a hole in the base of the spinous process and remain outside the spinal canal. Sublaminar wires require careful preparation of the cephalad and caudad interlaminar spaces to minimize the risk of neurologic injury as wires are passed beneath the lamina and dorsal to the neural elements.

12. Describe the use of pedicle screw anchors in posterior spinal contructs.

Pedicle screw anchors can be used throughout the thoracic and lumbar spinal regions and have become the most popular type of spinal anchor currently. Advantages of pedicle screws include secure fixation, the ability to apply forces to both the anterior and posterior columns of the spine from a posterior approach, and the capability to achieve fixation when lamina are deficient. The disadvantages of pedicle screws include technical challenges related to screw placement and the potential for neurologic, vascular, and visceral injury due to misplaced screws. Pedicle screws may be broadly classified as fixed head screws (monoaxial), mobile head screws (polyaxial), or bolts (require a separate connector for attachment to the longitudinal member) (Fig. 29-6).

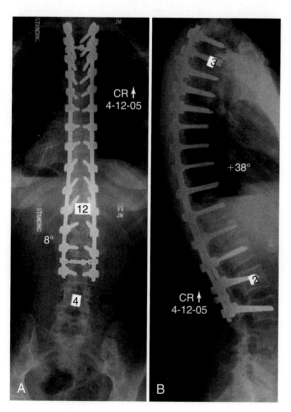

Figure 29-6. Pedicle screw-based instrumentation construct. (From Buchowksi JM, Kuhns CA, Bridwell KH, et al. Surgical management of posttraumatic thoracolumbar kyphosis. Spine J 2008;8:666–77.)

13. What are the anatomic landmarks for placement of pedicle screws in the thoracic and lumbar spine?

- In the thoracic region, screw placement is initiated at the lateral aspect of the pedicle. The pedicle entry site is determined by referencing the transverse process, the superior articular process, and the pars interarticularis. Exact position of the entry site is adjusted depending on the specific level of the thoracic spine and whether the screw trajectory is *straight-ahead* or *anatomic*

- In the lumbar region, the entry site for screw placement is located at the upslope where the transverse process joins the superior articular process just lateral to the pars interarticularis. This site can be approximated by making a line along the midpoint of the transverse process and a second line along the lateral border of the superior articular process. The crossing point of these two lines defines the entry site to the pedicle (Fig. 29-7)

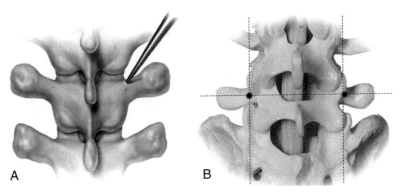

Figure 29-7. Landmarks for pedicle screw placement. **A,** Thoracic spine. **B,** Lumbar spine. (Courtesy of DePuy Spine, Inc.)

14. What is dynamic stabilization of the spine?

Dynamic stabilization is a concept of placing anchors (generally pedicle screws) into the spine and connecting these anchors with a flexible longitudinal member (e.g. rod, cable, spring). The goal of this type of implant is to constrain but not eliminate motion. Proponents of this concept believe this type of implant will produce less stress on the adjacent spinal segments and may prevent some of the complications observed following spinal fusion (e.g. adjacent-level degenerative changes). Opponents worry that without concurrent spinal arthrodesis, these implants may loosen or fail prematurely and require revision surgery. Currently, there are limited data to prove or disprove the scientific utility of this concept (Fig. 29-8).

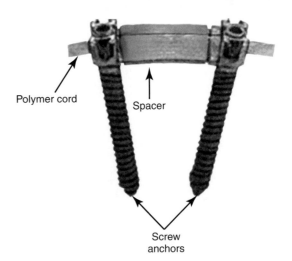

Polymer cord

Spacer

Screw anchors

Figure 29-8. Dynamic spinal fixation system. Pedicle screws are linked by a flexible rod, allowing constrained motion between the screws.

15. What are interspinous implants?

Interspinous implants are designed and indicated 1) for treatment of symptomatic lumbar spinal stenosis when fusion is not intended and 2) as a method for achieving lumbar segmental fixation when fusion of a spinal segment is intended. Interspinous implants indicated for the treatment of lumbar spinal stenosis are inserted between adjacent spinous processes to slightly distract the spinous processes apart and induce segmental kyphosis. Spinous process distraction results in slight enlargement of the cross-sectional area of the spinal canal and may relieve position-dependent spinal stenosis symptoms. Various materials (titanium, silicone, polyethylene) have been proposed for this category of implant. Patients who experience positional relief of leg pain symptoms due to lumbar spinal stenosis while in a sitting position are considered surgical candidates. This type of device is a motion-preserving implant that avoids the need for spinal fusion. Interspinous implants have also been utilized as a means of achieving segmental fixation when fusion of a motion segment is intended (Fig. 29-9).

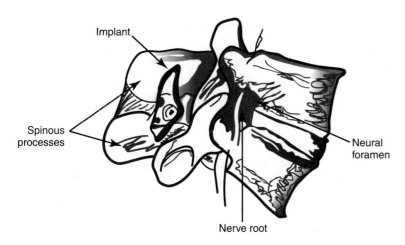

Implant

Spinous
processes

Neural
foramen

Nerve root

Figure 29-9. Interspinous implant.

ANTERIOR SPINAL INSTRUMENTATION

16. What are the two main types of anterior spinal instrumentation?

- Anterior spinal implants may be broadly classified as extracolumnar or intracolumnar implants. **Extracolumnar implants** are located on the external aspect of the vertebral body and span one or more adjacent vertebral motion segments. Extracolumnar implants consist of vertebral body screws connected to a longitudinal member consisting of either a plate or a rod. Extracolumnar implants are placed on the lateral aspect of the thoracic and lumbar vertebral bodies with screws directed in a coronal plane trajectory. An exception to this principle occurs at the L5–S1 level where implants are placed in an anterior midline location due to anatomic constraints created by the vascular structures at this level
- **Intracolumnar implants** consist of implants that reside within the contour of the vertebral bodies. Implant options include bone, metal, or synthetic materials that are capable of bearing loads. Intracolumnar implants may or may not possess potential for biologic incorporation within the anterior spinal column

17. Contrast the utility of anterior plate and rod systems.

- **Anterior plate systems** (Fig. 29-10A) are useful for short-segment spinal disorders (one or two spinal levels). Tumors, burst fractures, and degenerative spinal disorders requiring anterior fusion over one or two levels are indications for use of an anterior plate system. The use of a plate system is problematic when significant coronal or sagittal plane deformity exists or when multiple anterior vertebral segments require fixation. Technical difficulties arise because restoration of spinal alignment is required prior to plate application in the presence of significant spinal deformity
- **Anterior rod systems** (Fig. 29-10B) offer advantages in comparison to plate systems. In short-segment spinal problems, anterior rod systems permit corrective forces to be applied directly to spinal segments, thereby restoring spinal alignment. For example, in the presence of a kyphotic deformity secondary to a burst fracture, initial distraction provides deformity correction and facilitates subsequent placement of an intracolumnar implant. Subsequent compression of the anterior graft or cage restores anterior load sharing and enhances arthrodesis. In long-segment spinal problems (e.g. scoliosis) single or double rod systems can be customized to the specific spinal deformity requiring correction

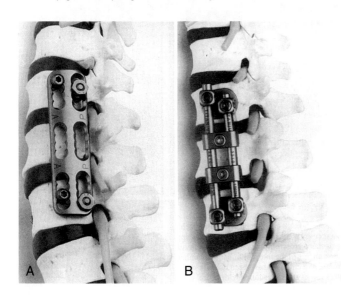

A   B

Figure 29-10. Anterior extracolumnar implants: plate system **(A)** and rod system **(B)**. (From Devlin VJ, Pitt DD. The evolution of surgery of the anterior spinal column. Spine State Art Rev 1998;12:493–528.)

18. What are some guidelines for placement of vertebral body screws when using an anterior plate or rod system?

The screws should be parallel to the vertebral endplates. In the axial plane, the screws should be parallel with or angle away from the vertebral canal. The screw tips should purchase the far cortex of the vertebral body but should not protrude more than 5 mm beyond this point (Fig. 29-11).

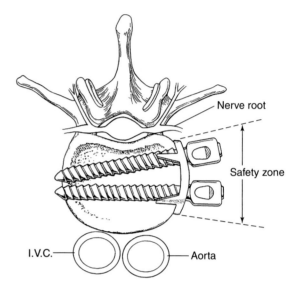

Figure 29-11. Correct placement of anterior vertebral body screws. (From Zindrick MR, Selby D. Lumbar spine fusion: different types and indications. In: Wiesel SW, Weinstein JN, Herkowitz H, et al., editors. The Lumbar Spine. 2nd ed. Philadelphia: Saunders; 1996.)

19. Describe three possible functions of intracolumnar implants.

Intracolumnar implants may be differentiated based on their intended function:

- **Promote fusion.** Intracolumnar implants that have potential for biologic incorporation include autograft bone (e.g. ilium, fibula), structural allograft bone (tibia, femur, humerus), and synthetic cages (titanium mesh, carbon fiber, polyether ether ketone) filled with bone graft. Such implants are typically used after discectomy or corpectomy to reconstruct the anterior spinal column and promote spinal fusion
- **Function as a spacer.** Certain intracolumnar implants (e.g. polymethylmethacrylate [PMMA]) are intended to function as an anterior column spacer despite lack of potential for biologic incorporation
- **Preserve motion.** An emerging concept is the use of a disc spacer to maintain segmental mobility, stability, and disc space height without fusion

20. What factors should be considered in choosing among autograft, allograft, and cage devices when an intracolumnar implant is indicated?

- **Autograft** remains the gold standard from the standpoint of fusion success. However, significant donor site morbidity is associated with procurement of a structural autograft
- **Allograft** provides good early strength and avoids donor site morbidity. However, allograft possesses a lower and slower fusion rate compared with autograft. In addition, use of allograft exposes the patient to the infectious risk associated with donor tissue
- **Cage devices** possess excellent strength and provide the advantage of mechanical interdigitation with vertebral receptor sites, thereby decreasing risk of dislodgement (Fig. 29-12). Cage devices can be filled with cancellous autograft, allograft, or biologic agents (e.g. bone morphogenetic proteins) to promote fusion. However, cage devices may subside into the vertebral bodies, resulting in loss of anterior column height. In addition, radiographic assessment of anterior column fusion can be difficult in the presence of cage devices. Cage devices are grouped into two main categories:
  - Static (cage dimensions determined prior to implantation)
  - Expandable (possess capacity for expansion following implantation to optimize stability)

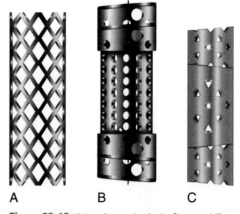

Figure 29-12. Intracolumnar implants. Commercially available vertebrectomy spacers: Titanium mesh **(A)**, expandable titanium cage **(B)**, and stackable modular polyetheretherketone (PEEK) **(C)**. (From Kim DH, Henn JS, Vaccaro AR, et al. Surgical Anatomy and Techniques to the Spine. Philadelphia: Saunders; 2006.)

21. When is it reasonable to use polymethylmethacrylate (PMMA) as a spacer to reconstruct an anterior spinal column defect?

Currently, PMMA is used in two situations:

- **Anterior spinal reconstruction of metastatic vertebral body lesions in patients with a finite lifespan.** When used for this purpose, PMMA is subject to tensile failure and loosening secondary to development of a fibrous membrane at the cement-bone interface
- **Reconstruction of osteoporotic compression fractures.** Vertebroplasty and kyphoplasty procedures involve the injection of PMMA into the vertebral bodies to alleviate pain secondary to acute and subacute fracture

22. What are the approach options for placement of an intracolumnar implant?

Intracolumnar implants may be placed through anterior, posterior, or lateral surgical approaches. The best approach depends on the location and type of spinal pathology requiring treatment. Recently, minimally invasive approaches have been popularized for placement of intracolumnar implants.

Key Points

1. Spinal implants function to maintain or restore spinal alignment, stabilize spinal segments, and enhance spinal fusion.
2. Short-term stabilization of the spine is provided by spinal implants and long-term stabilization of the spine is traditionally provided by fusion.
3. A posterior spinal instrumentation construct consists of:
   a. Vertebral anchors (hooks, wires, screws)
   b. Longitudinal elements (rods) on each side of the spine
   c. Transverse connectors (cross-linking devices)
4. Reconstruction of the load-bearing capacity of the anterior spinal column is critical to successful application of spinal instrumentation.
5. The safety and efficacy of motion preserving spinal implants is an area of active investigation.

Websites

History of surgery for correction of spinal deformity: http://www.medscape.com/viewarticle/448306
Thoracic pedicle screw fixation for spinal deformity: http://www.medscape.com/viewarticle/448311
Classification of posterior dynamic stabilization devices: http://www.medscape.com/viewarticle/555030

BIBLIOGRAPHY

1. Asher MA, Strippgen WE, Heinig CF, et al. Isola implant system. Semin Spine Surg 1992;4:175–92.
2. Cotrel Y, Dubousset J, Guillaumat M. New universal instrumentation in spine surgery. Clin Orthop 1988;227:10–23.
3. DiPaola CP, Molinari RW. Posterior lumbar interbody fusion. J Am Acad Ortho Surg 2008;16:130–9.
4. Harms J, Tabasso G. Instrumented Spinal Surgery: Principles and Techniques. New York: Thieme; 1999.
5. Harrington PR. The history and development of Harrington instrumentation. Clin Orthop 1988;227:3–5.
6. Kim DH, Albert TJ. Interspinous process spacers. J Am Acad Orth Surg 2007;15:200–7.
7. Kim DH, Henn JS, Vaccaro AR, et al. Surgical Anatomy and Techniques to the Spine. Philadelphia: Saunders; 2006.
8. Kim YJ, Lenke LG, Kim J, et al. Comparative analysis of pedicle screw versus hybrid instrumentation in posterior spinal fusion of adolescent idiopathic scoliosis. Spine 2006;31:291–8.
9. Lenke LG, Betz RR, Harms J. Modern Anterior Scoliosis Surgery. St. Louis: Quality Medical Publishing; 2004.
FDA Disclosure: Pedicle screw system clearance by the FDA is limited to use as an adjunct to fusion in skeletally mature patients. The use of pedicle screws is not FDA approved in the pediatric population as of 8/1/2010.

INSTRUMENTATION AND FUSION OF THE SPINE TO THE SACRUM AND PELVIS

Vincent J. Devlin, MD, Joseph Y. Margulies, MD, PhD, and William O. Shaffer, MD

1. When is fusion across the L5–S1 motion segment indicated?
- L5–S1 spondylolisthesis
- Symptomatic degenerative disorders involving the L5–S1 level
- Tumor, infection, or fractures involving the lumbosacral junction
- Spinal deformities (e.g. neuromuscular scoliosis with pelvic obliquity, adult idiopathic or de novo scoliosis with associated L5–S1 degenerative changes)
- Revision/salvage situations (e.g. distal extension of a prior scoliosis fusion due to degenerative changes below previously fused levels)

2. What complications are associated with fusion across the lumbosacral junction?
- Pseudarthrosis
- Loss of lumbar lordosis resulting in sagittal imbalance (flatback syndrome)
- Recurrent or progressive spinal deformity
- Implant loosening or failure
- Sacroiliac pain or arthrosis
- Pelvic stress fracture

3. Why is the L5–S1 level considered the most difficult level of the spine to fuse?
- **Unfavorable biomechanical conditions.** The lumbosacral junction is a transition zone between the highly mobile L5–S1 disc and the relatively immobile sacropelvis. Tremendous loads are transferred across the lumbosacral junction (up to 11 times body weight) as axial weight-bearing forces are transmitted from the vertebral column to the pelvis. In addition, the oblique orientation of the L5–S1 disc results in increased shear forces across this level
- **Unique anatomy of the sacrum and pelvis.** The sacrum is composed of cancellous bone and possesses limited sites for screw fixation. The large-diameter S1 pedicle provides less secure screw purchase compared with proximal vertebral levels

4. What is the *80–20 rule* of Harms? How is it relevant to L5–S1 fusion procedures?
Biomechanical studies of the lumbosacral region have demonstrated that approximately 80% of axial load is transmitted through the anterior spinal column, and the remaining 20% is transmitted through the posterior column. Spinal fusion and instrumentation procedures that do not restore anterior column load sharing across the lumbosacral junction are destined for failure.

5. Explain why it is more difficult to achieve successful fusion between T10 and the sacrum compared with fusion between L4 and the sacrum.
Long-segment fusion constructs (e.g. T10–S1) have a higher rate of failure than short-segment constructs (e.g. L4–S1) because of the following factors:
- **Increased risk of pseudarthrosis.** The pseudarthrosis rate increases as the number of levels undergoing fusion increases
- **Increased forces placed on distal sacral fixation.** Increasing the number of instrumented levels proximal to the sacrum increases the lever arm exerted by the proximal spine on the distal sacral implants. The degree of strain on S1 screws increases as the number of segments immobilized above the sacrum increases. These unfavorable biomechanical factors increase the risk of distal fixation failure

6. What types of anterior spinal implants are used when arthrodesis is performed across the lumbosacral junction?
The most common anterior implants utilized when arthrodesis is performed across the lumbosacral junction are *intracolumnar implants*. These include structural bone graft (autograft or allograft) and fusion cages (e.g. titanium mesh, carbon fiber, PEEK) used in combination with autograft, allograft, or biologics (e.g. bone morphogenic protein). Placement of *extracolumnar implants* is challenging due to proximity of vascular structures and the osseous anatomy

of the lumbosacral junction. Low-profile plates may be placed anteriorly distal to the bifurcation of the great vessels. Large-diameter cancellous screws may be used to secure bone grafts/cages between the L5 and S1 vertebral bodies.

7. What are the options for posterior implant fixation in the sacrum and pelvis when arthrodesis is performed across the lumbosacral motion segment?

Posterior implant fixation in the sacrum and pelvis can be categorized based on the three anatomic zones of the sacropelvic unit:

- **Zone 1**: Composed of the S1 vertebral body and upper margin of the sacral ala. Zone 1 fixation most commonly consists of *S1 pedicle screws* directed medially into the S1 pedicle and body. Alternate zone 1 fixation options for special situations include bilateral *L5–S1 transfacet screws* and *"S" rods* (as described by Dunn-McCarthy or Warner-Fackler).
- **Zone 2**: Composed of the sacral ala and the middle and lower sacrum. Fixation options in zone 2 include *S1 alar screws* (directed laterally into the sacral ala at the level of S1), *S2 alar screws* (directed laterally into the sacral ala at the level of S2), and *intrasacral (Jackson) rods.*
- **Zone 3**: Composed of the ilium bilaterally. Fixation is most commonly achieved with large-diameter (7–10 mm) screws placed in the lower iliac column. An alternative is placement of a solid rod (Galveston technique). Occasionally, the upper iliac column is utilized as a supplementary fixation site. Alternate zone 3 fixation techniques include the S2-alar-iliac screw fixation technique, transiliac (sacral) bar fixation, and sacroiliac screw fixation. Figure 30-1.

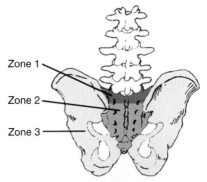

Figure 30-1. The fixation zones of the sacropelvic unit. (From O'Brien MF, Kuklo TR, Lenke LG. Sacropelvic instrumentation: anatomic and biomechanical zones of fixation. Semin Spine Surg 2004;16:76–90.)

8. Describe the technique of S1 pedicle screw placement.

The dorsal bony cortex at the base of the superior S1 articular process is removed with a rongeur or burr. A pedicle probe is directed perpendicular to the sacrum and directed medially and angled toward the S1 endplate. Careful penetration of the anterior cortex of the sacrum permits *bicortical* fixation and increases screw purchase. Screw purchase can be further enhanced by directing the S1 pedicle screw superiorly to engage the anterior margin of the endplate of S1and is termed *tricortical* fixation (posterior sacral cortex, anterior sacral cortex, and superior endplate cortex). Due to the cancellous nature of the S1 pedicle, *unicortical* screws (short screws that do not engage the anterior sacral cortex) provide less secure fixation and are prone to loosening and failure.

9. Describe the technique of laterally directed sacral screw placement.

Laterally directed sacral screws (alar screws) may be placed at the level of S1 and/or S2. The S1 alar screw entrance point is located just distal to the L5–S1 facet joint in line with the dorsal S1 neural foramen. The S2 alar screw entrance point is located between the dorsal S1 and S2 neural foramina. A starting point is created with a burr or drill in this area. A probe is placed through the sacrum until it contacts the anterior sacral cortex. The desired trajectory is 35° laterally and parallel with the S1 endplate. Length of this pilot hole is determined with a depth gauge. The anterior sacral cortex is then perforated in a controlled fashion to achieve bicortical fixation. Laterally directed sacral screws may be used in combination with medially directed S1 screws. Figure 30-2.

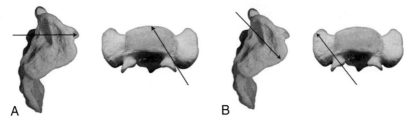

A   B

Figure 30-2. Sacral screw options. S1 pedicle screw **(A)** and S1 alar screw **(B)**. (From Kim DH, Henn JS, Vaccaro AR, et al. Surgical Anatomy and Techniques of the Spine. Saunders; 2006. p. 241.)

10. What structures are at risk when a screw is placed through the anterior cortex of the sacrum?

Medially directed S1 screws, which are directed parallel to the upper S1 endplate or toward the sacral promontory, do not endanger any neurovascular structures with the exception of the middle sacral artery and vein. If a screw is inserted in a straightforward direction without medial angulation, the L5 nerve root is at risk of injury where it crosses the anterior sacrum. Screws placed laterally at the S1 level have a greater potential to injure critical structures including the lumbosacral trunk, internal iliac vein, and sacroiliac joint. Laterally directed screws at the S2 level have potential to injure the colon, which may be adjacent to the lateral sacrum in this region (Fig. 30-3).

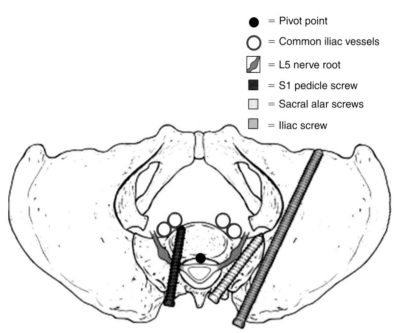

Figure 30-3. Sacropelvic fixation options in relation to the lumbosacral pivot point and adjacent critical structures. (From Polly DW, Latta LL. Spinopelvic fixation biomechanics. Semin Spine Surg 2004;16:101–6.)

11. When is it reasonable to perform a fusion across the sacrum with only bilateral S1 screw fixation?

Bilateral S1 screw fixation is effective for short-segment instrumentation and fusion across the lumbosacral junction (i.e. L4 or L5 to sacrum). A typical instrumentation construct consists of bilateral lumbar pedicle screws at each proximal level undergoing fusion. Supplemental anterior structural grafts and/or cages are utilized to provide anterior column load sharing as needed.

12. List situations where it is desirable to supplement S1 screw fixation with additional fixation strategies.

Indications for use of S1 screw fixation combined with additional sacropelvic fixation include:
- Long-segment scoliosis fusions that extend to the sacrum
- When correction of pelvic obliquity is required
- Stabilization and/or reduction and fusion of high-grade spondylolisthesis
- Lumbar revision surgery (e.g. osteotomy for sagittal imbalance syndrome; decompression and fusion for distal degeneration and stenosis below a long-segment fusion ending at L5)
- Multilevel fusion procedures in patients with osteopenia/osteoporosis

13. Describe the technique for placement of iliac fixation.

A rongeur is used to remove bone from the region of the posterior superior iliac spine (PSIS) at the level of S2–S3. A blunt probe or drill is used to develop a channel for insertion of a screw or rod between the cortices of the iliac bone along a trajectory extending from the posterior superior iliac spine and passing above the greater sciatic notch toward the anterior inferior iliac spine. Typically an anchor of at least 80 mm in length can be safely placed in adult patients. A rod-connector is often required to link the iliac screw with the longitudinal rod as the iliac screw is not colinear with the proximal screw anchors (Fig. 30-4).

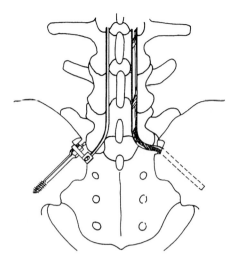

Figure 30-4. Iliac fixation. A rod is inserted on the right side and an iliac screw is inserted on the left side. (From Chewning SJ. Pelvic fixation. Spine State Art Rev 1992;6:359–68.)

14. What risks may be associated with iliac fixation?

- Need for extensive surgical exposure that can be associated with increased bleeding and prolonged operative time
- Injury to surrounding neurovascular structures including the superior gluteal artery, sciatic nerve, and cluneal nerves
- Potential for damage to the acetabulum or hip joint by misdirected anchor placement
- Implant prominence leading to the need to remove implants after fusion has occurred
- Sacroiliac pain

15. What is S2-alar-iliac fixation?

This technique for spinopelvic fixation is a modification of the traditional technique for iliac fixation (starting point in the posterior superior iliac spine). S2-alar-iliac fixation utilizes a modified starting point located 1 mm lateral and 1 mm distal to the S1 dorsal sacral foramen. The screw is directed laterally through the sacral ala, across the lower portion of the sacroiliac joint, and between the cortical tables of the ilium toward the anterior inferior iliac spine. As the starting point is colinear with an S1 pedicle screw, an offset connector is not required to link the screw to a longitudinal rod. As the starting point is more medial compared with traditional iliac fixation, there is decreased implant prominence.
A potential disadvantage of this technique is the unknown long-term consequence of placing a screw across the sacroiliac joint compared with traditional iliac fixation, which spans the posterior sacroiliac region without violation of the sacroiliac joint.

16. Describe the technique for placement of an intrasacral rod.

A rod is inserted into the lateral sacral mass through the canal of a previously placed S1 pedicle screw. The rod and screw interlock within the sacrum providing secure fixation. The implants are *buttressed* by the posterior ilium. Fixation provided by this technique is superior to fixation provided by S1 screws alone. Figure. 30-5.

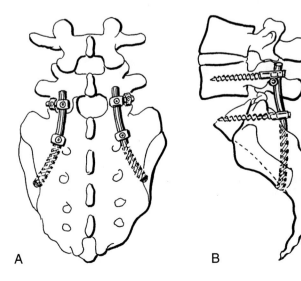

A   B

Figure 30-5. Anteroposterior **(A)** and lateral **(B)** views of the lumbosacral junction depicting an intrasacral rod construct. (From Margulies JY, Armour EF, Kohler-Ekstrand C. Revision of fusion from the spine to the sacropelvis: Considerations. In: Margulies JY, Aebi M, Farcy JP, editors. Revision Spine Surgery. St. Louis: Mosby; 1999. p. 623–30.)

17. What is transsacral fixation?

In cases of high-grade isthmic spondylolisthesis (grades 3 and 4) screws and/or bone grafts/cages may be placed obliquely across the L5–S1 disc space and obtain purchase in both the L5 and S1 vertebrae. Traditionally, a fibular graft is placed from either a posterior approach (from S1 into L5) or anterior approach (from L5 into S1). The addition of screw fixation from the upper sacrum across the L5–S1 disc space and into the L5 vertebral body increases distal screw fixation, increases the fusion rate, and decreases the risk of graft fracture.

18. What is a transiliac (sacral) bar?

This type of fixation uses rod(s) that spans the sacrum passing horizontally from ilium to ilium. Initially, sacral bars were used for fixation of sacral fractures. They have been modified to serve as an anchor within the pelvis to form the basis for complex reconstruction procedures involving fusion across the lumbosacral region. Specialized connectors have been developed to link the trans-iliac bar with longitudinal rods anchored to proximal spinal levels.

19. What is meant by the lumbosacral pivot point in relation to the biomechanics of lumbosacral fixation?

The stability provided by sacropelvic fixation devices has been conceptualized in relation to a pivot point located at the posterior aspect of the L5–S1 disc space (see Fig. 30-3). Iliac fixation provides the most stable method of sacropelvic fixation because it extends fixation for a greater distance anterior to the lumbosacral pivot point than any other technique. S1 screw fixation provides the least resistance to counteract flexion moments around the pivot point compared with other sacropelvic fixation techniques. The addition of a second point of sacral fixation provides improved fixation compared with use of S1 fixation alone.

20. What type of brace should be prescribed if the surgeon wishes to restrict motion across the lumbosacral junction?

The surgeon should prescribe a thoracolumbosacral orthosis (TLSO) with a thigh cuff. Lumbar orthoses that do not immobilize the thigh will increase rather than decrease motion across the L5–S1 level.

21. A 75-year-old woman with severe osteoporosis and adult degenerative scoliosis underwent treatment with posterior spinal instrumentation and fusion from T10 to sacrum 2 weeks ago. Distal fixation in the sacrum consisted of bilateral S1 screw fixation. Anterior column support at L5–S1 was provided with a structural femoral allograft. The patient complains of new-onset severe sacral pain, which has developed over the past several days. Radiographs show no obvious signs of sacral screw pull-out. What is the most likely explanation for the patient's severe sacral pain?

A fracture of the proximal sacrum at the level of the S1 screws should be suspected. If the fracture is nondisplaced, it may be overlooked on radiographs. A computed tomography (CT) scan of the sacrum with sagittal and coronal reconstructions should be obtained to confirm this diagnosis. Prompt treatment should be initiated before displacement of the fracture occurs and before traumatic spondyloptosis develops. Fixation distal to the fracture can be achieved with iliac fixation or S2-alar-iliac fixation.

22. Summarize the techniques that a surgeon can utilize to increase the rate of successful fusion across the L5–S1 segment.

- Perform an L5–S1 interbody fusion with a structural spacer (e.g. allograft, autograft, fusion cage) to restore anterior column load sharing and increase likelihood of successful arthrodesis
- Use multiple fixation points within the sacropelvic unit (iliac fixation is the most stable type of fixation)
- Cross-link the longitudinal members in the region of the sacrum
- Use an appropriate orthosis to restrict lumbosacral motion

Key Points

1. S1 pedicle fixation is the most common sacral fixation technique utilized when performing fusion to the sacrum.
2. For *high-risk* fusions to the sacrum, bilateral S1 pedicle screws supplemented with iliac fixation is the most reliable instrumentation technique.
3. Structural interbody support at the L4–L5 and L5–S1 levels increases the rate of fusion and decreases the risk of construct failure when performing fusion to the sacrum.

Websites

S2-alar-iliac pelvic fixation: http://thejns.org/doi/pdf/10.3171/2010.1.FOCUS09268
Comparison of pelvic fixation techniques in neuromuscular deformity correction: Galveston rod versus iliac and lumbosacral screws: http://www.medscape.com/viewarticle/545049
Spinopelvic fixation: http://www.bioline.org.br/pdf?ni05154

BIBLIOGRAPHY

1. Devlin VJ, Asher MA. Biomechanics and surgical principles of long fusions to the sacrum. Spine State Art Rev 1996;10:515–29.
2. Jackson R, McManus A. The iliac buttress: a computed tomographic study of sacral anatomy. Spine 1993;18:1318–28.
3. Lebwohl NH, Cunningham BW, Dmitriev A, et al. Biomechanical comparison of lumbosacral fixation techniques in a calf spine model. Spine 2002;27:2312–2320.
4. Lehman RA Jr, Kuklo TR, Belmont PJ Jr, et al. Advantage of pedicle screw fixation directed into the apex of the sacral promontory over bicortical fixation: a biomechanical analysis. Spine 2002;27:806–11.
5. Margulies JY, Floman Y, Farcy JP, et al, editors. Lumbosacral and Spinopelvic Fixation. Philadelphia: Lippincott-Raven; 1996.
6. Moshirfar A, Kebaish KM, Riley LH. Lumbosacral and spinopelvic fixation in spine surgery. Semin Spine Surg 2009;21:55–61.
7. McCord DH, Cunningham BW, Shono Y, et al. Biomechanical analysis of lumbosacral fixation. Spine 1992;17:S235–S243.
8. O'Brien MF, Kuklo TR, Lenke LG. Sacropelvic instrumentation: anatomic and biomechanical zones of fixation. Semin Spine Surg 2004;16:76–90.

31 | CHAPTER

INTRAOPERATIVE NEUROPHYSIOLOGIC MONITORING DURING SPINAL PROCEDURES

Robin H. Vaughan, PhD, DABNM, and Vincent J. Devlin, MD

1. What is intraoperative neurophysiologic monitoring?

Intraoperative neurophysiologic monitoring refers to the various neurophysiologic techniques used to assess functional integrity of the nervous system during surgical procedures that place these structures at risk.

2. What neurologic structures are at risk during spinal surgery?

- Spinal cord and/or nerve roots at the surgical site
- Spinal cord and/or nerve roots remote from the surgical site (e.g. placed at risk of injury from positioning of extremities, head, or neck)
- Optic nerve

3. What criteria need to be met if intraoperative neurophysiologic monitoring is used during spinal surgery?

Three criteria need to be met if monitoring is used during spinal surgery:

- Neurologic structures are at risk
- Those structures can be monitored reliably and efficiently by qualified personnel
- The surgeon is willing and able to alter surgical technique based on information provided

4. List common types of spinal procedures during which intraoperative neurophysiologic monitoring is commonly utilized.

- Correction of spinal deformities (scoliosis, kyphosis, spondylolisthesis)
- Insertion of spinal fixation devices (e.g. pedicle screw placement)
- Decompression at the level of the spinal cord
- Surgical treatment of spinal cord tumors

5. Which intraoperative personnel may perform intraoperative neurophysiologic monitoring? What are their qualifications?

A variety of personnel may provide spinal monitoring services:

- **Certified neurophysiologic intraoperative monitoring technologist (CNIM):** Usually a registered electroencephalography (EEG) technologist who has completed a course of study, demonstrated competence in acquiring intraoperative data over a number of cases, and passed a nationally recognized technologist examination. No state license is available
- **Audiologist (CCC-A, Certified Clinical Competence-Audiology):** Certified audiologist with a minimum of a master's degree in audiology and related neurophysiology. Passing a nationally recognized audiology examination is required. There is no requirement to document surgical case experience or intraoperative skills. A license is available in every state, although not every state recognizes intraoperative monitoring as within the scope of practice of audiology
- **Neurophysiologist:** Noncertified neurophysiologist with a minimum of a master's degree and often a doctorate in neurophysiology or neurosciences. Demonstration of intraoperative monitoring proficiency is not required. No state license is available
- **Neurophysiologist, D.ABNM (Diplomate of the American Board of Neurophysiologic Monitoring):** Neurophysiologist with a minimum of a master's and often a doctorate degree in audiology, neurophysiology, or neurosciences. Requirements include passing a written and oral nationally accredited board examination with a minimum of 300 documented monitored surgical cases. No state license is available
- **Physician:** Usually a neurologist who may work with or without technologists. The physician is not required to pass any nationally recognized or accredited board examinations. A state license is required

6. What mechanisms may be responsible for neurologic injury during spine procedures?

- **Direct injury** due to surgical trauma (e.g. during spinal canal decompression or placement of spinal implants)
- **Traction and/or compression** affecting neural structures. This may occur during spinal realignment and deformity correction using spinal instrumentation or as a result of epidural hematoma following corpectomy procedures

- **Ischemia** resulting in decreased perfusion of the spinal cord and/or nerve roots, resulting in ischemic injury to neurologic structures (e.g. following ligation of critical segmental vessels supplying the spinal cord or after an episode of sustained hypotension). Ischemia is the most common mechanism responsible for neurologic injury during scoliosis surgery
- **Compressive neuropathy** as a result of patient positioning prior to or during surgery (e.g. brachial plexus injury)

7. What techniques are available for monitoring spinal cord function?
- Stagnara wake-up test
- Ankle clonus test
- Somatosensory-evoked potentials (SSEPs)
- Transcranial electric motor-evoked potentials (tceMEPs)

8. What is the technique for monitoring nerve root function during spinal surgery?
Electromyographic (EMG) monitoring.

9. What is the Stagnara wake-up test?
The Stagnara wake-up test is used to assess the gross integrity of spinal cord motor tract function during spinal surgery. Discussing this test with the patient before surgery increases its success. During the procedure, anesthesia is temporarily reduced to a degree where the patient is able to follow simple commands (move both hands and then both feet). Most patients have no recollection of being awakened, and those who recall do not report the experience to be unpleasant. This test has significant limitations. It does not provide information about spinal cord sensory tract function or individual nerve root function. In addition, it cannot be administered in a continuous fashion during surgery. A spinal cord injury may not manifest immediately following a specific surgical maneuver and thus may not be detected with a wake-up test. In addition, impending spinal cord compromise due to ischemia cannot be detected using this test. Furthermore, during the wake-up test, patient movement may disrupt sterility of the operative field or displace the endotracheal tube. The limitations associated with clinically based tests, such as the wake-up test and ankle clonus test, stimulated the development of intraoperative neurophysiologic monitoring techniques.

10. What is the ankle clonus test?
Ankle clonus is the rhythmic contraction of the calf muscles following sudden passive dorsiflexion of the foot. Clonus is produced by elicitation of the stretch reflex. In the normal, awake person, clonus cannot be elicited because of central inhibition of this stretch reflex. The clonus test relies on the presence of central inhibition and clonus to confirm that the spinal cord and peripheral neurologic structures are functionally intact. Neurologically intact patients emerging from general anesthesia normally have temporary ankle clonus bilaterally. Absence of transient ankle clonus has been correlated with neurologic compromise.

11. What are SSEPs?
Somatosensory-evoked potentials (SSEPs) are a modification of the basic EEG in which a cortical or subcortical response to repetitive stimulation of a peripheral mixed nerve is recorded at sites cephalad and caudad to the operative field. Data including signal amplitude (height) and latency (time of occurrence) are recorded continuously during surgery and compared with baseline data. SSEPs provide direct information about status of the ascending spinal cord sensory tracts (located in the dorsal medial columns of the spinal cord). SSEPs provide only indirect information about the status of the spinal cord motor tracts (located in the anterolateral columns of the spinal cord). SSEP data do not provide real-time data regarding neurologic function because there is a slight delay (usually <1 minute) while the SSEP response is averaged for extraction from background noise.

12. Discuss important limitations of SSEPs.
SSEPs directly assess spinal cord sensory tracts but provide only indirect information about motor tracts. Damage to the spinal cord motor tracts can occur without a concomitant change in SSEPs. SSEPs are better for detecting mechanical damage than ischemic damage to motor tracts because these cord regions have different blood supplies. The spinal cord motor tracts are supplied by the anterior spinal artery, whereas the spinal cord sensory tracts are perfused by radicular arteries. SSEPs may be unrecordable in patients with severe myelopathy, peripheral neuropathy, or obesity. In addition, recording SSEPs is not a sensitive technique for monitoring individual nerve root function.

13. What factors other than neurologic injury can have an adverse effect on SSEP recordings?
Operating room power equipment (due to electrical interference), halogenated anesthetic agents, nitrous oxide, hypothermia, and hypotension.

14. When should the surgeon be notified about changes in SSEPs?
The surgeon should be notified when SSEPs show a persistent unilateral or bilateral loss of amplitude 50% or greater relative to baseline amplitude. Changes in latency are common and less significant, and spinal cord injury is unlikely if amplitude is unchanged.

15. What are tceMEPs?

Transcranial electric motor-evoked potentials (tceMEPs) are neuroelectric impulses elicited by transcranial application of a high-voltage stimulus to electrodes placed over specific scalp regions to excite specific areas of the motor cortex. These descending impulses stimulate corticospinal tract axons and are typically recorded from electrodes placed over key upper and lower extremity peripheral muscles as a compound muscle action potential (CMAP). Motor-evoked potentials can also be recorded directly from the spinal cord (D- and I-waves) via electrodes placed percutaneously or through a laminotomy.

16. What is the advantage of using tceMEPs?

tceMEPs can provide information about the functional integrity of the spinal cord motor tracts that cannot be obtained using SSEPs. They are extremely sensitive to alterations in spinal cord blood flow resulting from intraoperative hypotension or evolving vascular injury. In addition, alterations in tceMEPs present earlier than changes in SSEPs in patients with evolving neurologic injury, which permits earlier initiation of corrective action to prevent permanent neurologic compromise. tceMEPs are not a replacement for SSEPs but are used in combination with SSEPs to provide a direct measure of both spinal cord sensory and motor tract function, thereby increasing the efficacy of spinal monitoring.

17. When should the surgeon be notified about changes in tceMEPs?

The surgeon should be notified when tceMEPs show a persistent unilateral or bilateral loss of amplitude 65% or greater relative to baseline amplitude.

18. Is the use of tceMEPs associated with any dangers or complications?

Only rare and minor complications have been reported in association with the use of tceMEPs in spine surgery. The most common complication is a tongue or lip laceration. This complication is easily preventable by ensuring that a single or double bite block is placed following intubation. Transcranial stimulation can safely be applied in patients with cardiac disease, pacemakers, and a history of prior or active seizures. Movement-related injury has not been a problem even with patients who are positioned in tongs or with a Mayfield positioner.

19. What is the role of electromyographic monitoring during spinal procedures?

Electromyography is used to assess the functional integrity of individual nerve roots. Electromyographic techniques are classified into two categories based on method of elicitation: mechanical and electrical. **Mechanically elicited electromyograms (EMGs)** are used during the dynamic phases of surgery (pedicle screw preparation and insertion, nerve root manipulation). Mechanically elicited EMGs are also termed *spontaneous* or *free-running* EMGs. **Electrically elicited EMGs** should be used during the static phases of surgery (immediately before or after pedicle screw placement). An electrically elicited EMG is also termed a *stimulus-evoked* EMG or *triggered* EMG.

20. How does a surgeon use electromyography to check that screws have been properly placed within the lumbar pedicles?

The surgeon places an electromyographic probe onto the pedicle screw and electrically stimulates the screw. If the pedicle wall is intact, the passage of electrical current will be restricted and the adjacent nerve root will not be stimulated. If the pedicle wall has been fractured, current passes through the pedicle wall and stimulates the adjacent nerve root. This results in contraction of the associated peripheral muscle, which is recorded as an EMG. Electrical thresholds for electromyographic activity consistent with safe screw placement have been determined and provide a reference for clinical practice.

21. What is the difference between *burst* EMG and *train* EMG?

Burst EMG activity is indicative of a nerve root being mechanically irritated, resulting in a brief burst of muscle activity of a few seconds duration. Multiple irritations or insults result in the muscle going into spasm, which is termed *train*. **Train EMG** activity is consistent with nerve root injury and must be dealt with immediately because it often predicts postoperative motor nerve deficit.

22. How is intraoperative spinal monitoring used to prevent neurologic injury secondary to patient positioning?

Paraplegia or quadriplegia may result from hyperextension positioning of the stenotic cervical or lumbar spine. Spinal monitoring of both upper and lower extremity neurologic function can permit prompt recognition and repositioning, thereby preventing permanent neurologic deficit. Monitoring of ulnar nerve SEPs is performed to assess possible brachial plexopathy due to changes in arm positioning. During anterior procedures, monitoring of peroneal nerve and femoral nerve function is performed. Peroneal nerve monitoring can alert staff to the onset of an impending peroneal nerve palsy secondary to pressure of the leg against the operating room table. A permanent injury can be averted by moving the patient's leg or adjusting the padding. Monitoring of femoral nerve function can alert the surgeon to excessive traction on the iliopsoas muscle and the adjacent nerve roots during an anterior procedure and prevent femoral nerve injury.

23. What is the effect of the anesthetic agents on neurophysiologic signals?

Inhalational agents, nitrous oxide, and partial muscle relaxation depress signal amplitude, increase signal variability, and increase interpretative error. When transcranial electric motor and somatosensory evoked potentials are recorded, a total intravenous anesthesia regimen (TIVA) is optimal. Inhalational agents should be avoided after induction and intubation. All depolarizing and nondepolarizing paralytic agents should be avoided, except at the beginning of the procedure during spinal exposure, because these agents block neuromuscular junction transmission and preclude muscle contraction.

24. What protocol should be followed if a neuromonitoring alert (significant decrease or loss of neurophysiologic potentials) occurs during surgery?

The surgeon and anesthesiologist should remain calm and communicate with the spinal monitoring personnel as the following steps are taken:
1. Check that the electrodes have not become displaced
2. Elevate and maintain the mean arterial blood pressure between 85 and 95 mm Hg
3. Assess if there has been a change in anesthetic technique
4. Reverse any antecedent surgical event (e.g. strut graft/cage placement; surgical maneuvers including distraction, compression, or translation)
5. Inspect for an obvious source of neural compression (e.g. bone fragment, hematoma)
6. Elevate body temperature and irrigate the wound with warm saline
7. Send an arterial blood gas and laboratory tests to assess for an unrecognized metabolic abnormality or unrecognized low hemoglobin
8. If tceMEP/SSEP data fail to recover, a wake-up test and awake clinical examination are considered
9. Depending on the patient's response to the wake-up test and the specific spinal problem undergoing treatment, spinal instrumentation may require removal. The individual clinical scenario and stability of the spine must be considered in decision making
10. Use of steroids (spinal injury protocol) is an option

25. A 60-year-old man with cervical myelopathy is scheduled for C4 to C6 corpectomies, anterior fibula grafting, and posterior spinal instrumentation and fusion C2 to T1. What neurophysiologic monitoring modalities are appropriate for this case?

Monitoring of spinal cord function is performed with tceMEPs and SSEPs recorded from both upper and lower extremities. Upper extremity SSEPs will also provide monitoring for brachial plexopathy due to positioning. Cervical nerve roots can be monitored with spontaneous electromyography and tceMEPs recorded from the deltoid and hand muscles. Brainstem auditory-evoked responses (BAERs) can be considered to monitor brainstem perfusion because the vertebral artery is at risk with this surgical exposure.

26. A 50-year-old woman is undergoing surgical treatment for adult scoliosis, consisting of multilevel anterior discetomies and fusion (T12–S1) followed by posterior spinal instrumentation (pedicle screws) and fusion (T4–S1). What neurophysiologic monitoring modalities are indicated for this type of surgical procedure?

Multimodality, intraoperative neurophysiologic monitoring is indicated. A combination of SSEPs and tceMEPs is required to optimally assess spinal cord function. Electromyographic techniques are required to assess nerve root function. Upper extremity SSEPs are indicated to monitor for positional brachial plexopathy. A wake-up test can be performed if significant deterioration of SSEPs and/or tceMEPs occurs during surgery.

27. A 40-year-old man is scheduled for L2–L3 and L3–L4 transforaminal lumbar interbody fusion, allograft cages L2–L3 and L3–L4, and pedicle screw placement. What neurophysiologic monitoring modalities are indicated?

In lumbar procedures, monitoring modalities are determined by the level of surgery. The spinal cord extends distally to the L1–L2 region, and monitoring of both spinal cord (SSEPs, tceMEPs) and nerve root function (EMG) is recommended for procedures extending above the L3 level. Ulnar nerve SSEP monitoring is performed to assess the brachial plexus during surgery.

28. A 20-year-old man with grade 3 L5 to S1 isthmic spondylolisthesis is scheduled for L4 to S1 posterior spinal instrumentation and fusion, L5 to S1 interbody fusion, and reduction of the spondylolisthesis. What neurophysiologic monitoring modalities are indicated?

For procedures below L2, neurophysiologic monitoring is directed to assessment of nerve root function utilizing electromyographic techniques. Ulnar nerve SSEPs are indicated to permit identification of impending brachial plexus injury due to prolonged prone positioning. Addition of anal sphincter electromyography can be considered for intraoperative assessment of S2 to S4 nerve root integrity.

Key Points

1. Multimodality, intraoperative neurophysiologic monitoring permits assessment of the functional integrity of the spinal cord and nerve roots during spinal surgery.
2. Intraoperative assessment of spinal cord function is optimally achieved with a combination of transcranial electric motor-evoked potentials (tceMEPs) and somatosensory-evoked potentials (SSEPs).
3. Intraoperative assessment of nerve root function is achieved via electromyographic (EMG) monitoring techniques.
4. The optimal anesthesia maintenance protocol for successful intraoperative neurophysiologic monitoring of spinal cord function is a total intravenous anesthesia (TIVA) regimen with avoidance of muscle relaxation, nitrous oxide, and inhalational agents.

Websites

American Board of Registration of Electroencephalographic and Evoked Potential Technologists: http://abret.org/
American Society of Neurophysiologic Monitoring: http://www.asnm.org/default.aspx
Credentialing and competency policy statement for intraoperative neuromonitoring staff:
   http://www.asnm.org/PolicyStatement08.pdf
Scoliosis Research Society Information Statement, 2009, Neurophysiologic Monitoring:
   http://www.srs.org/UserFiles/Neuromonitoring%20Information%20statement%202%206%2009.doc

BIBLIOGRAPHY

1. Devlin VJ, Anderson PA, Schwartz DM, et al. Intraoperative neurophysiologic monitoring: focus on cervical myelopathy and related issues. Spine J 2006;6(6 Suppl):212S–224S.
2. Devlin VJ, Schwartz DM. Intraoperative neurophysiologic monitoring during spinal surgery. J Am Acad Ortho Surg 2007;15:549–60.
3. Hilibrand AS, Schwartz DM, Sethurasman V, et al. Comparison of transcranial electric motor and somatosensory evoked potential monitoring during cervical surgery. J Bone Joint Surg 2004;86A:1248–53.
4. Hoppenfeld S, Gross A, Lonner B. The ankle clonus test for assessment of the integrity of the spinal cord during operations for scoliosis. J Bone Joint Surg 1997;79A:208–12.
5. Lee JY, Hilibrand AS, Lim MR, et al. Characterization of neurophysiologic alerts during anterior cervical spine surgery. Spine 2006;31:1916–22.
6. Owen JH. Cost efficacy of intraoperative monitoring. Semin Spine Surg 1997;9:348–52.
7. Schwartz DM, Auerbach JD, Dormans JP, et al. Neurophysiological detection of impending spinal cord injury during scoliosis surgery. J Bone Joint Surg 2007;89A:2440–49.
8. Schwartz DM, Dormans JP, Drummond DS, et al. Transcranial electric motor evoked potential monitoring during spine surgery–is it safe? Presented at the 42nd annual meeting of the Scoliosis Research Society, Edinburg, Scotland, September 6, 2007.
9. Schwartz DM, Drummond DS, Schwartz JA, et al. Neurophysiological monitoring during scoliosis surgery: a multimodal approach. Semin Spine Surg 1997;9:97–111.
10. Schwartz DM, Sestokas AK. A systems-based algorithmic approach to intraoperative neurophysiological monitoring during spine surgery. Semin Spine Surg 2002;14:136–45.

ANESTHESIA AND RELATED INTRAOPERATIVE CONSIDERATIONS IN SPINE SURGERY

CHAPTER 32

Ashit C. Patel, MD, Vincent J. Devlin, MD, and William O. Shaffer, MD

1. What are the top 10 areas of concern in relation to perioperative anesthesia care for spinal surgery patients?
1. Assessment of patient-specific risk factors
2. Assessment of procedure-specific risk factors
3. Airway management
4. Invasive monitoring
5. Intraoperative neurophysiologic monitoring
6. Intraoperative positioning
7. Maintenance of normothermia
8. Fluid management (crystalloid, colloid, transfusion, autotransfusion)
9. Preparation for potential intraoperative disasters
10. Postoperative assessment and coordination of postoperative care

2. What patient-specific risk factors are emphasized during the preoperative anesthetic evaluation?
- **Cardiac:** Pediatric patients have a low incidence of coronary diseases unless neuromuscular disease or syndromic spinal deformities are present. In adult patients, risk stratification, beta-blockade, and noninvasive cardiac testing are implemented based on cardiac risk factors and symptoms according to American College of Cardiology/American Heart Association (ACC/AHA) guidelines
- **Pulmonary:** Restrictive lung disease may be present in patients with thoracic scoliosis/hyperkyphosis or spinal deformities secondary to neuromuscular disease. Smoking, chronic obstructive pulmonary disease, asthma, and sleep apnea are additional factors that influence perioperative management
- **Airway:** Unique challenges are posed by patients with rheumatoid arthritis, ankylosing spondylitis, cervical instability, and cervical myelopathy
- **Medications and allergies:** Cessation of antiplatelet agents (e.g. clopidogrel), aspirin, and anticoagulants must be coordinated with the patient's primary physicians prior to surgery. Nonsteroidal antiinflammatory medication is typically discontinued 7 to 10 days before surgery. Cardiac and diabetic medications are typically continued before surgery
- **Hemostasis:** A history of abnormal bruising or bleeding should be investigated. A laboratory coagulation profile is advised before surgery
- **Neurologic:** Important concerns include the presence/absence of neurologic deficit, stability of the cervical spine as it influences intubation technique, and possible need for an intraoperative wake-up test
- **Endocrine:** Diabetic patients are evaluated for adequacy of blood glucose control. Patients who are on long-term steroid therapy are administered perioperative (stress) steroids

3. What patient populations are at increased risk of latex allergy?
Prior exposure to latex as a result of medical treatment (e.g. multiple bladder catheterizations, multiple surgical procedures at a young age) or occupational exposure may lead to an IgE-mediated anaphylactic reaction with subsequent exposure to the latex antigen. Patient populations with an increased risk of latex allergy include patients with myelodysplasia, congenital genitourinary tract abnormalities, spinal cord injuries, cerebral palsy, ventriculoperitoneal shunts, and health care workers. Anaphylaxis secondary to latex allergy may occur intraoperatively (usually 20–60 minutes following induction) and must be included in the differential diagnosis of intraoperative emergencies. A detailed history is the best means of detecting patients at risk. Patients with a history of latex allergy may be treated with pharmacologic prophylaxis (diphenhydramine, ranitidine, prednisone), but this may not prevent an anaphylactic reaction. A latex-free environment must be provided in the operating room.

4. How do anesthesiologists estimate anesthetic risk and anticipate outcome associated with surgery?
Anesthesiologists perform a preanesthetic assessment and assign an American Society of Anesthesiologist (ASA) physical classification (Table 32-1).

Table 32-1. American Society of Anesthesiologists (ASA) Physical Status Classification System

CLASS	DESCRIPTION
1	Normal, healthy patient
2	Patient with mild systemic disease
3	Patient with severe systemic disease that limits activity but is not incapacitating
4	Patient with an incapacitating disease that is a constant threat to life
5	Moribund patient who is not expected to survive 24 hours without surgery
6	A declared brain-dead patient undergoing organ removal for donor purposes
E	Patient undergoing an emergency procedure

5. **What types of spinal procedures are associated with an increased risk of complications and perioperative morbidity?**
- Revision spinal deformity procedures
- Same-day multilevel anterior-posterior spinal procedures
- Multilevel anterior spinal instrumentation and fusion
- Fusions for spinal deformities in patients with neuromuscular scoliosis
- Emergent procedures for tumor, infection, and trauma

6. **What types of cervical pathology are associated with increased risk of neurologic injury with endotracheal intubation?**
Patients with an unstable cervical spine (e.g. fracture, rheumatoid arthritis, odontoid hypoplasia) or severe cervical stenosis are at risk for neurologic injury with endotracheal intubation. The most important factors for minimizing neurologic injury are recognizing cord compression and/or spinal instability, performing intubation with care, and avoiding neck movement. Many anesthesiologists prefer fiberoptic intubation in this setting. Monitoring of neurologic function can be performed directly if an awake intubation technique is utilized or indirectly with neurophysiologic monitoring if an unconscious fiberoptic-guided intubation is performed. A variety of alternative options for intubation in this setting have been described including manual inline cervical immobilization and orotracheal intubation, as well as use of specialized laryngoscope blades, video laryngoscopes, lighted stylets, and bronchoscopes.

7. **What types of spinal procedures require single lung ventilation?**
Thoracic spine procedures performed with the assistance of thoracoscopy require single-lung ventilation to maintain a safe working space within the thoracic cavity. Anterior thoracic spine procedures performed through an open thoracotomy approach for exposure of the spine above the level of T8 also benefit from single-lung ventilation. Single-lung ventilation decreases the difficulty of retracting the lung from the operative field in the upper thoracic region. For open procedures below the T8 level, the lung can more easily be retracted out of the operative field without the need for single-lung ventilation. Options for single lung ventilation include use of a double lumen endotracheal tube or a bronchial blocker tube.

8. **What complications have been reported in association with hypothermia during surgery?**
Complications reported in association with intraoperative hypothermia (core temperature < 35.5° C) include myocardial depression, cardiac arrhythmias, thrombocytopenia, decreased mobilization of calcium, prolongation of drug half-lives, and lactic acidosis.

9. **What steps can be taken to prevent hypothermia during spine surgery?**
- Use of forced-air warming systems
- Use of fluid warmers
- Use of humidified, warmed (40° C) inspired gases
- Use of warm lavage for wound irrigation
- Warming of the operating room

10. **What are the requirements for hemodynamic monitoring during spinal procedures?**
The minimum requirements for major spine procedures include two large-bore peripheral intravenous lines and intra-arterial blood pressure monitoring. Central venous pressure monitoring is considered when:
- Expected intraoperative blood loss is expected to exceed 50% of blood volume
- Major fluid shifts are anticipated
- Preoperative assessment suggests that traditional signs of fluid management will be difficult to assess
- Complex surgical procedures (e.g. multilevel instrumentation and fusion for spinal deformity) or complex postoperative management (e.g. hyperalimentation) is planned

11. What is the best way to monitor fluid administration during major spinal reconstructive procedures?
Careful fluid calculations and hourly recording of estimated blood loss are the most effective methods to monitor fluid administration. Fluid replacement calculations must account for deficit, maintenance, third-space loss, and blood loss. Initially crystalloid solution is administered. Administration of colloid solution (e.g. 5% albumin or 6% hetastarch) or blood should be considered for surgery exceeding 4 hours or blood loss exceeding 25% of blood volume. There is no universally accepted threshold at which to transfuse blood. Factors to consider include patient age, concomitant disease, and concerns regarding perfusion of the optic nerve and spinal cord. Monitoring of heart rate, direct arterial pressure, and urine output combined with central venous pressure in complex cases provides the necessary information regarding hemodynamics.

12. What methods can be used to reduce allogeneic blood transfusion during spine surgery?
- Preoperative autologous blood donation
- Preoperative marrow stimulation (erythropoietin)
- Acute normovolemic hemodilution
- Intraoperative salvage (use of cell saver)
- Hypotensive anesthesia technique (use limited by concerns regarding paralysis and blindness—restrict to young patients without neurologic deficits and patients without *at-risk* spinal cord)
- Accepting a lower threshold hemoglobin level before transfusion
- Use of pharmacologic agents (aminocaproic acid, transexamic acid, desmopressin)

13. What problems are associated with use of a cell saver?
- Improper suctioning technique can lead to hemolysis
- Coagulopathy (loss of fibrinogen and platelets in salvaged blood)
- Potentially toxic materials may be infused to the patient (e.g. thrombin)
- Pulmonary complications due to tissue debris that accompanies washed cells
- Hemoglobinuria
- Inability to remove cancer cells and bacteria

14. What are the options for monitoring neurologic function during spinal procedures?
A variety of methods may be used to monitor neurologic function during spinal surgery including:
- Somatosensory-evoked potentials (SSEPs)
- Transcranial electric motor-evoked potentials (tceMEPs)
- Electromyography (EMG)
- Stagnara wake-up test
- Ankle clonus test

15. What are the anesthesia requirements for the different spinal monitoring techniques?
For **surgery at the level of the spinal cord or conus medullaris,** multimodality monitoring with a combination of SSEPs and tceMEPs is indicated. The preferred anesthetic technique in this situation is total intravenous anesthesia (TIVA) utilizing propofol and a short-acting opioid infusion. If TIVA is not possible, anesthesia with a combined low-level (e.g. 0.3 minimum alveolar concentration [MAC]) volatile agent augmented by combination intravenous drugs is used, although even this low concentration of volatile anesthetic is known to compromise cortical SSEP and tceMEP amplitudes, as well as increase signal variability. Hence, use of any inhalational anesthetics should be viewed only as a "last resort" measure. When propofol is either precluded or is not readily available, TIVA alternatives include ketamine, etomidate, and/or dexmedetomidine.

For **surgery in the lumbar region below the level of the conus medullaris,** monitoring typically is directed toward assessment of lumbar nerve root function with recording of spontaneous and stimulus evoked EMG from lower extremity myotomes in conjunction with upper extremity SSEPs to identify impending positional brachial plexopathy. This permits a less restrictive anesthesia protocol and allows greater flexibility in the use of inhalational agents rather than TIVA. In such cases, it is critical to ensure that the neuromuscular junction is unblocked. Once decompression commences, there should be no muscle relaxants on-board as evidenced by a train-of-four ratio of at least 0.7, measured preferably from a foot versus a hand muscle. Recent studies have shown that absence or cessation of spontaneous neurotonic electromyographic activity provides limited information about the functional integrity of spinal nerve roots and appears to be insensitive to slow-onset traction injuries or vascular insult to the nerve root. Consequently, some centers have modified their neurophysiologic monitoring strategy during instrumented lumbosacral spine surgery to include tceMEPs in order to provide ongoing information regarding nerve root functional integrity. When tceMEPs are recorded, a TIVA protocol is preferred. In such cases, the anesthetic requirements for TIVA are the same as for cervical or thoracic spine surgery (propofol, opioid [preferably remifentanil], midazolam [low dose of 1–2 mg/hour if needed], and no neuromuscular blockade).

16. **In addition to use of intraoperative neurophysiologic monitoring, name two other issues that require consideration to minimize risk of intraoperative neurologic injury?**
    - *Careful patient positioning.* The neurologic injury related to positioning can be minimized with attention to details and technique. Use of a Jackson turning frame has been documented to generate significantly less spine motion compared with log-roll technique during supine to prone transfers onto the operating room (OR) table in unstable spines.
    - *Careful maintenance of systemic blood pressure.* In high-risk patients (e.g. severe myelopathy, preexistent neurologic deficit), maintenance of systemic blood pressure at preoperative levels or induction of mild hypertension is valuable in maintaining spinal cord perfusion

17. **What difficulties have been reported in association with use of the Stagnara intraoperative wake-up test?**
    - Extubation secondary to patient movement
    - Dislodgement of intravenous access
    - Air embolus
    - Dislodgement of spinal implants
    - Difficulty using the test in patients with reduced capacity (e.g. deafness, language barrier)
    - Contamination of the surgical field

18. **What ophthalmologic complications are encountered in relation to spine procedures?**
    Corneal abrasions, periorbital edema, and postoperative visual loss. Postoperative visual loss most commonly occurs due to ischemic optic neuropathy (ION) and less commonly due to central retinal artery or vein occlusion or occipital infarct. Risk factors associated with ION include anemia, intraoperative hypotension, and external orbital pressure.

19. **List important considerations in positioning patients for a spinal procedure in the prone position.**
    Most patients readily tolerate spine surgery in the prone position. Important considerations include:
    - The head should be kept at or slightly above the level of the heart to maintain brain perfusion. The head-down position should be avoided because it decreases intraocular perfusion pressure. The cervical spine should be kept in a neutral or slightly flexed position
    - Cushioning should be placed beneath the forehead and chin, to keep the eyes, chin, and face free of pressure. Alternatively, cervical tong traction may be used to suspend the head.
    - The upper extremities should be positioned with the shoulders and elbows flexed below 90° (for thoracic and lumbar procedures) or tucked at the patient's sides (for cervical procedures)
    - Padding should be placed beneath the elbow to protect the ulnar nerve from compression
    - The abdomen should be free of compression to reduce venous backflow through Batson's plexus with resultant vertebral venous plexus engorgement
    - The breast, chest, and iliac areas should be adequately padded to prevent compression injury
    - If the surgical procedure involves lumbar fusion, the hips should be extended to create a lordotic alignment of the lumbar spinal segments
    - Male genitalia should be checked to verify absence of compression
    - Sequential compression stockings should be placed to prevent venous pooling in the lower extremities
    - The Foley catheter should be secured to prevent dislodgement

20. **List important considerations in positioning a patient for a spinal procedure in the lateral decubitus position.**
    The lateral decubitus position is commonly used for surgical procedures involving the anterior aspect of the thoracic and lumbar spine. Important considerations include:
    - Neutral alignment of the head and cervical spine
    - Protection of the dependent eye and ear from pressure
    - Placement of an axillary roll to relieve pressure on the dependent shoulder and prevent compression of the neurovascular bundle by the humeral head
    - Protection of the peroneal nerve in the dependent leg with a pillow
    - Placement of a pillow between the legs to prevent pressure from bony prominences
    - Sequential compression stockings to prevent venous pooling in the lower extremities

21. **What are the major concerns when the kneeling or tuck position is used for spinal procedures?**
    The extreme degree of hip and knee flexion required to achieve this position is not feasible for many patients, especially those with total joint replacements or severe hip or knee arthritis. This position can significantly compromise perfusion to the lower extremities, resulting in ischemia, thrombosis, compartment syndrome, and neurologic deficits. Use of this position is restricted to brief spinal procedures such as lumbar discectomy.

22. What are the major concerns with use of the sitting position for spinal procedures?

The sitting position is preferred by some surgeons for procedures involving the posterior cervical spine. The major advantage of this position is reduced blood pooling in the surgical field and potentially reduced blood loss because of improved venous drainage. The airway is easily accessible, and optimal ventilation of lungs is facilitated. The disadvantages include systemic hypotension and the creation of a negative pressure gradient that may result in air entrainment and venous air embolus (VAE). Careful management and monitoring are essential to prevent serious complications associated with this operative position. Prior hydration and gradual transfer to the sitting position avoid undue systemic hypotension. Insertion of a central venous pressure catheter is recommended to monitor intravascular pressure, confirm the potential diagnosis of air embolism, and potentially retrieve air in the event that a large embolus obstructs cardiac outflow. A precordial Doppler placed on the right chest is a sensitive marker for sounds of air embolus.

23. What are some intraoperative disasters reported during spinal procedures?

- Excessive bleeding
- Disseminated intravascular coagulation (DIC)
- Malignant hyperthermia (MH)
- Extubation in prone position
- Deterioration in neurologic status
- Air embolus
- Tension pneumothorax
- Cardiac arrest in prone position

24. What is disseminated intravascular coagulation (DIC)?

DIC is the intravascular consumption of coagulation factors and platelets that leads to diffuse and excessive hemorrhage. Normally, tissue injury initiates hemostasis and results in the formation of thrombus. In DIC the inciting factors render the local control mechanisms inadequate, and intravascular clot formation is precipitated. The conversion of plasminogen to plasmin triggers the fibrinolytic mechanism, resulting in diffuse hemorrhage. Subsequent renal failure, liver dysfunction, respiratory distress, shock, and thromboembolic phenomenon can lead to multisystem failure and death.

25. How is DIC diagnosed?

If the surgeon encounters diffuse, excessive hemorrhage during surgery, a coagulation panel should be drawn. Decreased platelet count, decreased fibrinogen level, increased fibrin degradation products, increased D-dimer level, and elevated coagulation times support this diagnosis. Treatment includes immediate transfusion of fresh frozen plasma and platelets. Administration of fibrinogen concentrates or cryoprecipitate can be considered. In extreme cases, administration of heparin is considered but remains controversial.

26. Define venous air embolus (VAE).

VAE has been reported in association with spinal surgery in both the prone and sitting position. Visible air bubbling at the operative site during posterior spinal instrumentation and fusion surgery has been reported as the first sign of VAE. Air may enter the venous system during spine surgery, as multiple venous channels remain open above the level of the heart. VAE may occur if the venous pressure at the level of the wound is less than the surrounding atmospheric pressure. Turbulence on the Doppler monitor and sudden decrease in the end-tidal carbon dioxide, followed by compromise of vital signs, suggest VAE. If air continues to enter, hypotension, arrhythmias, hypoxemia, and cardiac arrest may occur. Treatment consists of discontinuing nitrous oxide from the gas mixture and flooding the wound with saline to prevent further air entrainment. If the patient is in the sitting position, the head of the table should be lowered to allow the patient to be placed in the supine position. An attempt can be made to aspirate air from a well-positioned central line catheter. VAE has been associated with a patent foramen ovale, but this lesion is not present in all cases.

27. What is malignant hyperthermia (MH)?

MH is an uncommon inherited disorder of skeletal muscle characterized by a hypermetabolic response of skeletal muscle to anesthetic agents (primarily halogenated agents and depolarizing muscle relaxants). An important pathophysiologic process in this disorder is intracellular hypercalcemia. Intracellular hypercalcemia activates metabolic pathways that, if left untreated, result in depletion of adenosine triphosphate, high temperature, acidosis, and cell death. No simple preoperative diagnostic test is available. Disorders associated with MH include myopathies (e.g. central core disease), Duchenne muscular dystrophy, and osteogenesis imperfecta.

28. How is MH diagnosed and treated?

Hypercarbia may be an early sign. Other signs include tachypnea, tachycardia, muscle rigidity, increased temperature, and decreased oxygen saturation. The following steps should be taken immediately when MH is diagnosed:

1. Discontinue inhalation agents and succinylcholine
2. Conclude surgery
3. Hyperventilate with 100% oxygen
4. Administer dantrolene intravenously at 2.5 mg/kg

5. Titrate dantrolene and bicarbonate to heart rate, body temperature, and $PaCO_2$
6. If significant metabolic acidosis is present, administer 2 to 4 mEq/kg bicarbonate
7. Change the anesthesia circuit
8. Treat arrhythmias with procainamide. (Avoid calcium channel blockers because they may induce hyperkalemia in the presence of dantrolene.)
9. Elevation of body temperature should be managed with external ice packs in addition to gastric, wound, and rectal lavage
10. Administer fluid and diuretics to maintain urine output
11. Transfer patient to an intensive care setting

Key Points

1. Spine surgery patients provide a wide range of challenges to the anesthesiologist in relation to airway management, positioning, blood loss, fluid management, and requirements for invasive monitoring.
2. Successful outcomes for complex spine procedures are dependent on coordination of anesthetic technique, intraoperative neurophysiologic monitoring, and surgical technique.

Websites

DIC: http://emedicine.medscape.com/article/779097-overview
Latex allergy: http://www.uam.es/departamentos/medicina/anesnet/gtoa/latex/manage.htm
Malignant hyperthermia: http://www.mhaus.org/
Useful anesthesia links: http://metrohealthanesthesia.com/links.htm#clin
Virtual anesthesia textbook: http://www.virtual-anaesthesia-textbook.com/vat/intubation.html

BIBLIOGRAPHY

1. Baron EM, Albert TJ. Medical complications of surgical treatment of adult spinal deformity and how to avoid them. Spine 2006;31:S106–18.
2. Dharmavaram S, Jellish WS, Nockels RP, et al. Effect of prone positioning systems on hemodynamic and cardiac function during lumbar spine surgery: an echocardiographic study. Spine 2006;31:1388–93.
3. DiPaola CP, Conrad BP, Horodyski MB, et al. Cervical spine motion generated with manual versus Jackson table turning methods in a cadaveric C1-C2 global instability model. Spine 2009;34:2912–18.
4. Faciszewski T, Winter RB, Lonstein JE, et al. The surgical and medical perioperative complications of anterior spinal fusion surgery in the thoracic and lumbar spine in adults. A review of 1223 procedures. Spine 1995;20:1592–9.
5. Hussain W, Gupta P. A rare anesthetic complication involving central line access during lumbar spine surgery: a case report and review. Spine 2009;35:E31–E34.
6. Narang J, Delphin E. Anesthesia in spinal deformity surgery. In: Heary RF, Albert TJ, editors. Spinal Deformity: The Essentials. New York: Thieme; 2007. p. 19–28.
7. Spessot GJ, Rosenberg AD. Anesthesia for spine surgery and management of blood loss. In: Errico TJ, Lonner BS, Moulton AW, editors. Surgical Management of Spinal Deformities. Philadelphia: Saunders; 2009. p. 421–32.
8. Tosi LL, Slater JE, Shaer C, et al. Latex allergy in spina bifida patients: prevalence and surgical implications. J Pediatr Orthop 1993;13:709–12.
9. Wills J, Schwend RM, Paterson A. Intraoperative visible bubbling of air may be the first sign of venous air embolism during posterior surgery for scoliosis. Spine 2005;30:E629–E635.

POSTOPERATIVE MANAGEMENT AND COMPLICATIONS AFTER SPINE SURGERY

CHAPTER 33

John M. Gorup, MD, Vincent J. Devlin, MD, and William O. Shaffer, MD

1. What types of complications may present in the early postoperative period following spinal procedures?

The spectrum of spine procedures ranges from outpatient lumbar discectomy to complex anterior and posterior multilevel fusion procedures. Health care providers must be knowledgeable regarding:

- Procedure-specific complications (e.g. problems related to the surgical approach, neural decompression, or spinal instrumentation)
- General postsurgical complications (may involve the neurologic, pulmonary, cardiovascular, or gastrointestinal systems. Nutritional and pain control issues are additional important considerations.)

2. List potential causes of neurologic deficits diagnosed after spine procedures.

- Direct intraoperative neural trauma (e.g. during decompression procedures, as a result of neural impingement by spinal implants)
- Spinal deformity correction (e.g. L5 root injury during L5–S1 spondylolisthesis reduction)
- Acute vascular etiology (e.g. intraoperative hypotension, disruption of crucial segmental vessels supplying the spinal cord during anterior surgical approaches)
- Subacute vascular etiology (neurologic deterioration may develop as late as 96 hours after spinal reconstructive surgery due to poor perfusion of the spinal cord and/or nerve roots)
- Patient positioning during surgery (e.g. brachial plexopathy, compressive neuropathy involving the peroneal nerve, compartment syndrome, cervical cord injury secondary to intraoperative neck positioning in a patient with cervical stenosis)
- Postoperative bleeding with resultant epidural hematoma and neural compression

3. What are the components of neurologic assessment after spinal surgery?

Initial neurologic assessment after spine surgery should include assessment of upper and lower extremity neurologic function (motor strength, sensation). Documentation of function of the major motor groups in both upper and lower extremities is required. It is not adequate to record that *the patient was able to wiggle toes* as documentation of intact lower extremity neurologic status. Instead, results of testing of iliopsoas, quadriceps, extensor hallucis, tibialis anterior, and gastrocnemius function should be documented. Neurologic examination is performed every 2 hours for the first 24 hours, every 4 hours for the next 48 hours, and then one time each shift until discharge.

4. Describe the clinical presentation of a postoperative epidural hematoma.

Epidural hemorrhage involving the cervical or thoracic region compresses the spinal cord and classically produces an acute, painful myelopathy. Epidural hematoma involving the lumbosacral region classically presents as cauda equina syndrome. Reports of pain unrelieved with narcotic analgesics or atypical neurologic symptoms or findings (e.g. unexplained numbness, balance difficulty, mild weakness) require careful evaluation because such symptoms may represent early manifestations of epidural hematoma. In addition to persistent bleeding at the operative site, coagulopathy-induced hemorrhage and spinal cord vascular malformations may lead to development of postoperative epidural hematoma. Additional risk factors include preoperative use of nonsteroidal antiinflammatory medications, multilevel laminectomies, intraoperative blood loss exceeding 1000 mL, and advanced age. Treatment is emergent spinal decompression.

5. What is cauda equina syndrome?

Cauda equina syndrome is a complex of low back pain, bilateral lower extremity pain and/or weakness, saddle anesthesia, and varying degrees of bowel and/or bladder dysfunction. Treatment is prompt surgical decompression. Complete neurologic assessment in the postoperative period includes evaluation of bowel and bladder function. Inadequate decompression of lumbar spinal stenosis is a risk factor for development of cauda equina syndrome in the postoperative period.

6. **After an uneventful posterior spinal instrumentation procedure for idiopathic scoliosis in a teenage patient, unilateral anterolateral thigh numbness and discomfort are noted. What is the most common cause of this problem?**
Pressure injury to lateral femoral cutaneous nerve (also known as meralgia paresthetica) secondary to intraoperative positioning. If there is no associated motor deficit and the sensory examination confirms a deficit limited to the distribution of the lateral femoral cutaneous nerve, the diagnosis is confirmed. The prognosis for recovery is good.

7. **An adult patient with grade 1 L5–S1 isthmic spondylolisthesis undergoes L5–S1 posterior spinal instrumentation (pedicle fixation), decompression, and fusion. Before surgery the patient experienced only right leg symptoms. After surgery the patient reports relief of right leg pain but has a new left L5 radiculopathy that was not present before surgery. What are the likely causes?**
A problem related to the left L5 pedicle screw with resultant neural impingement must be ruled out. The rates of screw malposition vary from 0% to 2%. However, most of these do not result in any long-term sequelae. Radiographs can be helpful in ruling out gross screw misplacement. However, a computed tomography (CT) scan is the best test because it can provide an axial view and depict the exact screw location in relation to the L5 nerve root. Other potential causes for new-onset left leg pain include intraoperative nerve root injury, inadequate L5 nerve root decompression, L5–S1 disc herniation, and postoperative hematoma.

8. **What is the incidence of ophthalmic complications after spinal surgery? What are the risk factors?**
The overall incidence of ophthalmic complications after spine surgery is 1 in 1000 procedures. The most common eye injury is a corneal abrasion. Postoperative visual loss may also occur and is due to a variety of mechanisms, which are not fully understood. These lesions may be classified as ischemic optic neuropathy, central retinal artery or vein occlusion, decreased visual acuity, and visual field deficits. Spine procedures performed in the prone position (i.e. scoliosis surgery, extensive lumbar spinal fusions) have the highest rates, but this complication may develop following procedures performed in the supine position. Additional risk factors include: extremes of age (<18 years, >84 years), anemia, peripheral vascular disease, hypertension, excessive blood loss, and hypotension during the procedure. An eye check should be included in the postoperative patient assessment. Symptoms or abnormal examination findings should prompt an ophthalmology consult.

9. **What pulmonary complications may occur after spine procedures?**
Atelectasis, pneumonia, pleural effusion, pneumothorax, acute respiratory distress syndrome (ARDS), pulmonary thromboembolism, hypoxemia, and respiratory failure.

10. **What factors are associated with an increased risk of pulmonary complications after spine surgery?**
Pulmonary complications are frequently noted in patients with nonidiopathic scoliosis, cognitive disability, advanced age, and chronic obstructive pulmonary disease. Patients undergoing anterior thoracic spine procedures and combined anterior and posterior spinal procedures associated with large blood loss and fluid shifts have an increased risk of postoperative pulmonary problems. Anterior cervical surgery, especially multilevel corpectomies, is associated with an increased risk of postoperative upper airway obstruction. Overnight intubation should be considered for high-risk patients.

11. **Can hemothorax or pneumothorax occur in association with posterior spinal procedures?**
Yes. During posterior surgical procedures, the chest cavity may be entered inadvertently if dissection is carried too deeply between the transverse processes. This complication is considered when a thoracoplasty is performed to decrease rib prominence as part of a posterior procedure for scoliosis. A tension pneumothorax may result from respirator malfunction or rupture of a pulmonary bleb. Insertion of a central venous pressure (CVP) line in the operating room may result in a pneumothorax that is not diagnosed before beginning the surgical procedure. Prompt diagnosis and chest tube insertion are required.

12. **After an anterior thoracic fusion performed through an open thoracotomy approach, a patient has persistent high chest tube outputs after the fourth postoperative day. The fluid has a milky color. What diagnosis should be suspected?**
Chylothorax. Injury to the thoracic duct or its tributaries may not be recognized intraoperatively and lead to leakage from the lymphatic system into the thoracic cavity. Treatment consists of continued chest tube drainage and decreasing the patient's fat intake. Hyperalimentation is of benefit during this period. Failure of these measures may require surgical exploration and repair of the lymphatic ductal injury.

13. **What is acute respiratory distress syndrome (ARDS)?**
ARDS results from diffuse, multilobar capillary transudation of fluid into the pulmonary interstitium, which dissociates the normal relationship of alveolar ventilation with lung perfusion. Persistent perfusion of poorly ventilated lung regions creates a shunt that results in hypoxia. ARDS has many causes including fluid overload, massive transfusion, sepsis,

malnutrition, and cardiac failure. Typically ARDS presents several days after surgery with fever, respiratory distress, reduced arterial oxygen, and diffuse bilateral infiltrates on chest radiographs. Treatment includes ventilator support with positive end-expiratory pressure (PEEP) to promote ventilation of previously trapped alveoli and minimize shunting.

14. **When should a chest tube be removed after an uncomplicated anterior thoracic spinal procedure?**
A chest tube is generally left in place for 48 to 72 hours after an anterior thoracic spinal procedure. No universal criteria define when a chest tube should be removed after anterior thoracic spine surgery. Unlike cardiac and pulmonary surgical procedures, anterior spinal procedures disrupt bony anatomy and stimulate a fracture-healing response with formation of serous fluid. This serous fluid can be absorbed by the pleura. Recommended criteria for chest tube removal range from 30 to 100 mL chest tube output in an 8-hour observation period. In addition, chest tube removal is generally deferred until the patient has been extubated after surgery.

15. **Are deep vein thrombosis and pulmonary embolism significant problems after spine procedures?**
Yes. The exact rate of these complications is difficult to define and ranges from 0.9% to 14%, depending on the patient population and type of spinal procedure. The application of sequential pneumatic compression stockings to the lower extremities before, during, and after surgery has been shown to reduce the rate of deep vein thrombosis. The use of pharmacologic agents for anticoagulation is not routinely used for posterior procedures because of potential complications of epidural bleeding, cauda equina syndrome, and wound hematoma. Patients at increased risk of deep vein thrombosis (e.g. prolonged immobility, paralysis, prior venous thromboembolism, cancer, obesity, staged adult scoliosis procedures) can be considered for additional preventive measures, including prophylactic placement of a vena cava filter or serial postoperative screening (e.g. duplex ultrasonography, magnetic resonance venography). The use of pharmacologic agents (e.g. low molecular weight heparin) can be considered for specific high-risk cases on an individual basis. The safe time for administration of anticoagulation following spinal procedures is controversial.

16. **You are called to assess a 49-year-old man in the recovery room immediately after an anterior L4 to S1 fusion performed via a left retroperitoneal approach. The nurse reports that the left leg is cooler than the right leg. The patient reports severe left leg pain. What test should be ordered?**
An emergent arteriogram and a vascular surgery consultation are indicated. The scenario is consistent with a vascular injury. The temperature change should not be attributed to the sympathectomy effect that is routinely noted following anterior lumbar surgery (in which case increased temperature is noted on the side of the exposure).

17. **A healthy 40-year-old woman underwent a 12-hour revision procedure consisting of anterior T10 to sacrum fusion and posterior spinal instrumentation and fusion from T2 to pelvis. Blood loss was 5000 mL, and the patient received 6 units of packed red cells, 2 units of fresh frozen plasma, and 12 L of crystalloid in the operating room. During the first 2 hours after surgery, this 60-kg patient had a urine output of 30 mL and CVP = 0. What is the problem?**
Hypovolemia. Decreased urine output in this otherwise healthy patient is a sign of fluid volume deficit due to third spacing as fluid volume is pulled out of the vascular space into the interstitial space. Complete blood count (CBC), platelet count, electrolyte panel, coagulation profile, and ionized calcium levels should be checked immediately. Transfusion of packed cells, fresh frozen plasma, platelets, calcium chloride, and additional crystalloid are administered based on these results. Cardiovascular status should be monitored with serial assessment of blood pressure, heart rate, urine output, and CVP measurements.

18. **Describe the pathophysiology of the syndrome of inappropriate antidiuretic hormone secretion (SIADH). What are the diagnostic findings and treatment?**
SIADH results in the retention of water by the body, causing serum hypoosmolality and urine hyperosmolality. Serum sodium is less than 130 mEq/L, serum osmolality is less than 275 mOsm/L, and urine sodium is greater than 50 mEq/L. Treatment is fluid restriction; if fluid must be given, it should be isotonic. In patients with SIADH, urine output generally returns to normal by the third postoperative day. There is approximately a 7% incidence of SIADH after spinal surgery. This condition must be differentiated from decreased urine output as a result of hypovolemia because the treatment for hypovolemia is fluid replacement. Decreased urine output due to hypovolemia is distinguished from SIADH because both urine and serum hyperosmolality are noted in the presence of hypovolemia.

19. **What is the most common gastrointestinal problem after spinal surgery? What are the causes?**
Ileus. Common causes include general anesthesia, prolonged use of narcotics, immobility after surgery, and significant manipulation of intestinal contents during anterior surgical procedures. Clinical findings include abdominal distention, abdominal cramping/discomfort, and pain. Diet restriction is the initial treatment. Nasogastric suction is instituted as needed for symptomatic relief.

20. What is Ogilvie's syndrome?

Acute massive dilation of the cecum and ascending and transverse colon in the absence of organic obstruction is termed Ogilvie's syndrome. Patients present with normal small bowel sounds and a colonic ileus. It is a dangerous entity that can result in cecal dilation and rupture. Death has been reported. The incidence appears to be increasing and may be related to use of patient-controlled analgesia (PCA). Diagnosis is made with an upright abdominal radiograph. Treatment consists of decompressing the colon with a rectal tube, colonoscopy, and, in some cases, cecostomy.

21. When should a patient be started on a diet after a spine fusion?

An abdominal assessment is performed. After bowel patency has been confirmed (presence of bowel sounds, absence of nausea and emesis), the patient may be given ice chips. If this is well- tolerated, the patient may progress to a clear liquid diet. This intake routine should be observed before advancing to a regular diet. With less invasive procedures, diet may be advanced more rapidly.

22. Define superior mesenteric artery syndrome.

This syndrome refers to bowel obstruction in the region where the superior mesenteric artery crosses over the third portion of the duodenum. In general, it is seen in thin patients who undergo significant correction of spinal deformity. Patients present with persistent postoperative emesis. Physical examination reveals hyperactive, high-pitched bowel sounds. Treatment includes complete restriction of oral intake, gastric decompression with a nasogastric tube, adequate intravenous hydration, and initiation of hyperalimentation if symptoms persist. Patients should be encouraged to lie in the prone or left lateral position. If symptoms persist, general surgery intervention is occasionally indicated.

23. What are the most common genitourinary complications after spine surgery?

Urinary retention is frequently seen after spine procedures. It is associated with the use of epidural analgesia and PCA. Urinary tract infection is the most common complication in spinal patients who are treated with a Foley catheter. This complication is readily treated with antibiotic therapy.

24. What is the most common non–life-threatening postoperative complication presenting in a patient older than 60 years who undergoes a spinal fusion?

Transient confusion and delirium. For acute control of delirium, doses of 0.25 to 2 mg of oral haloperidol 1 to 2 hours before bedtime is the preferred treatment.

25. A nurse reports that a patient has developed a small amount of wound drainage 5 days after a posterior lumbar decompression and fusion for spondylolisthesis. The discharge planner has already made arrangements to transfer the patient to a skilled nursing facility later that day. What should you advise?

The patient's transfer should be canceled, and the patient should remain hospitalized to permit evaluation by the surgical team. As a general principle, postoperative spine patients with wound drainage should not be discharged from the hospital because they generally require surgical exploration of the wound if drainage persists past the fourth or fifth postsurgical day. The differential diagnosis includes wound infection, seroma, and cerebrospinal fluid (CSF) leak. Expectant management and oral antibiotic treatment have little role in management.

Wound drainage is cultured. Routine laboratory tests including CBC with differential, erythrocyte sedimentation rate, and C-reactive protein levels are obtained. Aspiration of the wound may be performed under sterile conditions. Persistent wound drainage or aspiration of purulent fluid mandates operative exploration and debridement. Clinical findings associated with postoperative spine infections may be minimal or nonexistent. Potential clinical findings that suggest infection include general malaise, spinal pain out of proportion to the expected typical postoperative course, and a low-grade fever. If infection is suspected on clinical grounds, surgical exploration should be undertaken.

26. Describe steps involved in the surgical treatment of a patient with an acute wound infection 2 weeks after a lumbar posterior spinal instrumentation and fusion procedure. What is the role of vacuum-assisted wound closure?

In the operating room, the wound is opened sequentially with irrigation and debridement of the superficial and deep aspects of the wound. Specimens from both the superficial and deep levels of the wound are sent for aerobic and anaerobic cultures and Gram stain. Spinal implants are left in place if they are intact and appropriately placed. Loose bone graft is removed. All nonviable tissue is debrided. All layers of the wound are irrigated with multiple liters of saline. Broad-spectrum intravenous antibiotics that cover both gram-positive organisms (including methicillin-resistant *Staphylococcus aureus* [MRSA]) and gram-negative organisms (including *Pseudomonas*) are administered. Following debridement, the wound may be closed primarily or remain open in anticipation of future wound exploration and debridement procedures. In patients who develop infection following instrumented spine surgery, it is common to reexplore the wound in 24 to 72 hours to reassess the need for additional debridement versus wound closure.

Vacuum-assisted wound closure is a commonly used approach to manage such a wound following debridement. A reticulated polyurethane ether foam dressing is inserted, and the open wound is converted into a closed wound by use of an adhesive barrier. Subatmospheric pressure is maintained by the therapy device and provides a favored environment to promote wound healing. Wound drainage is directed into a specially designed canister and simplifies care. Alternative management options for an open wound following debridement include wound closure over drains, open wound packing, or use of a suction-irrigation system.

27. What is the incidence of dural tears associated with spinal decompression procedures? How are dural tears managed?

The incidence of dural tear is approximately 7% in primary cases, increasing to 16% in revision cases. Dural tears recognized in the operating room are best treated with water-tight closure of the dura and soft tissues at the time of the index procedure. Fibrin sealants and, more recently, synthetic dural substitutes can be used to augment the repair. When dural tear is suspected in the postoperative period (e.g. clear drainage on the postoperative surgical dressing), the patient can initially be maintained on strict bedrest. If drainage persists, a percutaneous lumbar subarachnoid catheter can be inserted to divert CSF into a closed sterile drainage system to permit healing of the dura. If this approach fails to resolve the problem, open surgical repair is required.

28. What is the most common method used for pain management after an extensive spinal fusion procedure?

Intravenous opioid injections are the most widely used method for postoperative pain management after spine surgery. In the alert and cooperative patient, opioids are typically administered by PCA. Meperidine (Demerol) should be avoided because of the potential for accumulation of the toxic metabolite normeperidine, which can lead to agitation, delirium, and seizures. Other options include opioids delivered in the epidural or intrathecal space. However, these techniques require additional surveillance of the patient to reduce the risk of side effects. Intercostal nerve blocks can provide substantial analgesia for thoracic and abdominal wall pain after anterior spinal procedures. Nonsteroidal antiinflammatories such as ketorolac (Toradol) can reduce opioid requirements in the immediate postoperative period, but a potential adverse effect on bone healing must be considered with longe-term use.

29. What complications are associated with early postoperative care of the quadriplegic patient?

Respiratory insufficiency, pneumonia, pressure ulceration, deep vein thrombosis, pulmonary embolism, gastric bleeding, urinary retention with bladder distention and calculus formation, joint contracture, autonomic dysreflexia, skeletal osteoporosis, and psychologic withdrawal.

30. Define reflexive dyssynergia.

Reflex dyssynergia is a reflex increase in blood pressure due to an obstructed viscus in a quadriplegic patient. A patient with a dangerously high blood pressure who is quadriplegic should be evaluated for an obstructed viscus (e.g. bladder or bowel obstruction).

31. How are steroids dosed after acute spinal cord injury? What is the most common complication of steroids in this setting?

A loading dose of 30 mg/kg of methylprednisolone is given within 8 hours of injury, followed by an infusion of 5.4 mg/kg/hr for 23 hours. If the loading dose is given within 3 hours of injury, the infusion is continued for 47 hours. The most common complication is wound infection (7% of patients).

32. Discuss mortality rates and complications in patients undergoing lumbar laminectomy, lumbar fusion, and adult spinal deformity surgery.

Mortality after spinal surgery is rare but may occur in the postoperative period. Recent studies cite perioperative mortality rates as 0.17% (lumbar laminectomy), 0.29% (lumbar fusion), and 2.4% (adult spinal deformity surgery). Mortality and complications are affected by a multitude of factors including age and medical comorbidities. In adult spinal deformity patients, mortality is most closely associated with increasing American Society of Anesthesiologists (ASA) physical status class. Opiate poisoning is responsible for more deaths among workers' compensation patients who undergo lumbar fusion than any other cause.

33. Discuss potential complications with usage of rhBMP-2 in spinal surgery.

To date, rhBMP-2 usage in spine surgery has been Food and Drug Administration (FDA) approved only for anterior lumbar interbody fusion. However, off-label physician-directed usage has expanded to other areas of the spine, including anterior cervical fusion and posterior lumbar procedures. Complications have been associated with rhBMP-2 use in the anterior cervical region, including severe soft tissue swelling, dysphagia, and respiratory difficulty requiring rehospitalization and additional treatment leading to a public health notification by the FDA. Complications associated with use in the posterior lumbar spine during posterior lumbar interbody fusion (PLIF) and transforaminal lumbar interbody fusion (TLIF) include heterotopic bone formation along the approach tract associated with nerve root compression, endplate resorption, radiculitis, and seroma formation.

34. Discuss potential complications associated with lumbar total disc replacement surgery.

Complications may arise due to the anterior surgical approach including vascular injury, ureteral injury, excessive blood loss, incisional hernia, retrograde ejaculation, neurologic injury, and infection. Device-related complications may occur and include implant subsidence and implant expulsion. With keeled implants, vertebral body fracture has been reported.

Key Points

1. Complications following spine surgery are unavoidable, but their negative effects can be lessened by prompt diagnosis followed by appropriate and expedient treatment.
2. Procedure-specific complications following spine surgery may be related to the surgical approach, neural decompression, or spinal instrumentation.
3. General postsurgical complications after spine surgery may involve the neurologic, pulmonary, cardiovascular, genitourinary, and gastrointestinal systems.

Websites

1. Cauda equina syndrome: http://www.caudaequina.org/index.html
2. Complications of spinal surgery:
   http://www.spineuniverse.com/displayarticle.php/article2541.html
3. Postoperative visual loss registry. Available at:
   http://www.asaclosedclaims.org
   http://depts.washington.edu/asaccp/eye/index.shtml
4. Vacuum-assisted wound closure: http://www.wheelessonline.com/ortho/wound_closure

BIBLIOGRAPHY

1. Devlin VJ, Williams DA. Decision making and perioperative care of the patient. In: Margulies JY, Aebi M, Farcy JP, editors. Revision Spine Surgery. St. Louis: Mosby; 1999. p. 297–319.
2. Emery SE, Akhavan S, Miller P, et al. Steroids and risk factors for airway compromise in multilevel cervical corpectomy patients: a prospective, randomized, double-blind study. Spine 2009;34:229–32.
3. Fujita T, Kostuik JP, Huckell CB, et al. Complications of spinal fusion in adult patients more than 60 years of age. Orthop Clin North Am 1998;29:669–78.
4. Glassman SD, Hamil CL, Bridwell KS, et al. The impact of perioperative complications on clinical outcome in adult deformity surgery. Spine 2007;32:2764–70.
5. Glotzbacher MP, Bono CM, Wood KB, et al. Thromboembolic disease in spinal surgery: a systematic review. Spine 2009;34:291–303.
6. Heck CA, Brown CR, Richardson WJ. Venous thromboembolism in spine surgery. J American Acad Ortho Surg 2008;16:656–64.
7. Juratli SM, Mirza SM, Fulton-Kehoe D, et al. Mortality after lumbar fusion surgery. Spine 2009;34:740–7.
8. Li G, Patil CG, Lad SP, et al. Effects of age and comorbidities on complication rates and adverse outcomes after lumbar laminectomy in elderly patients. Spine 2008;33:1250–5.
9. Pateder DB, Gonzales RA, Kebaish KM, et al. Short-term mortality and its association with independent risk factors in adult spinal deformity surgery. Spine 2008;33:1224–8.
10. Piasecki DP, Poynton AR, Mintz DN, et al. Thromboembolic disease after combined anterior posterior reconstruction for adult spinal deformity: a prospective cohort study using magnetic resonance venography. Spine 2008;33:668–72.

REVISION SPINE SURGERY

Joseph Y. Margulies, MD, PhD, Vincent J. Devlin, MD, and William O. Shaffer, MD

CHAPTER 34

GENERAL CONSIDERATIONS

1. **Why should the term *failed back surgery syndrome* be abandoned?**
   Failed back surgery syndrome is an imprecise term used to refer to patients with unsatisfactory outcomes after spine surgery. This term does not identify a diagnosis responsible for persistent symptoms and implies that additional treatment will not provide benefit. A better approach is to perform an appropriate assessment to differentiate problems amenable to additional surgical treatment from those problems unlikely to benefit from an operation. Additional surgery can be considered for appropriate candidates. Patients unlikely to benefit from additional surgery can be directed toward appropriate nonsurgical management strategies.

2. **Poor outcome after an initial spinal procedure is frequently attributed to one of the *three Ws*— what are they?**
   1. **Wrong patient:** Inappropriate patient selection for the initial surgical procedure led to a poor outcome. Examples include:
      - The patient indicated for spinal decompression or fusion had pathologic findings that could not be expected to benefit from the operation
      - The patient's psychosocial circumstances and expectations created a barrier to success (e.g. intravenous [IV] drug abuse, spousal abuse, litigation)
   2. **Wrong diagnosis:** Inadequate imaging studies or incomplete preoperative assessment led to misdiagnosis and selection of an inappropriate surgical technique not likely to benefit the patient (e.g. decompression at the wrong level or side for a disc herniation based on mislabeled diagnostic studies)
   3. **Wrong surgery:** Technical problems were associated with the initial procedure or the initial procedure was inadequate to address all aspects of the patient's spinal pathology. Examples include:
      - Incorrect placement of spinal implants resulting in neural impingement
      - Inadequate decompression of spinal stenosis
      - Unstable instrumentation construct with subsequent implant failure or dislodgement
      - Failure to maintain or restore lumbar lordosis resulting in flatback syndrome
      - Failure to stabilize and fuse when a decompression is performed at an unstable spinal segment (unstable spondylolisthesis with coexistent spinal stenosis)

3. **What additional factors may lead to a poor outcome after a spinal procedure?**
   - Unavoidable complication after appropriately performed surgery (e.g. infection, pseudarthrosis)
   - Failure to diagnose a significant surgically related complication (e.g. pseudarthrosis, instability, persistent neural compression)
   - Neurologic injury
   - Complications related to the surgical approach (e.g. vascular injury, recurrent laryngeal nerve injury)
   - Medical complications (myocardial infarction [MI], stroke, pulmonary embolus)
   - Recurrence or progression of an underlying disease process (e.g. metastatic disease, infection, myelopathy, rheumatoid arthritis)
   - Patient selection. Certain types of patients have a significantly increased risk of complications (e.g. Charcot spinal arthropathy, Parkinson's disease, neuromuscular spinal deformities, neurofibromatosis)
   - Inadequate postoperative rehabilitation
   - Surgeon inexperience. Surgeons who do not devote the majority of their practice to spine surgery are unlikely to master the sophisticated techniques of modern spine surgery

4. **What important factors should be assessed during the history and initial evaluation of a patient with continuing symptoms after spine surgery?**
   - Are the present symptoms the same, better, or worse after surgery?
   - Are the current symptoms similar to or different from those present before surgery?
   - Were the indications for the initial or most recent surgery appropriate?
   - Did intraoperative complications occur? (Review the operative report if possible.)
   - Was there a period during which the patient had relief of preoperative symptoms (pain-free interval)?

- Were any complications recognized in the postoperative period?
- Are the present symptoms predominantly radicular pain, axial pain, or both?
- Do ongoing legal entanglements exist?

5. What is the significance of a pain-free interval following a spinal decompression procedure?

The presence or absence of a pain-free interval following a spinal decompression procedure (e.g. lumbar laminectomy) can provide a starting point for determining the most likely causes of persistent symptoms:

- When the patient has no immediate relief, the wrong operation or wrong diagnosis should be suspected
- When the patient has immediate relief but symptoms recur within weeks to months after the operation, new pathology or a complication of the initial operation should be suspected
- When the patient has good relief initially but symptoms recur months to years later, new pathology or pathology secondary to an ongoing degenerative process should be suspected

6. What are important points to assess on physical examination in the patient being evaluated for possible revision spine surgery?

A general neurologic assessment and regional spinal assessment are performed. The presence of nonorganic signs (Waddell signs) should be assessed. Global spinal balance in the sagittal and coronal planes should be assessed. The physical examination is tailored to the particular spinal pathology under evaluation. For cervical spine disorders, shoulder pathology, brachial plexus disorders, and conditions involving the peripheral nerves should not be overlooked. For lumbar spine problems, the hip joints, sacroiliac joints, and prior bone graft sites should be assessed. Examination of peripheral pulses is routinely performed to rule out vascular insufficiency. Consider degenerative neurologic or muscle-based problems, such as amyotrophic lateral sclerosis or multiple sclerosis.

7. What diagnostic imaging tests are useful in the evaluation of patients following prior spinal surgery?

The sequence of imaging studies in the postoperative patient is similar to assessment for primary spine surgery. Imaging studies are indicated to confirm the most likely cause of symptoms based on a comprehensive history and physical examination.

- **Radiographs.** Upright posteroanterior (PA) and lateral spine radiographs are the initial imaging study. Lateral flexion-extension radiographs play a role in the diagnosis of postoperative instability or pseudarthrosis. Assessment of spinal deformities is best accomplished with standing 36-inch PA and lateral radiographs
- **Magnetic resonance imaging (MRI), computed tomography (CT), and CT-myelography.** The most appropriate study is selected based on the patient's symptoms, the presence or absence of spinal implants, and the specific spinal problem requiring assessment. MRI provides optimal visualization of the neural elements and associated bony and soft tissue structures. However, MRI is subject to degradation by metal artifact that may arise from microscopic debris remaining at the initial surgical site or from spinal implants (especially non-titanium implants). CT remains the optimal test to assess bone detail and is the preferred test for diagnosis of pseudarthrosis. CT-myelography is of great utility in evaluation of the previously operated spine. It provides excellent visualization of the thecal sac and nerve roots in addition to osseous structure even in the presence of spinal deformity or extensive metallic spinal implants
- **Technetium bone scans.** Although this study may provide valuable information for the diagnosis of infection and metastatic disease, it has little utility in planning revision spine procedures due to lack of spatial resolution
- **Discography.** May be helpful in confirming the disc as a pain generator for axial pain symptoms and can play a role in assessment of degenerative disc changes above or below a prior spinal fusion

8. What surgical options are available for patients who experience persistent symptoms following spine surgery?

- **Decompression** of neural elements (spinal cord, cauda equina, nerve roots)
- **Realignment** of spinal deformities
- **Spinal stabilization.** The load-bearing capacity of the vertebral column is restored in the short term by spinal implants and on a long-term basis by spinal fusion

Failure of a spinal procedure to improve a neurologic deficit, to correct a spinal deformity, to achieve a solid fusion, or to relieve associated pain is reason to assess the feasibility of revision spinal surgery.

9. What are the basic principles to follow when performing revision spinal surgery?

- Comprehensive preoperative assessment
- Optimization of the patient for spine surgery (smoking cessation, nutritional status)
- Perform definitive surgical procedures (combined anterior and posterior procedures often required)
- Adequate neural decompression
- Restoration or maintenance of sagittal spinal alignment
- Secure internal fixation
- Restoration of anterior spinal column load-sharing
- Use of autologous bone graft somewhere within the instrumentation construct
- Appropriate postoperative rehabilitation

10. **What treatment options are available for patients who fail to improve following spinal surgery in the absence of a surgically correctable spinal problem?**
    - Intensive rehabilitation
    - Spinal cord stimulation
    - Oral narcotics
    - Intrathecal narcotics (implantable drug pump)
    - Complementary and alternative medicine approaches

REVISION SURGERY AFTER PRIOR SPINAL DECOMPRESSION

11. **When a patient undergoes a spinal decompression procedure and reports no improvement in symptoms immediately after surgery, what are the most likely causes to consider?**
    Operation at the incorrect level, inadequate decompression, incorrect preoperative diagnosis, or psychosocial issues predisposing to failure.

12. **When a patient undergoes a spinal decompression procedure and reports temporary relief of symptoms followed by early recurrence of symptoms (within days to weeks), what are the most likely causes to consider?**
    Postoperative hematoma, infection (discitis, osteomyelitis, epidural abscess), meningeal cyst, and facet or pars fracture.

13. **When a patient undergoes a spinal decompression procedure and reports temporary relief of symptoms followed by recurrence of symptoms within weeks to months after the index procedure, what are the most likely causes to consider?**
    Recurrent disc herniation, perineural scarring, infection, and unrealistic patient expectations regarding surgical outcome.

14. **When a patient undergoes a spinal decompression procedure and reports temporary relief of symptoms followed by recurrence of symptoms more than 6 months after the index procedure, what are the most likely causes to consider?**
    Recurrent spinal stenosis and spinal instability. Recurrent spinal stenosis commonly presents as lateral stenosis secondary to disc space collapse after a discectomy. Risk factors for instability after lumbar decompression procedures include recurrent disc surgery at the L4–L5 level, multilevel decompression in patients with osteoporosis, and multilevel decompression in patients with scoliosis, especially if the deformity is flexible based on preoperative bending radiographs (Table 34-1).

15. **What is the incidence of recurrent lumbar disc herniation following lumbar microdiscotomy?**
    The reported incidence of recurrent lumbar disc herniation ranges from 5% to 27%.

16. **What is the incidence of postoperative wound infection after a lumbar microdiscectomy?**
    1% to 3%.

REVISION SURGERY AFTER PRIOR SPINAL FUSION

17. **What two factors obtained from the patient's history can be used to arrive at a differential diagnosis for persistent symptoms after spinal fusion surgery?**
    - Time of appearance of symptoms in relation to the most recent fusion procedure (Table 34-2)
    - Predominance of leg versus back pain symptoms

18. **Define pseudarthrosis.**
    Pseudarthrosis is defined as failure to obtain a solid bony union after an attempted spinal fusion. The time between initial surgery and diagnosis of pseudarthrosis is variable. One year following initial surgery is a reasonable and accepted interval for determining fusion success for short segment cervical and lumbar fusions. In certain cases, a patient's symptoms and imaging studies suggest the diagnosis of pseudarthrosis as early as 6 months following initial surgery. However, in patients undergoing multilevel spinal deformity instrumentation procedures, pseudarthrosis may not present until several years following index surgery. The diagnosis of pseudarthrosis is suggested by the presence of continued axial pain and the absence of bridging trabecular bone on plain radiographs. Other findings that suggest the presence of pseudarthrosis include abnormal motion on flexion-extension radiographs, loss of spinal deformity correction, and spinal implant loosening or failure.

Table 34-1. Classification of Problems after Spinal Decompression Procedures

1. LACK OF IMPROVEMENT IMMEDIATELY AFTER SURGERY WITH PERSISTENT OR UNCHANGED RADICULAR SYMPTOMS

A. Wrong Preoperative Diagnosis

Tumor	Psychosocial causes
Infection	Discogenic pain syndrome
Metabolic disease	Decompression performed too late

B. Technical Error

Surgery performed at wrong level(s)	Failure to treat both spinal stenosis and disc protrusion when necessary
Inadequate decompression performed	Conjoined nerve root
Missed disc fragment	

2. TEMPORARY RELIEF WITH RECURRENCE OF PAIN

A. Early Recurrence of Symptoms (within 6 Weeks)

Hematoma

Infection

Meningeal cyst

Facet or pars fracture

B. Midterm Failure (6 Weeks to 6 Months)

Recurrent disc herniation	Arachnoiditis
Stress fracture of pars interarticularis	Unrealistic patient expectations regarding surgical outcome
Battered root syndrome	

C. Long-Term Failure (> 6 Months)

Recurrent stenosis

Adjacent-level stenosis

Segmental spinal instability

Adapted from Kostuik JP. The surgical treatment of failures of laminectomy. Spine State Art Rev 1997;11:509–38.

Table 34-2. Classification of Problems after Spinal Fusion Procedures

TIME OF APPEARANCE	BACK PAIN PREDOMINANT	LEG PAIN PREDOMINANT
Early (Weeks)	**Infection**	**Neural Impingement by Fixation Devices**
	Wrong level fused	Foraminal stenosis due to change in spinal alignment (e.g. after spinal osteotomy)
	Insufficient levels fused	
	Psychosocial distress	
Midterm (Months)	**Pseudarthrosis**	**Neural Compression Due to Pseudarthrosis**
	Adjacent-level degeneration	Adjacent-level degeneration
	Sagittal imbalance	Graft donor site pain
	Graft donor site pain	
	Inadequate reconditioning	
	Implants loose, displaced or broken	
Long-Term (Years)	**Pseudarthrosis**	**Adjacent-Level Stenosis**
	Adjacent-level instability	Adjacent-level disc herniation
	Acquired spondylolysis	
	Compression fracture adjacent to fusion	
	Adjacent level degeneration	
	Abutment syndrome	

Adapted from Kostuik JP. Failures after spinal fusion. Spine State Art Rev 1997;11:589–650.

19. **What factors influence the rate of pseudarthrosis following a spinal fusion procedure?**
    - The number of levels fused
    - Fusion technique (anterior, posterior, transforaminal, combined approaches)
    - Use and type of spinal instrumentation
    - Use of autograft bone versus allograft bone or bone substitutes
    - Underlying pathologic condition for which the fusion was performed
    - Patient-related factors—age, smoking, osteoporosis, medications (e.g., nonsteroidal antiinflammatory drugs [NSAIDs])
    - Radiographic criteria used to define fusion

20. **What is the most reliable method for diagnosis of a pseudarthrosis?**
    The most reliable method for diagnosis of pseudarthrosis remains surgical exploration of the fusion mass. The most accurate imaging study for diagnosis of pseudarthrosis is a CT scan with two-dimensional and three-dimensional reconstructions. Plain radiography including flexion-extension views fail to detect pseudarthrosis in up to 50% of cases. Technetium bone scans have a poor predictive value for diagnosis of pseudarthrosis.

21. **What is the most reliable technique for achieving a successful fusion in a patient who develops a pseudarthrosis after a posterolateral L4–L5 fusion procedure?**
    The technique most likely to result in successful fusion is a combination of an L4–L5 interbody fusion and posterior fusion with pedicle fixation.

22. **What is a transition syndrome?**
    Spinal fusion causes increased stress on adjacent spinal motion segments that can lead to adjacent-level spinal instability, spinal stenosis, and/or disc herniation. This clinical scenario has been termed a **transition syndrome.** Treatment generally involves decompression and extension of the spinal fusion and spinal instrumentation.

REVISION SURGERY FOR SPINAL DEFORMITY

23. **What common problems may require revision surgery following an initial surgical procedure for spinal deformity?**
    - Pseudarthrosis
    - Back pain secondary to implant prominence or implant failure
    - Adjacent level disc degeneration, fracture or instability
    - Coronal plane imbalance
    - Sagittal plane imbalance (flatback syndrome)
    - Junctional kyphotic deformity
    - Residual rib prominence
    - Infection
    - Crankshaft phenomenon

24. **What is the crankshaft phenomenon?**
    Crankshaft phenomenon refers to continued anterior spinal growth after posterior spinal fusion in a skeletally immature patient, resulting in increased spinal deformity. Risk factors include skeletal immaturity (Risser stage 0, premenstrual, open triradiate cartilage), surgery before the peak growth period (prior to 10 years of age) and large residual curves after initial surgery. The traditional approach for prevention of crankshaft phenomenon is to perform an anterior spinal fusion in addition to posterior spinal fusion in high-risk patients. With use of modern segmental pedicle screw instrumentation, anterior surgery is no longer required in select patients.

25. **What procedure is advised to treat a severe rib prominence that persists after posterior spinal fusion and instrumentation for scoliosis?**
    An unsightly rib prominence can be treated with a *thoracoplasty.* This procedure involves resection of the medial portions of the ribs in the region of the prominence.

26. **Describe the surgical treatment for *flatback syndrome.***
    Fixed sagittal plane imbalance, or flatback syndrome, refers to symptomatic loss of sagittal plane balance primarily through straightening of the normal lumbar lordosis. Symptoms include pain and inability to stand upright with the head centered over the sacrum without bending the knees. Patients typically report a sense of leaning forward, thoracic pain, neck pain, and leg fatigue. Surgical treatment options include osteotomies (Smith-Petersen type or pedicle subtraction type), combined anterior and posterior procedures, or vertebral column resection procedures.

Key Points

1. Selection of appropriate candidates for revision spinal surgery depends on comprehensive assessment to determine the factors that led to a less than optimal outcome following initial surgery.
2. For poor surgical outcomes due to errors in surgical strategy or surgical technique associated with the index procedure, appropriate revision surgery may offer a reasonable chance of improved outcome.
3. For surgical failures due to errors in diagnosis or inappropriate patient selection for initial surgery, revision surgery offers little chance for improved outcome.
4. In the absence of relevant and specific anatomic and pathologic findings, pain itself is not an indication for revision surgery.

Websites

Complications of revision spinal surgery: http://www.medscape.com/viewarticle/462159
Revision anterior lumbar surgery: http://www.medscape.com/viewarticle/577213
Proximal fusion levels: http://www.medscape.com/viewarticle/566466
Sagittal imbalance: http://www.medscape.com/viewarticle/462179
Revision surgery for spinal deformity: http://www.orthospine.com/

BIBLIOGRAPHY

1. Albert TJ, Pinto M, Denis F. Management of symptomatic lumbar pseudarthrosis with anteroposterior fusion: a functional and radiographic outcome study. Spine 2000;25:129.
2. Bridwell KH. Decision-making regarding Smith-Petersen vs. pedicle subtraction osteotomy vs. vertebral column resection for spinal deformity. Spine 2006;31:S171–S178.
3. Devlin VJ, Anderson PA. Revision cervical spine surgery. In: Margulies JY, Aebi M, Farcy JP, editors. Revision Spine Surgery. St. Louis: Mosby; 1999. p. 52–88.
4. Dubousset J, Herring A, Shufflebarger H. Crankshaft phenomenon in spinal surgery. J Pediatr Orthop 1989;9:541–50.
5. Kostuik JP. The surgical treatment of failures of laminectomy. Spine State Art Rev 1997;11:509–38.
6. Kostuik JP. Failures after spinal fusion. Spine State Art Rev 1997;11:589–650.
7. Luhmann SJ, Lenke LG, Bridwell KH, et al. Revision surgery after primary spine fusion for idiopathic scoliosis. Spine 2009;34:2191–7.
8. Margulies JY, Aebi M, Farcy JP, editors. Revision Spine Surgery. St. Louis: Mosby; 1999.
9. Patel A, Brodke DS, Pimenta L, et al. Revision strategies in lumbar total disc arthroplasty. Spine 2008;33:1276–83.
10. Schwender JD, Casnellie MT, Perra JH, et al. Perioperative complications in revision anterior lumbar spine surgery: incidence and risk factors. Spine 2009;34:87–90.

SPINAL CORD STIMULATION AND IMPLANTABLE DRUG DELIVERY SYSTEMS

John W. Nelson, MD, FIPP

1. Where do spinal cord stimulation and implantable drug delivery systems fall along the continuum of management for treatment of chronic pain?

These modalities fall under the category of neuromodulation. Unlike surgery, which treats underlying spinal pathology, or neuroablative procedures, such as radiofrequency, that interrupt neural pathways, spinal cord stimulation and implanted drug infusion pumps act on neural receptors to decrease pain perception and transmission. These modalities have the advantage of being reversible and minimally invasive and permit a *trial implantation* to be performed to determine whether permanent implantation is appropriate. These modalities are a last resort and are only indicated for patients who have failed less complex and less invasive treatments.

2. What is spinal cord stimulation?

Modern spinal cord stimulators use epidural electrodes placed percutaneously, or through a limited open exposure, to stimulate the epidural space. The epidural electrodes are connected by lead wires to an implanted, programmable pulse generator that can have an internal or external power source. In a successful case, the electrical signals from the spinal cord stimulator reduce the sensation of pain by more than 50% and replace pain with a tingling sensation (paresthesia). Spinal cord stimulation is effective for neuropathic pain, which is defined as pain resulting from damage to the nervous system or secondary to abnormal processes of this system. Nociceptive pain, defined as pain from surgery or tissue damage, is not reliably relieved by spinal cord stimulation.

3. What are the mechanisms by which spinal cord stimulation exerts its effect?

The mechanism of spinal cord stimulation is conceptualized based on the gate control theory of pain. In simplistic terms, this theory states that peripheral nerve fibers carrying pain to the spinal cord may have their input modified at the spinal cord level prior to transmission to the brain. The synapses in the dorsal horns act as *gates* that can either close to keep impulses from reaching the brain or open to allow impulses to pass. Small-diameter nerve fibers (C-fibers and lightly myelinated A-delta fibers) transmit pain impulses. Excess small fiber activity at the dorsal horn of the spinal cord opens the gate and permits impulse transmission, leading to pain perception. Large nerve fibers (A-beta fibers) carry nonpainful impulses, such as touch and vibratory sensation, and have the capacity to close the gate and inhibit pain transmission. Spinal cord stimulation is thought to preferentially stimulate large nerve fibers because these fibers are myelinated and have a lower depolarization threshold than small-diameter nerve fibers.

Experimental evidence suggests a mechanism of action for spinal cord stimulation by increasing levels of gamma aminobutyric acid (GABA) within the dorsal horn of the spinal cord. GABA is an inhibitor of neural transmission in the spinal cord and suppresses hyperexcitability of wide dynamic range interneurons in the dorsal horn. Spinal cord stimulation may also exert a direct effect on brain activity, but this mechanism is not well understood at present.

4. Describe the two main types of epidural electrodes.

The two main types of electrodes are catheter-type electrodes and plate-type electrodes.

- **Catheter-type electrodes** (also known as percutaneous electrodes) are placed via a percutaneous needle approach under fluoroscopic guidance and are ideal for use in trial stimulation to determine whether permanent implantation is appropriate
- **Plate-type electrodes** (also known as laminotomy, paddle, or surgical electrodes) require a surgical laminotomy for placement. Advantages of plate-type electrodes include lower risk of migration in the epidural space and increased electrical efficiency. Lead systems have evolved from quadrapolar (four electrodes) or octapolar leads (eight electrodes) to current multilead systems
  See Figure 35-1.

5. Describe the two main types of pulse generators.

The two main types of pulse generator systems are totally implantable pulse generators and radiofrequency-driven pulse generators.

- **Totally implantable pulse generators** utilize an internal power source (lithium battery). Following activation, these pulse generators are controlled by transcutaneous telemetry and can be switched on-off with a magnet. The battery requires replacement in 2 to 5 years. Despite this disadvantage, totally implantable pulse generators are the most common type of system used.

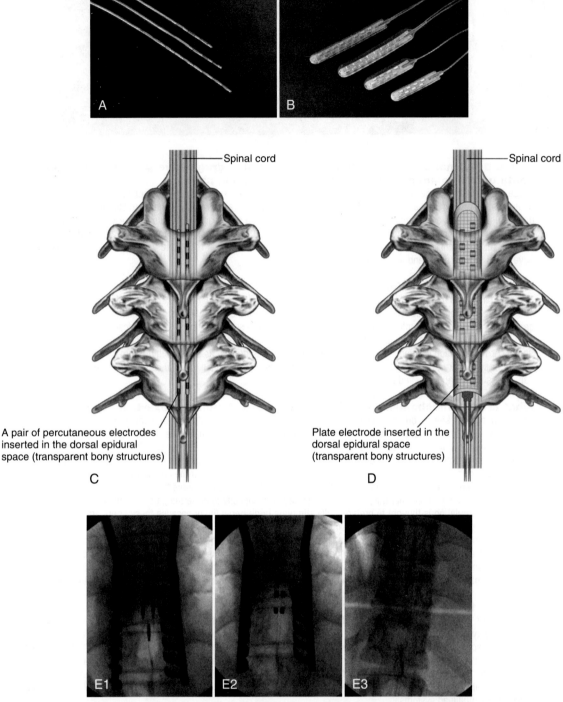

Figure 35-1. **A,** Advanced Neuromodulation Systems' percutaneous implantable lead types, demonstrating an eight-electrode Octrode lead and two four-electrode leads. The electrodes on all leads are 3 mm long. The eight-electrode and one of the four-electrode leads have an interelectrode distance of 4 mm. The other four-electrode lead has an interelectrode distance of 6 mm. **B,** Advanced Neuromodulation Systems' laminectomy implantable lead types. Four paddle-style leads are implanted via laminectomy. There are two wide leads and two narrow leads. One of the narrow leads has eight electrodes, and the other one has sixteen electrodes. There are two wide leads; one has eight electrodes and the other one has sixteen electrodes. **C,** Schematic drawing of two parallel octapolar percutaneous electrodes in the dorsal epidural space. **D,** Schematic drawing of a dual-plate electrode in the dorsal epidural space or of one dual octapolar plate electrode. **E,** Radiographs of different types of electrodes. **E1** and **E2,** Surgically implanted, via a laminotomy, electrodes of different configurations (Medtronic Inc.); **E3,** Percutaneously implanted dual quadrotapolar electrodes. (A-D from Slipman CW, Derby R, Simeone FA, Mayer TG (eds). Interventional Spine: An Algorithmic Approach. Philadelphia: Saunders; 2007. E1-E3 from McMahon: Wall and Melzack's Textbook of Pain, 5th ed, Churchill Livingstone.)

- **Radiofrequency-driven pulse generators** consist of a receiver implanted subcutaneously and a transmitter that is worn outside the body and utilizes an external power source. An antenna is applied to the skin and transmits the stimulation signals to the receiver. The radiofrequency-driven pulse generators have the ability to deliver more power than the totally implantable pulse generators and are appropriate for patients who have greater power requirements. Rechargeable systems are the newest type of pulse generators and are becoming popular.

6. **What parameters of neurostimulation are adjusted to optimize pain reduction?**

   Four basic parameters of the electrical signal are adjusted to optimize paresthesia and resultant pain reduction:
   - *Amplitude* refers to the strength of the stimulation and is measured in volts
   - *Pulse width* is the duration of the electric pulse and is measured in microseconds
   - *Rate* is measured in cycles per second or hertz (Hz)
   - *Electrode selection* is varied by computer-assisted programming with electrons flowing from cathodes (-) to anodes (+)

   Following programming of the device, the patient may adjust intensity and choose between different *programs* in the device, as well as turn the stimulator on and off.

7. **What pain problems are amenable to spinal cord stimulation?**

   Spinal cord stimulation has demonstrated effectiveness for many neuropathic pain conditions, including persistent radicular pain following failed spinal surgery, complex regional pain syndrome, limb ischemia, angina pectoris, and postherpetic neuralgia. Many experts consider the best candidates for spinal cord stimulation following failed spinal surgery as those patients with radicular pain greater than axial pain. However, patients with pure neuropathic pain following unsuccessful spine surgery are uncommon. Patients following unsuccessful spine surgery frequently present with mixed nociceptive/neuropathic pain. Advances in programming and electrode technology, including multilead systems, have improved outcomes in this patient population.

8. **What are contraindications to spinal cord stimulation?**

   Contraindications to spinal cord stimulation include uncontrolled bleeding/anticoagulation, systemic or local infection, inability to understand or communicate during trial placement, inability to understand and use technology, significant spinal stenosis or myelopathy, implanted cardiac pacemakers or defibrillators, metal allergy, and major psychiatric disease.

9. **How are trial spinal cord stimulation electrodes placed?**

   Most trial spinal cord stimulation electrodes are placed into the epidural space through epidural needles utilizing fluoroscopic guidance. The procedure is performed under mild sedation and local anesthetic, as the patient must be awake during electrode placement and testing. The wires from the trial electrode may be left protruding through the skin for direct connection to a trial stimulator. Alternatively, a small incision is made around the epidural needle insertion site and dissection is continued to the level of the thoracolumbar fascia to permit the electrode to be secured to fascia with a silastic anchor. Next, the trial electrode is connected to an extension wire, which is tunneled laterally toward the site where the pulse generator would be implanted if the trial is successful. A small incision is made to permit the extension wire to pass through the skin and permits the wire to connect to a trial stimulator.

   Some physicians prefer placing plate-type electrodes for the trial implant, especially if there is scarring in the epidural space following prior spinal surgery, which can make placement of catheter type electrodes challenging. Plate-type electrode placement can be performed either under mild sedation in combination with local anesthesia or under general anesthesia with the patient awakened during the procedure for testing. The trial period may last days to weeks, but trial periods beyond 3 to 5 days require that the leads be tunneled under the skin from the insertion site to decrease the risk of infection.

10. **How does the patient determine if trial spinal cord stimulation is effective?**

    The patient's report of subjective pain relief is documented. Spinal cord stimulation is intended to produce a fine/pleasant sensation of tingling, covering the area of pain. To be a candidate for implantation of a permanent stimulator, the patient must experience a minimum of 50% pain relief. Some clinicians prefer a minimum of 60% to 70% pain relief, believing such patients experience better long-term outcomes. Other measures of efficacy during a trial period include improved function and decreased medication use.

11. **If the spinal cord stimulation trial is successful, how is the implantation of a permanent spinal cord stimulator performed?**

    The patient undergoes a surgical procedure for placement of a pulse generator, which is most commonly implanted into a *pocket* in the posterior iliac area or lower abdominal region. If a previously placed catheter-type electrode will be used as the *permanent* electrode, the midline incision is reopened and the previously placed extension wire is discarded. The electrode is connected to a new extension wire, which is tunneled and connected to the pulse generator. If a plate-type electrode will be used as the permanent electrode, a midline spinal incision is made and dissection carried onto the lamina at the interspace below the level at which effective trial stimulation was achieved. A laminotomy is created, and the plate-type electrode is inserted over the dura and passed proximally to reach the desired level (usually the lower thoracic cord region for treatment of a lower extremity pain syndrome). The location of the electrode is confirmed with fluoroscopy, and the electrode is secured to the thoracolumbar fascia with a silastic anchor. If the procedure has been performed under general anesthesia, the patient is awakened intraoperatively to confirm electrode position through testing of the pattern of paresthesia generated by stimulation. Finally, extension wires are tunneled for connection to the pulse generator.

12. What are the complications associated with spinal cord stimulation?

The most common complication of spinal cord stimulation is lead migration. Lead migration is less common with plate-type electrodes. Modern catheter-type electrodes with eight electrode contacts per lead are programmable and allow flexibility in programming spinal cord stimulation to maintain effective stimulation should the leads move. Other complications of spinal cord stimulation include infection, lead breakage, implant malfunction, undesirable pattern/location of stimulation, seroma, and cerebrospinal fluid (CSF) leak. Paralysis as a result of lead insertion is extremely rare but has been reported.

13. What is the history of implanted spinal catheters and pumps?

The discovery in the 1970s of opioid receptors in the spinal cord led to injection and infusion of opioids into the epidural and subarachnoid space for acute and chronic pain due to cancer. In 1992, Medicare approved implanted pumps for chronic nonmalignant pain. By infusing opiates directly into the spine, the medication dosages required to treat pain are 30 to 300 times less than oral dosages.

14. What is an implantable drug delivery system?

An implantable drug delivery system consists of a pump that is surgically inserted into a pocket in the abdomen and delivers medication to the spinal canal through a catheter, which is tunneled under the skin. Pumps have a drug reservoir that can be refilled. Two main types of pumps exist:
- **Constant flow pumps** provide a fixed rate of drug delivery and require changing the drug concentration to adjust the drug dose
- **Programmable pumps** have the capacity to vary the rate and time of drug delivery to adjust drug dose

15. Which patients are potential candidates for an implantable drug delivery system?

Potential candidates for an implantable drug delivery system include:
- Patients with pain secondary to malignancy, which is not adequately relieved with oral or transdermal analgesics and who have a life expectancy in excess of 3 months
- Patients with nociceptive or neuropathic pain who do not experience relief with medication, spinal cord stimulation, or neuroablative procedures
- Patients who fail spinal cord stimulation trials
- Patients with spasticity of cerebral or spinal origin

Potential candidates for an implantable drug delivery system should have failed treatment with less complex and invasive therapies, including physical and occupational therapy, cognitive and behavioral therapy, and oral/transdermal opioid medications. In addition, documented pathology that correlates with the pain symptoms should exist. Indications for additional surgical intervention should be ruled out. Psychologic barriers to successful outcome should be examined. No absolute contraindications to implantation should be present. Prior to implantation, a trial should be performed to evaluate efficacy and rule out toxicity.

16. What are some contraindications for an implantable drug delivery system?

Contraindications to an implantable drug delivery system include:
- Intolerance to the medication that is infused
- Local or systemic infection
- Bleeding diathesis/anticoagulation
- Titanium allergy
- Pregnancy or desire to become pregnant
- Severe psychopathology

17. What medications are currently approved for infusion via an implantable drug delivery system?

The current Food and Drug Administration (FDA)-approved medications for infusion into the spinal canal are morphine (approved for intrathecal analgesia), ziconotide (Prialt, approved for intrathecal analgesia), and baclofen (approved for spasticity). Other medications have been used off-label, including Dilaudid, fentanyl, sufentanyl, bupivacaine, and clonidine. Although opioids are effective for nociceptive pain, they are less effective for neuropathic pain. Pain physicians may combine an opioid with clonidine or bupivacaine to enhance treatment of both nociceptive and neuropathic pain. In addition, combination drug therapy is believed to decrease the development of medication tolerance.

18. What are some risks and complications associated with an implantable drug delivery system?

- *Medical complications* may occur with therapy. For example, nausea, pruritus, urinary retention, oversedation, constipation, confusion, amenorrhea, and sexual dysfunction have been reported
- *Surgical complications* may occur and include CSF leak, infection, and neurologic injury
- *Device-related complications* may occur and include pump failure, catheter migration or occlusion, catheter dissociation, and catheter tip granuloma (may lead to neurologic deficit)

Key Points

1. Spinal cord stimulation is a minimally invasive treatment in select patients for persistent pain following spinal surgery, chronic regional pain syndrome, and other neuropathic pain syndromes.
2. Implantable drug delivery systems are considered for patients with nociceptive and/or neuropathic pain syndromes who do not experience relief with medication, spinal cord stimulation, or neuroablative procedures.
3. Successful outcomes with spinal cord stimulation or implantable drug delivery systems require careful preoperative evaluation, including a screening trial, to identify patients who are most likely to benefit from the procedure.

Websites

Implantable technologies:
   http://www.nationalpainfoundation.org/articles/340/implantable-technologies
Neuraxial analgesia by intrathecal drug delivery for chronic noncancer pain: http://cme.medscape.com/viewarticle/466349

BIBLIOGRAPHY

1. Barolat G. Spinal cord stimulation for chronic pain management. In: Slipman CW, Derby R, Simeone FA, et al, editors. Interventional Spine: An Algorithmic Approach. Philadelphia: Saunders; 2007.
2. Cohen SP, Dragovich A. Intrathecal analgesia. Anesthesiol Clin 2007;25:863–82.
3. Deer T, Chapple I, Classen A, et al. Intrathecal drug delivery for treatment of chronic low back pain: report from the national outcomes registry for low back pain. Pain Med 2004;5:6–13.
4. Harb M, Krames ES. Intrathecal therapies and totally implantable drug delivery systems. In: Slipman CW, Derby R, Simeone FA, et al, editors. Interventional Spine: An Algorithmic Approach. Philadelphia: Saunders; 2007.
5. North R. Spinal cord stimulation versus repeated lumbosacral spine surgery for chronic pain: a randomized, controlled trial. Neursurgery 2005;56:98–107.
6. Turner J, Loeser J, Deyo R, et al. Spinal cord stimulation for patients with failed back surgery syndrome or complex regional pain syndrome; a systematic review of effectiveness and complications. Pain 2004;108:137–47.

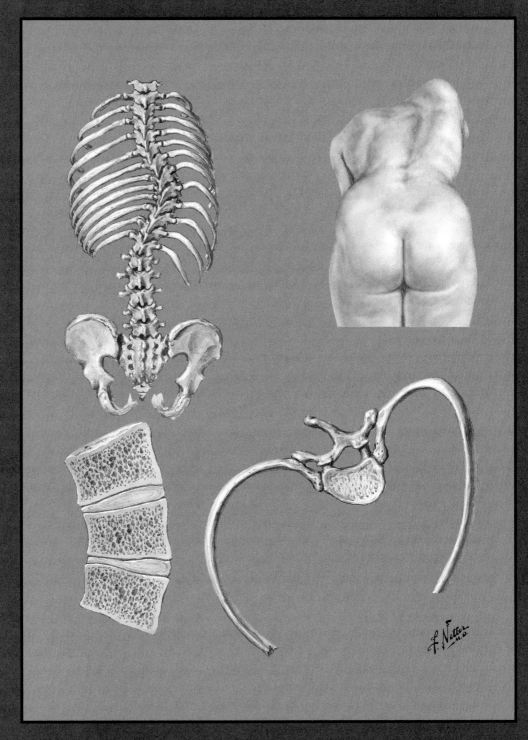

36 CHAPTER

PEDIATRIC BACK PAIN

Mary Hurley, MD, and Vincent J. Devlin, MD

1. Discuss the epidemiology of back pain in children compared with adults.

Traditionally, the prevalence of back pain in children is reported as less than in the adult population. In addition, among pediatric patients who seek evaluation for back pain, the likelihood of diagnosis of a definable cause of symptoms is traditionally considered higher than in adult patients. Complaints of back pain are less common before age 10 and increase between 12 and 15 years of age. Recent studies question these traditional beliefs and demonstrate that diagnosis of a definable cause of back pain symptoms is not possible for up to 75% of pediatric patients. The prevalence of idiopathic adolescent spinal pain approaches the reported rate of the adult population by age 18 years. Spinal pain in adolescence is considered to be a risk factor for spinal pain as an adult.

2. What is the differential diagnosis of back pain in children?

1. Mechanical disorders
   - Muscle strain
   - Overuse syndrome
   - Fracture
   - Herniated disc
   - Slipped vertebral apophysis
   - Spondylolysis/spondylolisthesis
2. Developmental disorders
   - Scheuermann's kyphosis
   - Spondylolysis/spondylolisthesis
3. Inflammatory disorders
   - Discitis
   - Vertebral osteomyelitis
   - Tuberculosis
   - Sacroiliac joint infection
   - Rheumatologic disorders
4. Neoplastic disorders
   - Benign primary spine tumors
   - Malignant primary spine tumors
   - Metastatic tumors
   - Spinal cord/canal tumors
   - Tumors of muscle origin
5. Psychogenic pain
6. Referred pain from visceral disorders
   - Pneumonia
   - Pyelonephritis
   - Retrocecal appendicitis
7. Idiopathic back pain

3. What are the most common causes of back pain in skeletally immature patients referred to a tertiary pediatric orthopedic clinic? To the emergency department?

- **In the clinic:** Idiopathic, spondylolysis or spondylolisthesis, Scheuermann's disease, spinal tumor or infection, and referred pain from visceral disorders
- **In the emergency room:** Trauma, muscle strain, sickle cell crises, urinary tract infection, viral syndrome and idiopathic

4. Why is the child's age often helpful in narrowing the diagnosis?

No diagnosis is unique to a single age group. However, some generalizations can help in determining the most likely diagnosis:

- **Younger than 10 years old:** Disc space infection, vertebral osteomyelitis, and certain tumors (Langerhans cell histiocytosis, leukemia, astrocytoma, neuroblastoma)
- **Older than 10 years:** Disorders involving repetitive loading and trauma, such as spondylolysis, spondylolisthesis, Scheuermann's kyphosis, fractures, lumbar disc herniation, and apophyseal ring injury.

5. What information should be obtained during a history for evaluation of back pain?

- Duration of pain symptoms (acute, >1 month, chronic)
- Location of pain (cervical vs. thoracic vs. lumbar)
- Frequency of symptoms (intermittent, constant)
- Aggravating and alleviating factors
- Timing
- History of trauma
- Recreational activities

Red flags that should prompt further workup include:
- A history of systemic symptoms (fever, weight loss)
- Neurologic complaints (numbness, weakness, bowel or bladder difficulty)
- Non-mechanical pain (night pain, pain at rest)

6. How should the physical examination be performed?

The physical examination must take place with the child undressed and appropriately gowned. All systems should be examined thoroughly. The child should be observed for posture, stance, and gait. The spine should be assessed for tenderness, alignment, and flexibility. A forward bend test should be performed to assess for symmetry and flexibility. Spinal deformity (kyphosis, scoliosis) should prompt further assessment. Suspicion of underlying disease is prompted by spinal tenderness, decreased spinal range of motion, spasticity, hamstring tightness, and skin abnormalities (hemangioma, midline hair patch). The single-leg hyperextension test is a useful provocative test for diagnosis of symptomatic spondylolysis and is performed by instructing the patient to stand on one leg while extending the lumbar spine. The neurologic examination should carefully document motor strength, sensation, deep tendon reflexes, and symmetry of abdominal reflexes. The musculoskeletal examination includes assessment of all muscle groups for tenderness or limited range of motion.

7. What laboratory tests are useful during the evaluation of back pain in children?

Useful laboratory tests include a complete blood count (CBC) with differential, erythrocyte sedimentation rate (ESR), and C-reactive protein. These tests are recommended for young children with a history of night pain or constitutional symptoms. If a rheumatologic disorder is considered in the differential diagnosis, additional potentially useful tests include a rheumatoid factor, antinuclear antibody (ANA), and HLA-B27.

8. What imaging studies play a role in evaluation of the child with back pain?
- Plain radiographs
- Technetium bone scans
- Computed tomography (CT)
- Magnetic resonance imaging (MRI)

9. When are radiographs indicated for evaluation of the child with back pain?

Anteroposterior (AP) and lateral spinal radiographs are the best first imaging test for a child with back pain. Spinal radiographs are indicated for initial evaluation of children 4 years old or younger, children who report pain symptoms for greater than 1 month, children who report that back pain awakens them from sleep, and children with constitutional symptoms.

10. When is a technetium bone scan indicated for evaluation of a child with back pain?

If a child with back pain has normal spinal radiographs and does not have a neurologic deficit, a technetium bone scan should be obtained. This test is quite sensitive for diagnosing spinal problems such as infections, tumors, and occult fractures. Single-photon emission computed tomography (SPECT) provides increase sensitivity and specificity compared with a planar bone scan. SPECT is especially helpful in the diagnosis of acute spondylolysis but is less helpful for diagnosis of chronic pars fractures as chronic injuries lack increased bone turnover.

11. When is an MRI scan indicated for evaluation of a child with back pain?

Children presenting with back pain and an abnormal neurologic examination require evaluation with a spinal MRI. MRI is the method of choice for evaluation of the spinal column and neural axis. It is useful for defining abnormalities such as tumor, infection, disc herniation, Arnold Chiari malformation, syrinx, and tethering of the spinal cord. Because it is a noninvasive test, it has largely replaced CT myelography.

Disadvantages of MRI include the need for anesthesia when the study is required in very young children and the danger of attributing symptoms to imaging findings that are clinically irrelevant.

12. When is a CT scan indicated for evaluation of a child with back pain?

CT is the method of choice for evaluation of a bone lesion diagnosed on plain radiographs or a technetium bone scan. Spinal CT provides the clearest depiction of bone detail and plays an important role in assessment of fractures, spondylolysis, spondylolisthesis, and tumors.

13. What guidelines exist to aid the practitioner in pursuing an effective and systematic approach to the child with back pain?

An algorithm has been developed to guide patient assessment on data obtained from clinical history and physical examination (Figure 36-1). The algorithm takes into account three factors:
1. Mechanism of injury: Clear or unclear
2. Nature of symptoms/physical findings: Local vs. systemic vs. neurologic
3. Duration of symptoms: Less than 1 month vs. greater than 1 month

The patient may enter into the algorithm at any stage on findings noted in the history and physical examination. The patient may progress from a lower to a higher level based on the above three factors. The algorithm has four levels:

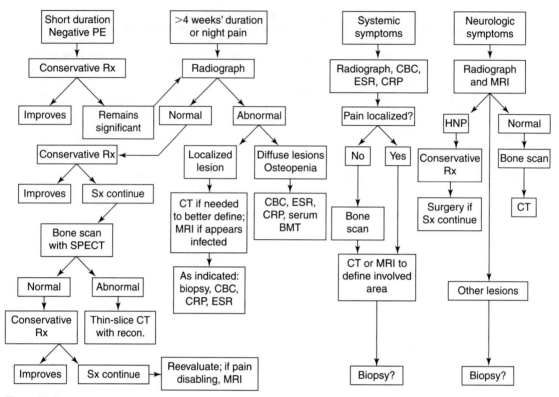

Figure 36-1. Diagnostic algorithm for back pain in children. BMT, bone mineral testing (DEXA) ; CBC, complete blood count; CRP, C-reactive protein; CT, computed tomography; ESR, erythrocyte sedimentation rate; HNP, herniated nucleus pulposus ; MRI, magnetic resonance imaging; PE, physical examination; Rx, therapy; SPECT, single-photon emission computed tomography; Sx, symptoms. (Redrawn from Ecker ML. Back pain. Spine State Art Rev 2000;14:236.)

LEVEL 1
- *Mechanism:* Clear history of specific injury
- *Nature of symptoms/findings:* Symptoms localized to back pain
- *Duration of symptoms:* Less than 1 month
- *Studies/action needed:* Symptomatic treatment (activity restriction, nonsteroidal antiinflammatory drugs [NSAIDs]) and follow-up in 1 month. If symptoms persist, advance to Level 2.

LEVEL 2
- *Mechanism:* History unclear
- *Nature of symptoms:* Back pain without systemic or neurologic signs, minor physical findings (spinal asymmetry, hamstring spasm), progression from level 1
- *Duration of symptoms:* Greater than 1 month
- *Studies/action needed:* PA and lateral radiographs of entire spine (lumbosacral [LS] spine radiographs if spondylolysis/ spondylolisthesis suspected). Positive radiographs (Scheuermann's disease, spondylolysis, significant scoliosis) can be referred to a specialist. Patients with negative radiographs can be observed or advanced to Level 3, depending on clinical judgment

LEVEL 3
- *Mechanism:* History unclear
- *Nature of symptoms:* Back pain with systemic symptoms (fever, weight loss)
- *Duration of symptoms:* Greater than 1 month
- *Studies/action needed:* CBC, ESR, C-reactive protein, and bone scan in addition to spinal radiographs. Patients with negative findings on these studies require only symptomatic treatment as most serious disorders have been excluded. Patients with positive studies require specialty referral

LEVEL 4
- *Mechanism:* History unclear
- *Nature of symptoms:* Back pain with neurologic deficit or patients advanced from Level 3
- *Duration of symptoms:* Generally greater than 1 month but not always
- *Studies/action needed:* MRI and/or CT is obtained in addition to Level 3 studies (radiographs, CBC, ESR, C-reactive protein, bone scan). Refer patient to surgeon for assessment for surgical treatment

14. How is a muscle strain diagnosed in children?

History and physical examination are usually sufficient to establish the diagnosis of muscle strain. A short history of localized pain, no neurologic findings, and association with physical activity are typical. The pain should resolve within a few weeks. The treatment for muscle strain is activity modification, ice, and NSAIDs. If the pain does not resolve with this treatment, reevaluation is needed.

15. Define spondylolysis.

Spondylosis is a defect in the pars interarticularis. The defect is unilateral in 20% and bilateral in 80% of cases.

16. Who is at risk for spondylolysis?

Children engaged in repetitive activities involving hyperextension of the spine. Commonly associated sporting activities include gymnastics, diving, dancing, wrestling, and football.

17. How is spondylolysis diagnosed?

History and physical examination are important indicators of spondylolysis. A history of hyperextension activities should alert the clinician to the possibility of the diagnosis. Patients typically present with back pain radiating into the buttocks. Physical examination may reveal tenderness to palpation, hamstring tightness, decreased forward flexion of the lumbar spine, a positive single-leg hyperextension test, or a stiff gait. Lateral radiographs may reveal a pars defect. Oblique views can more clearly delineate the pars interarticularis. Bone scan with SPECT can help diagnose pars defects but may be negative if the spondylolysis is chronic. CT scan delineates the defect most clearly.

18. How is spondylolysis treated?

Activity modification, bracing, physical therapy, and NSAIDs are the basis of nonoperative therapy. Surgical intervention is rarely necessary. Surgical options include repair of the pars defect or a posterolateral fusion.

19. Define spondylolisthesis. How is it diagnosed in children?

Spondylolisthesis is a forward slippage of a vertebra in relation to the adjacent inferior vertebra. The most common type of spondylolisthesis in children is the isthmic type, which occurs when bilateral pars defects allow the upper vertebra to slide forward on the lower vertebra, usually L5 on S1. A standing lateral lumbar radiograph is the best test for making the diagnosis. MRI plays a role when there is a need to assess the intervertebral disc or if a neurologic deficit is present. CT scan plays a role when details about formation of the posterior spinal elements (dysplasia) are required for surgical planning.

20. What treatment is recommended for spondylolisthesis?

Low-grade slips (30%–50%) do not require active treatment if the patient is asymptomatic. Such patients should be followed closely for slip progression through skeletal maturity. Symptomatic low-grade slips should undergo initial nonoperative treatment, including activity modification, physical therapy, NSAIDs, and bracing, before considering surgical treatment (spinal fusion). Higher-grade slips (50%) are generally treated with spinal fusion.

21. What is Scheuermann's disease? How does it present in children?

Scheuermann's disease is a disorder of endochondral ossification that alters the development of the vertebral endplate and ring apophysis. It may lead to intraosseous disc herniation, anterior wedging of the vertebral body, and kyphotic deformity. Scheuermann's disease may affect either the thoracic or lumbar region.

In the thoracic region, three consecutive wedged vertebra ($>5°$), irregular upper and lower vertebral endplates, apparent loss of disc space height, and increased thoracic kyphosis that does not correct when the patient lies supine are criteria for diagnosis. Patients typically are referred for assessment of the associated kyphotic deformity, which may be associated with pain over the apex of the kyphosis. Scheuermann's kyphosis should be differentiated from postural round back, which is a flexible deformity that reduces when the patient lies supine.

Patients with Scheuermann's disease in the lumbar region present with back pain. Spinal deformity is generally not a significant problem. Patients generally report a history of strenuous physical activity or acute injury. Radiographs show vertebral endplate irregularities, intraosseous disc herniation (Schmorl's nodes), and disc space narrowing.

22. What treatment is recommended for Scheuermann's disease?

Most patients with Scheuermann's disease involving the thoracic region can be successfully treated with exercise, bracing, and supportive care. Surgical intervention can be considered for persistent pain associated with a kyphotic deformity exceeding 75°. Scheuermann's disease involving the lumbar region is generally treated with activity modification and occasionally with an orthosis.

23. Is idiopathic scoliosis commonly associated with severe pain in children?

No. Idiopathic scoliosis is not a cause of severe back pain in children. Up to one third of patients with adolescent idiopathic scoliosis report mild, intermittent, and nonspecific back pain. When persistent severe back pain is noted in the presence of a spinal curvature, further workup is indicated to determine the source of pain. Conditions such as infection, tumor, syringomyelia, or disc herniation may cause secondary scoliosis.

24. What is the difference between discitis and vertebral osteomyelitis?

In the past, a distinction was made between discitis (infection involving the disc space) and osteomyelitis (infection in the vertebral body). Studies have shown that in children the vascular supply crosses the vertebral endplate from vertebral body to the disc space. As a result, discitis and vertebral osteomyelitis are considered to represent a continuum termed *infectious spondylitis.* Hematogenous seeding of the vertebral endplate leads to direct spread of infection into the disc space. Subsequently, infection involving the disc space and both adjacent vertebral endplates may progress to osteomyelitis. Vertebral fracture and epidural abscess may occur if the infection is permitted to progress without treatment. *Staphylococcus aureus* is the most frequently isolated bacteria. Tuberculosis is prevalent in developing countries and should be considered in children who have traveled outside of the United States to endemic areas.

25. Describe the presentation, workup, and treatment for spinal infection in a child.

Children may present with back, abdominal, or leg pain symptoms. The child may limp or refuse to walk. When asked to pick something up from the floor, the child generally avoids bending over and squats in an attempt to keep the spine straight. Some children may appear quite ill with a fever, whereas others are afebrile and report minimal pain.

Radiographs are typically normal during the first month. Bone scans demonstrate increased uptake even in the early stages of infection. MRI is the most sensitive and specific imaging test and demonstrates the extent of the lesion, as well as the presence or absence of an epidural abscess. Laboratory studies may be helpful in making the diagnosis. The white blood cell count is elevated in less than 50% of cases. The ESR is elevated in more than 90% of patients. C-reactive protein is a more specific indicator of infection and may be useful in diagnosis and evaluation of treatment. Blood cultures should be drawn before starting antibiotics, because 50% yield an organism. Disc space cultures are not necessary for diagnosis and yield positive results in only 60% of cases. *S. aureus* is the most commonly isolated organism.

Treatment consists of intravenous antibiotics, casting, or bracing as needed. Surgical treatment is rarely necessary. Early in the disease process with minimal tissue destruction, intravenous antibiotics may be sufficient treatment. In the presence of significant bony destruction, kyphotic deformity, or soft tissue abscess, surgical intervention is indicated.

26. How does a lumbar disc herniation present in children?

Lumbar disc herniation is less common in children than adults. In contrast to adults, children commonly have a history of acute injury or chronic repetitive injury. The child may present with back pain and/or radicular leg pain. Physical examination may reveal reduced lumbar range of motion and a positive Lasegue's sign. Neurologic changes and bowel and bladder compromise are rare in adolescents. Initial treatment includes activity reduction, NSAIDs, ice, and physical therapy. Surgery is reserved for prolonged symptoms or neurologic involvement. Whereas 85% of adult patients experience resolution of acute symptoms by 6 weeks, 75% of adolescents do not improve with nonsurgical treatment.

27. What is a slipped vertebral apophysis?

Slipped vertebral apophysis or apophyseal ring fracture is a fracture through the junction of the vertebral body and the cartilaginous ring apophysis. This injury is possible prior to complete fusion of the cartilaginous ring apophysis, which occurs at approximately 18 years of age. Most injuries occur at the L4–L5 or L5–S1 level. This traumatic injury presents most often in males who participate in sports requiring repetitive flexion combined with rotation. Patients present with symptoms similar to a central disc herniation. Surgery is frequently necessary to excise the bone fragment with attached cartilage and disc.

28. What benign spinal tumors are most commonly found in children?

The most common benign tumors involving the spine in children are osteoid osteoma, osteoblastoma, aneurysmal bone cyst, Langerhans cell histiocytosis, giant cell tumor, hemangioma, and osteochondroma. Aneurysmal bone cyst, osteoid osteoma, osteochondroma, and osteoblastoma typically involve the **posterior spinal column.** Langerhans cell histiocytosis, giant cell tumor, and hemangioma typically involve the **anterior spinal column.** Langerhans cell histiocytosis classically manifests as a vertebra plana.

29. What is the most common malignant condition in the pediatric population?

Acute leukemia is the most common malignancy in children. Back pain may be the presenting symptom. This condition should be suspected in a child younger than 10 years old with pain at night. Additional findings include anemia, increased white blood cell count, increased ESR, vertebral compression fractures, diffuse osteopenia, and metaphyseal bands.

30. What primary bone tumors are most likely to involve the spine in the pediatric population?

Osteosarcoma and Ewing's sarcoma.

31. What are the most common spinal cord tumors in children?

Astrocytoma and ependymoma.

32. What is the most prevalent malignant condition that produces skeletal metastases in children?
Neuroblastoma. Up to 80% of patients develop spinal metastases.

33. What soft tissue sarcoma is most likely to involve the spine in the pediatric population?
Rhabdomyosarcoma.

Key Points

1. The majority of pediatric patients presenting with back pain do not have an identifiable diagnosis.
2. Initial evaluation of the pediatric patient presenting with back pain consists of a detailed history and physical examination combined with plain radiography.
3. Technetium bone scan and MRI are indicated for evaluation of pediatric patients with a suspected organic spine disorder.

Websites

Back packs and back pain: http://pediatrics.about.com/cs/safetyfirstaid/l/aa090202a.htm
Back pain evaluation in children and adolescents: http://www.aafp.org/afp/2007/1201/p1669.html
Back pain in children:
   http://www.virtualpediatrichospital.org/providers/BackPainInChildren/BackPainChildren.shtml

BIBLIOGRAPHY

1. Auerbach JD, Ahn J, Zgonis MH, et al. Streamlining the evaluation of low back pain in children. Clin Ortho Relat Res 2008;466:1971–7.
2. Bhatia NN, Chow G, Timon SJ, et al. Diagnostic modalities for the evaluation of pediatric back pain: a prospective study. J Pediatr Orthop 2008;28:230–3.
3. Davids JR, Wenger DR. Back pain in children and adolescents. J Musculoskel Med 1994;11:19–32.
4. DeLuca PF, Mason DE, Weiand R, et al. Excision of herniated nucleus pulposus in teenage children and adolescents. J Pediatr Orthop 1994;14:318–22.
5. Epstein NE. Lumbar surgery for 56 limbus fractures emphasizing noncalcified type 3 lesions. Spine 1992;17:1489–96.
6. Garg S, Dormans JP. Tumors and tumor-like conditions of the spine in children. J Am Acad Ortho Surg 2005;13:372–81.
7. Ginsburg GM, Bassett GS. Back pain evaluation in children and adolescents: evaluation and differential diagnosis. J Am Acad Orthop Surg 1997;5:67–78.
8. Jeffries LJ, Milanese SF, Grimmer-Somers KA. Epidemiology of adolescent spinal pain—a systematic overview of the research literature. Spine 2007;32:2630–7.
9. Neuschwander TB, Cutrone J, Macias BA, et al. The effect of backpacks on the lumbar spine in children—a standing magnetic resonance imaging study. Spine 2009;35:83–8.
10. Selbst SM, Lavelle JM, Soyupak SK, et al. Back pain in children who present to the emergency department. Clin Pediatr 1999;38:401–6.

PEDIATRIC CERVICAL DISORDERS

Thomas R. Haher, MD

GENERAL CONCEPTS

1. What family of genes regulates development of the vertebral column?

The *Hox* (homeobox) and *Pax* (paired box) genes regulate embryonic differentiation and segmentation of the developing vertebral column.

2. What anatomic features differentiate the immature cervical spine from the adult cervical spine?

Unique anatomic features of the immature cervical spine include hypermobility, hyperlaxity of ligamentous and capsular structures, presence of epiphyses and synchondroses, incomplete ossification, unique configuration of the vertebral bony elements (e.g. wedge-shaped vertebral bodies, horizontally oriented facet joints), and variable sagittal alignment.

3. When does the immature cervical spine approach adult size and shape?

The immature cervical spine approaches adult size and shape around age 8 years.

4. How does a child's age affect the pattern of traumatic cervical spine injury?

Before age 8 years, most cervical injuries occur at C3 or above and are associated with a high risk of fatality. After age 8, cervical injury patterns are similar to adults and occur below the C4 level and are less likely to be fatal.

5. How does a child's age affect the position for immobilization during initial evaluation of a suspected traumatic cervical spine injury?

Up to age 8 years, children have a large cranium in relation to their thorax. If children younger than 8 years are immobilized on a routine backboard, the cervical spine will be flexed and fracture deformity may be increased. Use of a double mattress to elevate the thorax or use of a recess for the occiput is recommended.

TORTICOLLIS

6. Define torticollis.

Torticollis is a clinical diagnosis based on head tilt in association with a rotatory deviation of the cranium.

7. What is the most common type of torticollis?

Congenital muscular torticollis is the most common type of torticollis. It presents in the newborn period. Its cause is unknown, but it has been hypothesized to arise from compression of the soft tissues of the neck during delivery, resulting in a compartment syndrome. Radiographs of the cervical spine should be obtained to rule out congenital vertebral anomalies. Clinical examination reveals spasm of the sternocleidomastoid muscle on the *same* side as the tilt causing the typical posture of head tilt toward the tightened muscle and chin rotation to the opposite side. Initial treatment is stretching and is successful in up to 90% of patients during the first year of life. Surgery is considered for persistent deformity after 1 year of age. Common problems noted in patients with congenital muscular torticollis include congenital hip dysplasia and plagiocephaly (facial asymmetry).

8. What are some other causes of torticollis?

When torticollis presents after the newborn period, the etiology is wide-ranging and may result from pathology involving any structure in the head or neck region:

- Congenital anomalies of the craniocervical junction or upper cervical spine
- Ocular or auditory dysfunction
- Tumors involving the posterior fossa, brainstem, or spinal cord
- Osseous tumors (osteoid osteoma, aneurysmal bone cyst)
- Infection
- Inflammatory disorders (e.g. juvenile rheumatoid arthritis)
- Fracture
- Rotatory subluxation of the atlantoaxial joints
- Sandifer's syndrome (gastroesophageal reflux and torticollis)

9. **What features suggest that torticollis is due to atlantoaxial rotatory subluxation?**
Features that suggest that torticollis is due to atlantoaxial rotatory subluxation include prior normal cervical alignment and motion, history of recent upper respiratory infection (Grisel's syndrome), normal neurologic examination, and spasm in the sternocleidomastoid muscle on the side *opposite* the head tilt. This posture has been termed the "cock robin" deformity. It is distinct from congenital muscular torticollis, in which muscle spasm occurs on the same side as the head tilt. Plain radiographs are frequently difficult to interpret but typically show asymmetry of the C1 lateral masses on the anteroposterior (AP) odontoid view. A cervical computed tomography (CT) scan can be obtained to confirm the diagnosis. Recommendations for the optimal type of CT study include a cervical CT scan with standard sagittal and coronal reconstructions, a dynamic rotational CT scan, and a CT scan performed with the patient under general anesthesia.

10. **How is atlantoaxial rotatory subluxation classified?**
Type 1: Rotatory displacement without anterior shift of C1
Type 2: Rotatory displacement with C1 anterior shift of 5 mm or less
Type 3: Rotatory displacement with C1 anterior shift greater than 5 mm
Type 4: Rotatory displacement with C1 posterior shift

11. **Describe the treatment of atlantoaxial rotatory subluxation.**
When the problem is diagnosed early, many children respond well to immobilization with a soft cervical collar and activity restriction. If early follow-up shows persistent subluxation, inpatient treatment with traction via a head halter is indicated. If reduction occurs (confirmed clinically and by CT), immobilization is continued for at least 6 weeks with a Minerva cast or halo cast. Surgery is indicated for failure of reduction following traction treatment, recurrent subluxation, neurologic involvement, and deformities present for more than 3 months. Posterior C1–C2 arthrodesis is the most commonly performed surgical procedure. First-stage transoral or lateral retropharyngeal release of the atlantoaxial joints followed by posterior reduction, atlantoaxial fusion, and C1-C2 screw-rod fixation has been advocated for chronic subluxations by some experts.

CERVICAL ANOMALIES

12. **What serious problems are associated with congenital anomalies of the cervical region?**
Recognition of congenital anomalies involving the cervical region is important because of their association with spinal deformity, spinal instability, and spinal cord and brainstem compression resulting in myelopathy. Other organ system anomalies may be associated with cervical spine anomalies because these systems share common embryonic development.

13. **What are some commonly diagnosed cervical spine anomalies?**
Cervical anomalies may be broadly grouped into those located in the upper cervical region (occiput–C2) and those occurring in the subaxial cervical region (C3–C7).

OCCIPUT–C2 REGION
1. *Congenital anomalies associated with neural compression*
  - Basilar impression
  - Congenital cervical stenosis
  - Arnold-Chiari malformation
2. *Anomalies associated with cervical instability at occiput–C1*
  - Occipitalization of C1 (skeletal dysplasia)
  - Skeletal dysplasia (e.g. Kniest's dysplasia)
  - Down's syndrome
3. *Anomalies associated with C1–C2 instability*
  - Odontoid anomalies (aplasia, hypoplasia, os odontoideum)
  - Skeletal dysplasia (e.g. mucopolysaccharidosis)
  - Down syndrome

SUBAXIAL CERVICAL REGION
1. *Anomalies associated with deformity and instability*
  - Klippel-Feil anomaly
2. Miscellaneous disorders
  - Postlaminectomy kyphosis
  - Neurofibromatosis
  - Skeletal dysplasia (e.g. Larsen's syndrome)

14. **What is basilar impression?**
Basilar impression is a downward displacement of the base of the skull in the area of the foramen magnum. It is identified by the protrusion of the tip of the odontoid through the foramen magnum. The most significant clinical problems associated with congenital basilar impression are due to anterior or posterior brainstem compression with or without atlantoaxial instability. It is the most common congenital anomaly of the upper cervical spine.

15. **What are the different types of basilar impression?**
There are two main types of basilar impression: primary and secondary. The primary type is most common. It is frequently associated with other vertebral defects, including atlanto-occipital fusion, odontoid abnormalities, Klippel-Feil anomaly, and hypoplasia of the atlas. Vertebral artery abnormalities may also be present. Secondary basilar impression arises as the result of softening of osseous structures at the base of the skull. Diseases associated with secondary basilar impression include osteomalacia, rickets, Paget's disease, osteogenesis imperfecta, renal osteodystrophy, and rheumatoid arthritis.

16. What clinical problems result from basilar impression?

Patients present with a short neck, painful cervical motion, and asymmetry of the skull and face. Additional clinical problems include nuchal pain, vertigo, long tract signs with associated cerebellar ataxia, and lower cranial nerve involvement resulting in dysarthria and dysphagia.

17. How is the diagnosis of basilar impression confirmed radiographically?

Magnetic resonance imaging (MRI) or CT-myelography with sagittal reconstructions demonstrate the position of the dens in relation to the foramen magnum with precision and provide the definitive method for diagnosis. A lateral craniocervical radiograph can demonstrate the position of the tip of the dens in relation to the various skull base lines (McGregor, McRae, Chamberlain) but is less precise than MRI or CT.

18. What treatment is indicated for symptomatic basilar impression?

Treatment typically involves decompression and stabilization. Options for decompression include anterior transoral odontoid resection or posterior suboccipital craniectomy and C1 laminectomy. Stabilization typically includes posterior occipitocervical fusion. Associated neurologic conditions, such as hydrocephalus, also require treatment.

19. What is the Arnold-Chiari malformation?

The Arnold-Chiari malformation is a developmental anomaly in which the brainstem and cerebellum are displaced caudally into the spinal canal. In Type 1 Arnold-Chiari malformation, the cerebellar tonsils are displaced into the cervical spinal canal. This malformation is associated with other cervical anomalies including basilar impression and Klippel-Feil syndrome. Dense scarring at the level of the foramen magnum may lead to hydromyelia or syringomyelia. Type 2 Arnold-Chiari malformation is a more complex anomaly and is usually associated with myelomeningocele. Cerebellar displacement is accompanied by elongation of the fourth ventricle, as well as displacement of the fourth ventricle and cervical nerve roots.

20. How is atlantooccipital instability defined radiographically?

Atlantooccipital instability is defined as greater than 1 mm of translation measured from the basion to the posterior margin of the anterior arch of C1 on lateral flexion-extension views (Fig. 37-1).

21. What is Steel's *rule of thirds?*

Steel noted that the area of the spinal canal at the C1 level in a normal person could be divided into equal thirds with one third occupied by the odontoid process, one third by the spinal cord, and one third as empty space (Fig. 37-2). The empty space serves as a safe zone into which displacement can occur without neurologic impingement. In the presence of atlantoaxial instability, the safe zone may decrease resulting in spinal cord compression.

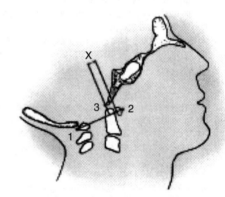

Figure 37-1. Method of measuring atlantooccipital instability according to Wiesel and Rothman. These lines are drawn on flexion and extension lateral radiographs, and translation should be no more than 1 mm. Atlantal line joins points 1 and 2. Line drawn perpendicular to atlantal line at posterior margin of anterior arch of atlas. Point 3 is basion. Distance from point 3 to perpendicular line (represented by X) is measured in flexion and extension. Difference represents anteroposterior translation. (From Gabriel KR, Mason DE, Carango P. Occipitoatlantal translation in Down's syndrome. Spine 1990;15:997.)

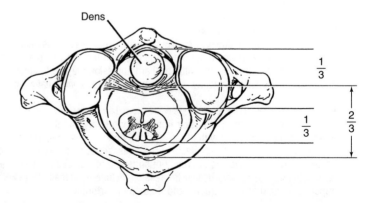

Figure 37-2. Steel's rule. (From Moskovich R. Atlanto-axial instability. Spine State Art Rev 1994;8:533, with permission.)

22. How is atlantoaxial instability defined radiographically?

Atlantoaxial instability is defined as an increased mobility between the anterior surface of the odontoid and the posterior aspect of the anterior arch of the atlas. This measurement is called the atlantodens interval (ADI) and is measured from lateral flexion-extension radiographs. The upper limit of normal for the ADI in children is 4 mm (some experts consider 5 mm as the upper limit of normal). An ADI greater than 4 mm is considered pathologic and represents failure of the transverse ligament. An ADI greater than 10 mm suggests failure of the secondary supporting ligaments, including the alar ligaments, with increased risk of neurologic compromise. In patients with chronic atlantoaxial instability, the odontoid may be hypermobile resulting in an increased ADI in the absence of clinical symptoms. In this situation, measurement of the space available for the cord (SAC) is more helpful in assessing pathologic instability. The SAC is measured from the posterior margin of the odontoid to the closest posterior structure, either the foramen magnum or the posterior ring of C1 (Fig. 37-3). A SAC of 13 mm indicates insufficient space for the spinal cord and may be associated with neurologic signs or symptoms.

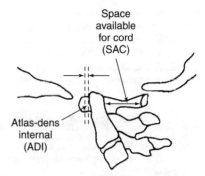

Figure 37-3. Measurements for atlas-dens interval (ADI) and the space available for the cord (SAC) as determined on lateral cervical radiographs. (From Herman MJ, Pizzutillo PD. Cervical spine disorders in children. Orthop Clin North Am 1999;320:457–75, with permission.)

23. What are the major causes of nontraumatic atlantoaxial instability?

The major causes can be categorized into three groups:
1. Anomalies of the odontoid process (e.g. os odontoideum)
2. Ligamentous laxity (e.g. Down's syndrome, juvenile rheumatoid arthritis, osteochondrodystrophies)
3. Synostosis at adjacent spinal levels (e.g. Klippel-Feil anomaly, occipitalization of the atlas)

24. Define os odontoideum and explain its likely etiology.

Os odontoideum is an anomaly of the odontoid process that appears as an ossicle with smooth cortical margins separate from the body of the axis. The atlantoaxial joint becomes unstable as the odontoid becomes unable to function as a peg. Associated symptoms range from mild neck pain to myelopathy and sudden death secondary to minor trauma. Surgery is considered in the presence of neurologic deficit, C1–C2 instability greater than 10 mm on flexion-extension radiographs, or persistent neck pain. Some experts advise surgical stabilization for all patients with os odontoideum due to the risk of catastrophic spinal cord injury from minor trauma. Recent data support two separate etiologies for os odontoideum: posttraumatic and congenital.

25. What patterns of upper cervical instability are seen in patients with Down's syndrome?

Patients with Down's syndrome may manifest instability of both the atlanto-occipital joints and the atlantoaxial joints. It is important to rule out atlanto-occipital instability prior to performing fusion of the atlantoaxial joints. In addition, atlanto-occipital instability may develop following a successful atlantoaxial fusion. The underlying problem is generalized ligamentous laxity. Hypoplasia of the posterior arch of C1, occipital condyle hypoplasia, and os odontoideum are also prevalent in this population. Caution is advised when surgical treatment is undertaken because of the high risk of surgical complications in this population.

26. What is the clinical triad described by Klippel-Feil syndrome?

Klippel-Feil syndrome has been classically described as the clinical triad of a short neck, low posterior hairline, and limitation of cervical motion. The spinal anomaly associated with Klippel-Feil syndrome is congenital fusion of the cervical spine. The classic triad is seen in less than 50% of cases. The number of fused segments may vary from two segments to fusion of the entire cervical spine.

27. Why is early recognition of Klippel-Feil syndrome important?

Klippel-Feil anomalies are a marker that should prompt investigation for a wide range of systemic anomalies. Because the embryologic development of cervical spine parallels the development of many other organ systems, a wide range of anomalies may be present, including anomalies involving the genitourinary, cardiovascular, auditory, gastrointestinal, skeletal, and neurologic systems. The most common neurologic abnormality is synkinesis (unconscious mirror movement of one extremity that mimics the opposite extremity). Associated skeletal system anomalies include scoliosis, Sprengel's deformity (failure of descent of the scapula), presence of an omovertebral bone, and cervical ribs.

28. What workup should be performed for a patient diagnosed with Klippel-Feil syndrome?

Diagnosis of a congenital cervical fusion should prompt assessment of the genitourinary system (renal ultrasound), cardiac system (echocardiogram, cardiology referral), and auditory system (hearing test). Neurologic symptoms should be evaluated with an MRI of the brainstem and cervical spine. Cervical instability is evaluated with flexion and extension radiographs.

29. Are any patterns of congenital cervical fusion in Klippel-Feil patients associated with an increased risk of neurologic deficit?

Three fusion patterns are considered to be associated with an increased risk of neurologic problems:

1. C2–C3 fusion with occipitalization of the atlas
2. A long cervical fusion in the presence of an abnormal occipital-cervical junction
3. A single open interspace between two fused spine segments

Key Points

1. A wide range of conditions may cause upper cervical instability.
2. Children younger than 8 years are predisposed to upper cervical injury due to their high head-to-body ratio and horizontal facet orientation.
3. Evaluation of C1–C2 instability should include assessment of both the atlantodens interval (ADI) and the space available for the spinal cord (SAC).
4. The presence of a Klippel-Feil anomaly should prompt investigation for associated organ system anomalies.

Websites

Atlantoaxial instability: http://emedicine.medscape.com/article/1265682-overview
Congenital and acquired anomalies of the cervical spine: http://www.sheddonphysio.com/cspine%20anomalies.pdf
Evaluation and treatment of congenital and developmental anomalies of the cervical spine: http://thejns.org/doi/pdf/10.3171/spi.2004.1.2.0188
Klippel-Feil syndrome: http://emedicine.medscape.com/article/1264848-overview

BIBLIOGRAPHY

1. Bedi A, Hensinger RN. Congenital anomalies of the cervical spine. In: Herkowitz HN, Garfin SR, Eismont FJ, et al, editors. The Spine. 5th ed. Philadelphia: Saunders; 2006. p. 630–74.
2. Copley LA, Dormans JP. Cervical spine disorders in infants and children. J Am Acad Orthop Surg 1998;6:204–14.
3. Drummond DS. Congenital anomalies of the pediatric cervical spine. In: Bridwell KH, DeWald RL, editors. Textbook of Spinal Surgery. 2nd ed. Philadelphia: Lippincott-Raven; 1997. p. 951–68.
4. Dubousset J. Torticollis in children caused by congenital anomalies of the atlas. J Bone Joint Surg 1986;68A:178–88.
5. Fielding JW, Hawkins RJ. Atlantoaxial rotatory fixation (fixed subluxation of the atlantoaxial joint). J Bone Joint Surg 1977;59A:37–44.
6. Hensinger RN, Lang JE, MacEwen GD. Klippel-Feil syndrome: a constellation of associated anomalies. J Bone Joint Surg 1974;56A:1246–53.
7. Herman MJ, Pizzutillo PD. Cervical spine disorders in children. Orthop Clin North Am 1999;30:457–75.
8. Herzenberg JE, Hensinger RN, Dedrick DK, et al. Emergency transport and positioning of young children who have an injury of the cervical spine: the standard backboard may be hazardous. J Bone Joint Surg 1989;71A:15–22.
9. Samartzis DD, Lubicky JP, Herman J. Classification of congenitally fused cervical patterns in Klippel-Feil patients: epidemiology and role in the development of cervical spine-related symptoms. Spine 2006;31:E798–804.
10. Sankar WN, Wills BP, Dormans JP, et al. Os odontoideum revisited: the case for a multifactorial etiology. Spine 2006;31:979–84.

SPONDYLOLYSIS AND SPONDYLOLISTHESIS IN PEDIATRIC PATIENTS

CHAPTER 38

Vincent J. Devlin, MD

1. Define spondylolysis.
Spondylolysis is a unilateral or bilateral defect in the region of the pars interarticularis that may or may not be accompanied by vertebral displacement. The origin of the term *spondylolysis* is from the Greek words *spondylo* (vertebra) and *lysis* (break or defect).

2. Define spondylolisthesis.
Spondylolisthesis refers to anterior displacement of a vertebra in relation to the subjacent vertebra. The origin of the term is from the Greek words *spondylo* (vertebra) and *olisthesis* (movement or slippage). The deformity not only involves the olisthetic vertebra but affects the entire spinal column above the level of slippage as the entire trunk moves forward with the displaced vertebra.

3. Define spondyloptosis.
Spondyloptosis refers to a slippage of the L5 vertebra in which the entire vertebral body of L5 is located below the top of S1. It is the most severe degree of slippage possible. Fortunately, this condition is quite rare. The origin of the term is from the Greek words *spondylo* (vertebra) and *ptosis* (to fall).

4. Describe the Wiltse classification of spondylolisthesis (Fig. 38-1).
- **Type 1:** *Dysplastic:* Associated with a congenital deficiency of the L5–S1 articulation
- **Type 2:** *Isthmic:* Associated with a lesion in the pars interarticularis
  - Subtype 2A: Lytic defect (stress fracture) of the pars
  - Subtype 2B: An elongated or attenuated pars
  - Subtype 2C: An acute pars fracture

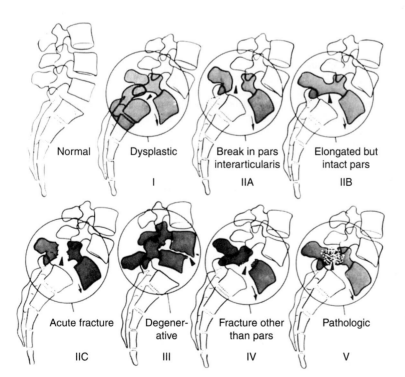

Normal   Dysplastic   Break in pars interarticularis   Elongated but intact pars
            I   IIA   IIB

Acute fracture   Degenerative   Fracture other than pars   Pathologic
     IIC   III   IV   V

Figure 38-1. Wiltse classification of spondylolisthesis. (From Neuwirth MG. Spondylolysis and spondylolisthesis in children and adults. In: Comins M, O'Leary P, editors. The Lumbar Spine. New York: Raven Press; 1987. p. 258, with permission.)

- **Type 3:** *Degenerative*: Disc degeneration and facet arthrosis lead to spondylolisthesis and associated spinal stenosis
- **Type 4:** *Traumatic*: An acute fracture in a region of the posterior elements other than the pars interarticularis (e.g. facets, pedicle, lamina) leads to spondylolisthesis
- **Type 5:** *Pathologic*: Generalized bone disease (e.g. metabolic, neoplastic) results in attenuation of the pars and/or pedicle region leading to spondylolisthesis
- **Type 6:** *Postsurgical*: Spondylolisthesis that develops following lumbar laminotomy or laminectomy

5. **Does the presence or absence of a pars defect unequivocally determine whether a spondylolisthesis is classified as an isthmic or dysplastic type of slippage?**
No. When a spondylolisthesis with dysplastic features increases in severity, a defect may develop in the region of the pars interarticularis that was not present when the slippage was first diagnosed. Use of the Wiltse classification for this type of patient is problematic. For this reason, it is preferable to classify spondylolisthesis into two major subgroups (developmental and acquired) based on the presence or absence of dysplasia (abnormal tissue development) at the level of spondylolisthesis. Some of the dysplastic changes that may be present include lumbosacral facet anomalies, deficient L5 and S1 lamina, elongation of the pars interarticularis, rounding of the dome of the sacrum, and a trapezoidal-shaped L5 vertebra. The classification of Marchetti and Bartolozzi recognizes these features and divides spondylolisthesis into two major subgroups: Developmental and acquired (Table 38-1).

Table 38-1. Marchetti and Bartolozzi Classification of Spondylolisthesis	
DEVELOPMENTAL	**ACQUIRED**
High dysplasia	Traumatic
Low dysplasia	Degenerative
	Post surgical
	Pathologic

6. **How common are spondylolysis and spondylolisthesis?**
The prevalence of spondylolysis and spondylolisthesis is approximately 4% at age 6 and 6% by age 14 years. Prevalence remains constant in adulthood. The male-to-female ratio is 2:1. Slip progression may occur during adolescence but is less common in the adult population.

7. **What causes spondylolysis and spondylolisthesis in children?**
Although the exact cause remains unknown in all cases, important factors include:
- **Biomechanics:** Mechanical factors play a role because these conditions are not seen in patients who are nonambulatory. Upright posture and lumbar lordosis lead to stress concentration in the region of the pars interarticularis
- **Growth:** These conditions are almost never seen at birth and are most common between 6 and 10 years of age. Recent studies of developmental type of spondylolisthesis suggest that sacral growth plate abnormalities are a primary cause of the deformity in contrast to the acquired traumatic type of spondylolisthesis where focus is directed toward pathology in the region of the pars interarticularis
- **Trauma:** Repetitive microtrauma such as the repetitive hyperextension experienced by young athletes (e.g. gymnasts, weightlifters) is considered to play a role in etiology in certain cases
- **Heredity:** These conditions do not occur in a uniform distribution across populations. Spondylolysis and spondylolisthesis are more common in males than females and in the offspring of first-degree relatives with these conditions. The familial predisposition is greater for the dysplastic type than for the isthmic type. There is an extremely high incidence in Alaskan Eskimos, but the reason is unclear

8. **When are children with spondylolysis and spondylolisthesis referred to the spine specialist for evaluation?**
The presentation of patients with spondylolysis and spondylolisthesis is varied. Symptomatic patients most commonly present with low back pain, which may radiate into the buttocks and thighs. Hamstring tightness or spasm is not uncommon. Some patients will recall an episode of inciting trauma. Occasionally a patient will report radicular symptoms due to nerve compression at the level of the slippage. Patients with severe degrees of spondylolisthesis may present with postural deformity, scoliosis, or gait abnormality. In some cases, spondylolysis and spondylolisthesis are diagnosed as incidental findings on lumbar or pelvic radiographs obtained for unrelated reasons in asymptomatic patients.

9. **What radiographic views should be obtained to evaluate spondylolysis and spondylolisthesis?**
The initial radiographic assessment should include posteroanterior (PA) and lateral lumbosacral radiographs obtained in the standing position. The standing position documents the alignment of the spine under physiologic loading. Oblique views of the lumbosacral region may be obtained to assess the pars interarticularis region more closely. On the oblique view, the posterior spinal elements create a figure resembling a "Scottie dog." Spondylolysis is noted as a break in the

neck of the dog (see Chapter 10, Figure 10-8). Additional useful radiographic views include lateral flexion-extension views, comparison of supine and standing lateral radiographs, and the Ferguson view (anteroposterior [AP] view with 30° cephalad tilt). A lateral long cassette radiograph is used to assess the sagittal vertical axis and pelvic parameters in patients with high-grade slips.

10. What radiographic measurements are most useful for describing spondylolisthesis?

The most useful radiographic measurements for describing spondylolisthesis are the *degree of slip* and the *slip angle* (Fig. 38-2).

The **degree of slip** refers to the amount of translation of the superior vertebra relative to the inferior vertebra. Translation is quantified into five grades (Meyerding system): Grade 1, 1% to 25%; grade 2, 26% to 50%; grade 3, 51% to 75%; grade 4, 76% to 100%; and grade 5, slippage of the L5 vertebra anterior and distal to the superior S1 endplate (spondyloptosis)

The **slip angle** measures the degree of lumbosacral kyphosis. It is calculated by measuring the angle between a line perpendicular with the posterior aspect of S1 and a line parallel to either the superior or inferior endplate of L5

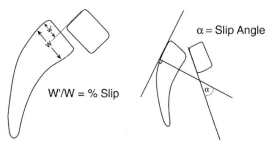

Figure 38-2. Radiographic measurements of spondylolisthesis. (From Ginsburg GM. Spondylolysis and spondylolisthesis. In: Brown DE, Neumann RD, editors. Orthopedic Secrets. 2nd ed. Philadelphia: Hanley & Belfus; 1999. p. 200–4, with permission.)

11. Discuss the role of bone scan in the assessment of spondylolysis and spondylolisthesis.

A technetium bone scan is helpful when clinical findings suggest a pars defect but radiographs are negative. A bone scan is helpful in the diagnosis of a stress reaction in the pars region. This finding represents an impending pars fracture. Bone scans are helpful in distinguishing acute from chronic pars interarticularis lesions. There are two types of bone scans: planar bone scans and single-photon emission computed tomography (SPECT). SPECT is more sensitive and specific than planar bone scans for the assessment of spondylolysis.

12. What is the role of computed tomography (CT) in the assessment of spondylolysis and spondylolisthesis?

CT plays a role when a pars defect is suspected on a clinical basis but is not evident on plain radiographs. CT remains the best test for assessment of osseous detail. It is useful for preoperative planning (e.g. evaluating the lumbar pedicles before screw placement), for assessment of osseous abnormalities, and for assessment of healing of spinal fusions.

13. What is the role of magnetic resonance imaging (MRI) in the assessment of spondylolysis and spondylolisthesis?

MRI is useful in the assessment of pediatric spondylolysis and spondylolisthesis in select cases. For example, it is invaluable for assessment of stress reaction involving the pars region, for assessment of high-grade slips with associated radiculopathy or neurologic deficit, and for evaluation of associated lumbar disc pathology. MRI is also useful to rule out other serious causes of back pain, such as tumor or infection.

14. What are the nonsurgical treatment options for an adolescent with spondylolysis or spondylolisthesis?

Asymptomatic spondylolysis or low-grade spondylolisthesis discovered as an incidental radiographic finding requires no specific treatment. Treatment of symptomatic patients begins with rest, nonsteroidal antiinflammatory medication, physical therapy, and activity modification. Avoidance of activities that require hyperextension of the spine is especially important. If symptoms persist, an orthosis that reduces lumbar lordosis can be prescribed. Athletic activities are avoided during the initial period of orthotic treatment and gradually resumed if back pain symptoms completely resolve.

15. When is surgery considered for spondylolysis?

Indications to consider surgical treatment include persistent or increasing pain lasting more than 6 months, persistent hamstring spasm, radiculopathy (rare), and failure of nonsurgical treatment.

16. What surgical options are advised for treatment of spondylolysis?

The surgical treatment options for spondylolysis are (1) an intertransverse fusion or (2) a direct repair of the pars interarticularis. In general, a **pars repair** is considered for defects between L1 and L4. An **intertransverse fusion** is most often considered for L5 pars defects, although pars repair remains an option at the L5 level.

17. What are the prerequisites for successful outcome with a pars repair? How is this procedure performed?

- Patients who are best suited for pars repair are younger than 25 years old, have no evidence of disc or facet pathology at the level of spondylolysis, and have a slippage less than 2 mm. The procedure requires careful debridement of the pars pseudarthrosis and application of autogenous bone graft to this region. Internal fixation across the pars defect is required (Fig. 38-3). Fixation options include:

- Direct screw fixation across the pars defect (Buck technique)
- Wire fixation between the transverse process and spinous process (Scott technique)
- Wire-screw or cable-screw construct (connects a pedicle screw via a wire or cable passing under the lamina and tightened around the spinous process)
- Screw-hook-rod fixation (ipsilateral pedicle screw and infralaminar hook are connected by a rod)
- An intralaminar link construct (V-shaped rod passes over the posterior aspect of the right and left lamina and underneath the spinous process to connect screws in the right and left pedicles)
- Pedicle screw-intralaminar screw-rod construct

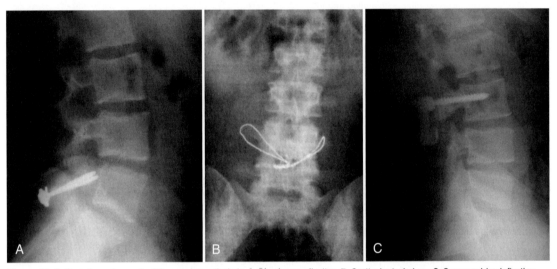

Figure 38-3. Techniques for repair of the pars interarticularis. **A,** Direct screw fixation. **B,** Scott wire technique. **C,** Screw-rod-hook fixation. (**A** from Reitman CA, Esses SI. Direct repair of spondylolytic defects in young competitive athletes. Spine J 2002;2:142–4; **B** from Ginsburg GM. Spondylolysis and spondylolisthesis. In: Brown DE, Neumann RD, editors. Orthopedic Secrets. 2nd ed. Philadelphia: Hanley & Belfus; 1999. p. 200–4, with permission; **C** from Benzon HT, Rathmell JP, Wu CL, et al. Raj's Practical Management of Pain. 4th ed. St. Louis: Mosby; 2008.)

18. **What clinical and radiographic factors suggest that a child with spondylolisthesis is likely to have persistent symptoms, slip progression, and spinal deformity?**
    See Table 38-2.

Table 38-2. Risk Factors for Symptomatic or Progressive Spondylolisthesis

CLINICAL FACTORS	RADIOGRAPHIC FACTORS
Young age	Dysplastic type of spondylolisthesis
Female sex	Unstable radiographic contour (dome-shaped sacrum, trapezoidal-shaped L5 vertebra)
Presence of back pain symptoms	Instability on dynamic radiographs Degree of slip > 50% Slip angle > 40°

19. **What are the indications to consider surgery for children with spondylolisthesis?**
    Surgical indications include intractable low back or radicular pain, progressive slippage, grade 2 or 3 slips in skeletally immature patients, and patients with neurologic symptoms, gait abnormality, and severe spinal deformity.

20. **What is the procedure of choice for treatment of children with low-grade (grade 1 and 2) spondylolisthesis?**
    The procedure of choice is an in situ posterolateral spinal fusion (Fig. 38-4). The procedure can be performed through either a midline approach or a paraspinal approach. Spinal implants are not routinely used by all surgeons because of the good potential for healing of posterolateral fusions in pediatric patients with low-grade slips. Many surgeons consider pedicle fixation advantageous if a decompression is performed at the time of fusion. Traditional teaching is to perform posterolateral fusion from L5 to S1 if the slip is less than 50% and to extend fusion to L4 if the slip is greater

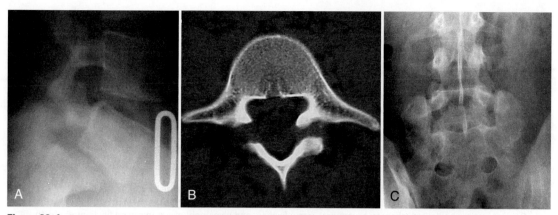

Figure 38-4. Treatment of low-grade isthmic spondylolisthesis with posterolateral in situ fusion using iliac crest autograft. **A,** Preoperative lateral radiograph. **B,** Preoperative computed tomography. **C,** Postoperative anteroposterior radiograph showing a healed fusion.

than 50%. Use of postoperative immobilization (brace, cast) is also controversial. To decrease motion at the L5–S1 level, an orthosis must incorporate the patient's thigh.

21. **What problems are associated with the treatment of high-grade (grade 3 and 4) spondylolisthesis with in situ posterolateral spinal fusion?**
Problems associated with in situ fusion for patients with high-grade spondylolisthesis include progressive slippage, pseudarthrosis, persistent lumbosacral deformity, and cauda equina syndrome.

22. **What type of procedure for pediatric high-grade spondylolisthesis has the highest rate of fusion?**
Circumferential fusion. A classic study (8) showed that the rate of fusion in pediatric high-grade spondylolisthesis depends on the type of fusion procedure:

Procedure	Fusion Rate (%)
Posterior fusion without spinal implants	55
Posterior fusion with posterior spinal implants	71
Circumferential fusion with posterior implants	100

In the circumferential fusion group, bilateral S1 and iliac screw fixation and interbody fusion using anterior structural grafts or cages were utilized. Interbody fusion via a transforaminal lumbar interbody (TLIF) approach has been documented as an alternative approach for achieving circumferential fusion in this setting (Fig. 38-5).

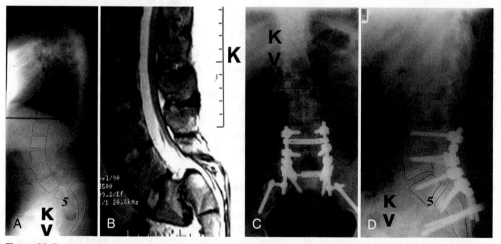

Figure 38-5. Treatment of high-grade isthmic spondylolisthesis with reduction and circumferential fusion from a posterior approach. **A,** Lateral radiograph. **B,** Magnetic resonance imaging show grade 4 developmental spondylolisthesis. Treatment included reduction of the spondylolisthesis utilizing bilateral S1 and iliac screws, reduction screws in L3, L4, and L5, sacral dome osteotomy and posterior lumbar interbody fusion with cortical bone interbody spacers and iliac crest autograft. **C,** Postoperative anteroposterior radiograph. **D,** Lateral radiograph. (From O'Brien MF, Kuklo TR, Mardjetko SJ, et al. The sacropelvic unit: creative solutions to complex fixation and reconstruction problems. Semin Spine Surg 2004;16:134–49.)

23. What problems are associated with spondylolisthesis reduction procedures?

Spondylolisthesis reduction procedures are technically complex and associated with numerous potential complications:

- Increased operative time compared with nonreductive techniques
- L5 nerve root injury
- Cauda equina injury
- Proximal lumbar plexus neural injury
- Sacral fixation failure

24. What are the potential advantages of spondylolisthesis reduction procedures compared with in situ fusion?

- Increased fusion rate
- Potential to correct spinal deformity
- Potential to limit fusion to a single spinal motion segment in high-grade slips
- Potential to achieve complete neural decompression
- Prevention of deformity progression
- Restoration of body posture and mechanics

25. What is the role of transfixation, decompression, and transsacral interbody fusion using a fibula graft in the treatment of high-grade spondylolisthesis?

Decompression, partial reduction, transvertebral screw fixation, and placement of a transsacral fibula graft are an attractive treatment option for patients with high-grade spondylolisthesis. This technique permits reduction of the slip angle, which is the major component of the deformity. It minimizes the risks associated with attempting complete correction of vertebral translation (spondylolisthesis reduction) and provides a circumferential fusion through a single-stage posterior approach (Fig. 38-6).

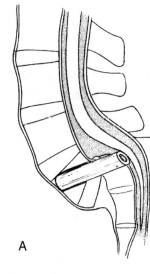 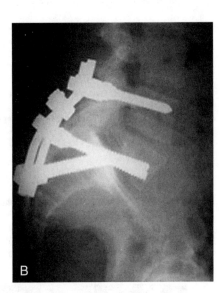

Figure 38-6. Decompression, transfixation, and transsacral interbody fusion. **A,** A fibula graft is placed across the sacrum, L5–S1 disc and into the L5 vertebral body. **B,** Pedicle screws are subsequently placed via the S1 pedicle from S1 into L5. (**A** from Winter RB, Lonstein JW, Denis F, Smith MD, editors. Atlas of Spine Surgery. Philadelphia: Saunders; 1995. p. 461, with permission.)

26. How does a surgeon choose whether to perform in situ fusion, partial reduction and transfixation, or an instrumented reduction procedure for a pediatric patient with high-grade spondylolisthesis?

This decision remains controversial because no universally accepted guidelines exist. Decision making is based on correlation of clinical examination and radiologic studies taking into account neurologic compression, global sagittal balance, spino-pelvic parameters, posterior element dysplasia, and lumbosacral kyphosis. The risk of pseudarthrosis is weighed against the neurologic risk associated with reduction, as well as the risks associated with a more complex procedure. Reduction procedures for high-grade developmental spondylolisthesis are generally favored in the presence of global spinal imbalance and high degrees of lumbosacral kyphosis.

27. What are the treatment options for spondyloptosis?

Fortunately, spondyloptosis is a rare condition. Treatment options include a reduction procedure or L5 vertebral resection (Gaines procedure). The Gaines procedure is generally preferred and is performed in two stages. In the first stage, an anterior approach to the spine is performed and the L4–L5 disc, L5–S1 disc, and L5 vertebra are removed. In the second stage, the lamina and pedicles of L5 are removed to complete the L5 resection and the L4 vertebra is placed on top of the sacrum and held in place with pedicle fixation (Fig. 38-7).

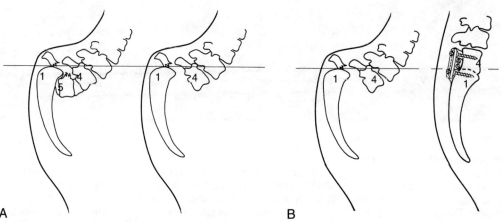

Figure 38-7. Gaines procedure. **A,** First stage. **B,** Second stage. (From Grobler LJ, Wiltse LL. Classification and nonoperative treatment of spondylolisthesis. In: Fryomer JW, editor. The Adult Spine: Principles and Practice. 2nd ed. Philadelphia: Lippincott-Raven; 1997. p. 1889, with permission.)

Key Points

1. Pediatric patients with spondylolysis usually respond to nonsurgical treatment, and the need for surgical treatment is uncommon.
2. Spondylolisthesis may be classified into two main types: developmental and acquired.
3. Circumferential fusion provides the highest likelihood of successful arthrodesis in patients with high-grade spondylolisthesis.

Website

Spondylolysis: http://www.posna.org/education/StudyGuide/spondylolysis.asp
Spondylolisthesis: http://www.posna.org/education/StudyGuide/spondylolisthesis.asp

BIBLIOGRAPHY

1. Abdu WA, Wilber RG, Emery SE. Pedicular transvertebral screw fixation of the lumbosacral spine in spondylolisthesis. Spine 1994,19:710–15.
2. Beutler WJ, Fredrickson BE, Murtland A, et al. The natural history of spondylolysis and spondylolisthesis—45 year follow-up evaluation. Spine 2003;28:1027–35.
3. Boachie-Adjei O,Twee Do, Rawlins B. Partial lumbosacral kyphosis reduction, decompression and posterior lumbosacral transfixation in high grade isthmic spondylolisthesis. Spine 2002;27:E161–E168.
4. Bradford DS, Boachie-Adjei O. Treatment of severe spondylolisthesis by anterior and posterior reduction and stabilization: a long-term follow-up study. J Bone Joint Surg 1990;72A:1060–6.
5. Gaines RW. L5 vertebrectomy for the surgical treatment of spondyloptosis: thirty cases in 25 years. Spine 2005;30:S66–S70.
6. Hammerberg KW. New concepts on the pathogenesis and classification of spondylolisthesis. Spine 2005;30:S4–S11.
7. Hu SS, Tribus CB, Diab M, et al. Spondylolisthesis and spondylolysis. J Bone Joint Surg 2008;90A:656–71.
8. Molinari RM, Bridwell KH, Lenke LH. Complications in the surgical treatment of pediatric high-grade dysplastic spondylolisthesis. Spine 1999;24:1701–11.
9. Ruf M, Koch H, Melcher RP, et al. Anatomic reduction and monosegmental fusion in high-grade developmental spondylolisthesis. Spine 2006;31:269–74.
10. Sasso RC, Shively KD, Reilly TM. Transvertebral transsacral strut grafting for high-grade isthmic spondylolisthesis L5-S1 with fibular allograft. J Spinal Disord 2008;21:328–33.
11. Ulibarri J, Anderson PA, Escarcega T, et al. Biomechanical and clinical evaluation of a novel technique for surgical repair of spondylolysis in adolescents. Spine 2006;31:2067–72.

39 | CHAPTER

IDIOPATHIC SCOLIOSIS

Vincent J. Devlin, MD

1. What is idiopathic scoliosis?

Idiopathic scoliosis is the most common type of scoliosis. At present it is uncertain whether this deformity represents a single disease entity or reflects a similar clinical expression of several different disease states. Idiopathic scoliosis is defined as a spinal deformity characterized by lateral bending and fixed rotation of the spine in the absence of any known cause. The criterion for diagnosis of scoliosis is a coronal plane spinal curvature of 10° or more as measured by the Cobb method. Curves less than 10° are referred to as *spinal asymmetry.* Idiopathic scoliosis is classified according to age at onset into *infantile* (birth–3 years), *juvenile* (3–10 years), and *adolescent* (after 10 years) subtypes. An alternative classification distinguishes *early-onset scoliosis* (0–5 years) from *late-onset scoliosis* (after 5 years) due to increased cardiopulmonary risk associated with early-onset scoliosis. In general, the younger the age at diagnosis, the more likely the deformity will progress and require treatment.

2. What causes idiopathic scoliosis?

The cause of idiopathic scoliosis is the focus of ongoing research. A significant problem associated with this research is the challenge in distinguishing whether observed changes are secondary to spinal deformity or whether they are the cause of the deformity. Areas under investigation include:

- Genetic factors: A genetic basis has been confirmed and genetic testing for adolescent idiopathic scoliosis is currently available. Clinicians have long been aware of the higher incidence of idiopathic scoliosis within families compared with the general population
- Central nervous system (CNS) factors: CNS asymmetry, vestibular dysfunction
- Collagen, muscle, and platelet defects
- Growth and hormonal factors: Asymmetric spinal growth patterns, melatonin
- Biomechanical factors

3. List characteristic features of infantile idiopathic scoliosis.

- Common in Europe but rare in the United States (<1% of cases in United States)
- Male predominance (vs. adolescent idiopathic scoliosis, which is more common in females)
- Left thoracic curve pattern is most common (vs. adolescent idiopathic scoliosis, in which right-sided thoracic curves are typical)
- Association with plagiocephaly, developmental delay, congenital heart disease, and developmental hip dysplasia
- Two types have been identified: a resolving type (85%) and a progressive type (15%)

4. How are resolving and progressive infantile curve types distinguished?

Resolving and progressive curve types are distinguished by analyzing the relationship between the apical vertebra of the thoracic curve and its ribs on an anteroposterior (AP) radiograph in order to determine the **rib-vertebral angle difference (RVAD)** and **rib phase.** The *rib vertebral angle* is determined by a line perpendicular to the endplate of the apical vertebra and a line drawn along the center of the rib (Fig. 39-1A). The rib vertebral angle difference is calculated by subtracting the angle of the convex side from the concave side. An RVAD greater than 20° indicates that curve progression is likely. *Rib phase* is assessed by determining the amount of overlap between the convex rib head and the apical vertebral body. If the convex rib does not overlap the vertebral body (phase 1), progression is unlikely (Fig. 39-1B). As the curve increases, the apical convex rib overlaps the vertebral body (phase 2) and further curve progression is likely (Fig. 39-1C).

5. How is infantile idiopathic scoliosis treated?

Resolving curves are observed with serial physical examinations and radiographic monitoring. Sleeping in the prone position is recommended because supine positioning has been associated with infantile curves by some investigators. **Progressive curves** are treated with serial casting followed by orthotic treatment with a Milwaukee brace. Curves that continue to progress despite orthotic treatment require surgery. Options include posterior spinal instrumentation without fusion or the vertically expandable prosthetic titanium rib (VEPTR). These are growth-preserving procedures that permit delay of definitive fusion until the child has achieved additional growth. Posterior spinal instrumentation and fusion are not recommended due to: 1) restriction of thoracic cage and lung development, and 2) the risk of crankshaft phenomenon (persistent anterior spinal growth in the presence of a posterior fusion, leading to recurrent and increasing spinal deformity). In extreme cases, a combined anterior and posterior fusion procedure is an option but will limit development of the thorax, lungs, and normal trunk height.

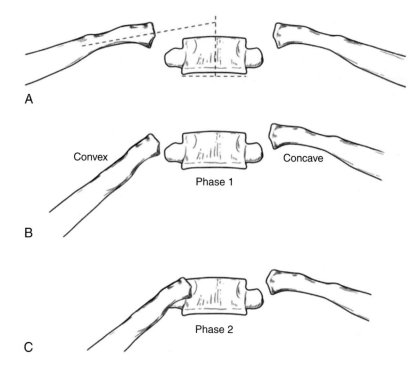

A

Convex

Concave

Phase 1

B

Phase 2

C

Figure 39-1. The rib-vertebral angle difference (RVAD) and rib phase. **A,** The rib vertebral angle is determined by a line perpendicular to the endplate of the apical vertebra and a line drawn along the center of the rib. **B,** Phase 1, the convex rib does not overlap the vertebral body. **C**, Phase 2, the convex rib overlaps the vertebral body. (From Errico TJ, Lonner BS, Moulton AW. Surgical Management of Spinal Deformities. Philadelphia: Saunders; 2009. p. 90.)

6. **What are the characteristic features of juvenile idiopathic scoliosis?**
   Juvenile idiopathic scoliosis represents a gradual transition from the characteristics of infantile idiopathic scoliosis to those of adolescent idiopathic scoliosis. Characteristic features include:
   * Less common than adolescent idiopathic scoliosis (12%–16% of all patients with idiopathic scoliosis)
   * Increasing female predominance is noted with increasing age (female-to-male ratio is 1:1 from 4–6 years and increases to 8–10:1 from 6–10 years)
   * Most common curve patterns are right thoracic and double major curve types
   * Approximately 70% of curves progress and require some forms of treatment (bracing or surgery)
   * Magnetic resonance imaging (MRI) of the entire spine to visualize from the craniocervical junction to the sacrum is appropriate (also in infantile idiopathic scoliosis) because spinal deformity may be the only clue to the presence of a coexistent neural axis abnormality potentially requiring treatment (e.g. syrinx, Arnold-Chiari malformation, tethered spinal cord)

7. **How is juvenile idiopathic scoliosis treated?**
   Orthotic treatment is initiated for curves in the 25° to 50° range. Surgical treatment is considered when curve magnitude exceeds 50° to 60°. Surgical decision making is complex in view of the wide age range of patients presenting in this group. Major concerns include the effect of treatment on remaining growth and potential for development of crankshaft if a single-stage posterior fusion procedure is performed. Dual growing rod instrumentation is considered for early juvenile scoliosis patients. Combined anterior and posterior fusion with posterior instrumentation is an option for older patients. More recently, single-stage posterior spinal instrumentation and fusion using segmental pedicle fixation has been reported as an effective alternative for select juvenile patients. In larger patients with single curves, single-stage anterior instrumentation and fusion are options. Innovative growth modulation techniques such as convex disc stapling and anterior tethering procedures are under investigation and may offer an option for fusionless correction of scoliosis in the future.

8. **List characteristic features of adolescent idiopathic scoliosis.**
   * The most common type of scoliosis in children (prevalence is 3% in the general population)
   * Few adolescent patients (0.3%) develop curves requiring treatment
   * A female predominance is noted, which increases substantially for larger curves requiring treatment
   * Thoracic curve patterns are generally convex to the right (atypical curve patterns are an indication for MRI)
   * Idiopathic scoliosis in adolescence is not typically associated with severe pain

9. **Describe the initial evaluation for a patient referred for assessment for adolescent idiopathic scoliosis.**
   Patient history: Includes menstrual history, birth and developmental history, and inquiry regarding family history of scoliosis
   PHYSICAL EXAMINATION
   * Height and weight assessment
   * Observation (look for shoulder, thorax, or waist asymmetry)

- Adams forward bend test. The right and left sides of the trunk should be symmetrical. Presence of a thoracic or lumbar prominence suggests scoliosis. Use a scoliometer to quantitate asymmetry
- Neurologic assessment. Includes motor strength testing, deep tendon reflexes, abdominal reflexes (abnormalities may indicate intraspinal pathology such as syringomyelia), plantar reflexes, clonus testing
- Upper and lower extremity assessment. Include gait and leg length evaluation

RADIOGRAPHIC ASSESSMENT

- A standing posteroanterior (PA) long cassette radiograph is the initial view obtained
- Lateral radiographs are indicated when sagittal plane abnormalities are noted on physical examinations, for patients with back pain, when spondylolisthesis is suspected, and for presurgical planning prior to scoliosis correction
- Side-bending radiographs are indicated for defining curve type for presurgical planning prior to scoliosis surgery but are not required for a routine initial patient evaluation

10. **What radiographic parameters should be assessed on the PA radiograph?**
   Identify the end vertebra, apical vertebra, curve location, curve direction, curve magnitude, and Risser sign.
   - **End vertebra.** The top and bottom vertebra that tilt maximally into the concavity of the curve are termed the end vertebra. They are typically the least rotated and least horizontally displaced vertebra within the curve
   - **Apical vertebra.** The apical vertebra is the central vertebra within a curve. It is typically the least tilted, most rotated, and most horizontally displaced vertebra within a curve
   - **Curve location.** The curve location is defined by its apex

Curve	Apex
Cervicothoracic	C7 or T1
Thoracic	Between T2 and T11–T12 disc
Thoracolumbar	T12 or L1
Lumbar	Between L1–L2 disc and L4
Lumbosacral	L5 or S1

   - **Curve direction.** Curve direction is determined by the side of the convexity. Curves convex toward the right are termed right curves, while curves convex to the left are termed left curves
   - **Curve magnitude.** The Cobb-Lippman technique is used to determine curve magnitude. Perpendicular lines are drawn in relation to reference lines along the superior endplate of the upper end vertebra and along the inferior endplate of the lower end vertebra. The angle created by the intersection of the two perpendicular lines is termed the Cobb angle and defines the magnitude of the curve (also see Chapter 10, Fig. 10-12)
   - **Risser sign.** The Risser sign describes the ossification of the iliac apophysis. The iliac crest is divided into quarters, and the stage of ossification is used as a guideline to assess skeletal maturity: grade 0: absent, grade 1 (0–25%), grade 2 (26%–50%), grade 3 (51%–75%), grade 4 (76%–100%), grade 5 (fusion of apophysis to the ilium). Risser stage 4 correlates with the end of spinal growth in females, and Risser stage 5 correlates with the end of spinal growth in males (Fig. 39-2)

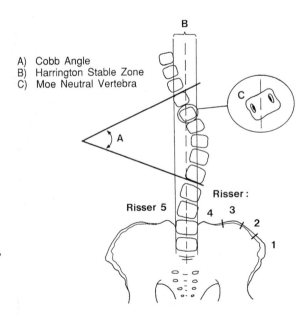

A) Cobb Angle
B) Harrington Stable Zone
C) Moe Neutral Vertebra

Figure 39-2. Measurement for idiopathic scoliosis. **A,** Note the Cobb angle. **B,** Harrington's stable zone. **C,** Moe's neutral vertebra, Risser staging, and the center sacral line (dashed line). (From Stefko RM, Erickson MA. Pediatric orthopaedics. In: Miller MD, editor. Review of Orthopaedics. 3rd ed. Philadelphia: Saunders; 2000.)

11. Define nonstructural curve, structural curve, major curve, minor curve, full curve, and fractional curve.

Patients typically present with a combination of fixed and flexible spinal deformities. Side-bending radiographs are used to assess the flexibility of curves that comprise a spinal deformity.

- Curves that correct completely when the patient bends toward the convexity of the curve are termed **nonstructural curves.** Nonstructural curves permit the shoulders and pelvis to remain level to the ground and permit the head to remain centered in the midline above the pelvis. For this reason, nonstructural curves are also referred to as compensatory curves. Over time, compensatory curves may develop structural characteristics
- Curves that do not correct completely are termed **structural curves**
- The **major curve** is the curve with the largest Cobb measurement and is always a structural curve
- All other curves are termed **minor curves** and may be either structural or nonstructural, depending on classification criteria
- Curves in which both end vertebrae are tilted from the horizontal are termed **full curves**. Full curves and fractional curves are distinguished by assessing the angular displacement of the end vertebra of the curve
- Curves that have one end vertebra parallel to the ground are termed **fractional curves**

12. What are the neutral and stable vertebrae?

- The **neutral vertebra** is the first nonrotated vertebra at the caudal and cranial end of a curve. Rotation is assessed based on the radiographic appearance of the vertebral pedicle shadow in reference to the lateral margins of the vertebral body (Nash-Moe classification). In a neutrally rotated vertebra the pedicle shadows will be equidistant from the lateral vertebral margins
- The **stable vertebra** is the vertebra bisected by the center sacral line (a vertical line extending cephalad from the center of the sacrum and through the S1 spinous process)

13. What is the King-Moe classification?

The **King-Moe classification** (Fig. 39-3) of thoracic curve patterns in idiopathic scoliosis distinguishes five curve types as a guide to surgical treatment:

- **Type 1:** S-shaped curve in which both the thoracic and lumbar curves cross the midline. Both curves are structural, and the lumbar curve may be larger or less flexible than the thoracic curve
- **Type 2:** S-shaped curve in which the thoracic curve is larger or less flexible than the lumbar curve (also called a "false" double major curve)
- **Type 3:** Single thoracic curve without a structural lumbar curve
- **Type 4:** Long thoracic curve in which L5 is centered over the sacrum and L4 is tilted into the thoracic curve
- **Type 5:** Double thoracic curve with T1 tilted into the convexity of the upper curve

The King classification does not address lumbar curves, thoracolumbar curves, or triple major curves. It does not evaluate sagittal plane alignment. It was developed to guide surgical treatment in the era of Harrington instrumentation.

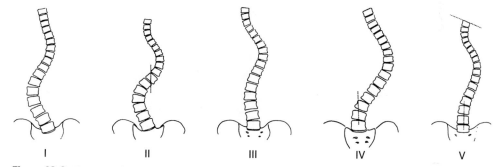

Figure 39-3. Five types of idiopathic scoliosis as defined by King, Moe, Bradford, and Winter. (From Roach JW. Adolescent idiopathic scoliosis. Orthop Clin North Am 1999;30:353–65.)

14. What is the comprehensive classification system for idiopathic scoliosis described by Lenke and colleagues?

As decision making for scoliosis surgery has become increasingly complex, a more comprehensive classification system has been developed. The **Lenke classification** is based on assessment of PA, lateral, and side-bending radiographs. Six curve types are identified:

- Primary thoracic
- Double thoracic
- Double major
- Triple major
- Primary thoracolumbar or lumbar
- Primary thoracolumbar or lumbar with a secondary thoracic curve

The **basic steps** in curve classification include:

- **Determine curve type:** Measure all curves. Identify the major curve. Determine whether the minor curves are structural or nonstructural (see Fig. 39-4)
- **Determine the lumbar spine modifier:** The six main curve types are subclassified as A, B, or C on relationship of the center sacral vertical line (CSVL) to the lumbar spine
- **Determine the thoracic sagittal modifier:** "-", "N", or "+" is determined on, the T5 to T12 sagittal Cobb angle

This **triad** of radiographic information (curve type + lumbar modifier + sagittal modifier) is required to determine the *curve classification* (e.g. 1B+).

Curve Type

Type	Proximal Thoracic	Main Thoracic	Thoracolumbar/ Lumbar	Curve Type
1	Non-Structural	Structural (major*)	Non-Structural	Main Thoracic (MT)
2	Structural	Structural (major*)	Non-Structural	Double Thoracic (DT)
3	Non-Structural	Structural (major*)	Structural	Double Major (DM)
4	Structural	Structural (major*)	Structural	Triple Major (TM)
5	Non-Structural	Non-Structural	Structural (major*)	Thoracolumbar/Lumbar (TL/L)
6	Non-Structural	Structural	Structural (major*)	Thoracolumbar/Lumbar-Main Thoracic (TL/L - MT) Lumbar Curve>Thoracic by ≥5°

STRUCTURAL CRITERIA
(Minor Curves)

Proximal Thoracic: - Side Bending Cobb ≥ 25°
- T2 - T5 Kyphosis ≥+20°

Main Thoracic: - Side Bending Cobb ≥ 25°
- T10 - L2 Kyphosis ≥20°

Thoracolumbar/Lumbar: - Side Bending Cobb ≥ 25°
- T10 - L2 Kyphosis ≥+20°

*Major = Largest Cobb Measurement, always structural
Minor = All other curves with structural criteria applied

LOCATION OF APEX
(SRS definition)

CURVE	APEX
THORACIC	T2 - T11-12 DISC
THORACOLUMBAR	T12 - L1
LUMBAR	L1-2 DISC - L4

Modifiers

Lumbar Spine Modifier	CSVL to Lumbar Apex
A	CSVL Between Pedicles
B	CSVL Touches Apical Body(ies)
C	CSVL Completely Medial

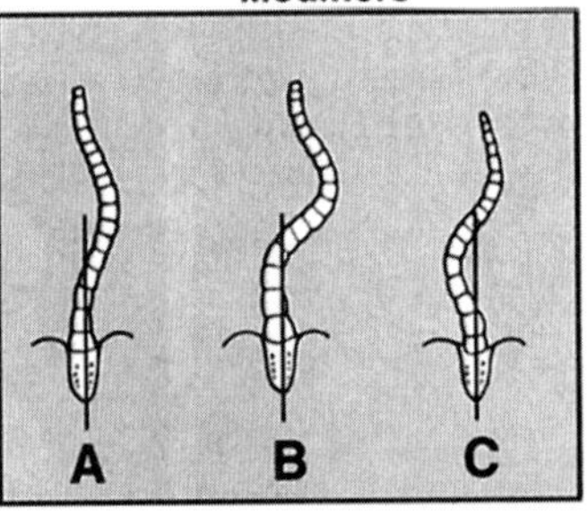

	Thoracic Sagittal Profile T5 - T12	
-	(Hypo)	< 10°
N	(Normal)	10° - 40°
+	(Hyper)	> 40°

Curve Types (1- 6) + Lumbar Spine Modifier (A, B, or C) + Thoracic Sagittal Modifier (-, N, or +)

Classification (e.g. 1B+):_____

Figure 39-4. Lenke's system of classification for idiopathic scoliosis. (From Hurley ME, Devlin VJ. Idiopathic scoliosis. In: Fitzgerald RH, Kaufer H, Malkani AL, editors. Orthopaedics. St. Louis: Mosby; 2000.)

15. What are the treatment options for adolescent idiopathic scoliosis?

The treatment options for adolescent idiopathic scoliosis include observation, orthoses, and operation (*the three O's*). There is no evidence that exercise programs, electrical stimulation, special diets, chiropractic adjustment, acupuncture, or other nontraditional treatment methods are effective in preventing curve progression or correcting established curves.

16. What is the purpose of observation for adolescent idiopathic scoliosis?

The purpose of observation for adolescent idiopathic scoliosis is to identify and document curve progression and thereby facilitate timely intervention. Curves less than 20° are observed.

17. What are the risk factors for curve progression in skeletally immature patients with idiopathic scoliosis?

- Future growth potential of the patient (assessed by a variety of factors, including age at presentation, Risser stage, Tanner stage, menarche, peak height velocity, triradiate physeal closure, skeletal age as determined by hand radiographs)
- Curve magnitude at the time of diagnosis

- Curve pattern (double curves progress more frequently than single curves)
- Female sex (curves in females are more likely to progress than curves in males)
- Genetic risk score (ScoliScore Prognostic Test, Axial Biotech)

18. What patients with adolescent idiopathic scoliosis are likely to experience progression of untreated curves in adulthood?
Curves measuring less than 30° at maturity are least likely to progress. Curves measuring 30° to 50° degrees are likely to progress an average of 10° to 15° over the course of a normal lifetime. Curves measuring 50° to 75° at maturity progress steadily at a rate of approximately 1° per year. Lumbar and thoracolumbar curves are more likely to progress than thoracic curves because they lack the inherent stability provided by the rib cage.

19. What are the consequences of untreated adolescent idiopathic scoliosis?
Natural history studies of untreated adolescent idiopathic scoliosis in adult patients focus on:
- **Mortality rate.** The mortality rate of untreated adult patients with adolescent idiopathic scoliosis is comparable with that of the general population. Patients with untreated adolescent idiopathic scoliosis do not typically develop respiratory failure and premature death. Patients with adolescent idiopathic scoliosis must be distinguished from patients with early-onset scoliosis (before age 5) who develop severe curves (>90°). Patients with early-onset scoliosis may develop cor pulmonale and right ventricular failure, resulting in premature death
- **Pulmonary and cardiac function.** Marked limitation of forced vital capacity does not occur until thoracic curves approach 90° in the absence of marked hypokyphosis. Only in thoracic curve patterns is there a direct correlation between curve magnitude and negative effects on pulmonary function
- **Back pain.** The incidence of back pain in adult scoliosis patients is comparable with the general population. Patients with large lumbar curves report an increased incidence of low back pain, particularly if a significant lateral translation develops
- **Self-image.** Spinal deformity and its negative effect on self-image remain a significant issue for many adult scoliosis patients. These issues are frequently the reason adult patients seek treatment for idiopathic scoliosis

20. When is bracing indicated for adolescent idiopathic scoliosis?
Patients who are Risser stage 0 to 1 and premenarchal with curves 20° to 29° are candidates for immediate bracing. In the Risser stage 2 patient with a curve of 20° to 29°, progression of 5° should be documented before bracing is initiated. Patients presenting with curves of 30° to 40° should be braced immediately if they are skeletally immature. Patients and families should be advised that a spinal orthosis is used to prevent curve progression and generally does not lead to permanent curve improvement. The best predictor of successful brace treatment is the initial correction achieved in the brace. If a curve is corrected by 50% or more upon initiation of bracing, there is a good chance brace treatment will be successful.

21. When is brace treatment contraindicated?
Contraindications to brace treatment include:
- Skeletally mature patients
- Curves greater than 40°
- Thoracic lordosis (bracing potentiates cardiopulmonary restriction)
- Patients unable to cope emotionally with treatment

22. What types of braces are used?
The general types of orthoses used for adolescent idiopathic scoliosis are:
- CTLSO (Milwaukee brace). Used less commonly due to its cosmetic appearance. However, for curves with an apex above T8, it remains most efficacious
- TLSO (e.g. Boston brace). These lower-profile orthoses are better accepted by patients and are indicated for curves with an apex at T8 or below
- Bending brace (e.g. Charleston brace). This type of brace holds the patient is an acutely bent position in a direction opposite to the curve apex. It is worn only during sleep. It has been advocated as an alternative to full-time bracing regimens
- Flexible brace (e.g. SpineCor brace)

23. When is surgery indicated for adolescent idiopathic scoliosis?
It is not possible to indicate patients for surgery based solely on the coronal Cobb angle. Additional factors to consider in decision making include sagittal plane alignment, rotational deformity, the natural history of the patient's curve, and the patient's skeletal maturity. In general, for the immature adolescent patient, surgery is indicated for curves greater than 40° that are progressive despite brace treatment. In the mature adolescent, surgery is considered for curves greater than 50°.

24. What treatment options exist when surgery is indicated?
- Posterior spinal instrumentation and posterior fusion
- Anterior spinal instrumentation and anterior fusion
- Anterior spinal fusion combined with posterior spinal instrumentation and fusion

25. Explain what is involved in a posterior spinal instrumentation and fusion procedure for adolescent idiopathic scoliosis.

The posterior surgical approach is applicable to all idiopathic scoliosis curve types. During the surgical procedure the posterior spinal structures are exposed, the facet joints are excised, and graft material is packed into the facet joints and over the decorticated posterior spinal elements. Posterior spinal instrumentation is placed and utilized to realign and stabilize the spinal deformity. A typical instrumentation construct consists of two parallel rods attached to the spine at multiple sites (posterior segmental spinal instrumentation). The rods are connected at their cephalad and caudad ends by cross-link devices, thereby creating a rigid rectangular construct. Contemporary spinal instrumentation constructs for scoliosis may be classified into two main types:

- Hybrid constructs. In a hybrid construct, the spinal implants used to achieve fixation to the posterior spinal elements include a combination of hooks, wires (cables), and/or pedicular screws (Fig. 39-5)
- Pedicle screw constructs. Pedicle screw constructs utilize screw fixation over multiple levels as the primary means of deformity correction (Fig. 39-6)

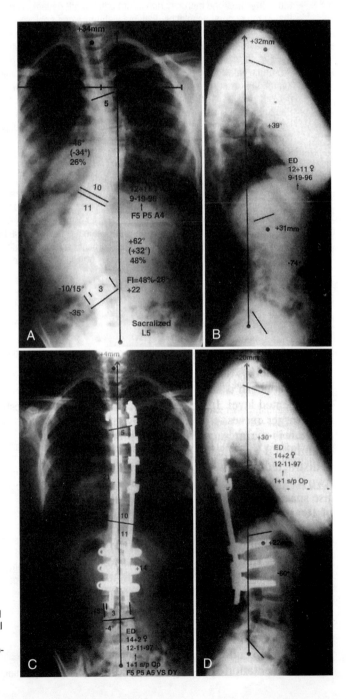

Figure 39-5. Posterior spinal instrumentation and fusion. **A,** Preoperative posteroanterior (PA) radiograph. **B,** Lateral radiographs of a 13-year-old girl. The curve may be classified as a Lenke 6CN or a King-Moe type 1 curve. **C** and **D,** Postoperative radiographs show a typical hybrid posterior segmental spinal instrumentation construct. (From Asher MA. Anterior surgery for thoraco-lumbar and lumbar idiopathic scoliosis. Spine State Art Rev 1998;12:708–9.)

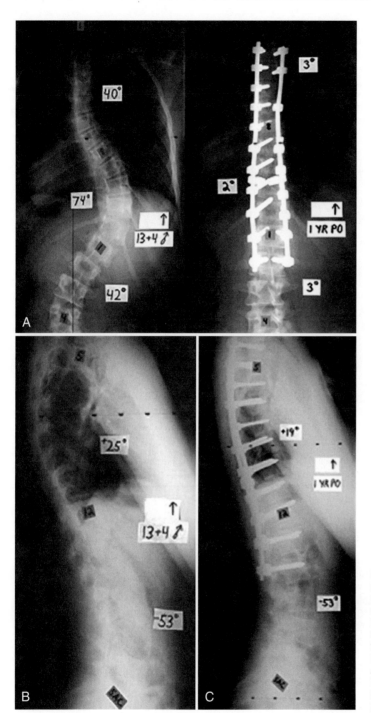

Figure 39-6. Posterior spinal instrumentation and fusion. Preoperative and postoperative radiographs of a 13-year-old girl treated with posterior spinal instrumentation and fusion utilizing an all-pedicle screw instrumentation construct. The curve may be classified as a Lenke 1AN or a King-Moe type 4 curve. **A,** Posteroanterior (PA) radiographs. **B,** Lateral radiographs. (From Silva FE, Lenke LG. Adolescent idiopathic scoliosis. In: Errico TJ, Lonner BS, Moulton AW, editors. Surgical Management of Spinal Deformities. Philadelphia: Saunders; 2009. p. 107.)

26. **Explain what is involved in an anterior spinal instrumentation and fusion procedure for adolescent idiopathic scoliosis.**

    Anterior spinal instrumentation and fusion procedures (Fig. 39-7) are most commonly indicated for single thoracic, thoracolumbar, or lumbar curve types. The convex side of the curve is exposed. The thoracic spine is approached via an open thoracotomy or minimally invasive thoracoscopic approach. The disc, annulus, and cartilaginous vertebral endplates are excised over the levels undergoing fusion. The disc spaces are packed with nonstructural bone graft. Structural spacers are placed in the disc spaces in the lumbar region. This structural spacer may be an allograft cortical ring (femur or humerus) or a synthetic fusion cage. Vertebral body screws are placed to engage the opposite vertebral cortex and achieve bicortical fixation. The screws are subsequently linked to rod(s), and corrective forces are applied to the spine. Single- or double-rod systems may be used, depending on a variety of factors such as patient body habitus, curve location, and patient willingness to wear a postoperative orthosis. Minimally invasive approaches utilizing thoracoscopic instrumentation and fusion have been documented to decrease approach-related morbidity in select cases.

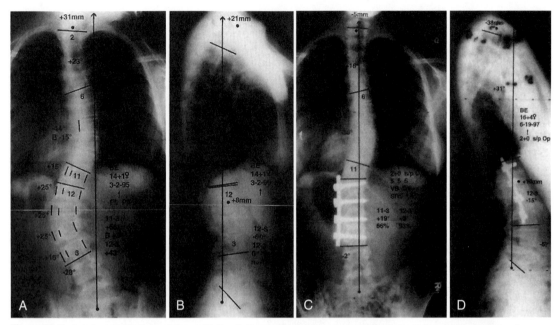

Figure 39-7. Anterior spinal instrumentation and fusion. **A,** Preoperative posteroanterior (PA) radiograph. **B,** Lateral radiographs of a 14-year-old girl with left thoracolumbar major and right thoracolumbar compensatory scoliosis. **C** and **D,** Postoperative radiographs show correction following anterior spinal instrumentation and fusion. (From Asher MA. Anterior surgery for thoracolumbar and lumbar idiopathic scoliosis. Spine State Art Rev 1998;12:706–7.)

27. When are combined anterior and posterior spinal procedures indicated for adolescent idiopathic scoliosis?

Combined anterior and posterior spinal procedures for adolescent idiopathic scoliosis are rarely required for uncomplicated adolescent idiopathic scoliosis. With the use of modern segmental instrumentation including all pedicle screw constructs in combination with Smith-Petersen osteotomies, Ponte osteotomies or a posterior vertebral column resection procedure, most severe curves can be treated with a single-stage posterior approach. Circumstances where combined anterior and posterior procedures are occasionally considered include:

- Extremely large stiff curves (e.g. >100° depending on curve flexibility and location)
- To address coexistent rigid sagittal plane deformities (e.g. excessive thoracic lordosis, hyperkyphosis)
- To prevent the crankshaft phenomenon in the situation of a patient younger than age 10 who has open triradiate cartilages, especially if surgery is performed prior to peak height velocity
- Revision procedures following unsuccessful prior scoliosis surgery

28. What is a thoracoplasty?

Thoracoplasty is a procedure performed during a spinal instrumentation and fusion operation for scoliosis to decrease the magnitude of the convex thoracic rib prominence. The medial portions of the convex ribs are excised in order to restore symmetry to the posterior thoracic cage. The procedure may be performed from either an anterior or posterior surgical approach. The excised rib segments provide an excellent source of bone graft for arthrodesis.

29. What potential complications are associated with scoliosis surgery?

The risks of perioperative complications have diminished with modern techniques of anesthesia, intraoperative neurophysiologic monitoring, improved spinal instrumentation systems, and enhanced postoperative intensive care and pain management. However, patients must be informed of the most common complications, including but not exclusively limited to hemorrhage, infection, pseudarthrosis, implant misplacement or construct failure, trunk imbalance, neurologic injury, and the possible need for future surgery to treat these problems.

Key Points

1. Idiopathic scoliosis is classified according to age at onset into *infantile* (birth–3 years), *juvenile* (3–10 years), and *adolescent* (after 10 years) subtypes.
2. Idiopathic scoliosis is a diagnosis of exclusion and requires thorough evaluation to rule out an underlying congenital, neurologic, or syndromic etiology.
3. The management options for patients diagnosed with idiopathic scoliosis include observation, orthoses, and operative treatment.

Websites

Spinal deformity: http://www.boneandjointburden.org/pdfs/BMUS_chpt3_spinal%20deformity.pdf
Idiopathic scoliosis: http://www.posna.org/education/StudyGuide/idiopathicScoliosisGreaterThan40.asp
Adolescent idiopathic scoliosis: http://www.srs.org/professionals/education/adolescent/idiopathic/
Genetic test for scoliosis: http://www.scoliscore.com/

BIBLIOGRAPHY

1. Asher MA, Burton DC. A concept of idiopathic scoliosis deformities as imperfect torsion(s). Clin Orthop Rel Res 1999;364:11–25.
2. Collis DK, Ponsetti IV. Long-term follow-up of patients with idiopathic scoliosis not treated surgically. J Bone Joint Surg 1969;51:425–45.
3. King HA, Moe JH, Bradford DS, et al. The selection of fusion levels in thoracic idiopathic scoliosis. J Bone Joint Surg 1983;65A:1302–13.
4. Lenke LG, Betz RR, Harms J, et al. Adolescent idiopathic scoliosis—a new classification to determine extent of spinal arthrodesis. J Bone Joint Surg 2001;83A:1169–81.
5. Lenke LG, Dobbs MB. Management of juvenile idiopathic scoliosis. J Bone Joint Surg 2007;89A:S55–S63.
6. Lenke LG, Kuklo TR, Ondra S, et al. Rationale behind the current state of the art treatment of scoliosis in the pedicle screw era. Spine 2008;33:1051–4.
7. Lonstein JE, Carlson JM. The prediction of curve progression in untreated idiopathic scoliosis during growth. J Bone Joint Surg 1984;66A:1061–71.
8. Sanders JO. Maturity indicators in spinal deformity. J Bone Joint Surg 2007;89A:S14–S20.
9. Suk SI, Lee SM, Chung ER, et al. Selective thoracic fusion with segmental pedicle screw fixation in the treatment of thoracic idiopathic scoliosis: more than 5-year follow-up. Spine 2005;30:1602–9.
10. Sponseller PD, Betz R, Newton PO, et al. Differences in curve behavior after fusion in adolescent idiopathic scoliosis patients with open triradiate cartilages. Spine 2009;34:827–31.

SAGITTAL PLANE DEFORMITIES IN PEDIATRIC PATIENTS

Munish C. Gupta, MD, and Vincent J. Devlin, MD

1. What are the common types of pediatric sagittal plane deformities?

Common types of pediatric sagittal plane deformities include Scheuermann's kyphosis, postural round back, and congenital kyphosis and lordosis. Additional etiologies responsible for sagittal plane deformities include myelomeningocele, idiopathic scoliosis, achondroplasia, postlaminectomy kyphosis, postirradiation kyphosis, tuberculosis, trauma, and spondylolisthesis.

2. What are Cobb angles? How are they measured?

Cobb angles are used to define the magnitude of curves on posteroanterior (PA) and lateral radiographs of the spine. Vertebral bodies at the top and bottom of the curve are called the **end vertebrae.** Cobb angles are measured from the top of the upper end vertebra to the bottom of the lower end vertebra. Curve progression is evaluated by measuring the same end vertebra on serial radiographs. Thoracic kyphosis is measured from T2 to T12 and lumbar lordosis from L1 to S1. There is approximately 6° of error in the Cobb angle measurement.

3. What is the normal sagittal plane alignment of the cervical, thoracic, and lumbar spine?

Normal thoracic kyphosis is between 20° and 40°. The thoracolumbar junction (T10–L2) has neutral sagittal plane alignment, and any degree of kyphosis in this region is considered abnormal. Normal lumbar lordosis is between 55° and 65°, with most of the curvature occurring between the fourth lumbar vertebra and the sacrum. Cervical lordosis is variable and adjusts to maintain the head over the sacrum in the sagittal plane. Thoracic kyphosis increases with age while lumbar lordosis decreases with aging. In the normal state, a line from the center of the C7 vertebral body passes anterior to the thoracic spine, through the center of the L1 vertebral body, posterior to the lumbar spine, through the lumbosacral disc, and between S2 and the femoral heads.

4. What is the differential diagnosis in evaluating an adolescent with excessive thoracic kyphosis with or without pain?

Scheuermann's kyphosis, postural round back, fractures of the thoracic spine, infection with vertebral body collapse, congenital kyphosis, and tumor.

5. What are the subtypes of Scheuermann's kyphosis?

- **Type I** Scheuermann's kyphosis is a rigid, angular thoracic kyphosis and has a hereditary component
- **Type II** is located in the thoracolumbar region, is more painful, and affects predominantly athletes and laborers.
  Endplate anomalies and loss of disc space height are common to both types I and II
    See Figure 40-1.

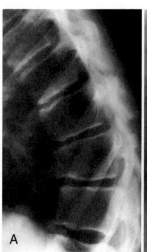 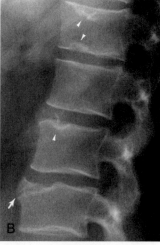

Figure 40-1. Scheuermann's disease. **A,** Thoracic spine lateral radiograph. Findings include irregularity in vertebral contour, reactive sclerosis, intervertebral disc space narrowing, anterior vertebral wedging, and kyphosis. **B,** Lumbar spine lateral radiograph. Observe the cartilaginous nodes *(arrowheads)* creating surface irregularity, lucent areas, and reactive sclerosis. Anterior disc displacement *(arrow)* has produced an irregular anterosuperior corner of a vertebral body, which is termed a *limbus vertebra.* (From Resnick D, Kransdorf MJ. Bone and Joint Imaging. 3rd ed. Philadelphia: Saunders; 2005.)

6. **Describe the typical presentation of a patient with thoracic Scheuermann's kyphosis.**

A male or female approaching the end of skeletal growth (12–15 years old) presents with complaints of thoracic deformity and/or back pain. The patient has an increased thoracic kyphosis, which is accentuated with forward-bending. Patients are not able to correct the kyphotic deformity by active extension. Thirty percent of patients have mild scoliosis in addition to increased kyphosis. A compensatory increase in cervical lordosis causes the head to translate forward. Patients often have tight hamstrings.

7. **How does the presentation of postural (asthenic) kyphosis differ from Scheuermann's kyphosis?**

The kyphosis associated with postural round back is less severe ($< 60°$). The patient is able to actively correct the thoracic kyphosis and may appear more athletically active. Parents may also have some round-back deformity. Focal wedging and endplate changes are absent on the lateral radiograph.

8. **Are symptoms of neural compression common in patients with Scheuermann's kyphosis?**

Myelopathy and radiculopathy are uncommon in pediatric patients and more likely in adult patients. The spinal cord drapes over the focal kyphosis and is predisposed to pressure from a subsequent fracture or disc herniation. Nevertheless, in symptomatic pediatric patients and prior to surgical intervention, it is important to obtain a magnetic resonance imaging (MRI) of the spine to evaluate for potential neural compression.

9. **What is the incidence of Scheuermann's disease?**

Reports range from less than 1% to $> 8\%$ of the general population. Studies also differ on male and female predominance; near-equal male and female ratios have been reported.

10. **Describe the standard radiographic evaluation of a patient with suspected Scheuermann's disease.**

Standing long cassette **posteroanterior (PA)** and **lateral views** of the spine are examined for excessive thoracic kyphosis, vertebral wedging, endplate changes, narrowing of the disc spaces, and scoliosis. The PA view should include the iliac apophyses and triradiate cartilages for evaluation of skeletal maturity. The patient should stand with his or her hips and knees fully extended. The elbows are flexed and the hands supported in the supraclavicular fossa so the arms neither flex nor extend the spine. PA radiographs decrease the radiation exposure to the breasts and heart compared with anteroposterior views. A **hyperextension lateral view** taken with the patient supine over a radiolucent wedge placed just caudal to the apex of the kyphosis is used to assess flexibility of the kyphotic deformity.

11. **What are the accepted radiographic criteria for diagnosis of thoracic Scheuermann's disease?**

The commonly accepted criteria—5° of wedging of three adjacent vertebrae—were popularized by Sorenson. Thoracic kyphosis greater than 50°, vertebral endplate irregularities, Schmorl's nodes, and decreased disc space height are additional radiographic findings that may be present. Scheuermann's kyphosis is structural and does not correct to within normal limits with maximal extension.

12. **How may radiographic findings differ between early and late stages of Scheuermann's disease?**

Early radiographic changes may be limited to irregular vertebral endplates, anterior disc space narrowing, and Schmorl's nodes (protrusion of intervertebral disc material through the vertebral endplate). Because the vertebral ring apophysis does not appear until approximately 10 years of age, the vertebral body appears rounded, and diagnosis of Scheuermann's disease is difficult. In skeletally mature patients, osteophytes, facet hypertrophy, and compression fractures may develop and accentuate the spinal deformity.

13. **What causes Scheuermann's disease?**

The exact cause is unknown. In 1921, Holger Scheuermann associated the disorder with avascular necrosis of the vertebral body ring apophysis. Abnormal growth plate cartilage, mechanical decompensation after endplate disc herniation (Schmorl's nodes), hormonal variation (increased growth hormone), osteoporosis, and malabsorption have been proposed as possible causes. Associations with Legg-Calvé-Perthes disease, hypovitaminosis, dystonia, dural cysts, and endocrine disorders have been described. There appears to be a familial tendency. Evidence suggests that Scheuermann's disease is autosomal dominant with high penetrance and variable expressivity. However, the genetics of this disorder are not well defined.

14. **What histologic findings are reported in patients with Scheuermann's disease?**

Despite the association with avascular necrosis of the ring apophysis, alteration in the growth plate cartilage without osteoporosis or necrosis of the ring apophysis has been observed. Both matrix and cells are altered. Collagen fibers are thinner and sparser. Proteoglycan content is increased.

15. Describe the natural history of Scheuermann's disease.

There is disagreement about both pain and functional limitations. Pain increases with age in some studies and decreases with age in others. Some studies suggest significant functional limitations, whereas others do not. The deformity may have profound psychosocial effects in terms of social stigma and poor self-esteem.

16. What are the indications for orthotic treatment for Scheuermann's kyphosis?

Extension bracing is appropriate for curves between 45° and 74° with 2 years of growth remaining and greater than 5° wedging. An apex at T9 or above is traditionally treated with a Milwaukee type brace. A thoracolumbar orthosis (TLSO) is considered if the apex is below T9. Braces should be updated every 4 to 6 months to maximize deformity correction and weaned with skeletal maturity.

17. Identify the indications for surgery for Scheuermann's kyphosis.

Immature adolescent patients with painful kyphosis greater than 75° with more than 10° of local wedging that is resistant to at least 6 months of bracing may be considered for surgery. Skeletally mature patients with painful deformity unresponsive to nonoperative treatment may also be considered for surgery.

18. What are the indications for single-stage posterior instrumentation and fusion for Scheuermann's kyphosis?

Traditionally, kyphosis correcting to less than 50° on hyperextension lateral radiographs is treated with posterior instrumentation and fusion. The instrumentation should include the entire kyphotic area proximally and extend distally to include one lordotic disc. Pedicle screws in the distal thoracic and lumbar spine provide better anchors and more powerful correction than hook fixation. Dual rods are secured proximally with claw hook configuration or pedicle screws. The deformity is corrected with cantilever bending and compression force securing the rods distally with screws (Fig. 40-2).

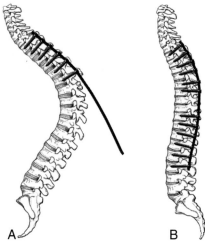

Figure 40-2. Correction of Scheuermann's kyphosis. **A,** Rods are contoured to reflect the degree of kyphosis correction desired and connected to screws in the vertebra above the apex of the deformity. **B,** Rods are cantilevered into screws in the vertebra distal to the deformity apex to achieve correction. (From Errico TJ, Lonner BS, Moulton AW. Surgical Management of Spinal Deformities. Philadelphia: Saunders; 2009.)

19. When is anterior release and fusion prior to posterior spinal instrumentation and fusion indicated in the surgical treatment of Scheuermann's kyphosis?

Kyphotic deformities that do not correct to less than 50° on hyperextension lateral radiographs traditionally have been treated with anterior release and anterior fusion via a transthoracic or thoracoscopic approach prior to performing the posterior fusion and instrumentation. However, over the past decade anterior surgery has been utilized less frequently due to advances in surgical techniques including the popularization of thoracic pedicle screw fixation combined with posterior column shortening osteotomies (Ponte osteotomies). For treatment of kyphotic deformities, multilevel Ponte osteotomies (Fig. 40-3) are performed and involve wide facetectomies, partial laminectomies, and spinous process resection. Closure of the osteotomies by application of compression forces is facilitated by segmental pedicle screw fixation. In appropriate cases, this technique permits correction of severe kyphotic deformities with a single-stage posterior surgical approach and avoids the morbidity associated with a separate anterior surgical procedure.

Figure 40-3. Ponte osteotomies. **A,** Broad posterior resection (shaded parts) at every intersegmental level extending over the entire area of fusion and instrumentation. **B,** Posterior view showing levels of completed resections. Correction is achieved by closing gaps. (From Canale ST, Beaty J. Campbell's operative orthopaedics. 11th ed. Philadelphia: Mosby; 2008. [Redrawn from Ponte A. Posterior column shortening for Scheuermann's kyphosis. An innovative one-stage technique. In: Haher TR, Merola AA: Surgical Techniques for the Spine. New York: Thieme; 2003.])

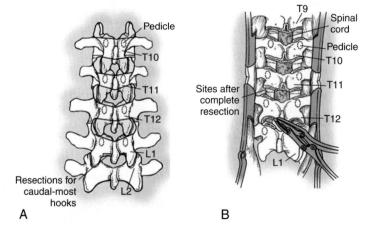

20. Define the surgical goals in terms of curve correction and balance for Scheuermann's kyphosis.

The goal of surgical treatment is restoration of normal and harmonious thoracic kyphosis and lumbar lordosis while relieving pain through successful arthrodesis. Approximately 50% correction is desired. Overcorrection of the deformity can lead to proximal or distal junctional kyphotic deformities, which may require additional surgical procedures for correction. Appropriate selection of fusion levels is critical for achieving long-term correction of sagittal deformity and a successful spinal fusion (Fig. 40-4).

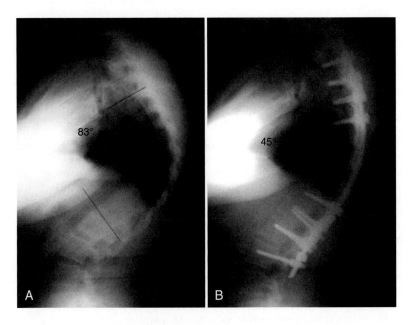

Figure 40-4. **A,** Preoperative standing lateral radiograph of a 16-year-old boy with an 80° thoracic kyphosis due to Scheuermann's disease. **B,** Postoperative standing lateral radiograph. (From Shah SA, Takemitsu M, Westerlund LE, et al. Pediatric kyphosis: Scheuermann's disease and congenital deformity. In: Herkowitz HN, Garfin SR, Eismont FJ, et al, editors. Rothman– Simeone The Spine. 5th ed. Philadelphia: Saunders; 2009. p. 573.)

21. Describe the different types of congenital kyphosis.

Type I is a defect of vertebral body formation (hemivertebra), type II is a defect of vertebral body segmentation (block vertebra or bar), and type III is a mixed or combined lesion. Type 1 defects are more common and more serious because they lead to a sharp angular kyphosis that may cause paraplegia.

22. Does bracing play a role in treatment of congenital kyphosis?

No. Bracing does not prevent deformity progression or provide long-term correction of a congenital kyphotic deformity. Nonsurgical management does not play a role in the treatment of congenital kyphosis.

23. What surgical procedures are indicated for congenital kyphosis?

Congenital kyphosis does not respond to nonoperative treatment. Posterior in situ fusion should be considered for a young child (1–5 years old) with a kyphosis measuring less than 50°. Kyphosis greater than 50° and older children require an anterior and posterior fusion. Symptomatic neural compression at the apex of the kyphosis requires decompression. In select deformities, circumferential decompression and fusion may be achieved through a single-stage posterior surgical approach. Extensive preoperative evaluation is required, including cardiopulmonary assessment, evaluation of the genitourinary system, detailed neurologic examination, MRI of the neural axis, and a computed tomography (CT) scan to define osseous abnormalities.

24. What is the cause of congenital lordosis?

Congenital lordosis is a rare disorder caused by failure of posterior segmentation, typically spanning multiple segments, with persistent anterior growth. Progressive thoracic lordosis causes diminution of the spine-sternal distance and restriction of pulmonary function.

25. Describe treatment options for congenital lordosis.

When congenital lordosis is diagnosed early in life, surgical treatment consists of anterior spinal fusion to eliminate anterior growth potential. Patients presenting later in life require more complex surgery. Moderate deformities may be treated with wide posterior release followed by segmental instrumentation and fusion. Severe deformities require anterior and posterior spinal surgery. Anterior closing wedge osteotomies and posterior segmental spinal fixation are required. Rib resections may be required as well. Preoperative pulmonary function tests are necessary. Associated pulmonary hypertension increases mortality and may be a contraindication to surgery.

26. Is thoracic hypokyphosis commonly present in adolescent idiopathic scoliosis?

Yes. Decreased thoracic kyphosis is ubiquitous among patients with idiopathic scoliosis. Thoracic lordosis is a contraindication to bracing. There is a subgroup of patients with severe hypokyphosis or actual lordosis of the thoracic spine. In patients with progressive thoracic lordosis or lordosis of −10° or more, surgical treatment should be considered, even if the coronal plane Cobb measurement is less than 40°.

27. What are the indications for surgical correction of a gibbus (severe short-segment kyphosis) associated with myelomeningocele?

Inability to maintain an acceptable sitting posture and skin breakdown over the apex of the deformity are reasons to correct the deformity surgically.

28. What is the most common sagittal plane deformity associated with achondroplasia?

Thoracolumbar kyphosis is the most common sagittal plane deformity among achondroplastic dwarfs. The kyphosis is generally evident at birth, progresses as the child begins to sit, and resolves in approximately 70% of cases with ambulation. Radiographs show anterior wedging at the apex of the deformity. Progression can lead to a focal kyphosis and possible neural compression, which may be masked by the lumbar stenosis associated with achondroplasia.

29. What are the nonoperative and surgical options for achondroplastic thoracolumbar kyphosis?

Newborn infants with achondroplasia typically demonstrate a thoracolumbar kyphosis in the range of 20° that resolves in many patients by age 12 to 18 months. Parents are advised regarding measures to prevent deformity progression including avoidance of unsupported sitting. A thoracolumbar orthosis is optional for children 3 years of age and older in whom the kyphosis does not resolve with ambulation. Anterior and posterior fusion is reserved for children with progressive deformity, thoracolumbar kyphosis greater than 50° at age older than 5 years, or neural compromise attributed to compression in the kyphotic region. Spinal instrumentation and arthrodesis with pedicle fixation is indicated. Spinal implants that enter the spinal canal (hooks, wires) are contraindicated due to associated spinal stenosis and lack of space in the spinal canal. Additional spinal problems requiring consideration in achondroplasia include foramen magnum stenosis, lumbar spinal stenosis, and hyperlordosis.

30. What factors contribute to the development of postlaminectomy kyphosis?

In the pediatric population, laminectomies are performed most commonly for treatment of children with tumors and dysraphism. Instability after facetectomy, hypermobility associated with removal of the posterior osteoligamentous structures, and growth disturbance contribute to the development of postlaminectomy kyphosis. Postlaminectomy kyphosis is associated with younger age, multilevel laminectomies, and surgery in the upper thoracic and cervical spine.

31. How can postlaminectomy deformity be avoided or treated?

Maintenance of the facet joints, laminoplasty in lieu of laminectomy, and postoperative bracing may help stabilize the spine following surgery. If wide decompression is required or if progressive spinal deformity develops, posterior fusion and stabilization are required.

32. How is tuberculosis of the spine uniquely associated with thoracolumbar kyphosis in children?

The three patterns of spinal involvement by tuberculosis are central, peridiscal, and anterior. Among the three patterns of tuberculosis involvement, central lesions are most common in children while peridiscal involvement is most common among adults. Central lesions generally involve the whole vertebral body and lead to bony collapse and kyphotic deformity. The thoracolumbar junction is the most common location affected by spinal tuberculosis. When multiple levels are involved, healing can lead to anterior bony bridging and worsening of the kyphotic deformity with growth.

33. What types of fractures lead to posttraumatic kyphosis in children?

Flexion-compression, burst, and flexion-distraction (seat-belt) type injuries can cause acute kyphosis in the pediatric spine. Growth disturbances may lead to late deformity. The risk of disrupting growth potential must be considered in planning operative versus nonsurgical treatment. Traumatic paralysis often results in neuromuscular kyphosis that does not respond to brace treatment. Posterior fusion is recommended for kyphotic deformities greater than 60°. Curves that are more rigid may require anterior release and fusion combined with posterior spinal instrumentation and fusion.

Key Points

1. Normal thoracic kyphosis ranges between 20° and 40°.
2. Common causes of pediatric kyphotic deformities include Scheuermann's disease, postural roundback, trauma, postlaminectomy deformity, congenital anomalies, infection, and achondroplasia.

Websites

Scheuermann's kyphosis: http://emedicine.medscape.com/article/1266349-overview
Scheuermann's kyphosis treatment: http://www.orthosupersite.com/view.aspx?rid=23486
Vertebral column resection: http://www.spinal-deformity-surgeon.com/vcr-paper.html
Scheuermann's kyphosis: http://www.spineuniverse.com/conditions/kyphosis/scheuermanns-kyphosis-scheuermanns-disease

BIBLIOGRAPHY

1. McMaster MJ, Singh H. The surgical management of congenital kyphosis and kyphoscoliosis. Spine 2001;26:2146–55.
2. Murray PM, Weinstein SL, Spratt KF. The natural history and long-term follow-up of Scheuermann kyphosis. J Bone Joint Surg 1993;75A:236–48.
3. Ponte A. Posterior column shortening for Scheuermann's kyphosis. In: Haher TR, Merola AA, editors. Surgical Techniques for the Spine. New York: Thieme; 2003. p. 107–13.
4. Shah SA, Takemitsu M, Westerlund LE, et al. Pediatric kyphosis: Scheuermann's disease and congenital deformity. In Herkowitz HN, Garfin SR, Eismont FJ, et al, editors. Rothman–Simeone The Spine. 5th ed. Philadelphia: Saunders; 2006. p. 565–85.
5. Shirley ED, Ain MC. Achondroplasia: Manifestations and treatment. J Am Acad Ortho Surg 2009;17:231–41.

CHAPTER 41

NEUROMUSCULAR SPINAL DEFORMITIES

Steven Mardjetko, MD, FAAP, and Vincent J. Devlin, MD

1. Why do patients with neuromuscular diseases develop spinal deformities?

The most plausible cause of the vast majority of neuromuscular spinal deformities is spinal muscle imbalance acting in concert with gravity in a growing child. Alteration of vertebral loading patterns creates secondary changes in the vertebrae and soft tissues around the spine, according to the Heuter-Volkmann principle (increased loading across an epiphyseal growth plate inhibits growth and decreased pressure tends to accelerate growth). A wide spectrum of spinal deformities may develop including scoliosis (most common), hyperkyphosis, hyperlordosis, and complex multiplanar deformities.

2. What are the different types of neuromuscular scoliosis?

The various diseases associated with neuromuscular scoliosis are categorized as **neuropathic** (affecting either the upper or lower motor neurons) or **myopathic.** Certain conditions such as myelodysplasia and spinal trauma may have both upper and lower motor neuron involvement.

MYOPATHIC DISORDERS
1. Arthrogryposis multiplex congenita
2. Muscular dystrophy
   - Duchenne type
   - Limb-girdle
   - Fascioscapulohumeral
3. Fiber-type disproportion
4. Congenital hypotonia
5. Myotonia dystrophica

NEUROPATHIC DISORDERS
1. Upper motor neuron lesions
   - Cerebral palsy
   - Spinocerebellar degeneration: Friedreich's ataxia, Charcot-Marie-Tooth disease, Roussy-Levy disease
   - Syringomyelia
   - Quadriplegia secondary to spinal cord trauma or tumor
2. Lower motor neuron lesions
   - Spinal muscular atrophy: Werdnig-Hoffman disease, Kugelberg-Welander disease
   - Poliomyelitis
   - Dysautonomia (Riley-Day syndrome)

3. What is the prevalence of spinal deformities in different neuromuscular diseases?

The prevalence of spinal deformities in different neuromuscular diseases is variable: cerebral palsy (25%), myelodysplasia (60%), spinal muscular atrophy (67%), Friedreich's ataxia (80%), Duchenne muscular dystrophy (90%), and spinal cord injury before 10 years of age (100%).

4. List important differences between neuromuscular scoliosis and idiopathic scoliosis.

- Evaluation of neuromuscular scoliosis requires assessment of the underlying neuromuscular disease in combination with the spinal deformity. In contrast, idiopathic scoliosis is a spinal deformity occurring in otherwise normal patients
- Multidisciplinary evaluation is required for problems associated with the underlying neuromuscular disease (e.g. contractures, hip dislocations, seizures, malnutrition, cardiac and pulmonary disease, urinary tract dysfunction, developmental delay, pressure sores, insensate skin)
- Neuromuscular scoliosis develops at an earlier age than most cases of idiopathic scoliosis, often before age 10
- Neuromuscular spinal deformities are more likely to progress in severity due to the early age of onset of neuromuscular disease
- Neuromuscular curves tend to be longer and involve more vertebrae than idiopathic curves
- Neuromuscular curves are frequently accompanied by pelvic obliquity, which may compromise sitting ability and upper extremity function
- Neuromuscular curves do not respond well to orthotic treatment
- Spinal surgery is frequently required for neuromuscular spinal deformities

5. How are neuromuscular spinal deformities diagnosed?

Diagnosis is based on clinical examination and confirmed with long cassette radiographs. Upright radiographs are obtained in patients who are able to stand. Patients who are able to sit without hand support are assessed in the sitting position. Patients who are unable to sit are evaluated with recumbent anteroposterior (AP) and lateral radiographs. The examiner should assess curve magnitude, curve progression, spinal balance, pelvic obliquity (if present), and curve flexibility. Spinal magnetic resonance imaging (MRI) is required if intraspinal disease (e.g. syrinx, tethered cord) is suspected. After a child is diagnosed with neuromuscular disease, the patient should have yearly examinations to assess for development of spinal deformity.

6. **What radiographic features are characteristic of typical neuromuscular curves?**
Neuromuscular curves are typically long, sweeping C-shaped curves that extend to the pelvic region. The curve apex is usually in the thoracolumbar or lumbar region. When secondary curves develop, they are usually unable to restore coronal balance. Significant sagittal plane deformity often accompanies coronal plane deformity. Pelvic obliquity is common and poses a major problem because it creates an uneven sitting base.

7. **What treatment options exist for managing neuromuscular scoliosis?**
Three options exist for managing neuromuscular scoliosis: observation, orthotic management, and surgical treatment with spinal instrumentation and fusion.

8. **When is observation indicated?**
Observation is reasonable for patients with small curves (<30°), patients with severe developmental disability who develop large curves not associated with functional loss, and patients in whom medical comorbidities make them poor candidates for major spinal reconstructive surgery.

9. **What is the role of orthotic treatment?**
The role of orthotic treatment is two fold: (1) to help nonambulatory patients to sit with the use of a seating support, and (2) to attempt to control spinal deformity.
In most cases of neuromuscular scoliosis, a spinal orthosis will not prevent curve progression. However, orthotic treatment is valuable in slowing progression of spinal deformities until the onset of puberty and permits growth of the spine prior to definitive treatment with spinal instrumentation and fusion. Orthotic management is challenging in neuromuscular disorders because of poor muscle control, impaired sensation, pulmonary compromise, impaired gastrointestinal function, obesity, and difficulty with cooperating with brace wear.

10. **What are the indications and options for surgical treatment?**
There is no absolute minimum age at which to consider spinal surgery. In general, operative treatment is considered when progressive curves exceed 40° or when patients develop trunk decompensation. Earlier surgical treatment is advised for patients with Duchenne's muscular dystrophy (when curves reach 20°) due to predictable pulmonary deterioration associated with further curve progression. It is not necessary to delay surgery until skeletal maturity. Curves up to 90° are most commonly treated with posterior spinal instrumentation and fusion. Curves exceeding 90° or curves with severe stiffness are considered for more complex procedures. Anterior release and anterior fusion or posterior-based osteomies/vertebral resection in combination with posterior spinal instrumentation and fusion are options for surgical treatment of severe curves.

11. **List important preoperative considerations in evaluation of patients with neuromuscular spinal deformity.**
   - **Functional status:** Ambulatory function, sitting ability, hand function, mental ability, visual acuity
   - **Pulmonary assessment:** Ask about history of upper respiratory infection or pneumonia; assess for chronic aspiration; perform pulmonary function testing if possible
   - **Gastrointestinal assessment:** Assess for gastroesophageal reflux and intraabdominal volume compromise
   - **Cardiac assessment:** Critical in disorders such as Duchenne's muscular dystrophy, Friedreich's ataxia, myotonic dystrophy due to associated cardiac anomalies
   - **Nutritional status:** Address deficits to help prevent impaired wound healing and decrease infection risk
   - **Seizure disorders:** Require assessment by a neurologist and confirmation of appropriate levels of antiseizure medications
   - **Metabolic bone disease:** Osteopenia is common secondary to disuse, poor nutrition, and anticonvulsants. It is an important influence regarding strategy for spinal instrumentation

12. **List the goals of surgical treatment for neuromuscular spinal deformities.**
   - Prevent curve progression
   - Correct spinal deformities safely
   - Obtain a solid arthrodesis
   - Balance the spine in the coronal and sagittal planes above a level pelvis
   - Correct pelvic obliquity
   - Prevent progressive respiratory compromise due to increasing spinal deformity
   - Optimize functional ability (e.g. permit the patient to sit without using the arms for trunk support)
   - Decrease trunk fatigue and pain. Fatigue is associated with maintaining an upright posture in the presence of severe spinal deformity. Pain may result from facet arthrosis or impingement of the ribs on the pelvis in severe deformities

13. What are the basic principles of posterior spinal instrumentation and fusion for treatment of neuromuscular scoliosis?

The classic procedure for neuromuscular scoliosis is a long posterior fusion from the upper thoracic spine to the pelvis. Segmental spinal fixation consisting of sublaminar wires placed at every spinal level provides secure fixation and excellent deformity correction. Distal implant fixation is achieved by insertion of rods between the tables of the ilium along a path extending from the posterior superior iliac spine toward the anterior inferior iliac spine (Galveston technique). The rods are connected with a cross-link or a specially designed unit rod may be utilized. The fixation achieved with this technique is sufficiently secure to permit mobilization of the patient without the need for a postoperative orthosis. Allograft bone is commonly used for long fusions for neuromuscular scoliosis due to the excellent healing potential of the pediatric spine and because the ilium does not provide a sufficient amount of bone graft. See Figure 41-1.

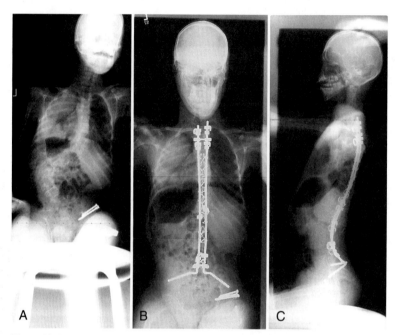

Figure 41-1. A, Anteroposterior (AP) radiograph shows a large thoracolumbar curve with pelvic obliquity in a 12-year-old patient with cerebral palsy. Postoperative AP **(B)** and lateral **(C)** radiographs after combined anterior and posterior procedures. Anterior surgery included multi-level anterior discectomies and fusion. An apical vertebrectomy was performed to enhance deformity correction. Posterior instrumentation and fusion was performed using proximal hooks, multiple sublaminar wires, and Galveston iliac fixation.

14. How does the surgeon select the appropriate distal level for spinal instrumentation and fusion?

The instrumentation and fusion should extend to the sacropelvis if the curve involves the sacrum, if there is significant pelvic obliquity, or if the patient has poor sitting balance. Ambulatory patients who lack pelvic obliquity and have mild curves that do not involve the sacrum may be considered candidates for ending the instrumentation and fusion proximal to sacropelvis to avoid potential compromise of ambulatory ability.

15. What is the rationale to perform combined anterior and posterior spinal surgery?

- **To enhance deformity correction.** Correction of rigid spinal deformities is improved following anterior discectomy and fusion. Indications include patients with fixed pelvic obliquity, large rigid curves with limited flexibility on bending or traction radiographs, as well as significant kyphotic deformities
- **To enhance the fusion rate.** Indications include patients with deficient posterior elements (e.g. myelodysplasia) and adults who require long fusions to the sacropelvis
- **To avoid the crankshaft phenomenon.** An important indication for skeletally immature patients in whom the presence of a posterior fusion acts as a tether to prevent elongation of the spine. As the vertebral bodies increase in height, the spine rotates out of the sagittal plane leading to a recurrent and increasing spinal curvature. Anterior fusion destroys the anterior growth plates of the vertebral bodies and prevents this phenomenon

16. Discuss recent advances in the surgical treatment of neuromuscular spinal deformities. See Figure 41-2.

- **Pedicle screw constructs.** Pedicle screws provide fixation across all three spinal columns and are biomechanically superior to hook or sublaminar wire fixation. Screw fixation enhances curve correction and provides a means of achieving secure fixation in patients with congenital or acquired laminectomy defects
- **Iliac screw fixation.** Modular implant components facilitate linkage of longitudinal members to the ilium and eliminate the need for complex rod bends. The combination of a bicortical S1 pedicle screw and an iliac screw provides a secure foundation for correction of severe neuromuscular deformities with pelvic obliquity
- **Hook fixation at the proximal end of instrumentation constructs.** Use of sublaminar wires at the proximal end of instrumentation constructs has been associated with development of a proximal junctional kyphotic deformity following surgery. Use of hook fixation at the proximal end of implant constructs can decrease the incidence of this problem. Hybrid instrumentation constructs combining hooks, wires, and screws can be customized to optimize spinal fixation and maximize deformity correction
- **Osteotomy/vertebral column resection procedures for rigid deformities.** Multilevel osteotomies or excision of vertebrae in the apical region of a severe rigid curve can enhance multiplanar correction of severe spinal deformities
- **Intraoperative halo-femoral traction.** Use of this adjunctive technique has been shown to facilitate treatment of severe neuromuscular spinal deformity using a posterior-only approach and avoids complications associated with circumferential procedures
- **Temporary internal distraction technique.** Gradual deformity correction using the temporary internal distraction technique performed with spinal cord monitoring has been shown to obviate the need for an anterior procedure in the treatment of select severe deformities

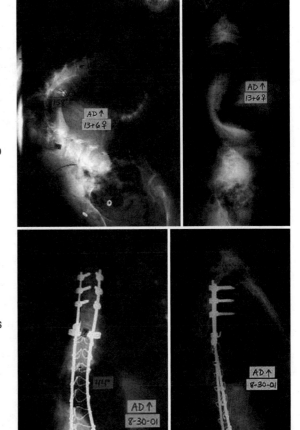

Figure 41-2. A 13-year-old girl with neuromuscular scoliosis. Preoperative anteroposterior (AP) and lateral images with 1-year follow-up utilizing iliac screws, proximal and distal pedicle screws, and sublaminar wires. (From Lenke LG, Kuklo TR. Sacropelvic fixation techniques in the treatment of pediatric spinal deformity. Semin Spine Surg 2004;16:114–18.)

17. What intraoperative problems should be anticipated during spinal procedures for neuromuscular spinal deformity?

Problems not uncommonly encountered during operations on children with neuromuscular spinal deformities include excessive blood loss, malignant hyperthermia, cardiac dysfunction, hypotension, coagulopathy, latex allergy, and difficulty with monitoring neurologic function.

18. What type of spinal cord monitoring is ideal in patients with neuromuscular spinal deformity?

The Stagnara wake-up test requires patient cooperation and is not a realistic option in most patients. An ideal combination of spinal cord monitoring modalities consists of somatosensory evoked potentials (SSEPs) in combination with transcranial evoked motor-evoked potentials. Intraoperative spinal monitoring is utilized if the patient has substantial preoperative neurologic function. In the presence of profound motor impairment, the indications for monitoring are less clear.

19. What postoperative problems should be anticipated after spinal procedures for neuromuscular spinal deformities?

- **Pulmonary dysfunction.** Atelectasis, pneumonia, and aspiration are common. Postoperative ventilator support is frequently required. Bilevel positive airway pressure (BiPAP) can be helpful. Postop management in an intensive care unit (ICU) setting is anticipated.

- **Fluid shifts.** Careful monitoring is necessary. Maintain hemoglobin levels at 9 g/dL or greater and urine output of 0.5 to 1 mL/kg/hour.
- **Gastrointestinal problems.** Ileus is common. Use of hyperalimentation can be considered until adequate gastrointestinal feeding can be resumed. Additional problems include pancreatitis, superior mesenteric artery syndrome, and cholelithiasis.
- **Wound infection.** The incidence of postoperative wound infection is much higher in neuromuscular patients than in other types of spinal deformity surgery. Prophylactic antibiotics should be administered for 24 hours following surgery. Addition of antibiotics to the allograft bone used for fusion is an option.

20. Discuss important considerations for surgical treatment of scoliosis secondary to cerebral palsy.

Cerebral palsy, the most common neuromuscular disorder, is frequently accompanied by scoliosis. Progression of scoliosis beyond 40° is the most common indication for surgical stabilization. Curves have been classified into two groups:

- **Group 1**, which includes single or double curves in ambulatory patients with a level pelvis. Group 1 patients are generally treated with posterior spinal fusion and instrumentation. Fusion to the sacrum is not usually required
- **Group 2**, which includes lumbar or thoracolumbar curves in nonambulatory patients, typically associated with pelvic obliquity. Group 2 patients are typically treated with fusion to the sacropelvis. If the pelvis becomes level on a traction radiograph, the deformity can be treated with a posterior spinal instrumentation and fusion from T2 to the pelvis using iliac fixation. If the deformity is rigid on the traction radiograph, combined anterior and posterior fusion or adjunctive posterior procedures (osteotomies, intraoperative traction, temporary internal distraction) are considered

21. What is the role of surgery for scoliosis associated with Duchenne muscular dystrophy?

Duchenne muscular dystrophy is the most common form of muscular dystrophy. It is X-linked recessive disorder resulting from mutation in the dystrophin gene. Ninety-five percent of patients with this disease develop scoliosis. Patients typically become wheelchair bound by the age of 13 and develop scoliosis at this time. Because these curves progress rapidly and are associated with loss of vital capacity, surgical stabilization is advised to prevent pulmonary impairment once the curve is greater than 20°. Typically, posterior spinal instrumentation and fusion are performed from T2 to the pelvis with segmental fixation, including iliac fixation. Some surgeons limit the distal extent of fusion to L5 in select patients with mild curves that are not associated with pelvic obliquity. Recent studies suggest a potential role for steroids (deflazacort) in prolongation of ambulatory ability and scoliosis prevention in this population.

22. Discuss important aspects of spinal deformities associated with spinal muscular atrophy.

Spinal muscular atrophy is a group of autosomal recessive disorders due to mutation in the *SMN1* gene. The disorders are characterized by degeneration of the anterior horn cells of the spinal cord resulting in trunk and proximal muscle weakness. The severity of the disease is variable. In general, the earlier the clinical onset, the worse the prognosis. Posterior spinal fusion should be performed before spinal deformities become severe and pulmonary function becomes compromised.

23. What curve pattern is most commonly noted in patients with Friedreich's ataxia who develop scoliosis?

Friedreich's ataxia is a spinal cerebellar degenerative disorder resulting from a mutation in the gene encoding for the protein *frataxin* and transmitted in an autosomal recessive pattern. Scoliosis develops in approximately 80% of patients. The curve pattern is similar to idiopathic scoliosis and is not usually accompanied by pelvic obliquity. Posterior spinal instrumentation and fusion are performed for curves that approach 40°. Fusion to the pelvis is rarely necessary.

24. A teenager presents with a painful 45° left thoracic curve pattern associated with thoracic kyphosis of 50°. Neurologic examination reveals asymmetric abdominal reflexes and dissociated pain and temperature loss in the extremities. What is the most likely diagnosis?

The radiographic and clinical findings are typical for syringomyelia. Syringomyelia, a fluid-filled cavity within the spinal cord, may lead to a spinal curvature that can be mistakenly attributed to idiopathic scoliosis. Idiopathic thoracic curves typically are not associated with severe pain in adolescence, are convex to the right, and are associated with normal or decreased thoracic kyphosis. MRI is indicated to confirm this diagnosis. A symptomatic syrinx requires surgical treatment, which may improve neurologic deficits and prevent curve progression. Severe curves require surgical correction and fusion.

25. What is the most significant risk factor for the development of spinal deformity in a patient who sustains a traumatic complete spinal cord injury?

The *age at injury* is the most significant risk factor for development of spinal deformity. The incidence of spinal deformity after spinal cord injury has been reported as 100% in patients injured before 10 years of age. Various studies have reported that scoliosis developed in 97% of patients injured before the adolescent growth spurt and 50% of those injured after the growth spurt. Prophylactic bracing should be used to attempt to slow deformity progression in young patients. Surgical treatment utilizing the surgical principles for treatment of neuromuscular spinal deformities is indicated for large or progressive deformities.

26. What types of spinal deformities may occur with myelomeningocele?
Myelomeningocele, the most common form of neural tube defect, is the result of failed closure and abnormal differentiation of the embryonic neural tube. Its exact cause remains uncertain but has been linked to folic acid deficiency. Spinal deformities are common in myelomeningocele patients and include severe kyphosis, scoliosis, and lordosis. Spinal deformities may be developmental (paralytic) or congenital (due to anomalous vertebra).

27. What underlying problems may be responsible for progressive scoliosis in a child with myelomeningocele?
Deformities and anomalies in a child with myelomeningocele may involve the spinal canal and its contents (neural axis) and influence the behavior and management of a spinal deformity. Progressive scoliosis in a child with myelomeningocele warrants further workup, including spinal and brain MRI to rule out problems such as a tethered cord, syringomyelia, or decompensated hydrocephalus.

28. What is the principal factor responsible for difficulty achieving successful spinal fusion in the patient with myelomeningocele and spinal deformity?
The lack of normal posterior vertebral elements makes achieving a solid spinal fusion difficult. In general, both anterior and posterior fusion should be performed in regions of the spine where the posterior elements are deficient in order to maximize fusion success.

29. What procedure is indicated to treat congenital lumbar kyphosis in a child with spina bifida?
Kyphectomy. Indications to resect a kyphosis include skin breakdown over the kyphosis and inability of the child to use their hands due to the need to support himself or herself on the thighs. The procedure includes resection of vertebrae in the region of the apex of the deformity, segmental fixation to any remaining posterior bony structures, and placement of S-shaped rods inserted distally through the L5–S1 neural foramen. This technique involves placement of a rod with two 90° bends at the distal end of the rod. The most distal limb of the rod rests on the anterior sacrum. The short limb of the rod between the two 90° bends rests on the top of the sacrum. The instrumentation construct provides excellent distal fixation and permits cantilever reduction of the kyphotic deformity. Posterior skin coverage is frequently a problem in these patients. Soft tissue procedures including the use of tissue expanders or muscle flaps may be required to provide adequate coverage of the spinal implants. See Figure 41-3.

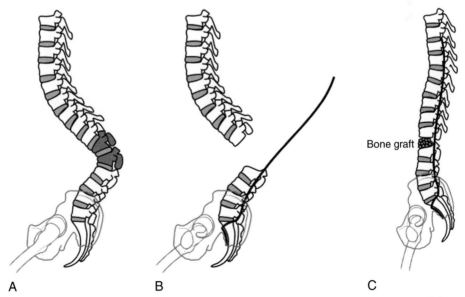

Bone graft

A   B   C

Figure 41-3. Sagittal diagram describing the sequence for performing kyphectomy. **A,** The spine is exposed, the dural sac is mobilized or tied off, and the kyphotic segment of the spine is excised. **B,** To improve mobility of the remaining segments, the discs can be excised and the lower two or three pairs of ribs sectioned from their origins. **C,** The two segments of the spine are then "folded inward," bone grafted (from the excised segments), and wired to previously contoured rods. (From Newton PO, Faro F, Wenger D, et al. Neuromuscular scoliosis. In: Herkowitz HN, Garfin SR, Eismont FJ, et al, editors. Rothman and Simeone The Spine. 5th ed. Philadelphia: Saunders; 2009. p. 557.)

Key Points

1. Neuromuscular disorders frequently result in severe spinal deformities that are challenging to treat and associated with high complication rates following surgery.
2. Evaluation of the patient with a neuromuscular spinal deformity requires assessment of the underlying disease process in combination with the spinal deformity.
3. Surgical treatment of neuromuscular spinal deformities has the potential to improve the patient's functional ability and quality of life, as well as provide improved caregiver satisfaction.

Websites

Neuromuscular scoliosis: http://emedicine.medscape.com/article/1266097-overview
Neuromuscular scoliosis: http://www.uwtv.org/programs/displayevent.aspx?rID=9384&fID=497

BIBLIOGRAPHY

1. Arlet V, Ouellet J. Myelomeningocele spinal deformities. In: Errico TJ, Lonner BS, Moulton AW, editors. Surgical Management of Spinal Deformities. Philadelphia: Saunders; 2009. p. 277–93.
2. Buchowski JM, Bhatnagar R, Skaggs DL, et al. Temporary internal distraction as an aid to correction of severe scoliosis. J Bone Joint Surg 2006;88A:2035–41.
3. Borkhuu B, Borowski A, Shah SA, et al. Antibiotic-loaded allograft decreases the rate of acute deep wound infection after spinal fusion in cerebral palsy. Spine 2008;33:2300–4.
4. Keeler KA, Lenke LG, Good CR, et al. Spinal fusion for spastic neuromuscular scoliosis—is anterior releasing necessary when intraoperative halo-femoral traction is used? Spine 2010;35:E427–E433.
5. Lonstein JE. Neuromuscular spinal deformities. In: Weinstein SL, editor. The Pediatric Spine: Principles and Practice. Philadelphia: Lippincott; 2001. p. 789–96.
6. Miller F. Spinal deformity secondary to impaired neurologic control. J Bone Joint Surg 2007;89A:S143–S147.
7. Newton PO, Faro F, Wenger D, et al. Neuromuscular scoliosis. In: Herkowitz HN, Garfin SR, Eismont FJ, Bell GR, Balderston RA, editors. Rothman and Simeone The Spine. 5th ed. Philadelphia: Saunders; 2006. p. 535–64.
8. Shook JF, Lubicky JP. Paralytic scoliosis. In: Bridwell KH, DeWald RL, editors. The Textbook of Spinal Surgery. 2nd ed. Philadelphia: Lippincott-Raven; 1997. p. 839–80.

CONGENITAL SPINAL DEFORMITIES

Lawrence I. Karlin, MD

CHAPTER 42

1. Define congenital scoliosis.
A lateral curvature of the spine is caused by vertebral anomalies that produce a frontal plane growth asymmetry. The anomalies are present at birth, but the curvature may take years to become clinically evident.

2. What genes are thought to be responsible for the congenital spinal malformations?
Homeobox genes of the Hox class.

3. When do congenital vertebral anomalies form?
During weeks 4 to 6 of the embryonic period.

4. What are the two main categories of congenital scoliosis?
Defects of segmentation and defects of formation. Some congenital abnormalities cannot be placed into this classification scheme.

5. What are the common defects of segmentation?
Block vertebra, unilateral bar, and unilateral bar and hemivertebra (Fig. 42-1).

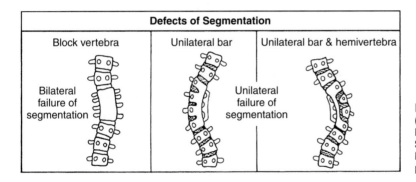

Figure 42-1. Defects of segmentation. (From McMaster MJ. Congenital scoliosis. In: Weinstein SL, editor. The Pediatric Spine: Principles and Practice. New York: Raven Press; 1994. p. 227–44, with permission.)

6. What are the common defects of formation?
Hemivertebra and wedge vertebra (Fig. 42-2).

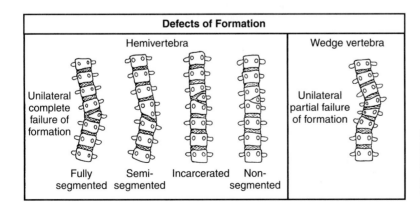

Figure 42-2. Defects of formation. (From McMaster MJ. Congenital scoliosis. In: Weinstein SL, editor. The Pediatric Spine: Principles and Practice. New York: Raven Press; 1994. p 227–44, with permission.)

7. What are the types of hemivertebra?

Fully segmented, semisegmented, nonsegmented, and incarcerated.

8. What is the anatomic cause of progressive deformity?

Unbalanced growth. The greater the disparity in the number of healthy growth plates between the left and right sides of the spine, the greater the deformity and the more rapidly spinal deformity develops.

9. What factors are used to prognosticate the rate of progression and ultimate deformity due to a congenital spinal anomaly?

1. The **anatomic type** helps determine the risk and rate of progression.
2. The **location** of the defect affects spinal balance and difficulty of treatment. A hemivertebra located at the lumbosacral junction causes far more spinal imbalance than one located at the mid-thoracic level. In addition, a hemivertebra at the cervicothoracic junction is more difficult to treat surgically due to limited approach options, and timing of intervention may be altered based on this consideration.
3. The **age** of the patient determines the risk of progression. Spinal deformities are more likely to progress during times of rapid growth, such as the first 2 years of life and during the adolescent growth spurt.

10. What forms of congenital scoliosis cause the most rapidly progressive deformities?

- Unilateral unsegmented bar with contralateral hemivertebra (an average of 6° progression per year)
- Unilateral unsegmented bar (an average of 5° progression per year)

11. What is the accepted initial treatment for a unilateral unsegmented bar?

Early in situ fusion because this deformity can only progress.

12. What is the risk of progression of the various types of hemivertebra?

- **Fully segmented.** There are two extra growth plates on one side of the spine. Unbalanced growth occurs, producing a scoliosis that worsens at a rate of 1 to 2° per year. Two fully segmented hemivertebra on the same side of the spine produce a more rapid deterioration (about 3° per year).
- **Semisegmented.** One border is synostosed to its neighbor, producing a balanced number of growth plates on either side. The hemivertebra produces a tilting of the spine, and a slowly progressive curvature may occur.
- **Nonsegmented.** No growth plates are associated with this type of hemivertebra, and a progressive deformity does not occur.
- **Incarcerated.** The vertebral bodies above and below accommodate the hemivertebra, and little or no deformity is produced. The growth plates tend to be narrow with little growth potential. This form of hemivertebra causes little or no deformity.

13. What percentage of people with vertebral malformations have associated anomalies?

Sixty percent have malformations either within or outside the spine. A relatively benign vertebral abnormality may be associated with a life-threatening (but initially asymptomatic) problem. The importance of a thorough search for associated abnormalities cannot be overemphasized.

14. What common malformations are associated with congenital spinal anomalies?

- **Vertebral abnormalities at another level.** For example, cervical vertebral anomalies are detected in 25% of people with congenital scoliosis or kyphosis.
- **Urinary tract structural abnormalities.** Up to 37% of people with congenital vertebral anomalies have urinary tract anomalies, such as renal agenesis, duplication, ectopia, fusion, ureteral anomalies, and reflux.
- **Intraspinal abnormalities.** Up to 38% of people with congenital vertebral anomalies have intraspinal abnormalities detectable by magnetic resonance imaging (MRI), including tethered cord, diastematomyelia, diplomyelia, and syringomyelia.
- **Other associated anomalies.** Cranial nerve palsy (11%), upper extremity hypoplasia (10%), clubfoot (9%), dislocated hip (8%), congenital cardiac disease (7%).

15. Define diastematomyelia.

A *diastematomyelia* is a congenital bony or fibrocartilaginous septum in the spinal canal that impinges on or splits the neural tissue.

16. What is the incidence of diastematomyelia associated with congenital vertebral abnormalities?

5% to 20%.

17. What are the clinical findings in diastematomyelia?
- Cutaneous lesions, such as hair patch, dimple (55%–75%)
- Anisomelia (52%–58%)
- Foot deformity usually cavus, usually unilateral (32%–52%)
- Neurologic deficits (58%–88%)
- Scoliosis (60%–100%)

18. What radiographic findings are associated with diastematomyelia?
- Spina bifida occulta (76%–94%)
- Widened interpedicular distance (94%–100%)

19. What is the normal level of the conus in the pediatric population according to age?
The L2–L3 disc in the neonate and the L1–L2 disc or cephalad at 1 year and older.

20. What vertebral malformation is most often associated with an abnormality of the neural axis?
A unilateral unsegmented bar and a same-level contralateral hemivertebra. Approximately 50% of people with this vertebral abnormality have been reported to have an associated neural axis abnormality.

21. What is the VATER association?
VATER is the acronym for the association of the following congenital anomalies: **v**ertebral, **a**norectal, **t**racheo-**e**sophageal fistula, and **r**adial limb dysplasia and **r**enal anomalies. This acronym has now been expanded to **VACTERLS**, adding **c**ardiac and **s**ingle umbilical artery. Trill the *L*, and you will remember **l**ung abnormalities, another associated problem.

22. What tests should be performed to screen a patient with congenital scoliosis for renal abnormalities?
Urinalysis and renal ultrasound are sufficient.

23. When should an MRI be performed to screen for intraspinal abnormalities when a patient presents with a congenital vertebral anomaly?
Perhaps a controversial answer: A number of studies now place the incidence of associated intraspinal abnormalities in the 30% range. The standard recommendation is to perform an MRI if surgery is planned or when clinical symptoms or physical findings are suggestive of intraspinal pathology. The author believes, as do others, that an MRI should be part of the initial evaluation of congenital scoliosis. The 30% incidence is too high to ignore when clinical manifestations are frequently initially absent.

24. What is the accuracy of measurement of congenital spinal deformities on plain radiographs?
The abnormally shaped vertebrae make it difficult to be consistent with radiographic measurements. One study revealed an intraobserver variability of $\pm 9.6°$ and an interobserver variability of $\pm 11.8°$. Another study reported an average intraobserver variance of $2.8°$ and an interobserver variance of $3.4°$.

25. What is the role of brace treatment for congenital scoliosis?
The role is limited. Orthoses will not halt the progression of a rigid congenital structural abnormality. A brace may control a compensatory curvature or a long flexible curvature in which the rigid congenital deformity comprises a small section of the entire spinal deformity. Total contact braces may restrict chest wall development and should not be used. A Milwaukee brace (cervicothoracolubosacral orthosis, CTLSO) is preferable.

26. What are the surgical treatment options for congenital spinal deformities?
- Posterior fusion without spinal instrumentation
- Posterior fusion with spinal instrumentation
- Combined anterior and posterior fusion
- Convex growth arrest procedures
- Hemivertebra excision
- Vertebrectomy
- Combinations of the above procedures
- Vertical expandable prosthetic titanium rib instrumentation (VEPTR)
- Growing rods (intermittent rod distraction techniques)

27. In treating congenital scoliosis, what is the indication for in situ posterior spinal arthrodesis without instrumentation?
This procedure is indicated for a small curvature that is anticipated to worsen (e.g. scoliosis due to a unilateral unsegmented bar). However, bending of the fusion (crankshaft) can occur with significant anterior growth. Anterior and posterior arthrodesis is indicated in the very young patient or when significant anterior growth (healthy anterior growth plates) is anticipated.

28. In treating congenital scoliosis, what is the indication for posterior fusion with instrumentation?

This procedure is indicated in the older child when some correction of the deformity is desired. The correction will occur not through the rigid congenital deformity but through the adjacent flexible spine segments.

29. In treating congenital scoliosis, what is the indication for convex hemiepiphyseodesis and hemiarthrodesis? What levels should be fused?

This procedure is designed to produce a gradual correction of curvatures due to hemivertebra. The prerequisites for success include a curvature with concave growth potential, limited length (5 or fewer vertebral bodies), limited magnitude ($< 70°$), no kyphosis, and young age (younger than 5 years). The entire curvature should be fused on the convex side. The benefit of the procedure is safety. The disadvantage of the procedure is the unpredictability of final curve correction.

30. What is the indication for hemivertebra excision?

Hemivertebra excision is indicated for a fully segmented hemivertebra, causing significant trunk imbalance (Fig. 42-3). This is theoretically a more dangerous procedure than in situ fusion or hemiepiphyseodesis. However, it produces dramatic curve correction while maintaining maximal spinal flexibility. It is the treatment of choice for a lumbosacral hemivertebra, causing significant oblique take-off. A number of surgical series using a simultaneous anterior and posterior approach for hemivertebra excision have documented excellent results with few complications. More recently, posterior-only techniques have been advocated as an alternative technique.

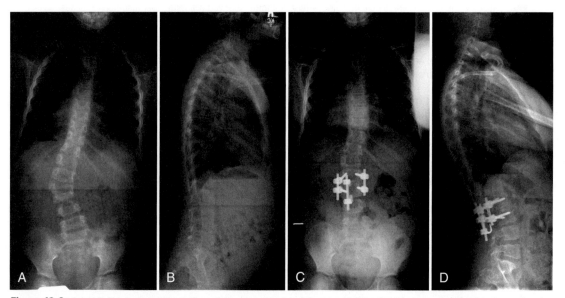

Figure 42-3. A and **B,** This 2-year-old boy with scoliosis, secondary to a fully segmented hemivertebra, progressed 12° in 1 year. **C** and **D,** A hemivertebra resection performed through a single-stage posterior approach produced a significant improvement in both the curvature and coronal balance without an appreciable loss of flexibility or growth. In a small child, the bones may not tolerate the stresses produced by instrumented manipulation, and fixation to maintain the correction may be lost. Here the correction was obtained by manual pressure over the ribs and flank and compression of the laminar hooks. The correction was then fine-tuned and maintained by the pedicle screw-rod construct.

31. What is the indication for transpedicular anterior and posterior convex hemiepiphyseodesis or transpedicular hemivertebra excision?

These procedures were initially described for cases in which hemiepiphyseodesis or hemivertebra excision is appropriate, but the anterior approach is difficult (e.g. the upper thoracic spine) or not desired. The anterior growth areas are accessed from a posterior approach via the pedicle. Posterior transpedicular techniques have subsequently been applied to all levels of the thoracic and lumbar spine.

32. Does the crankshaft phenomenon occur after the surgical treatment of congenital scoliosis?

The crankshaft phenomenon results when a scoliotic deformity previously treated by posterior arthrodesis demonstrates progressive increase in curve magnitude and rotational deformity. The cause is thought to be anterior growth tethered by the posterior fusion. This phenomenon, documented in idiopathic scoliosis, has been reported in children with congenital scoliosis treated by posterior fusion alone before age 10 years. It has not been reported when anterior and posterior arthrodesis were performed together in this population.

33. How is congenital kyphosis classified (Fig. 42-4)?

Type I: Failure of formation
Type II: Failure of segmentation
Type III: Mixed anomalies

Defects of Vertebral Body Segmentation	Defects of Vertebral Body Formation		Mixed Anomalies
Partial	Anterior and unilateral aplasia	Anterior and median aplasia	
Anterior unsegmented bar	Posterolateral quadrant vertebra	Butterfly vertebra	Anterolateral bar and contralateral quadrant vertebra
Complete	Anterior aplasia	Anterior hypoplasia	
Block vertebra	Posterior hemivertebra	Wedged vertebra	

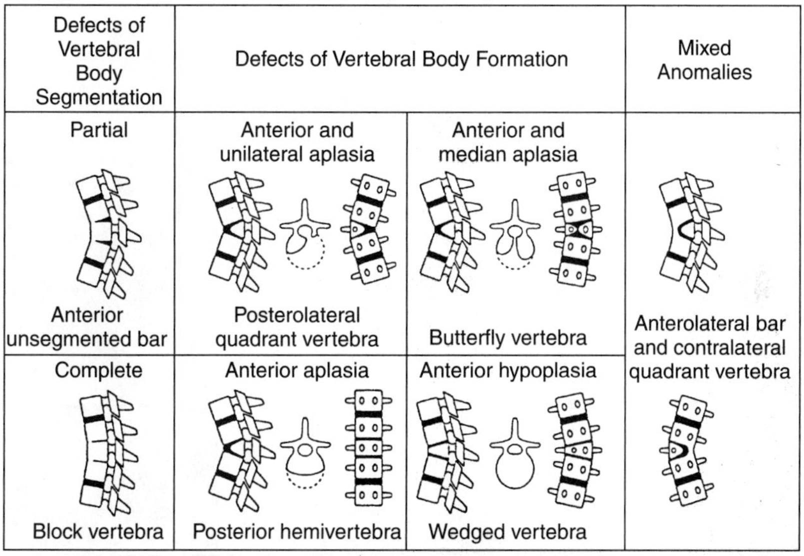

Figure 42-4. Classification of congenital kyphosis. (From McMaster MJ, Singh H. Natural history of kyphosis and kyphoscoliosis: A study of one hundred and twelve patients. J Bone Joint Surg 1999;81A:1367–83, with permission.)

34. What forms of congenital kyphosis are associated with spontaneous neurologic deterioration?

Type I (failure of formation) and type III (mixed anomalies).

35. In congenital kyphosis, when is posterior surgery alone sufficient?

Posterior surgery is reasonable in the absence of anterior neural compression, kyphosis correcting to 50° or less on supine radiographs, and age younger than 5 years.

36. What is the treatment of type I congenital kyphosis?

Arthrodesis by age 5 years. An aggressive surgical approach is indicated due to the substantial risk of neurologic deficit without treatment.

37. What is the treatment for type II congenital kyphosis?

Observation. Fusion should be performed if deformity progression is noted. The prognosis for deformity progression is greater when there is an anterolateral bar producing kyphoscoliosis than when a midline bar produces a pure kyphotic deformity.

38. What is the treatment for type III congenital kyphosis?

Arthrodesis by age 5.

39. Lumbar hypoplasia is an unusual cause of congenital thoracolumbar kyphosis. Define this entity and describe the clinical significance of this deformity.

Lumbar hypoplasia is a kyphotic deformity of the upper lumbar spine in which the anatomic defect is limited to the superior aspect of the anterior half of a single affected vertebral body. Unlike congenital kyphosis due to anterior failure of formation, the natural history of lumbar hypoplasia is spontaneous resolution (Fig. 42-5).

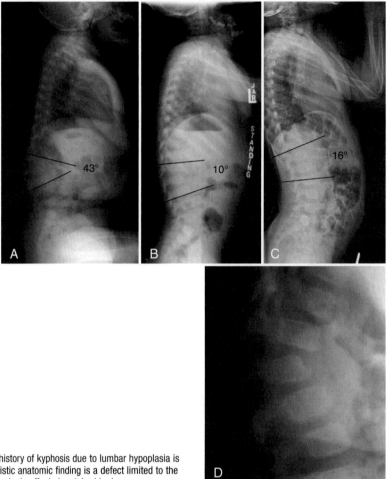

Figure 42-5. **A, B,** and **C,** The natural history of kyphosis due to lumbar hypoplasia is spontaneous resolution. **D,** The characteristic anatomic finding is a defect limited to the anterior half of the superior portion of the single affected vertebral body.

40. What characteristics distinguish congenital spinal dislocation from congenital kyphosis?

The *congenitally dislocated spine* is the most severe form of congenital kyphosis and is distinguished by a sudden sagittal vertebral displacement designated as the *step-off* sign. Multiplanar displacements have been reported. The deformity is frequently associated with instability and neurologic compromise. Stabilization by circumferential fusion at the time of diagnosis is recommended.

41. Define segmental spinal dysgenesis and describe treatment of this deformity.

Segmental spinal dysgenesis is a congenital spinal deformity characterized by focal dysgenesis or agenesis of the lumbar or thoracolumbar spine and a focal abnormality of the underlying spinal cord and nerve roots. The bony defects include canal stenosis, hypoplastic vertebrae, and spinal column subluxation and instability. Neural pathology includes narrowing of the thecal sac and absent nerve roots. Early spinal stabilization, usually by anterior and posterior arthrodesis, is required to prevent progressive deformity and neurologic deterioration.

42. What is the role of the VEPTR procedure in congenital spinal deformity?

The vertical expandable prosthetic titanium rib instrumentation (VEPTR) was developed to treat the thoracic insufficiency syndrome (defined as the inability of the thorax to support normal respiration and lung growth) associated with fused ribs. Following thoracoplasty of the fused ribs, the device lengthens and expands the hypoplastic hemithorax. When used in congenital scoliosis associated with fused ribs, growth of the concave and convex sides of the spine, including growth through unilateral unsegmented bars, may occur in addition to hemithorax enlargement.

Key Points

1. The prognosis for a congenital spinal deformity depends on three factors: type of anomaly, patient age, and location of the defect.
2. A wide range of intraspinal and extraspinal anomalies is associated with congenital spinal deformities, and thorough workup for associated abnormalities is critical.
3. MRI of the spine is an integral part of the evaluation of a patient with congenital spinal deformity.
4. Orthoses have little effect on progression of congenital spinal deformities.
5. Early surgical intervention is advised for progressive congenital spinal deformities to balance spinal growth and avoid development of rigid deformity and secondary structural curvatures.

Websites

Classification of congenital scoliosis and kyphosis: http://www.medscape.com/viewarticle/707687
Congenital scoliosis: http://www.srs.org/professionals/education/congenital
Congenital spinal deformity: http://members.medscape.com/article/1260442-overview

BIBLIOGRAPHY

1. Andrew T, Piggot H. Growth arrest for progressive scoliosis: Combined anterior and posterior fusion of the convexity. J Bone Joint Surg 1985;67B:193–7.
2. Campbell RM Jr, Smith MD, Mayes TC, et al. The effect of opening wedge thoracoplasty on thoracic insufficiency syndrome associated with fused ribs and congenital scoliosis. J Bone Joint Surg 2004;86A:1659–74.
3. Campos MA, Fernandes P, Dolan LA, et al. Infantile thoracolumbar kyphosis secondary to lumbar hypoplasia. J Bone Joint Surg 2008;90A:1726–9.
4. Hedequist DJ. Instrumentation and fusion for congenital spine deformities. Spine 2009;34:1783–90.
5. Hughes LO, McCarthy RE, Glasier CM. Segmental spinal dysgenesis: A report of three cases. J Pediatr Orthop 1998;18(2):227–32.
6. Keller PM, Lindseth RE, DeRosa P. Progressive congenital scoliosis treatment using a transpedicular anterior and posterior convex hemiepiphyseodesis and hemiarthrodesis: A preliminary report. Spine 1994;19:1933–9.
7. Lazar RD, Hall JE. Simultaneous anterior and posterior hemivertebra excision. Clin Orthop Rel Res 1999;364:76–84.
8. McMaster MJ, Singh H. The surgical management of congenital kyphosis and kyphoscoliosis. Spine 2001;26:2146–54.
9. Ruf M, Jensen R, Letko L, et al. Hemivertebra resection and osteotomies in congenital spine deformity. Spine 2009;34:1791–9.
10. Terek RM, Wehner J, Lubicky JP. Crankshaft phenomenon in congenital scoliosis: A preliminary report. J Pediatr Orthop 1991;11:527–32.
11. Yazici M, Emans J. Fusionless instrumentation systems for congenital scoliosis. Expandable spinal rods and vertical expandable prosthetic titanium ribs in the management of congenital spine deformities in the growing child. Spine 2007;34:1800–7.
12. Zeller RD, Ghanem I, Dubousset J. The congenital dislocated spine. Spine 1996;21:1235–40.

CHAPTER 43

SPECIAL SURGICAL TECHNIQUES FOR THE GROWING SPINE

Gregory M. Mundis, Jr., MD, and Behrooz A. Akbarnia, MD

1. How is scoliosis classified in the growing child?

Scoliosis is most commonly classified according to **etiology** and **age at diagnosis.** Idiopathic scoliosis has traditionally been categorized according to age at diagnosis as *infantile* (birth–3 years), *juvenile* (age 3–10 years), or *adolescent* (age beyond 10 years). Currently there is a trend to classify scoliosis according to age into two categories: *early onset* and *late onset.* This classification is intended to more accurately reflect the physiologic stages of thoracic development. Growth of the thorax and lungs is greatest in the first 5 years of life, slows from age 5 to 10 years, and demonstrates a second less intense growth phase during the adolescent growth spurt. *Early-onset scoliosis (EOS)* includes curves diagnosed between 0 and 5 years, and *late-onset scoliosis (LOS)* includes curves diagnosed beyond 5 years of age.

2. Summarize the four main categories of early onset scoliosis (EOS).

- **Idiopathic:** A comprehensive workup must be completed in order to rule out an identifiable cause as a prerequisite for diagnosis of early-onset idiopathic scoliosis
- **Neuromuscular:** Etiologies include spinal dysraphism, cerebral palsy, muscular dystrophy
- **Congenital:** Anomalies associated with spinal deformities include hemivertebrae, vertebral bars, syrinx, and tethered cord
- **Syndromic:** Common diagnoses include neurofibromatosis and Marfan's syndrome

3. Why is the age of onset of scoliosis important?

Unrecognized and untreated, early-onset scoliosis may result in significant impairment of growth of the thorax, lungs, and spinal column. This may be associated with significant pulmonary dysfunction, including restrictive lung disease, pulmonary hypertension, and thoracic insufficiency syndrome.

4. Describe the different periods of spine growth during childhood.

The growth of the immature spine can be conceptualized in terms of **three phases:**

- **Early phase (0–5 years):** A phase of early rapid growth. Average height gained is 2 cm per year. By age 5, two thirds of sitting height is achieved. Thoracic volume grows from 5% of adult lung volume to 30% (six-fold increase) at age 5 years
- **Middle phase (5–10 years):** A phase of slow to moderate growth. Growth slows to 0.9 cm per year and thoracic volume reaches 50% by age 10. By age 8, most alveolar growth is complete and respiratory branching is complete
- **Adolescent phase (>10 years):** A phase of increasing growth during the adolescent growth spurt. Growth rate increases to 1.8 cm per year but never reaches the rapid velocity of early spine growth. Alveolar volume is stable and thoracic volume reaches that of adulthood around age 15 (the last 50%)

5. What is the significance of the rib vertebral angle difference (RVAD) and rib phase?

The **RVAD** measures the amount of rotation at the apex vertebra and has prognostic value regarding curve progression. The angle is determined by a line perpendicular to the endplate of the apical vertebra and a line drawn through the center of the adjacent rib on both the concave and convex side of the apical vertebra (see Fig 39-1). The RVAD equals the difference between the convex and concave angles. If the difference is greater than 20°, curve progression is likely. The **phase of the rib** is determined by ascertaining whether the head of the convex rib overlaps the apical vertebral body. If there is no overlap (phase 1), then the RVAD is calculated to determine the likelihood of progression. If there is overlap (phase 2), the risk of progression is high and measuring the RVAD is unnecessary.

6. What are the nonoperative treatment options for early-onset scoliosis?

- **Observation:** Curves of 25° or less and RVAD of 20° or less are observed due to the low risk of curve progression. Clinical and radiographic monitoring is continued every 4 to 6 months.
- **Active treatment:** Orthotic treatment is indicated for progressive curves. Patients who present with curves greater than 35° are considered for immediate treatment.

7. Describe orthotic treatment for early-onset scoliosis.

Orthotic treatment typically consists of initial cast treatment to obtain maximum deformity correction followed by brace treatment. A cast is applied under general anesthesia and changed every 6 to 12 weeks until ultimate correction is achieved. In the next treatment phase, a Milwaukee brace is continued for 2 years until the Cobb angle and RVAD are stable. A Milwaukee brace (cervicothoracolumbar orthosis, CTLSO) is preferred over an underarm thoracolumbosacral orthosis (TLSO) due to the tendency of underarm braces to cause chest wall deformity secondary to rib cage compression.

8. **When is surgery indicated for early-onset scoliosis?**
   - Progressive curves greater than 45°
   - Failure of nonoperative management
   - Thoracic insufficiency syndrome

9. **What are the surgical treatment options for early-onset scoliosis?**
   Current surgical treatment options for early-onset scoliosis include spinal fusion with or without spinal instrumentation, hemiepiphysiodesis, and spinal instrumentation without fusion (growing rods). The vertical expandable prosthetic titanium rib (VEPTR) is an additional potential treatment option for specific indications.

10. **What are the drawbacks of spinal fusion for treatment of early-onset scoliosis?**
    Multilevel spinal fusion is a less than ideal option for treatment of scoliosis in the very young child because the procedure inhibits future growth. Early spinal fusion will limit future increase in spinal height and restrict development of the thoracic cage and lung parenchyma. An additional concern is the risk of recurrent scoliosis and rib deformity following posterior spinal fusion due to continued anterior spine growth (crankshaft phenomenon). The ideal operative procedure would provide curve correction, prevent future curve progression, and facilitate normal growth of the spine, thoracic cage, and lungs.

11. **Explain the rationale and evolution of growing rod surgical techniques.**
    Harrington formulated the concept of instrumentation without fusion for children younger than 10 years. Moe and colleagues pioneered the technique utilizing a single Harrington rod placed subcutaneously through small incisions. Patients were immobilized in a brace and underwent periodic rod lengthenings until definitive fusion was indicated based on curve magnitude and patient age. The dual rod technique was introduced and popularized by Akbarnia to address problems encountered with use of a single rod that included hook dislodgement, rod breakage, and the need for brace immobilization. In this technique, the spine is exposed at only the upper and lower ends of the implant construct. Proximal and distal fixation is achieved with hooks or screws placed over two or three spinal levels. Limited fusions are performed at the fixation sites. Dual rods are placed proximally and distally and linked by a tandem connector placed in the thoracolumbar region to complete the four-rod construct. Lengthenings are performed at the site of the tandem connectors at 6-month intervals until the time of definitive spinal fusion. See Figures 43-1 and 43-2.

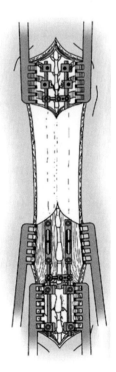
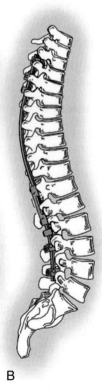

Figure 43-1. Technique of dual-rod instrumentation. **A,** Anteroposterior view. **B,** Lateral view showing construct contoured to maintain sagittal alignment. Extended tandem connectors are placed in thoracolumbar spine to minimize profile. (Redrawn from Akbarnia B, McCarthy R. Pediatric Isola instrumentation without fusion for the treatment of progressive early onset scoliosis. In: McCarthy R, editor. Spinal Instrumentation Techniques. Chicago: Scoliosis Research Society; 1998. From Canale ST, Beaty JH, editors. Campbell's Operative Orthopaedics. 11th ed. Philadelphia: Mosby; 2007.)

A   B

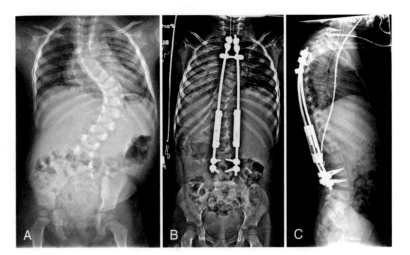

Figure 43-2. A, A 29-month-old patient with progressive early-onset scoliosis. Nonoperative treatment failed to control the curve progression. Postoperative radiographs. **B,** Antero-posterior view and **C,** lateral view. Patient underwent dual growing rods instrumentation from T2 to L4. Four hooks and a cross connector were used at the upper foundation (T2–T4) and four screws were used at the lower foundation (L3–L4).

12. List the key steps procedural steps in the placement of dual growing rods.
- Two incisions are required: one cephalad at the proximal foundation and one caudally at the distal foundation. These are the only sites of subperiosteal dissection. Rods and tandem connectors are passed smoothly under the fascia
- The proximal foundation consists of bilateral supralaminar and infralaminar hooks (claw formation) in combination with a cross connector. Alternatively four pedicle screws may be used
- The caudal foundation consists of four pedicle screws
- Rods (after appropriate contouring) are passed below the fascia underneath the long skin bridge
- Cephalad and caudal rods are connected via a tandem connector through which lengthening will be performed
- Initial lengthening is performed through the tandem connector at time of index surgery. Subsequent lengthenings are planned at 6 month intervals
- In rigid curves, preoperative traction, apical anterior release, or osteotomy are considered

13. Does it make a difference whether the rods are placed in a subcutaneous location or a submuscular location?
Yes. Subcutaneous rod placement is associated with a higher number of complications compared with submuscular placement. Subcutaneous placement is associated with an increased incidence of wound problems, prominent implants, and implant-related unplanned returns to the operating room.

14. What are the principles to follow for exposure of the spine for placement of dual growing rods?
- Avoid subperiosteal dissection except at the levels of the foundation where fusion is the primary goal
- Use careful blunt dissection beneath the skin bridge to avoid inadvertent pleural violation during passage of growing rod

15. What are the principles to follow during placement of implants for the dual growing rod technique?
- Use fluoroscopy to identify the correct surgical levels and confirm proper screw placement
- Perform meticulous rod contouring to achieve correction of both sagittal and coronal plane deformity
- Place tandem connectors with the set screws facing medially to permit access through single incision
- Place tandem connectors at the thoracolumbar junction because the connectors will match the sagittal contour of the spine in this region

16. Describe the common complications associated with dual growing rods and strategies to minimize or avoid these complications.
- **Wound problems/infection:** The best strategy is prevention. Dissection should include thick tissue flaps, minimal tissue disruption, and meticulous closure in layers. If wound dehiscence occurs, it is recommended to involve a plastic surgeon to assist in providing early wound coverage. Infections should be treated with irrigation and debridement and culture-specific antibiotics.
- **Implant-related complications:** Complications include screw loosening, hook dislodgement, and rod breakage. Early recognition and early intervention are critical. Usually revision of instrumentation will address implant complications. This can be performed at the time of a preplanned 6-month lengthening or as an unplanned trip to the operating room. Careful attention should be paid to parental concerns and changes in the child's demeanor during treatment because this frequently indicates an issue related to the implants.
- **Alignment/balance problems:** Occasionally patients will be left with a situation in which their coronal or sagittal balance is unacceptable (>5 cm deviation). Coronal imbalance can be corrected with asymmetric lengthening if

dual growing rods are used. Sagittal balance is more difficult to address because growing rods are posterior-based implants and naturally induce kyphosis. Sagittal imbalance can be addressed with revision of the rods and modifying rod contour prior to reimplantation

- **Neurologic complications:** Neurologic complications are rare in treatment of EOS with a distraction-based construct. Case reports describe neurologic deficits developing postoperatively that have responded to immediate construct shortening

17. What is a SHILLA procedure?

This surgical technique is intended to permit control of the patient's curve and preservation of spinal growth while avoiding the need for additional rod lengthening procedures. In the SHILLA procedure, the apex of the deformity is treated with a first-stage short segment anterior fusion. Deformity correction is achieved during a second procedure consisting of posterior instrumentation using extraperiosteally placed pedicle screws combined with a limited apical fusion. The remainder of the spine is not fused and specially designed screws at the ends of the rods permit the spine to continue to grow over the nonfused levels.

18. When should alternative treatments other than growing rods be considered?

- Very stiff curves (consider apical fusion, osteotomy, or anterior release)
- Poor bone quality
- Older children with limited growth potential
- Children too young to support internal fixation
- Congenital curves with fused ribs or thoracic insufficiency syndrome

19. What is thoracic insufficiency syndrome?

Thoracic insufficiency syndrome is defined as the inability of the thorax to support normal respiration or lung growth (due to inadequate space available). In the presence of a deformed spine and severe chest wall deformity (e.g. fused or absent ribs, hypoplastic thorax, lateral flexion contracture of the thorax associated with early-onset spinal deformity) normal respiration is altered because the thorax is unable to expand and contract normally. If the thorax does not grow at a normal pace, normal lung and pulmonary development is severely affected because lung alveolar development is not complete until 8 years of age. Without treatment, these children require supplemental oxygen, variable/bilevel positive airway pressure (VPAP/BiPAP), or ventilatory support to maintain life-sustaining oxygen levels in their blood.

20. How is the surgical strategy different for a patient with thoracic insufficiency syndrome?

Treatments utilizing posterior spinal instrumentation are not sufficient for these patients because surgical treatment requires addressing the thorax. This particular group of patients is treated with a vertically expandable prosthetic titanium rib (VEPTR, Synthes Spine).This is a growth-directed device that attaches to ribs at the cephalad foundation and to the ribs, spine, or pelvis at its caudal foundation. It has been shown that VEPTR treatment results in improved thoracic volume and fusionless correction of thoracic and spine deformities. See Figure 43-3.

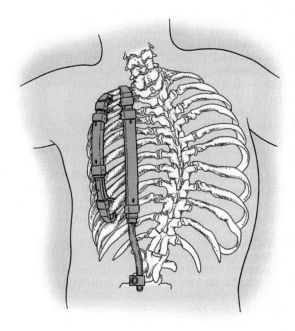

Figure 43-3. Expandable prosthetic rib device. (Redrawn from Campbell RM, personal communication. From Canale ST, Beaty JH, editors. Campbell's Operative Orthopaedics. 11th ed. Philadelphia: Mosby; 2007.)

21. What are the indications for VEPTR?

The VEPTR device was pioneered by Campbell and Smith and is currently approved in the United States under a Humanitarian Device Exemption (HDE). The device has been used for treatment of:

- Flail chest syndrome
- Constrictive chest wall syndrome, including rib fusion and scoliosis
- Hypoplastic thorax syndrome (e.g. Jeune's syndrome, achondroplasia, Jarcho-Levin syndrome, Ellis van Creveld syndrome)
- Progressive scoliosis of congenital or neurogenic origin without rib anomaly

See Figure 43-4.

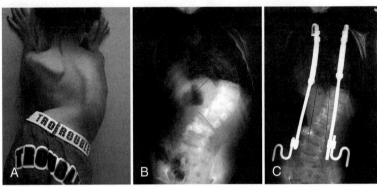

Figure 43-4. **A,** Five-year-old girl with a history of an omphalocele and progressive early-onset scoliosis resulting in pelvic obliquity. She had failed brace treatment. **B,** Standing posteroanterior view of the spine showing scoliosis and pelvic obliquity. **C,** Standing posteroanterior view of the spine after placement of bilateral percutaneous rib to pelvis vertical expandable prosthetic titanium rib (VEPTR) constructs. (From Smith JT. The use of growth-sparing instrumentation in pediatric spinal deformity. Orthop Clin North Am 2007;38:547–52.)

22. Describe the key procedural steps involved in placement of the VEPTR device.

- The procedure is performed with the patient in the lateral decubitus position
- A long J-shaped thoracotomy incision is made along the medial border of the scapula and curved anteriorly
- Additional incisions are required if a *rib to spine* or a *rib to iliac crest* construct is utilized in combination with or instead of a *rib to rib* construct
- The proximal site of attachment to the rib cage (superior cradle) is completed
- The distal site of attachment (rib cage, lumbar lamina, iliac crest) is completed
- Additional required procedures are performed as indicated including opening wedge thoracostomy and rib osteotomy
- The expandable portion of the device is inserted over the rib cage and underneath the skin and muscle and attached at the proximal and distal sites
- The device is expanded using distraction pliers. The devices are expanded on a regular schedule every 6 months

23. What complications are associated with use of the VEPTR device?

The most common complications are wound infection, skin slough, and device migration.

Key Points

1. Multilevel spinal fusion limits future increase in spinal height and restricts development of the thoracic cage and lung parenchyma in patients with early-onset scoliosis.
2. Growth-preserving surgical treatment options for early-onset scoliosis include dual growing rods and a vertically expandable prosthetic titanium rib (VEPTR).
3. Thoracic insufficiency syndrome is defined as the inability of the thorax to support normal respiration or lung growth.

Websites

Infantile scoliosis: http://emedicine.medscape.com/article/1259899-overview
Early-onset scoliosis: http://early-onset-scoliosis.com/default.aspx
Dual growing rod technique: http://www.cmj.org/periodical/PDF/201012058784220.pdf
VEPTR: http://www.synthes.com/html/uploads/media/080902-VEPTR_Montage_EN.pdf

BIBLIOGRAPHY

1. Akbarnia BA. Management themes in early onset scoliosis. J Bone Joint Surg 2007;89:S42–S54.
2. Akbarnia BA, Marks DS, Boachie-Adjei O, et al. Dual growing rod technique for the treatment of progressive early-onset scoliosis: A multicenter study. Spine 2005;30:S46–S57.
3. Bess S, Akbarnia BA, Thompson GH, et al. Complications in 910 growing rod surgeries: Use of dual rods and submuscular placement of rods decreases complications. J Child Orthop 2009;3:145–68.
4. Campbell RM, Smith MD, Mayes TC, et al. The characteristics of thoracic insufficiency syndrome associated with fused ribs and congenital scoliosis. J Bone Joint Surg 2003;85:399–408.
5. Campbell RM, Smith MD. Thoracic insufficiency syndrome and exotic scoliosis. J Bone Joint Surg 2007;89:S108–S122.
6. Dimeglio A. Growth of the spine before age 5 years. J Pediatr Orthop B 1993;1:102–7.
7. Gillingham BL, Fan RA, Akbarnia BA. Early onset idiopathic scoliosis. J Am Acad Orthop Surg 2006;14:101–12.
8. Sankar W, Skaggs D, Yazici M, et al. Growing Spine Study Group, Lengthening of dual growing rods: Is there a law of diminishing returns? J Child Orthop 2009;3:503–33.
9. Smith JR, Samdani AF, Pahys J, et al. The role of bracing, casting and vertical expandable prosthetic titanium rib for the treatment of infantile idiopathic scoliosis: A single-institution experience with 31 consecutive patients. J Neurosurg Spine 2009;11:3–8.

FDA Disclosures: The use of posterior spinal instrumentation for use in nonfusion constructs is not FDA approved.

PEDIATRIC SPINAL TRAUMA

Burt Yaszay, MD, and Behrooz A. Akbarnia, MD

GENERAL CONSIDERATIONS

1. **What are some anatomic differences between the immature and the adult spine that influence patterns of spinal injury presenting in the pediatric population?**
   Unique anatomic features of the immature spine include:
   - Hypermobility
   - Hyperlaxity of ligamentous and capsular structures
   - Presence of epiphyses and synchondroses
   - Incomplete ossification
   - Unique configuration of the vertebral bony elements (e.g. wedge-shaped vertebral bodies, horizontal cervical facet joints)
     The young child has a high head-to-body ratio that predisposes the polytraumatized child to cervical injury. The capacity for growth and the potential for injury to the growth plate contribute to the complexity of evaluation of the pediatric spine trauma patient.

2. **Why is it important to understand the normal growth and development of the spine when evaluating a child with a suspected spinal injury?**
   Knowledge of the developmental anatomy of the spine is important to avoid misdiagnosis of normal physes or synchondroses as acute fractures.
   - The **atlas (C1)** is formed from three ossification centers: the anterior arch and two posterior neural arches. The anterior arch is ossified in only 20% of newborns.
   - The **axis (C2)** is formed from five primary ossification centers. The area between the odontoid process and C2 body (dentocentral synchondrosis) commonly fuses by 6 years of age and may be confused with a fracture before this age. The tip of the odontoid (ossiculum terminale) typically fuses by age 12
   - The **subaxial cervical spine (C3–C7)** and the **thoracic** and **lumbar spine** develop in a similar pattern from three primary ossification centers. Secondary ossification centers can form at the tips of the spinous processes, transverse processes, and superior and inferior vertebral margins and may be misdiagnosed as fractures

3. **What are the most common injury mechanisms in children who sustain significant spine trauma?**
   Motor vehicle collisions, falls, and sports-associated injuries. Birth injuries and nonaccidental injury (child abuse) are less common but important injury mechanisms to consider.

4. **What are the relative strengths and weaknesses of plain radiographs, computed tomography (CT) scan, and magnetic resonance imaging (MRI) in the detection of cervical spine injuries in children?**
   Plain radiographs are typically the initial imaging test evaluated in the spine-injured child. A cervical spine series consists of a lateral film (the most diagnostic view of the series), an anteroposterior film (AP), and an open-mouth odontoid view. Anteroposterior (AP) and lateral radiographs of the thoracic and lumbar spine are obtained if there is concern regarding injury to these spinal regions. If faced with equivocal films or an uncooperative child with a mechanism of injury or physical examination that is suspicious for spinal injury, more advanced imaging is indicated. Plain radiographs can miss up to 25% of spinal injuries in children, typically those involving unossified tissues, such as the cartilaginous endplate. CT scanning is superior for the detection of bony injuries. The use of helical CT scans for evaluation from the head to pelvis in the polytrauma patient is commonplace and is more sensitive than plain radiograph for screening for spinal injury. MRI is superior for the detection of soft tissue injuries that may be missed by plain films and CT scans.

5. **What is SCIWORA?**
   SCIWORA is an acronym for **s**pinal **c**ord **i**njury **w**ithout **r**adiographic **a**bnormality. The spinal column in children is more elastic than the spinal cord. It has been demonstrated that the spinal column of an infant can be stretched up to 2 inches, whereas the spinal cord can be stretched only 0.25 inches before rupturing. SCIWORA injuries occur when a traction force (such as during difficult deliveries) is applied to the spine and accommodated by the spinal column but

exceeds the elastic limit of the spinal cord. This mechanism causes a damaging stretch injury to the cord that may result in complete tetraplegia. The typical site of injury is the cervicothoracic junction. SCIWORA is defined as an injury to the spinal cord without visible changes on plain radiographs or CT. This acronym was described prior to the widespread availability of MRI and is no longer accurate, as the presence of abnormalities on MRI is a common feature of this syndrome. MRI is the imaging study of choice to diagnose injury to the spinal cord and unossified tissues. Typical findings include acute hemorrhage and edema of the spinal cord, ligamentous injury, disc herniation, and physeal injuries.

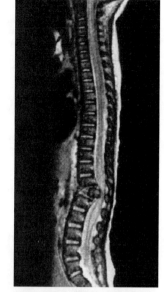

6. What common radiographic findings are noted in a child who has sustained a spine injury as a result of child abuse?

Most of these injuries involve the vertebral bodies, with varying degrees of anterior compression. Other findings include anterior notching of the vertebral body near the superior endplate, decreased disc height caused by disc herniation, as well as fracture-dislocation (Fig. 44-1). Injuries of the cervical region may occur, but injuries to the thoracolumbar and lumbar region are more common. Although vertebral body fractures and subluxations are injuries with moderate specificity for child abuse, if a history of trauma is absent or inconsistent with these injuries, they become high-specificity lesions.

7. How does the addition of a shoulder harness to a lapbelt influence the type of spinal injury sustained by a pediatric motor vehicle passenger?

Use of a lapbelt in isolation permits the belt to act as an anterior fulcrum leading to a flexion-distraction injury mechanism in the thoracolumbar spine. The additional of a shoulder harness to a lapbelt reduces this injury pattern by limiting forward flexion of the thorax during impact and reducing flexion-distraction forces on the lumbar spine. However, by restraining the thorax, a shoulder harness can increase the risk of cervical spine injuries in severe accidents. Children have a large head size relative to their body length and a higher center of gravity compared with adults. During impact, the forces acting on the unrestrained head are transmitted to the cervical spine when the thorax is restrained with a shoulder harness.

Figure 44-1. Magnetic resonance image of a fracture-dislocation of the spine occurring in a 10-month-old infant who was the victim of child abuse. The image reveals cord compression in this patient with incomplete paraplegia. (From Akbarnia BA. Pediatric spine fractures. Orthop Clin North Am 1999;30:531, with permission.)

CERVICAL SPINE

8. What is the correct way to immobilize a child during initial evaluation of a suspected traumatic cervical spine injury?

Because children have a large cranium in relation to their thorax, immobilization on a standard spine board will place the cervical spine in a flexed position. Use of a double mattress to elevate the thorax or use of pediatric spine board with a recess for the occiput is recommended to avoid undesirable displacement of cervical injuries.

9. What unique anatomic features of the immature cervical spine can lead to confusion during the evaluation of cervical radiographs following spine trauma?

Ten anatomic features of the pediatric cervical spine commonly cause confusion during spine trauma evaluation (Fig. 44-2).

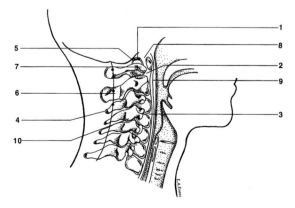

Figure 44-2. Ten unique features of the pediatric cervical spine that can cause confusion during the trauma evaluation: (1) the apical ossification center can be mistaken for a fracture; (2) the synchondrosis at the base of the odontoid can be mistaken for a fracture; (3) vertebral bodies appear rounded-off or wedged, simulating a fracture; (4) secondary centers of ossification at the tips of the spinous processes can be mistaken for a fracture; (5) the odontoid may angulate posteriorly in 4% of children; (6) C2–C3 pseudosubluxation (can be assessed with Swischuk's line); (7) the ossification center of the anterior arch of C1 may be absent in the first year of life; (8) the atlantodens interval may be as wide as 4.5 mm and still be normal; (9) the width of the prevertebral soft tissues varies widely, especially with crying, and may be mistaken for swelling; and (10) horizontal facets in young children can be mistake for a fracture. (From Flynn JM. Spine trauma in the pediatric population. Spine State Art Rev 2000;14:249–62, with permission.)

10. How does a child's age affect the pattern of traumatic cervical spine injury?

Before age 8 years, most cervical injuries occur at *C3 or above* and are associated with a high risk of fatality. After age 8, cervical injury patterns are similar to adults, occur *below the C4 level*, and are less likely to be fatal. Injuries in patients younger than 2 years are very rare and usually due to birth trauma or child abuse.

11. What is pseudosubluxation?

This is normal anterior translation that can occur between C2 and C3 and less frequently between C3 and C4 in patients younger than 8 years. This displacement is secondary to the increased ligamentous laxity and transverse facet orientation seen in young children. The *posterior cervical line (spinolaminar line of Swischuk)* is used to distinguish pathologic displacement from normal anterior displacement. A line is constructed connecting the anterior aspect of the spinous processes of C1 to C3. If the anterior aspect of the spinous process of C2 is more than 1.5 mm from this line, an injury should be suspected.

12. What is the most common cervical spine injury in children?

Odontoid fractures are the most common cervical spine injuries in children, with 4 years being the mean age of injury. The injury usually occurs as an epiphyseal separation of the growth plate at the base of the odontoid. Minimally displaced fractures are difficult to diagnose on plain film, making CT scan with reconstructions and MRI important diagnostic studies (Fig. 44-3).

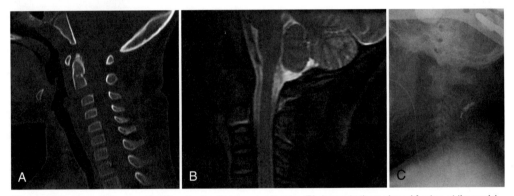

Figure 44-3. Computed tomography **(A)** and magnetic resonance imaging **(B)** demonstrating a physeal fracture at the caudal end of C2 with distraction between C2 and C3. This occurred in a 5-year-old unrestrained passenger involved in a motor vehicle accident. **C,** The patient was neurologically intact and was treated with C2–C3 posterior fusion and spinous process wiring followed by placement of a halo orthosis.

13. What is an os odontoideum?

An *os odontoideum* appears as a rounded piece of bone at the apex of the odontoid with a radiolucent gap separating it from the remainder of the axis and body of C2. Many consider os odontoideum to arise from a previously unrecognized injury. Unrestricted motion following this initial fracture leads to the development of a pseudoarthrosis. Clinical presentation may mimic an acute fracture.

14. Injury to what spinal ligament will result in atlantoaxial instability?

Injury to the transverse atlantal ligament will result in atlantoaxial (C1–C2) instability. This injury is suspected if the **atlanto-dens interval** is greater than 5 mm on a lateral cervical radiograph. Treatment remains controversial. A trial of nonoperative treatment for 10 to 12 weeks consisting of immobilization in a Minerva brace or halo is advocated by some experts. Other experts advocate immediate C1–C2 fusion. Surgery is required for patients with persistent instability despite orthotic treatment.

15. How is an occipitoatlantal dislocation diagnosed and treated?

This is generally a catastrophic and fatal injury, although survival is possible with early diagnosis and treatment. The dislocation may spontaneously reduce and remain unrecognized until traction is applied to the skull. Determining the **Powers ratio** on a lateral plain radiograph can reveal an anterior occipitoatlantal dislocation but is insensitive to posterior dislocation (Fig. 44-4). This ratio is calculated by dividing the distance from the basion (anterior margin of foramen magnum) to the posterior arch of the atlas by the distance from the opisthion (posterior margin of foramen magnum) to the anterior arch of the atlas. Ratios less than one are normal, whereas ratios equal to or greater than one indicate anterior occipitoatlantal dislocation. Additional reference lines that should be assessed are **Wackenheim's line** and **Harris lines**. Halo immobilization is recommended as soon as this injury is recognized. Definitive treatment consists of a posterior occipital-cervical fusion with halo vest immobilization.

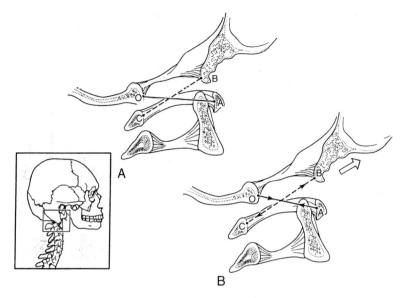

Figure 44-4. The Powers ratio is determined by means of drawing a line from the basion (B) to the posterior arch of the atlas (C) and a second line from the opisthion (O) to the anterior arch of the atlas (A). The length of the line BC is divided by the length of line OA. **A,** Values less than 0.9 are normal. **B,** A ratio greater than 1.0 suggests the diagnosis of anterior occipitoatlantal dislocation. (From Lebwohl NH, Eismont FJ. Cervical spine injuries in children. In: Weinstein SL, editor. The Pediatric Spine: Principles and Practice. 2nd ed. Philadelphia: Lippincott, Williams & Wilkins; 2001. p. 557, with permission.)

16. **What special measures should be taken when considering halo placement in a pediatric patient?**
    Special considerations are necessary, especially in very young patients, and include:
    - **Appropriate size halo ring:** a custom ring is often required and should be 2 cm larger than skull diameter
    - **Appropriate size halo vest or halo cast:** custom fabrication is often necessary
    - **Preapplication skull CT scan:** to assess skull thickness and location of cranial suture lines
    - **General anesthesia:** frequently required in the very young patient
    - **Appropriate number of pins:** less than 2 years use 10 to 12 pins; 2 to 7 years use 6 to 8 pins; and 8 year and older use 4 pins
    - **Appropriate pin torque:** less than 2 years use 2 in-lbs; 2 to 7 years use 4 to 5 in-lbs; 8 years and older use 8 in-lbs

THORACIC AND LUMBAR SPINE

17. **What are the common injury mechanisms and types of thoracic and lumbar fractures seen in the pediatric population?**
    Thoracic and lumbar fractures are rare in the pediatric population. Motor vehicle accidents, pedestrian-vehicle accidents, and falls are the most common injury mechanisms. The common fracture types are described as:
    - **Compression fractures:** present with isolated loss of anterior vertebral body height due to an injury mechanism associated with flexion and axial loading.
    - **Burst fractures:** present with loss of anterior and posterior vertebral body height due to an injury mechanism associated with axial loading. Retropulsion of bone into the spinal canal, posterior element fractures, posterior ligamentous injuries, and neurologic deficits may occur depending on the severity of injury.
    - **Flexion-distraction injuries:** present as a three-columns spinal injury due to application of flexion-distraction forces relative to a fixed axis (e.g. seat-belt). Neurologic injury and abdominal injury are frequently associated with this injury pattern.
    - **Fracture-dislocations:** present as the result of high-energy injury that completely disrupts the integrity of all three spinal columns and results in displacement of the spine in one or more planes. Severe neurologic injuries are associated with this fracture pattern.

18. **What is the appropriate treatment for a child with a Risser sign of 0 or 1 who sustains multiple compression fractures with less than 10 degrees of deformity in each vertebra and no neurologic compromise?**
    Studies following these patients to skeletal maturity have shown that no treatment is necessary in such patients. Children, especially those younger than 10 years of age, have excellent healing potential and usually reconstitute lost vertebral height in the sagittal plane in mild compression fractures. Patients who are older, have more than 10 degrees of deformity per vertebra, or have deformity in the coronal plane usually require treatment.

19. How are flexion-distraction injuries treated in children?

Injuries confined to bone both anteriorly and posteriorly generally heal without instability if treated nonoperatively in a thoracolumbosacral orthosis (TLSO) for 2 to 3 months. Bracing is usually successful if the initial kyphosis is less than 20°. Surgical treatment is indicated for:

- Unstable, purely ligamentous injuries
- Very unstable fractures that cannot be managed in a brace
- Fractures with significant kyphosis that cannot be reduced or maintained in a brace
- Fractures associated with neurologic injury or abdominal injury

The guiding surgical principle is to reconstitute a sufficient posterior tension band either with posterior wiring in small children or posterior compression constructs in older or larger children.

20. What are the two primary surgical indications for the treatment of pediatric burst fractures?

The first indication is partial or progressive neurologic deficit caused by spinal canal compromise. The mere presence of bone in the canal is not a sufficient indication for surgery because bone remodeling and reabsorption occur over time. The second indication is the prevention of late kyphotic deformity. More than 25° of localized kyphosis is generally accepted as an indication for surgery.

21. How does the treatment of burst fractures differ in children and adults?

Children and adolescents have strong bones with excellent healing potential. Late kyphotic deformity is less likely in children. Combined anterior and posterior fusions, which are commonly used for highly comminuted adult burst fractures, are rarely necessary in children. Children also have greater potential to remodel bone within the spinal canal than adults. In addition, children are less likely to suffer the detrimental effects of immobilization compared with adults. Otherwise, the basic principles of adult burst fracture treatment can be applied to children and adolescents.

22. What is the treatment for a fracture-dislocation of the thoracic or lumbar spine?

Posterior spinal instrumentation and fusion is the treatment of choice for all fracture-dislocations with or without neurologic deficit.

23. What is the risk of scoliosis following pediatric spinal cord injury?

The risk of scoliosis is dependent on the patient's age at the time of spinal cord injury and the timing of the injury in relation to the adolescent growth spurt. The prevalence of spinal deformity approaches 100% in patients who sustain a spinal cord injury prior to age 10. Surgical treatment typically involves a long spinopelvic fusion.

24. What is a limbus fracture? Where does it occur?

Fractures crossing the vertebral endplate in the immature spine are called **limbus fractures.** These fractures often traverse through the growth plate (hypertrophic zone) of the physis, in the same pattern seen in immature long bone injuries. This region is biomechanically weak and thus susceptible to injury. A limbus fracture should not be confused with a limbus vertebra, which represents herniation of nucleus pulposus through the vertebral endplate and beneath the ring apophysis.

25. What are the most common clinical and imaging findings in children with limbus fractures?

Most limbus (vertebral endplate) fractures occur in the lumbar spine at the L4–L5 and L5–S1 levels. Clinical presentation is similar to that of a herniated nucleus pulposus. Most patients have symptoms of stiffness and spasm, numbness, weakness, and occasionally neurogenic claudication. Infrequently, limbus fractures present with a cauda equina syndrome. Many patients have a positive Lasègue sign. Limbus fractures are difficult to visualize on plain radiographs. MRI, CT, or CT-myelography can be used to confirm the diagnosis.

26. What are the four types of vertebral endplate fractures? (See Fig. 44-5)

- **Type I:** Pure cartilage avulsion of the entire posterior cortical vertebral margin without attendant osseous defect
- **Type II:** Large central fracture of portions of the posterior cortical margin and cancellous bony rim
- **Type III:** More localized, lateral fracture of the posterior cortical margin of the vertebral body
- **Type IV:** Fracture that involves the entire length and breadth of the posterior vertebral body

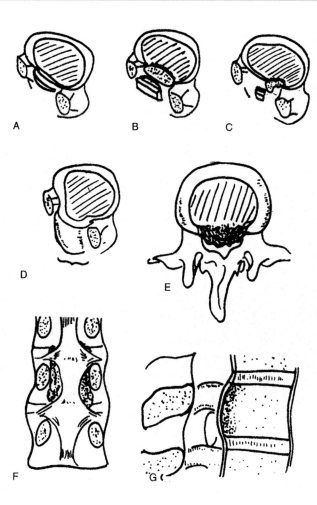

Figure 44-5. Fractures of the vertebral limbus. **A,** Type I—pure cartilage avulsion of the entire posterior cortical vertebral margin without attendant osseous defect. **B,** Type II—large central fracture of portions of the posterior cortical margin and cancellous bony rim. **C,** Type III—more localized, lateral fracture of the posterior cortical margin of the posterior vertebral body. **D–G,** Type IV—fracture that involves the entire length and breadth of the posterior vertebral body. The type IV fracture effectively displaces bone in the posterior direction, filling the floor of the spinal canal with a combination of reconstituted cortical bone and cancellous bone accompanied in part by scar formation. (From Akbarnia BA. Pediatric spine fractures. Orthop Clin North Am 1999;30:525, with permission.)

27. What treatment is advised for acute traumatic spondylolysis?

Treatment of traumatic spondylolysis is usually nonoperative. Nonoperative treatment consists of immobilization with a corset or TLSO, restriction from vigorous activity, and physical therapy for stretching of the hamstring muscles and strengthening of the abdominal musculature. If nonoperative treatment fails, various surgical options exist, including posterolateral fusion or direct bony repair of the pars defect supplemented with screw, wire, or screw-rod fixation.

Key Points

1. Up to age 8 years, children have a large cranium in relation to their thorax. The size of the cranium must be accommodated when pediatric patients are immobilized on a spine board to prevent excessive cervical flexion.
2. Normal variation and development must be considered when evaluating pediatric spine radiographs to avoid interpreting these findings as spinal injuries.
3. The elasticity of the immature spinal column exceeds the elasticity of the spinal cord. Pediatric spinal trauma may lead to tension-distraction injury with associated neurologic deficit.
4. Odontoid fractures are the most common pediatric cervical spine fracture.
5. In pediatric patients with symptoms suggestive of a disc herniation, the diagnosis of an apophyseal ring fracture should be considered.
6. Skeletally immature patients who sustain a spinal cord injury require surveillance for the development of spinal deformities.

Websites

1. Lumbar fractures: http://www.posna.org/education/StudyGuide/lumbarFractures.asp
2. Pediatric cervical spine: http://radiographics.rsnajnls.org/cgi/content/full/23/3/539?maxtoshow=&HITS=10&hits=10&RESULTFOR MAT=&fulltext=spine&andorexactfulltext=and&searchid=1&FIRSTINDEX=0&sortspec=relevance&resourcetype=HWCIT
3. Pediatric spinal cord and spinal column trauma: http://www.neurosurgery.org/sections/section.aspx?Section=PD&Page= ped_spine.asp
4. Pediatric spine trauma: http://www.orthonurse.org/portals/0/spinal%20cord%20injury%208.pdf
5. Thoracic fractures: http://www.posna.org/education/StudyGuide/thoracicFractures.asp

BIBLIOGRAPHY

1. Akbarnia BA. Pediatric spine fractures. Orthop Clin North Am 1999;30:521–36.
2. Antonacci MD. Spinal cord injury. In: Errico TJ, Lonner BS. Moulton AW, editors. Surgical Management of Spinal Deformities. Philadelphia: Saunders; 2009. p. 295–304.
3. Arlet V, Fassier F. Herniated nucleus pulposus and slipped vertebral apophysis. In: Weinstein SL, editor. The Pediatric Spine: Principles and Practice. 2nd ed. Philadelphia: Lippincott Williams & Wilkins; 2001. p. 576–83.
4. Bollini G. Thoracic and lumbar spine injuries in children. In: Floman Y, Farcy JC, Argenson C, editors. Thoracolumbar Spine Fractures. New York: Raven Press; 1993. p. 307–25.
5. Chambers HG, Akbarnia BA. Thoracic, lumbar, and sacral spine fractures and dislocations. In: Weinstein SL, editor. The Pediatric Spine: Principles and Practice. 2nd ed. Philadelphia: Lippincott Williams & Wilkins; 2001. p. 576–83.
6. Ferguson RL. Thoracic and lumbar spinal trauma of the immature spine. In: Herkowitz HN, Garfin SR, Eismont FJ, Bell GR, Balderston RA, editors. Rothman-Simeone The Spine. 5th ed. Philadelphia: Saunders; 2006. p. 603–12.
7. Flynn JM. Spine trauma in the pediatric population. Spine State Art Rev 2000;14(1):249–62.
8. Lebwohl NH, Eismont FJ. Cervical spine injuries in children. In: Weinstein SL. editor. The Pediatric Spine: Principles and Practice. 2nd ed. Philadelphia: Lippincott Williams & Wilkins; 2001. p. 553–66.
9. Limbrick DD, Leonard JC, Wright NM, et al. Cervical spine trauma in children including spinal cord injury without radiographic abnormality. In: Kim DH, Betz RR, Huhn SL, Newton PO, editors. Surgery of the Pediatric Spine. New York: Thieme Medical Publishers; 2008. p. 489–500.
10. Pouliquen JC, Kassis B, Glorion C, et al. Vertebral growth after thoracic or lumbar fracture of the spine in children. J Pediatr Orthop 1997;17(1):115–20.

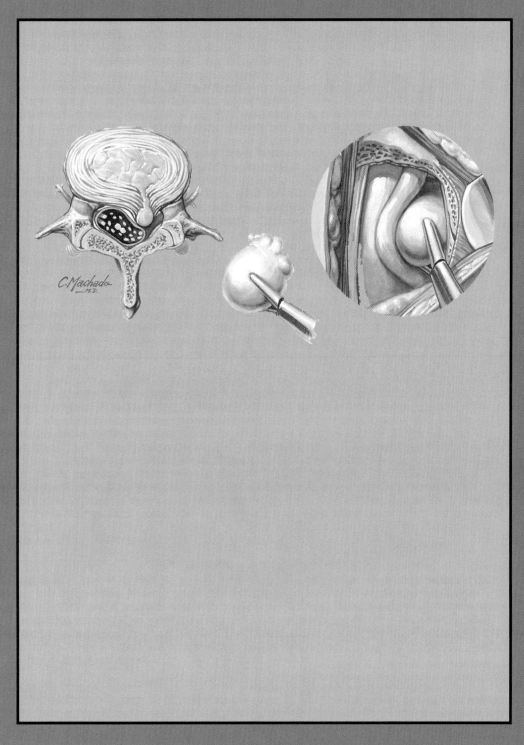

PATHOPHYSIOLOGY AND PATHOANATOMY OF DEGENERATIVE DISORDERS OF THE SPINE

Vincent J. Devlin, MD

1. What factors play a role in the development of degenerative disorders of the spine?

Spinal column degenerative changes are associated with increasing age but remain asymptomatic in many individuals. Mechanical, traumatic, nutritional, biochemical, and genetic factors interact and contribute to development of spinal degeneration. The relative importance of these factors varies among individuals and remains incompletely understood. Recent evidence suggests that disc degeneration is genetically determined.

2. Describe the morphology of the normal intervertebral disc.

The intervertebral disc consists of **three distinct regions:**

- The **annulus fibrosus** comprises the outer aspect of the disc and is composed of concentric rings (lamellae) of predominantly type 1 collagen. Fibroblast-like cells and elastin fibers are located between adjacent lamellae. Collagen fibers penetrate the endplate and attach the disc to the vertebral body
- The **nucleus pulposus** comprises the central disc region and consists of type 2 collagen and elastin embedded in a hydrated proteoglycan matrix that contains chondrocytes
- The **vertebral endplate** is the interface between the disc and the adjacent vertebral body and consists of a layer of condensed cancellous bone and an adjacent thin layer of hyaline cartilage. Disc metabolism and nutrition is dependent on diffusion of nutrients across the vertebral endplate (Fig. 45-1)

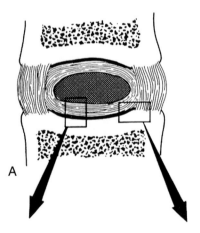

A

Figure 45-1. Intervertebral disc structure. **A,** Fibers of the annulus fibrosus are arranged in a concentric lamellar fashion and surround the nucleus pulposus. **B,** Magnified view of the central part of the disc. 1, nucleus pulposus; 2, annulus fibrosus; 3, horizontal disposition of the collagen fibers of the cartilaginous endplate; 4, bony endplate; 5, vascular channel in direct contact with cartilaginous endplate. **C,** Magnified view of the peripheral part of the disc. 6, outer fibers of the annulus fibrosus; 7, anchoring of the fibers to the bony endplate (Sharpey-type fibers). (From Kirkaldy-Willis WH, Bernard TH. Managing Low Back Pain. 4th ed. Philadelphia: Churchill Livingstone; 1999. Fig. 2-8 on p. 15.)

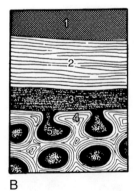

B

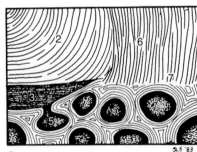

C

3. **What pathoanatomic changes occur in the spinal motion segment in association with the degenerative process?**
   There is loss of distinctness between the nuclear and annular regions in the disc. Loss of hydration of the nucleus pulposus occurs. Fissures develop in the annulus fibrosus. Thinning of the vertebral endplate occurs. Disc resorption and loss of disc space height develop. Disc function is compromised as the disc is no longer able to function hydrostatically under load resulting in abnormal force distribution across the spinal segment. This results in an increase in loading of the facet joints and may ultimately lead to facet arthrosis. Facet joint cartilage thinning, facet capsule laxity, hypermobility, facet subluxation, and facet joint hypertrophy may develop.

4. **What changes occur in the biochemistry of the disc with disc degeneration?**
   - **Annulus.** The ratio and relative distribution of type 1 to type 2 collagen changes in the outer annulus. A decrease in collagen cross-links occurs, making the annulus more susceptible to mechanical failure
   - **Nucleus.** Matrix changes occur including fragmentation of proteoglycans (mainly aggrecan), increase in the ratio of keratin sulfate to chondroitin sulfate, decreases in proteoglycan and water concentrations, and decrease in number of viable cells
   - **Endplate.** Thickening and calcification in the endplate region leads to decreased blood supply and impaired disc nutrition, which contributes to tissue breakdown in the endplate region and nucleus (Fig. 45-2)

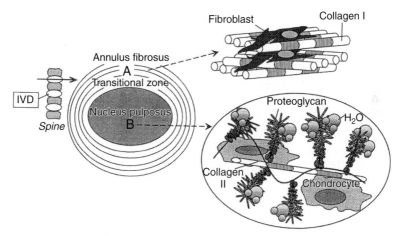

Figure 45-2. Microstructure of the intervertebral disc. The annulus fibrosus consists of densely packed layers of collagen type 1 fibers maintained by fibroblast cells. The fiber direction of each layer is perpendicular to the adjacent layer. The nucleus pulposus contains collagen type 2 fibers providing support, proteoglycan aggregates that attach water molecules, and chondrocytes that maintain the type 2 collagen and the proteoglycan matrix in which it is embedded. (From Chung SA, Khan SN, Diwan AD. The molecular basis of disc degeneration. Orthop Clin North Am 203;34:209–19. Fig. 1 on p. 210.)

5. **What are the clinical manifestations of degenerative spinal disorders?**
   The clinical manifestations of degenerative spinal disorders are wide ranging and may include axial pain syndromes, radiculopathy, myelopathy, and spinal instabilities. Spinal deformities may develop as the structural integrity of the motion segment is compromised by the degenerative process. Unisegmental spinal deformities (e.g. degenerative spondylolisthesis) or multisegmental spinal deformities (e.g. degenerative scoliosis or kyphosis) may develop.

6. **What are the major factors to evaluate in association with degenerative disease involving the cervical spine?**
   The important anatomic structures in the cervical spine involved by the degenerative process include the intervertebral disc, facet joints, neurocentral joints of Luschka, and ligamentum flavum. The adverse effects of the degenerative process may be exacerbated by abnormal motion segment mobility, congenital narrowing of the cervical spinal canal, ossification of the posterior longitudinal ligament (OPLL), and kyphotic deformity. The degree and extent of neurologic compression requires detailed evaluation with high-quality neurodiagnostic imaging studies. The common clinical syndromes associated with cervical degenerative disease include neck pain, radiculopathy, and myelopathy.

7. **Why are symptomatic thoracic disc herniations less common compared with cervical or lumbar disc herniations?**
   Symptomatic thoracic disc herniations represent less than 1% of all symptomatic disc herniations. Less than 2% of operations performed for disc herniation involve the thoracic spine. The low rate of symptomatic disc herniation is attributed to the limited mobility of the thoracic spine. Stability provided by the rib cage, costovertebral joints, and vertical orientation of the thoracic facet joints limits force application to the thoracic region and decreases the risk of disc degeneration. Thoracic disc herniations most commonly occur at the thoracolumbar junction, where the transition from a more stiff thoracic spine to a more mobile lumbar spine occurs.

8. **What is the degenerative cascade?**

The term **degenerative cascade** was introduced by Dr. Kirkaldy-Willis to explain the typical progression of lumbar spine degeneration. This process is conceptualized in terms of a **three-joint complex** composed of the intervertebral disc and two zygoapophyseal joints that comprise a **functional spinal unit,** the smallest anatomic unit of the spinal column that demonstrates its basic functional characteristics. The progression of degenerative changes involving the three-joint complex is conceptualized in terms of **three phases:** dysfunction, instability, and stabilization.

In the **first phase, dysfunction,** minor trauma or unusual activity leads to back pain. Segmental spinal muscles become tender and spastic. Circumferential tears in the annulus and degeneration of the nucleus occur. Synovitis and cartilage degeneration in the facet joints develop. Disc material may herniate into the spinal canal through an annular tear.

In the **second phase, instability,** progressive facet capsule laxity and internal disc disruption lead to segmental instability. Degenerative spondylolisthesis and dynamic lateral nerve root entrapment may develop during this phase.

In the **third phase, stabilization,** osteophytes develop around and within the facet joints and intervertebral disc. The ligamentum flavum may thicken and cause narrowing of the spinal canal. Central spinal stenosis and fixed lateral nerve root entrapment may occur (Fig. 45-3).

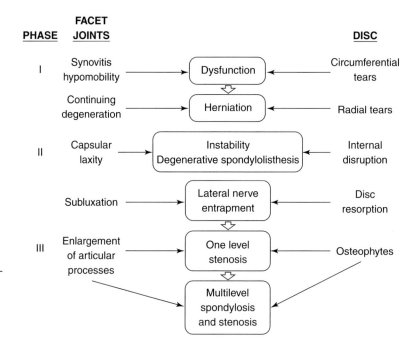

Figure 45-3. The degenerative cascade. Interactions between the facet joints and intervertebral disc during the three phases of degenerative spondylosis. (Adapted from Kirkaldy-Willis WH, Bernard TH. Managing Low Back Pain. 4th ed. Philadelphia: Churchill Livingstone; 1999. Fig. 13-2 on p. 250.)

9. **Explain why spinal deformities develop in the aging thoracic and lumbar spine?**

As an individual patient's spine passes through the degenerative cascade, the rate of degeneration may exceed the patient's ability to autostabilize the spinal column by formation of osteophytes around the facet joints and intervertebral disc. Risk factors remain incompletely understood but include osteoporosis, female sex, poor connective tissue quality, diabetes, and obesity. Disc height loss, facet subluxation, and asymmetric disc space collapse may occur. These changes may lead to deformity in the sagittal plane due to decrease in lumbar lordosis. Deformity may develop in the frontal and axial planes due to asymmetric disc space narrowing and development of rotatory subluxations and lateral listhesis between adjacent vertebrae. Narrowing of the central and lateral spinal canal may lead to lower extremity symptoms due to spinal stenosis. Deformity magnitude ranges from mild curvatures causing minimal symptoms to major deformities presenting with severe coronal and sagittal imbalance and symptomatic lumbar stenosis.

10. **What mechanical factors have been associated with disc degeneration?**

Disc degeneration has traditionally been linked to mechanical factors such as excessive or repetitive loading resulting in structural injury and subsequent development of axial pain symptoms. Factors traditionally associated with the occurrence of disc degeneration according to this *injury model* include age, occupation, male gender, cigarette smoking, and exposure to vehicular vibration. An observation cited to support a mechanical basis for disc degeneration is the development of degenerative changes adjacent to previous spinal fusions.

11. **How does genetics explain the development of disc degeneration?**

Finding from multiple studies including the Twin Spine Study have shown that disc degeneration is a condition that is *genetically determined* to a large degree. Research from the 1990s through the present has demonstrated familial patterns of disc degeneration. Genetic influences combined with yet unidentified factors play a significant role as risk factors for disc degeneration. The traditional factors associated with disc degeneration in the *injury model* had only a modest influence on disc degeneration in these recent studies. A variety of genes have been implicated in the development of disc degeneration including vitamin D receptor genes (Taq1 and Fok1), metalloproteinase-3-genes, and collagen type IX genes.

12. **Can psychosocial factors influence a patient's perception of axial pain associated with degenerative spinal disorders?**
Yes. A variety of factors have been shown to influence a patient's perception of axial pain associated with degenerative spinal disorders. When pathologic processes stimulate pain sensitive structures in the lumbar spine and pelvis, neural signals are transmitted through the dorsal root ganglion (DRG) to the spinal cord and ultimately to the brain for processing. Perception of these stimuli may be modulated by a variety of factors along the pathway of signal transmission. Psychologic and social factors have been demonstrated to influence this process. Such factors include chronic pain illness, depression, somatization (expression of emotional and psychologic symptoms in physical terms), and secondary gain (e.g. worker's compensation claims, litigation claims following motor vehicle accidents). One of the most challenging aspects in the evaluation and treatment of patients with degenerative spinal disorders is our poor understanding of why similar appearing degenerative changes may be asymptomatic in one patient but cause severe pain and impaired function in other individuals.

13. **What are some predictions regarding future therapeutic strategies for intervention in patients with degenerative spinal disorders?**
With increased understanding of the interplay of mechanical, biochemical, and genetic factors in the development of spinal degeneration, strategies that permit earlier intervention in the degenerative cascade will evolve. Current surgical technologies including instrumented spinal fusion will remain an option for treatment of the severe end-stage degenerative pathology. Clinical and basic science research efforts will lead to development of new treatment strategies that specifically target individual stages of the degenerative cascade:
- **Phase 1 (Dysfunction):** Genetic tests and/or blood markers for disc degeneration will be identified. Interventions for early degeneration of the nucleus pulposus to reverse the degenerative process may include injection of growth factors, gene therapy, or cell transplantation to the intervertebral disc. More advanced degeneration may be addressed by replacement of the disc nucleus. Interventions to address structural failure of the annulus fibrosus may include augmentation or repair of the annulus using laser, thermal, or tissue engineering technologies.
- **Phase 2 (Instability):** Segmental instability secondary to progressive disc degeneration and facet capsule laxity may be addressed by posteriorly implanted tethering devices to guide motion of the degenerated motion segment, thereby avoiding the need for fusion. Static or dynamic interspinous implants may provide a similar function. Use of artificial disc replacement technologies may become more widespread as technology evolves. Facet joint replacement technology may evolve and extend the indications for artificial disc replacement to patients with combined facet joint and disc degeneration.
- **Phase 3 (Restabilization):** Spinal stenosis requiring surgical decompression will be treated using advanced minimally invasive surgical techniques. Spinal stenosis associated with instability will be treated with minimally invasive decompression and fusion in combination with biologic agents to achieve high fusion rates with minimal approach-related morbidity.

Key Points

1. Mechanical, traumatic, nutritional, biochemical, and genetic factors interact and contribute to development of spinal degeneration.
2. Spinal degeneration occurs in all individuals and remains asymptomatic in many patients.
3. There is a poor correlation between the severity of degenerative changes on spinal imaging studies and the severity of spine-related symptoms.
4. The clinical manifestations of degenerative spinal disorders may include axial pain syndromes, radiculopathy, myelopathy, spinal instabilities, and spinal deformities.

Websites

Lumbar facet arthropathy: http://emedicine.medscape.com/article/310069-overview
Intervertebral disc degeneration: http://www.biomedcentral.com/content/pdf/ar629.pdf
Genetics of intervertebral disc degeneration: ftp://ftp.energy.wsu.edu/usr/EriHam/Genetics%20of%20disc%20degeneration.pdf

BIBLIOGRAPHY

1. Battié MC, Videman T, Kaprio J, et al. The twin spine study: Contributions to a changing view of disc degeneration. Spine J 2009;9:47–59.
2. Carragee EJ, Alamin TF, Miller JL, et al. Discographic, MRI and psychosocial determinant of low back pain disability and remission: A prospective study in subjects with benign persistent back pain. Spine J 2005;5:24–35.
3. Frymoyer JW. Lumbar disk disease: Epidemiology. Instr Course Lect 1992;41:217–23.
4. Polatin PB, Kinney RK, Gatchel RJ, et al. Psychiatric illness and chronic low back pain: the mind and the spine—which goes first? Spine 1993;18:66–71.
5. Singh K, Phillips FM. The biomechanics and biology of the spinal degenerative cascade. Semin Spine Surg 2005;17:128–36.
6. Urban JPG, Roberts S. Degeneration of the intervertebral disc. Arthritis Res Ther 2003;5:120–30.

CERVICAL DEGENERATIVE DISORDERS

Paul A. Anderson, MD, and Vincent J. Devlin, MD

1. Define cervical spondylosis. What causes it?

Cervical spondylosis is a nonspecific term that refers to any lesion of the cervical spine of a degenerative nature. Cervical spondylosis results from an imbalance between formation and degradation of proteoglycans and collagen in the disc. With aging, a negative imbalance with subsequent loss of disc material results in degenerative changes. Factors such as heredity, trauma, metabolic disorders, certain occupational exposures, and other environmental effects (e.g. smoking) can influence the severity of degeneration.

2. Describe the clinical conditions associated with cervical spondylosis.

Patients with symptomatic cervical spondylosis may present with neck pain (axial pain), cervical radiculopathy, or cervical myelopathy. Most patients with spondylosis have little or no pain. In patients who present with neck pain symptoms, it is unclear whether the spondylotic changes are responsible for pain.

3. Describe the degenerative changes seen on radiographs in patients with cervical spondylosis.

Degenerative changes noted on radiographs include narrowing of the intervertebral disc, sclerosis of the vertebral endplates, and osteophyte formation. As a result, the segmental range of motion is decreased. Similar changes may occur in the facet joints. Rarely, facet degeneration is advanced compared with degeneration of the intervertebral disc. Degenerative changes are observed most frequently at the C5–C6 and C6–C7.

4. Describe the relationship between facet degeneration and disc degeneration.

In the majority of cases, disc degeneration is thought to precede or occur simultaneously with facet degeneration. However, in some cases isolated facet degeneration may be present. Facet-mediated pain is especially prevalent in patients with hyperextension injuries such as rear-end motor vehicle accidents. Extension moments create high-contact forces in the facet joints, which can lead to chronic facet-mediated pain even in the absence of radiographic findings.

5. What is the prevalence of cervical spondylosis noted on radiographs obtained in *asymptomatic* patients?

Table 46-1

Table 46-1. Percent of Asymptomatic Population with Radiographic Changes by Age Group

20–30 years	31–40 years	41–50 years	51–60 years	61–70 years
5%	25%	35%	80%	95%

6. What is the prevalence of cervical spondylosis (i.e. cervical disc herniation, degenerative disc changes, cervical stenosis) noted on magnetic resonance imaging (MRI) in asymptomatic patients?

Table 46-2

Table 46-2. Percent of Asymptomatic Population with Spondylosis on MRI by Age Group

	AGE	
	<40 years	>40 years
Cervical disc herniation	5%	10%
Degenerative disc changes	25%	60%
Cervical stenosis	4%	20%

7. List common causes of chronic neck pain.
Common causes of neck pain include:
1. Degenerative disc and/or facet disease
2. Neurologic compression syndromes secondary to herniated discs or cervical stenosis
3. Cervical instability
4. Posttraumatic soft tissue or facet injury after whiplash
5. Inflammatory arthritis, such as rheumatoid arthritis or ankylosing spondylitis

8. Do patients with chronic neck pain improve with the passage of time?
A natural history study by Gore showed that, at 10 years, 79% of patients had less pain. Overall, 43% were pain-free, 25% had mild pain, 25% had moderate pain, and 7% had severe pain. The level of pain did not correlate with degenerative changes or other radiographic parameters. However, the pain level was correlated with the severity of the initial pain and whether onset was due to an injury. Chronic disabling symptoms were seen in 18% of patients.

9. Define cervical spinal instability.
Instability is present when the spine is unable to withstand physiologic loads, resulting in significant risk for neurologic injury, progressive deformity, and long-term pain and disability. Instability is not common in patients with cervical spondylosis except in those with stiffness in the middle and lower segments who develop compensatory hypermobility at C3–C4 or C4–C5. This condition can result in degenerative spondylolisthesis and lead to symptomatic cervical myelopathy. Cervical spinal instability may be diagnosed according to the radiographic criteria of White (>11° angulation, > 3.5 mm translation of adjacent subaxial cervical spine segments).

10. Is surgery indicated for chronic neck pain?
Indications for surgical treatment of patients with axial neck pain are uncommon. Surgery may be indicated for conditions such as instability, posttraumatic facet injuries, and C1–C2 osteoarthritis. Patients with discogenic-mediated neck pain secondary to degenerative disc disease can occasionally be treated surgically. Whitecloud has shown that 60% to 70% of patients improve following anterior discectomy and fusion. Before surgery, patients are evaluated by provocative cervical discography to confirm the source of pain. Poorer results are seen in litigation cases and cases involving more than two cervical levels.

11. List the typical signs and symptoms present in a patient with a symptomatic cervical disc herniation.
Signs and symptoms may include neck pain, radicular arm pain, weakness in a specific myotome, diminished sensation in a specific dermatome, and altered reflexes.

12. Which nonoperative treatment options are effective for cervical disc herniations?
Few studies evaluating the effectiveness of nonoperative treatment are available. A commonly accepted treatment is to decrease the associated inflammatory response with the use of nonsteroidal antiinflammatory drugs, oral corticosteroids, or epidural and selective nerve root steroid injections. Rest by use of an orthosis such as a soft collar and reduction of activities may be useful. Traction, physical therapy, and manipulation are frequently attempted but are often poorly tolerated in patients with acute cervical disc herniations.

13. List the surgical indications for patients with herniated cervical discs.
Indications for surgical treatment for a symptomatic cervical disc herniation include intractable radicular pain and neurologic changes, especially if they are progressive and interfere with quality of life. Neuroimaging studies should correlate with clinical symptoms.

14. What are potential surgical treatment options for a patient with a cervical herniated nucleus pulposus?
Surgical treatment options include:
- Posterior foraminotomy with discectomy
- Anterior discectomy and fusion
- Artificial disc replacement

15. Discuss the indications and results of posterior foraminotomy and discectomy for a herniated cervical disc.
Patients who have acute radiculopathy without long-standing chronic neck pain and posterolateral or intraforaminal soft tissue disc herniation are excellent candidates for posterior foraminotomies. The disc space height should be well preserved, and there should be no associated spinal instability. The advantages of this technique are avoidance of fusion and early return to function. The disadvantages are difficulty in removing pathology ventral to the nerve root, especially an osteophyte, and the potential for instability if more than 50% of the facet is removed. Satisfactory outcomes are seen in 85% to 90% of properly selected cases (Fig. 46-1).

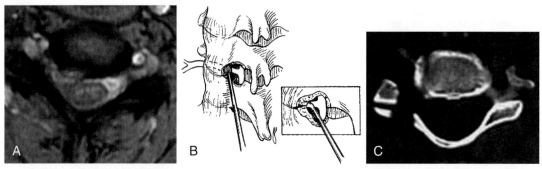

Figure 46-1. **A,** Magnetic resonance imaging shows a C5–C6 disc herniation. **B,** Posterior foraminotomy and discectomy were performed. **C,** Postoperative computed tomography scan shows extent of foraminotomy. (**B** and **C** from Herkowitz HN, Garfin SR, Eismont FJ, et al. The Spine. 5th ed. Philadelphia: Saunders; 2006. p. 843–4).

16. What are the advantages of using an anterior cervical plate after anterior discectomy and fusion?

Anterior cervical plate stabilization prevents graft collapse, maintains alignment (prevents local kyphosis), decreases postoperative brace requirements, and usually allows earlier return to activities such as work or driving. When fusion is performed at more than one level, fusion success and clinical outcome are improved with the use of an anterior cervical plate (Fig. 46-2).

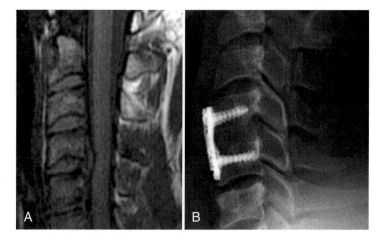

Figure 46-2. **A,** Sagittal magnetic resonance imaging shows a C4–C5 disc herniation. **B,** Surgical treatment with C4–C5 anterior cervical discectomy and fusion with allograft bone graft and anterior cervical plate.

17. What is the rate of pseudarthrosis after an anterior cervical discectomy and fusion procedure?

Pseudarthrosis rates strongly correlate to number of levels arthrodesed and whether anterior cervical fusion is performed with or without anterior plate fixation (Table 46-3).

Table 46-3. Pseudarthrosis Rates Following Anterior Cervical Fusion

Pseudarthrosis When Anterior Plate Is Not Used	
One-level fusion	0–5%
Two-level fusion	10%–20%
Three-level fusion	30%–60%
Pseudarthrosis When Anterior Plate Is Used	
One-level fusion	0–5%
Two-level fusion	0–3%
Three-level fusion	0–7%

18. Have allograft or interbody cage devices replaced autograft in the treatment of patients requiring cervical fusion?

Interbody spacer devices and allografts have been developed and used to avoid the morbidity of autogenous bone grafting. Similar fusion rates using autograft or allograft are reported for one-, two-, or three-level anterior cervical fusions performed with plate fixation. The efficacy of interbody cage devices is currently under investigation.

19. What are the indications for discectomy and interbody fusion versus corpectomy in patients requiring treatment of two-level cervical disc pathology?

Patients with two-level disease may be treated by discectomy and interbody fusion at both sites or by discectomies and removal of the intervening vertebral body (corpectomy), followed by strut grafting. Radiographic results in retrospective series are conflicting. Biomechanical studies strongly favor two-level discectomy over corpectomy. The authors' current recommendation is to perform corpectomy only when it is required to complete a neural decompression and when it enhances safety during removal of disc and bone pathology from a narrow spinal canal.

20. List common complications associated with anterior cervical discectomy and fusion.

Table 46-4

Table 46-4. Common Complications Associated with Anterior Cervical Discectomy and Fusion

Dysphagia	
Acute (<3 weeks)	35%
Chronic	8%–18%
Graft-related complications	
Collapse	10%–25%
Dislodgement	5%–10%
Nonunion	5%–30%
Implant-related problems	1%–5%
Neurologic injury	1%–3%
Spinal cord or nerve root injury	<1%
Recurrent laryngeal nerve injury	1%–2%
Superior laryngeal nerve injury	1%–2%
Horner's syndrome	<1%
Vertebral artery injury	<1%
Airway obstruction	<1%
Esophageal injury	<1%
Thoracic duct injury	<1%

21. Why does degeneration occur at spinal segments adjacent to a prior cervical fusion?

The causes of adjacent segment degeneration are:
1. Progression of the underlying degenerative disease process, which would occur regardless of whether spinal surgery was performed
2. Increased load and stress transfer, resulting in accelerated degeneration of the motion segment adjacent to a cervical fusion.

No clear evidence determines which process is the more important one.

22. What is the potential for development of degenerative changes adjacent to fused cervical spine segments?

Long-term studies after anterior cervical discectomy and fusion indicate that progressive radiographic degenerative changes occur in up to 50% of cases. The incidence of degenerative changes after anterior cervical fusion has been reported to exceed the rate predicted if fusion was not performed. Hilibrand documented development of new symptomatic radiculopathy or myelopathy in adjacent segments at a rate of 3% per year. Within 10 years after anterior cervical decompression and fusion, 26% of patients developed symptomatic radiculopathy or myelopathy.

23. What are the advantages and disadvantages of cervical disc replacement compared with anterior cervical discectomy and fusion in the treatment of cervical radiculopathy?

Cervical disc replacement is a motion-preserving procedure that uses the identical surgical approach and requires similar neural decompression as anterior cervical discectomy and fusion. Short-term results of cervical disc replacement (2–4 years) are at least equivalent to anterior cervical discectomy and fusion in appropriately selected patients. Longer term studies are necessary to determine whether cervical disc replacement will have a lower rate of adjacent segment degenerative changes than anterior cervical discectomy and fusion. Contraindications to cervical disc replacement include patients with facet arthrosis, kyphosis, prior laminectomy, metabolic bone disease, inflammatory arthritis, and insulin-dependent diabetes. Currently, cervical disc replacement is approved by the United States Food and Drug Administration (FDA) for use at a single disc level for treatment of cervical radiculopathy and select cases of cervical myelopathy (Fig. 46-3).

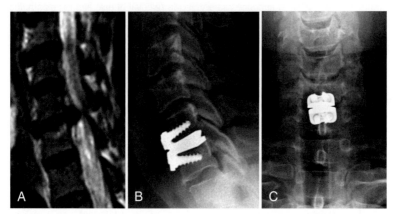

Figure 46-3. A, Sagittal magnetic resonance imaging shows a C6–C7 disc herniation. Treatment was anterior cervical discectomy and cervical disc arthroplasty. **B,** Lateral postoperative radiograph. **C,** Anteroposterior postoperative radiograph.

24. What is cervical myelopathy and how does it develop?

Cervical myelopathy is the most common cause of spinal cord dysfunction in patients older than age 55. Spinal cord dysfunction arises secondary to spinal cord compression, a diminished vascular supply, or both. In some patients, spinal cord compression occurs due to a congenitally narrowed spinal canal. In the majority of patients, spinal cord dysfunction occurs secondary to compression by degenerative changes associated with the normal aging process. Progressive cervical spondylosis may lead to spinal cord compression, which may be exacerbated by spinal instability (e.g. spondylolisthesis), especially at C3–C4 or C4–C5, kyphotic deformity, ossification of the posterior longitudinal ligament (OPLL), and large central disc herniations. Rheumatoid arthritis with associated instability involving the craniocervical, atlantoaxial, or subaxial spinal regions is an additional cause of cervical myelopathy.

25. What are the physical findings in patients with cervical spondylotic myelopathy?

Cervical spondylotic myelopathy is often slowly progressive. It is associated with nonspecific symptoms such as generalized fatigue, weakness, clumsiness of hands, loss of balance, gait disturbance, and rarely bladder or bowel impairment. Pain may be lacking or minimal. Physical findings include reduced neck motion, especially in extension; atrophy and weakness of muscles; muscle fasciculation; poor hand coordination; increased muscle tone; ataxia of gait; and the Romberg sign. Reflexes in the upper extremity are variable but are usually increased in the legs. Pathologic reflexes (e.g. Hoffman's sign, Babinski's sign) and clonus may be present. Abnormal pinprick and vibratory sensation indicates severe involvement.

26. Discuss the natural history of cervical myelopathy.

The natural history of patients with established cervical myelopathy is poor. Often there is a slow stepwise worsening with periods of neurologic plateau preceding another episode of deterioration. Rarely, patients present with acute deterioration or even quadriplegia.

27. Describe the typical radiographic and imaging findings associated with cervical spondylotic myelopathy.

A variety of spinal pathologies may result in cord compression and lead to subsequent development of myelopathy. Spinal pathology may occur at a single level or, more commonly, involve multiple spinal levels. Patterns of cord encroachment vary and include anterior-based compression, posterior-based compression, or circumferential compression. Many patients with myelopathy have a congenitally small spinal canal with a mid-sagittal diameter measuring less than 10 mm. Associated imaging findings may include anterior and posterior osteophytes, retrolisthesis (especially at C5–C6 and C6–C7), anterolisthesis (most common at C3–C4 and C4–C5), and acute soft tissue disc herniation. MRI may demonstrate focal or diffuse cord compression. Plastic deformation of the cord with decreased anteroposterior diameter and increased medial-lateral diameter may be noted. In 20% to 40% of cases, signal changes in the cord are present on MRI. If high signal is present only on T2-weighted images, this represents a broad range of pathology (e.g. edema) and may be reversible. It does not necessarily indicate a poor potential for recovery following surgery. If high signal is present on T2-weighted images and low signal is present on T1-weighted, this represents a severe gray matter lesion with a poor prognosis.

28. What are the indications for surgery for patients with cervical myelopathy?

Most patients with cervical myelopathy should be treated surgically, unless intervention is contraindicated by age or medical conditions. Increasing numbers of patients with cord compression on MRI but without neurologic symptoms or evidence of myelopathy are being evaluated. In the absence of objective findings or symptoms of myelopathy, such patients are best treated nonoperatively. However, they should be monitored with periodic examinations for the development of cervical myelopathy.

29. List the surgical options for patients with cervical myelopathy.

POSTERIOR PROCEDURES
- Laminectomy
- Laminectomy and posterior fusion combined with posterior spinal instrumentation
- Laminoplasty

ANTERIOR PROCEDURES
- Anterior discectomy or corpectomy and fusion combined with anterior spinal instrumentation

COMBINED ANTERIOR AND POSTERIOR PROCEDURES
- Anterior decompression and fusion combined with posterior fusion and posterior spinal instrumentation

The number of levels requiring treatment, anatomic location and cause of neural compression, cervical spinal alignment, presence/absence of instability, surgeon preference, and patient preference are the important factors that determine the surgical approach.

30. Why is laminectomy associated with poorer outcomes compared with anterior cervical decompression for the treatment of cervical myelopathy?

Outcomes after laminectomy deteriorate over time secondary to development of spinal instability and cervical kyphosis.

31. Discuss advantages and disadvantages of cervical laminectomy combined with posterior fusion and screw-rod instrumentation.

The addition of instrumentation and fusion can prevent postlaminectomy instability and improve neck pain. In addition, patients with flexible kyphotic deformities can undergo correction of their deformities following laminectomy by surgical repositioning and fusion in a more lordotic posture. Laminectomy and fusion provides a good alternative for select patients who require multilevel treatment for myelopathy associated with mechanical neck pain. Disadvantages of this approach include a higher rate of complications than alternative procedures such as laminoplasty (Fig. 46-4).

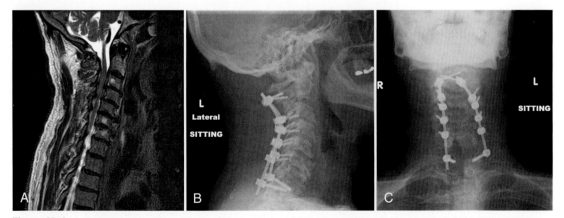

Figure 46-4. A 60-year-old man with severe progressive cervical myelopathy. **A,** Sagittal magnetic resonance imaging shows severe multilevel cervical stenosis, loss of lordosis and C4–C5 spondylolisthesis. Treatment consisted of C3 to C7 laminectomy and posterior spinal fusion with instrumentation C2 to T1. **B,** Lateral postoperative radiograph. **C,** Anteroposterior postoperative radiograph. Lateral mass screws were used from C3-C6 and pedicle screws were used at T1. *Continued*

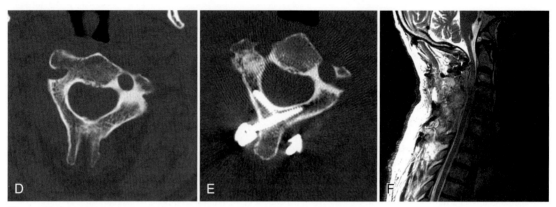

Figure 46-4, cont'd. D, Anatomy of the vertebral artery at the C2 level precluded safe C2 pedicle screw placement (note location of the vertebral artery foramen). **E,** C2 translaminar screws were utilized as an alternative for C2 fixation. **F,** Postoperative MRI shows adequate decompression of the spinal cord.

32. Discuss the indications for and results of cervical laminoplasty.

Laminoplasty increases the midsagittal diameter and cross-sectional area of the spinal canal. This procedure directly decompresses dorsal aspect of the spinal cord. It also allows posterior displacement of the cord, which indirectly decompresses its ventral surface. Accepted indications for laminoplasty are a straight or lordotic cervical spine, a stable spine, and multilevel cord compression. It is the preferred technique when only dorsal cord compression is present. Long-term improvement is seen in 60% to 75% of patients (Fig. 46-5).

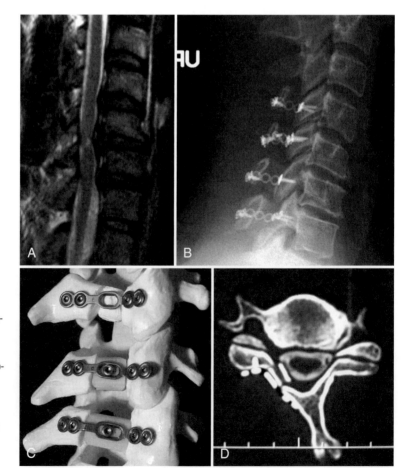

Figure 46-5. A 55-year-old man with cervical myelopathy. **A,** Sagittal magnetic resonance imaging shows severe multilevel stenosis due to congenital spinal canal narrowing and superimposed multilevel disc herniations. **B,** Lateral radiograph following C4 to C7 laminoplasty. **C,** Model demonstrates use of laminoplasty miniplates and allograft spacers that are used to hold open the hinge and maintain expansion of the spinal canal. **D,** Postoperative computed tomography myelogram demonstrates expansion of the spinal canal via allograft bone spacers and miniplate fixation. (**C** and **D** from Feigenbaum F, Henderson FC. A decade of experience with expansile laminoplasty: Lessons learned. Semin Spine Surg 2006;18(4):207–10.)

33. List the long-term morbidities associated with laminoplasty.

The limitations and morbidity of laminoplasty include loss of range of motion, chronic neck pain (up to 30% of patients), and recurrent stenosis. Acutely, 3% to 5% of patients develop a C5 motor neurapraxia. This complication may have a delayed onset and occur within 24 to 48 hours postoperatively. This complication resolves in two thirds of cases.

34. What are the indications for anterior cervical decompression and fusion for treatment of cervical myelopathy?

Anterior decompression and fusion is the most accepted treatment for cervical spondylotic myelopathy for patients with ventral cord compression. Reports indicate that 60% to 70% of patients experience improvement in neurologic function following surgery. Most surgeons perform anterior decompression for up to three levels of compression, although successful results have been reported with anterior decompression for four-or-five level pathology. Complications related to reconstruction increase significantly as more levels are treated.

35. What pitfalls are associated with the use of anterior cervical plates in conjunction with multilevel corpectomies?

Multilevel corpectomy constructs stabilized by anterior plates without use of supplemental posterior fixation are at high risk of failure due to:
1. Screw pullout at the inferior segment
2. Subsidence of the strut graft or cage into the vertebral body receptor sites
3. Graft or cage dislodgement
4. Pseudarthrosis

Biomechanical studies have shown that excessive forces occur at the caudal vertebral body screws. In multiple-level corpectomy constructs, subsidence from 1 to 3 mm at each level results in increased screw contact forces caudally. Resultant loss of fixation can lead to graft dislodgement with catastrophic failure of the construct. Additionally, graft resorption commonly occurs at the proximal and distal extent of the graft, where it contacts the vertebral body. If the construct is splinted by a plate, nonunion may result. For these reasons, anterior decompression and fusion combined with posterior spinal instrumentation (typically a screw-rod system) are recommended when multilevel cervical corpectomy procedures are performed—specifically, all three-level corpectomies and certain two-level corpectomies.

36. Are there any techniques that can be used to decrease the risk of construct failure when cervical corpectomies are performed and posterior instrumentation is not utilized?

Depending on the pattern of neurologic compression, a hybrid corpectomy-discectomy construct may be a feasible option and can increase the stability of the construct by increasing the number of screw fixation points below the corpectomy (Fig. 46-6).

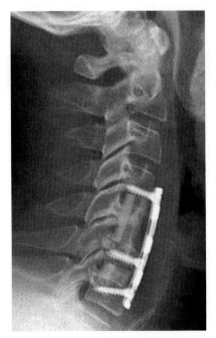

Figure 46-6. A corpectomy-discectomy construct. This patient with cervical myelopathy from three disc level disease was treated with C5 corpectomy and a C6–C7 anterior discectomy and fusion. This construct allowed for additional fixation into the intervening segment at C6 and provided greater stability compared with a two-level corpectomy of C5 and C6. (From Rhee JM, Riew KD. Evaluation and management of neck pain, radiculopathy and myelopathy. Semin Spine Surg 2005;17(3):174–185. p. 182.)

37. When are combined anterior and posterior procedures indicated for the treatment of cervical myelopathy ?

Common indications for combined anterior and posterior procedures are:
1. Postlaminectomy kyphotic deformities
2. Complex spinal deformities and instabilities
3. All three-level corpectomies and some two-level corpectomies (e.g. corpectomies ending at C7, patients with osteopenia)
4. Treatment of complex pseudarthroses

See Figure 46-7.

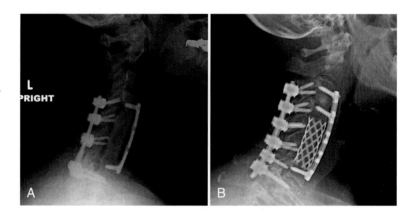

Figure 46-7. Circumferential cervical procedures. **A,** Anterior reconstruction following C5 and C6 corpectomy with fibula allograft and anterior plate combined with posterior instrumentation and fusion C4 to T1. **B,** Anterior reconstruction following two-level corpectomy and single-level discectomy using a hybrid anterior construct with titanium mesh C4 to C7 and allograft bone at C3–C4. Posterior instrumentation was extended from C3 to T1 to complete this circumferential construct.

Key Points

1. Cervical spondylotic changes are common with increasing age and may or may not be responsible for clinical symptoms.
2. To ensure optimal results for surgical treatment of radiculopathy, it is important that the patient's history, physical findings, and imaging studies correlate.
3. Surgical treatment is indicated for moderate or severe cervical spondylotic myelopathy unless medically contraindicated because there is no good nonsurgical treatment.

Websites

Cervical Spine Research Society. Patient information section: "Surgical indications and procedures for cervical myelopathy, radiculopathy and axial neck pain" www.csrs.org
American Academy of Orthopaedic Surgeons. Patient information section: "Cervical Spondylosis" www.aaos.org

BIBLIOGRAPHY

1. Gore DR. Roentgenographic findings in the cervical spine in asymptomatic persons: A ten-year follow-up. Spine 2001;26:2463–6.
2. Heller JG, Sasso RC, Papadoupoulos SM, et al. Comparison of BRYAN cervical disc arthroplasty with anterior cervical decompression and fusion: clinical and radiographic results of a randomized, controlled clinical trial. Spine 2009;34:101–7.
3. Hilibrand AS, Carlson GD, Palumbo MA, et al. Radiculopathy and myelopathy at segments adjacent to the site of a previous anterior cervical arthrodesis. J Bone Joint Surg 1999;81A:519–28.
4. Papadopoulos EC, Huang RC, Girardi FP, et al. Three-level anterior cervical discectomy and fusion with plate fixation—radiographic and clinical results. Spine 2006;31:897–902.
5. Rao RD, Currier BL, Albert TJ, et al. Degenerative cervical spondylosis: clinical syndromes, pathogenesis and management. J Bone Joint Surg Am 2007;89:1360–78.
6. Rao RD, Gourab K, David KS. Operative treatment of cervical spondylotic myelopathy. J Bone Joint Surg Am 2006;88:1619–40.
7. Rhee JM, Yoon T, Riew KD. Cervical radiculopathy. J Am Acad Orthop Surg 2007;15:486–94.
8. Samartzis D, Shen FH, Matthews DK, et al. Comparison of allograft to autograft in multilevel anterior cervical discectomy and fusion with rigid plate fixation. Spine J 2003;3:451–9.
9. Troyanovich SJ, Stroink AR, Kattner KA, et al. Does anterior plating maintain cervical lordosis versus conventional fusion techniques?: A retrospective analysis of patients receiving single-level fusions. J Spin Disord Tech 2002;15:69–74.

CHAPTER 47

THORACIC DISC HERNIATION AND STENOSIS

Jeffrey E. Deckey, MD, and Vincent J. Devlin, MD

1. Is thoracic disc herniation a common clinical problem?

No. The incidence of symptomatic thoracic disc herniation has been reported as 1 per million patients. It is estimated that 0.15% to 4% of all symptomatic disc protrusions occur in the thoracic spine. However, magnetic resonance imaging (MRI) and computed tomography (CT) myelogram studies have shown a prevalence of thoracic disc herniation ranging between 11% and 37% based on imaging studies performed in asymptomatic patients. Imaging studies alone cannot be used to select patients for operative treatment because more than 70% of asymptomatic adults will have positive anatomic findings on thoracic spine MRI studies (disc herniation, disc bulging, annular tear, spinal cord deformation, Scheuermann end plate irregularities, or kyphosis).

2. Describe the clinical presentation of a symptomatic thoracic disc herniation.

Peak incidence occurs in the fifth decade. Males and females are equally affected. Degenerative changes are considered to be the major factor responsible for thoracic disc herniation. An association between Scheuermann's disease and thoracic disc herniation has been reported. Trauma plays a role as a precipitating or aggravating factor in a small percentage of cases. The clinical presentation is variable and can include axial pain, radicular pain, and/or myelopathy. Axial thoracic pain is typically mechanical in nature but is sometimes confused with cardiac, pulmonary, or abdominal pathology. Radicular complaints most commonly consist of pain radiating around the chest wall along the path of an intercostal nerve but occasionally may include groin pain or lower extremity pain. Myelopathy may develop as a result of spinal cord compression. Careful examination for upper motor neuron signs can lead to the diagnosis of myelopathy. Findings may include a Romberg sign, Babinski reflex, clonus, ataxic gait, lower extremity motor weakness, loss of rectal tone, or decreased perianal sensation. T1–T2 disc herniations may mimic a cervical disc herniation and lead to intrinsic hand weakness and a Horner's syndrome.

3. At what spinal level do thoracic disc herniations most commonly occur?

Thoracic disc herniation can occur at any level in the thoracic spine. Disc herniation is most common in the lower third of the thoracic spine with the highest percentage reported at the T11–T12 level.

4. Which imaging modalities are useful in the diagnosis of a thoracic disc herniation?

Standard plain radiographs should be performed to rule out osseous abnormalities such as tumors, deformities, or fractures. In addition, plain radiographs are essential as an intraoperative reference to determine if the surgeon is operating at the correct level. MRI is the best imaging modality for assessment of the thoracic vertebra, intervertebral discs, and neural elements. CT myelography is helpful for assessment of patients who are unable to undergo MRI. CT myelography can complement MRI in patients who require surgical intervention by providing accurate assessment of the degree of spinal cord compression and determining whether calcification of the disc or posterior longitudinal ligament is present.

5. What are some important features of thoracic disc herniations to describe when reviewing a thoracic MRI?

A thoracic disc herniation is present when disc material extends beyond the posterior margin of the vertebral endplate and encroaches on the space available for the spinal cord and/or nerve roots. Important features to describe include level of herniation; disc location with respect to the spinal canal (central, paracentral, lateral), presence/absence of spinal cord compression, and the presence/absence of calcification within the disc herniation. See Figure 47-1.

6. How is treatment for a thoracic disc herniation determined?

Treatment of a thoracic disc herniation is individualized based on the patient's symptoms, physical examination, and radiologic findings.

7. What treatment is recommended for an asymptomatic thoracic disc herniation noted on thoracic MRI?

Asymptomatic disc herniations require no treatment. The natural history of asymptomatic disc herniations is not fully defined.

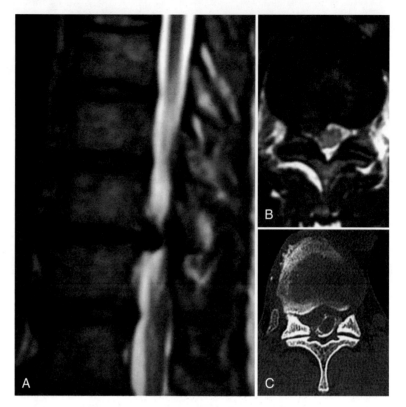

Figure 47-1. Preoperative imaging demonstrating a right paracentral disc herniation at the T11–T12 level. **A,** T2-weighted sagittal view of magnetic resonance imaging (MRI). **B,** T2-weighted axial view of MRI. **C,** Computed tomography myelogram. (From Sasai K, Adachi T, Togano K, et al. Two level disc herniation in the cervical and thoracic spine presenting with spastic paresis in the lower extremities without clinical symptoms or signs in the upper extremities. Spine J 2006;6:464–7.)

8. **What treatment is recommended for a symptomatic thoracic disc herniation without myelopathy?**
   Symptomatic disc herniations without myelopathy are initially treated nonoperatively. Clinical presentations vary, and symptoms are often vague. Acute disc herniations resulting in axial pain may be treated with activity modification, nonsteroidal antiinflammatory drugs, and short-term opiates. In patients with radicular complaints, oral corticosteroids, nerve blocks, and/or epidural steroid injections are considered. This approach often provides sufficient pain relief to permit initiation of physical therapy.

9. **When is surgical treatment considered for thoracic disc herniation?**
   Surgery is indicated for thoracic disc herniations associated with myelopathy and for select thoracic disc herniations associated with radiculopathy in patients who fail to improve with nonoperative treatment. Surgery for axial back pain associated with thoracic disc disease is controversial.

10. **What are the surgical approach options for treatment of a symptomatic thoracic disc herniation?**
    Surgical approach options include the anterior transthoracic approach, posterolateral approaches (transfacet, transpedicular, transforaminal, costotransversectomy), and lateral approaches (lateral extracavitary). The exposure of the thoracic disc provided by each approach is shown in Figure 47-2. The posterior laminectomy approach has been abandoned due to poor outcomes and associated high rate of neurologic injury.

11. **What factors are considered in selection of the most appropriate approach for treatment of a thoracic disc herniation?**
    Various factors are considered when selecting the most appropriate surgical approach for a thoracic disc herniation including:
    1. Location of the herniation in relation to the spinal cord (central, paracentral, lateral)
    2. Level of the herniation (the upper and lower ends of the thoracic region are more challenging to approach via thoracotomy)
    3. Patient's underlying medical condition
    4. Number of disc levels requiring treatment
    5. Surgeon's familiarity with various spinal approaches
    An anterior approach is preferred for central disc herniations and can be used for any type of disc herniation as direct access to the entire disc space is possible. In the middle and distal thoracic region, a standard thoracotomy approach is used. Exposure of the upper thoracic spine is more challenging. The T1–T2 and T2–T3 discs are typically exposed

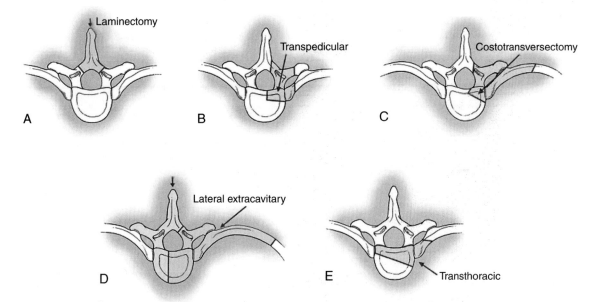

Figure 47-2. **A,** Exposure of thoracic disc provided by standard laminectomy. **B,** Transpedicular approach. **C,** Costotransversectomy approach. **D,** Lateral extracavitary approach. **E,** Transthoracic approach. (Redrawn from Fessler RG, Sturgill M. Review: complications of surgery for thoracic disc disease. Surg Neurol 1998;49:609. From Canale ST, Beaty J, editors. Campbell's Operative Orthopaedics. 11th ed. Philadelphia: Mosby; 2007. Fig. 39-90.)

via a low anterior cervical approach, but modifications such as resection of the medial clavicle or manubrium may be necessary depending on body habitus. Other anterior approach options in the upper thoracic region include a third rib thoracotomy or a transsternal approach. Video-assisted thoracoscopic surgery (VATS) is an additional approach option for appropriately trained and experienced surgeons.

Posterolateral approaches are an option for lateral or paracentral disc herniations but are suboptimal for central disc herniations because the spinal cord cannot be retracted or mobilized without injury. A transfacet approach provides good access to foraminal disc herniations by creating an approach window in the facet joint at the level and side of the disc herniation. Minimally invasive thoracic microdiscectomy is an additional option that utilizes a more lateral approach to access the thoracic disc via the neural foramen and lateral aspect of the facet complex. This approach has been reported to minimize approach-related morbidity and permits preservation of the majority of the facet complex.

12. How does the surgeon determine the correct surgical level intraoperatively?
Intraoperative determination of the correct surgical level is crucial. Often MRI scout films number the spine counting from C1 downward. Intraoperatively, however, it is often easier to count vertebrae upward from the sacrum or to use the ribs as a reference. Preoperatively, a scout film on MRI should be performed counting from the lumbar spine upward. In addition, anteroposterior and lateral radiographs of the thoracic and lumbar spine should be obtained to determine the number of thoracic and lumbar vertebra present. The ribs should be numbered to correspond with appropriate thoracic levels. In the thoracic spine, the first, eleventh, and twelfth ribs usually articulate only with their corresponding vertebral bodies. Between T2 and T10, the rib heads articulate with the corresponding vertebral body, as well as the proximal vertebral body, and overlie the intervening disc space.

13. At which level should a thoracotomy be performed for a transthoracic disc resection?
A chest radiograph can be used to determine the slope of the ribs in the thoracic spine. Usually, a thoracotomy is performed one or two levels above the target disc space. This strategy allows a parallel approach to the disc space, thus permitting the use of a microscope if desired. Alternatively, a minithoracotomy can be performed to attempt to decrease approach-related morbidity. The posterior portion of the rib leading to the target disc space is removed (e.g. remove the posterior portion of the ninth rib to access a T8–T9 disc herniation).

14. Is a fusion necessary after thoracic discectomy?
Fusion after thoracic discectomy is controversial. Currently, the addition of a fusion should be considered in cases of multilevel discectomy or underlying Scheuermann's disease with kyphosis and when a significant amount of the vertebral body must be resected to decompress the spinal cord. Instrumentation should be considered when instability is present and when a significant portion of a vertebral body is removed to access the spinal canal.

15. What complications can occur after surgery for thoracic disc herniation?

Complications can include death, deterioration of neurologic function (including complete paralysis), kyphotic deformity, pseudarthrosis, instrumentation failure, and infection, as well as medical and anesthetic complications.

16. Can spinal stenosis occur in the thoracic region?

Yes. Spinal stenosis can occur in the thoracic region although it is much less common than cervical or lumbar spinal stenosis. Thoracic spinal stenosis occurs most commonly in the T10 to T12 region due to acquired degenerative changes superimposed on preexisting developmental canal narrowing. Hypertrophic spondylosis and ossification of the posterior longitudinal ligament and ligamentum flavum may lead to circumferential narrowing of the lower thoracic spinal canal. A wide range of neurologic dysfunction may occur as the lower thoracic spinal canal contents include the lumbosacral spinal cord segments, conus medullaris, as well because the lower thoracic and lumbosacral nerve roots. Symptoms may include both upper and lower motor neuron lesions, claudication, lower extremity pain, back pain, and cauda equina symptoms.

17. What are the surgical treatment options for thoracic spinal stenosis?

Surgical treatment requires decompression of all stenotic levels diagnosed on preoperative imaging studies. If stenosis is the result of predominantly anterior pathology (e.g. disc-based osteophytes) and limited to one or two spinal segments, anterior decompression and fusion is an option. If stenosis is predominantly due to facet and/or ligamentum hypertrophy or extends over multiple levels, a posterior approach with laminectomy is reasonable. Posterior fusion and instrumentation are added when decompression involves multiple levels and especially when decompression crosses the thoracolumbar junction.

Key Points

1. Thoracic disc herniations associated with neurologic deficit are rare lesions with an estimated incidence of one per million population.
2. There is a high prevalence of anatomic abnormalities noted on thoracic spine MRI studies in asymptomatic patients.
3. An anterior transthoracic surgical approach is preferred for central thoracic disc herniations.
4. Posterolateral surgical approaches are an option for paracentral and lateral thoracic disc herniations.
5. Spinal stenosis can present in the thoracic region and typically occurs at the thoracolumbar junction.

Websites

Treatment of thoracic disc herniation: http://www.medscape.com/viewarticle/405650
Guidelines for treatment of thoracic disc herniation: http://www.mdguidelines.com/displacement-thoracic-intervertebral-disc-without-myelopathy

BIBLIOGRAPHY

1. Anand N, Regan JJ. Video-assisted thoracoscopic surgery for thoracic disc disease: classification and outcome study of 100 consecutive cases with a two year minimum follow-up period. Spine 2002;27:871–9.
2. Awwad EE, Martin DS, Smith KR Jr, et al. Asymptomatic versus symptomatic herniated thoracic discs: their frequency and characteristics as detected by computed tomography after myelography. Neurosurgery 1991;28:180–6.
3. Currier BL, Eismont FJ, Green BA. Transthoracic disc excision and fusion for herniated thoracic discs. Spine 1994;19:323–8.
4. Palumbo MA, Hilibrand A, Hart R, et al. Surgical treatment of thoracic spinal stenosis: two to nine year follow-up. Spine 2001;26:558–66.
5. Sheikh H, Samartzis D, Perez-Cruet MJ. Techniques for the operative management of thoracic disc herniation: minimally invasive thoracic microdiscectomy. Orthop Clin North Am 2007;38:351–61.
6. Simpson JM, Silveri CP, Simeone FA, et al. Thoracic disc herniation: re-evaluation of the posterior approach using a modified costotransversectomy. Spine 1993;18:1872–7.
7. Vanichkachorn JS, Vaccaro AR. Thoracic disk disease: diagnosis and treatment. J Am Acad Orthop Surg 2000;8:159–69.
8. Wood KB, Blair J, Aepple D, et al. The natural history of asymptomatic thoracic disc herniations. Spine 1997;22:525–9.
9. Wood KB, Garvey TA, Gundry C, et al. Magnetic resonance imaging of the thoracic spine. J Bone Joint Surg 1995;77A(11):1631–8.

LOW BACK PAIN: ASSESSMENT AND INITIAL MANAGEMENT

Maury Ellenberg MD, FACP, and Michael Ellenberg, MD

CHAPTER 48

1. Is low back pain (LBP) a common problem?

Yes. Epidemiologic studies show that by the age of 20, 50% of the population has experienced LBP. By age 60, the cumulative incidence is over 80%. It is present in all societies and cultures, although it may be experienced differently.

2. Define acute, subacute, and chronic LBP.

Acute LBP is defined as LBP lasting less than 3 months. The term **subacute** LBP is sometimes used to refer to LBP with a duration of 6 to 12 weeks. LBP lasting more than 3 months is defined as **chronic** LBP. The distinction between acute and chronic LBP is important because their natural history, treatment, and prognosis are different. Traditionally, 90% of patients with acute LBP experience resolution of symptoms while 5% to 10% of patients progress to chronic LBP. Recent studies report that a significant percentage of patients who present with acute LBP continue to experience recurrent or persistent symptoms.

3. What are the most common diagnoses in patients who present with LBP?

A specific abnormality or disease is not identified in up to 85% of patients who present with LBP resulting in the diagnosis of **nonspecific** LBP. In another subset of patients, LBP is associated with **specific spine pathology** such as compression fracture, spondylolisthesis, ankylosing spondylitis, malignancy, or infection. LBP may be a presenting symptom in patients with spinal stenosis or lumbar disc herniation. LBP may also originate from **nonspinal causes** such as:

- Visceral disease (e.g. renal stones, pancreatitis, aortic aneurysm)
- Myofascial disease (e.g. fibromyalgia)
- Hip joint arthritis
- Sacroiliac joint pathology

4. Are there really no detectable abnormalities in people with so-called nonspecific LBP?

There are many spinal abnormalities in patients who present with LBP. However, there is no conclusive evidence that these abnormalities are responsible for the patient's complaints. Clinical studies have shown a poor correlation between spinal radiographic abnormalities and LBP. More recently, as computed tomography (CT) and magnetic resonance imaging (MRI) of the spine evolved, additional abnormalities became visible including facet arthrosis, disc desiccation, and anular tears. In an attempt to determine whether these findings reflect natural progression of aging or symptomatic pathology, a variety of interventional techniques were introduced to sort out which anatomic structure is the pain generator. These techniques include discograms, zygapophyseal joint (z-joint) injections, medial branch injections, and sacroiliac joint injections. These techniques remain controversial and may only be able to differentiate a specific pain generator in a reliable patient who does not have psychologic, legal, or monetary reinforcers.

5. What is the most important tool to assess patients with LBP?

Believe it or not, the history and physical examination remain the mainstays of evaluation of LBP despite the many new expensive technologies that are available.

6. What elements of the patient's history are most important?

The patient's medical history is vital and should be comprehensive. Determine the onset and duration of the problem; the reason it occurred (if any); its relation to work, automobile, or other injury; if litigation is involved; and if there is financial remuneration. Define the pain carefully: its location, relationship to position and activity, and time of day it is most prominent. Determine if there are associated symptoms such as pain in an extremity, numbness, or tingling. *Red flags* that may indicate serious pathology include bowel or bladder dysfunction, history of cancer, and generalized disorders such as end-stage renal disease, osteoporosis, Paget's disease, HIV/AIDS, or intravenous drug abuse. Red flags warrant consideration of further investigation such as laboratory tests or imaging studies. See red flags on next page.

LOW BACK PAIN RED FLAGS

- Fever
- Unexplained weight loss
- Cancer history
- Significant trauma
- Alcohol or drug abuse

- Osteoporosis
- Age older than 50 years
- Failure to improve with treatment
- Nonmechanical pain

7. **Describe the key points in the physical examination of a patient with LBP.**
   Examination should assess the lumbar spine, pelvis, and lower extremities. Key examination points include:
   - **Lumbar range of motion (ROM),** for asymmetric movement, re-creation of pain, and areas of limited or guarded motion (spasm)
   - **Tenderness**, especially percussion tenderness over bony areas in the back and pelvis, palpate for tenderness over the sacroiliac joint and greater trochanter
   - **Gait and balance,** include heel-toe walking and squatting and returning to the upright position. Evaluate for Trendelenburg gait
   - **Lower extremity ROM,** assess for symmetry of motion and muscle tightness, especially in the hamstrings and quadriceps. Painful and limited hip motion is a tip-off for hip osteoarthritis
   - **Neurologic examination,** assess reflexes, strength, and sensation
   - **Peripheral vascular examination**, assess dorsalis pedis and posterior tibial pulses
   - **Abdominal examination,** back pain accompanied by additional symptoms such as abdominal pain, nausea, vomiting, or groin pain requires further evaluation to rule out problems such as renal stones, hernia, or abdominal aortic aneurysm

8. **When are imaging and laboratory studies important in the evaluation of patients with LBP?**
   Imaging studies are utilized to exclude severe disease. They are indicated if red flags or neurologic deficits are present or if there is little improvement after several weeks of treatment. The initial study is often plain radiography, which has low sensitivity and specificity in identifying symptomatic spinal pathology. MRI is the best study for comprehensive evaluation of the lumbar spine, but patients should be cautioned regarding the high incidence of age-appropriate degenerative changes that will be detected. Other imaging tests that can be considered are CT scans and technetium bone scans. Laboratory studies including complete blood count (CBC), erythrocyte sedimentation rate (ESR), and C-reactive protein (CRP) are important in the evaluation of suspected infection or tumor.

9. **Is disability from LBP common?**
   Patients with disability from LBP present a very different picture than patients with acute, acute recurrent, or even chronic LBP who are still functioning in daily life. Despite improvement in diagnostic and treatment techniques, disability from LBP has risen astronomically in the past few decades (as much as 2500%). The medical community must look beyond a purely physical explanation for this rise. Patients with disability from LBP that occurred either spontaneously, or more commonly from an injury, must also be assessed from a psycho-emotional, social, and vocational viewpoint.

10. **What are signs to look for in identifying the *disability syndrome*?**
    The most common associations that indicate disability from an injury are *not* physical ones. The best predictors are history of prior injury with time off work, high Minnesota Multiphasic Personality Inventory (MMPI) scale 3 (hysteria), and high work dissatisfaction scales. History and physical examination features that may help identify this syndrome include past episodes of back pain that led to disability, a long history of tests and surgical procedures, and a very detailed description of the event that generated the problem. Usually the patient reports that someone or something is at fault (e.g. oil on the floor, extra work that the patient was not supposed to do). Pain is often rated as very severe, such as 9 or 10 on a 0 to 10 scale, with 10 being excruciating pain. The patient may indicate a 10-level pain while sitting comfortably in no apparent distress. Certain patients may be very demonstrative, grimace, position their body in unusual ways, complain of pain with minor movements, and exhibit bizarre gait patterns. Evaluation of Waddell's signs is useful and indicates that organic abnormality is not the sole factor responsible for the patient's symptoms. These signs do not prove malingering but show that factors other than physical issues are significant contributors.

SIGNS (WADDELL AND OTHERS) THAT LBP IS NOT ORGANIC

- Simulated axial loading—pressure on the neck leading to LBP
- Simulated rotation—neck extension or rotation with back motion leading to LBP
- General overreaction to physical examination
- Superficial tenderness

- Regional weakness (not following anatomic patterns)
- Widespread nonanatomic distribution of pain
- Regional sensory deficit (not following anatomic patterns)
- Distracted straight-leg raising (e.g. sitting position vs. supine)

11. How does the physician treat a patient with acute LBP?

Generally, the offending structure is not known and the natural history is to improve regardless of (or despite) treatment. Few treatments have been proven to be beneficial, but several things may hasten the recovery process. **Reassurance** is vitally important. Advise the patient that the process is *benign* and unlikely to lead to long-term impairment, and major intervention is not anticipated. First-line **medication** options to consider include acetaminophen and nonsteroidal antiinflammatory medication. Opioids, tramadol, and muscle relaxants are options for symptoms refractory to first-line medications. **Educate** the patient to remain active and return to activities as soon as symptoms permit. Bedrest should be discouraged. Application of heat is a potentially helpful **self-care** option. Spinal manipulation may potentially decrease symptoms. Other treatments for acute LBP are usually not necessary.

12. What if the pain persists for several weeks after the initial treatment?

If the pain still does not resolve, the patient should be provided with reassurance. If not already performed, imaging studies are appropriate. MRI should be interpreted cautiously and correlated with clinical findings. If serious spinal pathology requiring referral to a spine specialist is not identified, supportive treatment is continued. Determine the severity of pain perception and how it interferes physically, psychosocially, and psycho-emotionally with function. Treatment options at this point include active physical therapy, medication, manipulation, and alternative medicine techniques such as acupuncture or yoga.

13. What about the patient whose pain becomes chronic and disabling?

Other factors contributing to the pain must be identified. There has been a large movement toward treating "benign" or "nonmalignant pain" problems with opioid medications and various injections, disc dissolution techniques, device insertion (spinal stimulators, intrathecal drug delivery systems), and surgery. However, these are unlikely to treat the entire problem. In addition, these treatments are invasive, associated with high complication rates, and unlikely to resolve disabling pain or restore functional ability. When the etiology of the pain is not clearly defined and there are multiple inorganic signs, treatment is directed at the functional loss and disability. This type of patient is best served by an interdisciplinary team (not multidisciplinary) approach, such as a **functional restoration program**. This approach uses cognitive-behavioral methods together with physical methods and is guided by a biopsychosocial approach to the patient's pain and disability. Acceptance of pain and restoring function is paramount to success with this type of program.

14. When is it appropriate to refer a patient with nonspecific LBP to a spine specialist?

When patients with nonspecific LBP fail to improve with noninvasive treatment after a minimum period of 3 months, it is reasonable to refer the patient to a spine specialist for further evaluation. A spine specialist can assist by providing recommendations regarding exercise therapy, interdisciplinary care, and spinal injections. Surgical intervention is generally deferred until symptoms have persisted for at least 1 year.

Key Points

1. Low back pain is ubiquitous in the human race and is not a disease.
2. Low back pain is a symptom and not a diagnosis.
3. There is poor correlation between anatomic abnormalities on imaging studies and clinical symptoms reported by patients with nonspecific low back pain.
4. Acute low back pain and chronic low back pain are completely different disorders and require distinct treatment algorithms.
5. *Red flag* findings suggest serious underlying pathology and may warrant further investigation with imaging studies and laboratory testing.

Websites

Cochrane reviews for LBP online: http://www.cochrane.iwh.on.ca/rev_comp.htm
Low back pain guidelines: http://www.annals.org/cgi/content/full/147/7/478
Acute LBP in adults: http://www.ncbi.nlm.nih.gov/bookshelf/br.fcgi?book=hsarchive&part=A25870

BIBLIOGRAPHY

1. Bigos SJ, editor. Agency for Health Care Policy & Research clinical practice guideline #14: acute low back problems in adults. Rockville, MD: U.S. Department of Health & Human Services Public Health Service; December 1994.
2. Chou R, Huffman L. Medications for acute and chronic low back pain for an American Pain Society/American College of Physicians clinical practice guideline. Ann Intern Med 2007;147:505–14.
3. Chou R, Qaseem A, Snow V, et al. Diagnosis and treatment of low back pain: a joint clinical practice guideline from the American College of Physicians and the American Pain Society. Ann Intern Med 2007;147:478–91.
4. Dagenais S, Haldeman S, editors. Special issue on evidence-informed management of chronic low back pain without surgery. Spine J 2008;8:1–277.
5. Waddell G. The Back Pain Revolution. 2nd ed. New York: Churchill Livingstone; 2004.

LUMBAR DISC HERNIATION

Vincent J. Devlin, MD

1. Describe the prevalence and natural history of lumbar disc herniations. How do they differ from the prevalence and natural history of low back pain?

The lifetime prevalence of a *lumbar disc herniatio*n is approximately 2%. The natural history of sciatica secondary to lumbar disc herniation is spontaneous improvement in the majority of cases. Among patients with radiculopathy secondary to lumbar disc herniation, approximately 10% to 25% (0.5% of the population) experience persistent symptoms. These statistics are in sharp contrast to *low back pain,* which has a lifetime prevalence of 60% to 80% in the adult population. Although the natural history of acute low back pain is favorable in the majority of patients, successful management of patients with chronic symptoms remains an enigma.

2. What is the typical history of a patient with a lumbar disc herniation?

Typically there is an attempt to link the onset of back and leg pain with a traumatic event, but frequently patients have experienced intermittent episodes of back and leg pain for months or years. Factors that tend to exacerbate symptoms include physical exertion, repetitive bending, torsion, and heavy lifting. Pain typically begins in the lumbar area and radiates to the sacroiliac and buttock regions. Radicular pain typically extends below the knee in the distribution of the involved nerve root. Radicular pain may be accompanied by paresthesia and weakness in the distribution of the involved nerve root. Patients with a disc herniation generally report that pain in the leg is worse than low back pain. Pain tends to be exacerbated by sitting, straining, sneezing, and coughing and relieved with standing or bed rest.

3. Define cauda equina syndrome.

Cauda equina syndrome is defined as a complex of low back pain, sciatica, saddle hypoesthesia, and lower extremity motor weakness in association with bowel or bladder dysfunction. The mode of onset may be slow or rapidly progressive. The most common cause of cauda equina syndrome is a central lumbar disc herniation at the L4–L5 level. Prompt surgical treatment is advised.

4. Outline key points in the physical examination of a patient with a suspected lumbar disc herniation.

The patient should be undressed. Observation may reveal the presence of a limp or a list (sciatic scoliosis). Spinal range of motion is assessed. A complete neurologic examination (sensory, motor, reflex testing) is performed to identify the involved nerve root. Nerve root tension signs are evaluated. Hip and knee range of motion are assessed to rule out pathology involving these joints. Peripheral pulses (dorsalis pedis and posterior tibial) are assessed to rule out peripheral vascular problems. A rectal examination is performed in patients suspected of having cauda equina syndrome.

5. What are nerve root tension signs?

Tension signs are maneuvers that tighten the sciatic or femoral nerve and in doing so further compress an inflamed nerve root against a lumbar disc herniation. The supine straight leg raise test (Lasegue's test) and its variants (sitting straight leg raise test, bowstring test, contralateral straight leg raise test) increase tension along the *sciatic nerve* and are used to assess the L5 and S1 nerve roots. The femoral nerve stretch test (reverse straight leg raise test) increases tension along the *femoral nerve* and is used to assess the L2, L3, and L4 nerve roots.

6. Compare and contrast sciatica with other common clinical syndromes presenting with low back and/or lower extremity pain symptoms.

- **Sciatica:** Leg pain rather than low back pain is the predominant symptom. Neurologic symptoms and signs are found in a specific nerve root distribution. Nerve root tension signs are present
- **Nonmechanical back and/or leg pain:** Pain is constant and minimally affected by activity and unrelieved with rest. Pain is usually worse at night or early morning (e.g. spinal tumor, infection)
- **Mechanical back and/or leg pain:** Pain is exacerbated by activity, changes in position, or prolonged sitting. Pain is relieved with rest, especially in the supine position (e.g. degenerative disc pathology, spondylolisthesis)
- **Neurogenic claudication:** Low back and buttock pain, radiating leg or calf pain, worse with ambulation, worse with spinal extension, relieved with flexion maneuvers, absent nerve root tension signs (e.g. spinal stenosis)

7. **When clinical examination suggests the presence of an acute lumbar disc herniation, what is the preferred imaging test to confirm the diagnosis?**

Magnetic resonance imaging (MRI) is the preferred imaging test because it provides the greatest amount of information about the lumbar region. It is unparalleled in its ability to visualize pathologic processes involving the disc, thecal sac, epidural space, neural elements, paraspinal soft tissue, and bone marrow. However, caution is indicated when interpreting results of MRI scans due to the high frequency of disc abnormalities in asymptomatic patients. It is critical to correlate imaging findings with clinical examination. Although lumbar radiographs cannot show a lumbar disc herniation, standing radiographs are advised prior to referral for MRI in order to define regional lumbar anatomy and diagnose other potential pathologies such as spondylolisthesis.

8. **At what spinal level are symptomatic lumbar disc herniations most commonly diagnosed?**

Most lumbar disc herniations occur at the L4–L5 and L5–S1 levels (90%). The L3–L4 level is the next most common level for a symptomatic lumbar disc herniation.

9. **What terms are used to describe lumbar disc pathology noted on MRI?**

Terms used to describe lumbar disc pathology noted on MRI include degeneration, annular tear, bulge, protrusion, extrusion, and sequestration (Fig. 49-1).

- **Degeneration:** Decreased or absent T2-weighted signal is noted from the intervertebral disc. It is not possible to distinguish symptomatic from asymptomatic degeneration based on MRI
- **Disc bulge:** Disc material is noted to extend beyond the disc space with a diffuse, circumferential, nonfocal contour. Disc bulges are caused by early disc degeneration and infrequently cause symptoms in the absence of spinal stenosis
- **Protrusion:** Displaced disc material extends focally and asymmetrically beyond the disc space. The displaced disc material is in continuity with the disc of origin. The diameter of the base of the displaced portion, where it is continuous with the disc material within the disc space of origin, has a greater diameter than the largest diameter of the disc tissue extending beyond the disc space
- **Extrusion:** Displaced disc material extends focally and asymmetrically beyond the disc space. The displaced disc material has a greater diameter than the disc material maintaining continuity (if any) with the disc of origin
- **Sequestration:** Refers to a disc fragment that has no continuity with the disc of origin. By definition all sequestered discs are extruded. However, not all extruded discs are sequestered

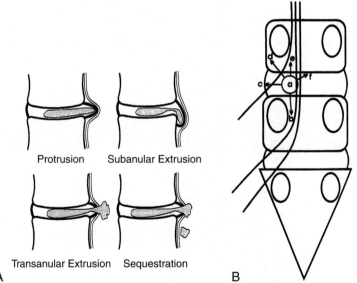

Figure 49-1. **A,** The four varieties of disc herniation. *Top row*, contained by anulus or ligament. *Bottom row*, non-contained by anulus or ligament. **B,** Potential patterns of migration of disc material away from typical posterior/lateral position (a) Migratory positions include (b) distal beside the pedicle of the level below; (c) lateral; (d) upward into neural foramen; (e) upward into axilla of exiting nerve root; and (f) medial. (From McCullough JA. Least invasive spine surgery at the L5–S1 level in adults. Spine State Art Rev 1994;11:215–238, with permission.)

10. How is the location of a disc herniation within the spinal canal described?

The location of a disc herniation within the spinal canal is described in terms of a *three-floor anatomic house* (story 1 = disc space level, story 2 = foraminal level, story 3 = pedicle level) (Fig. 49-2). The spinal canal is also divided in terms of *zones*—central, foraminal, and extraforaminal. The *central zone* is located between the pedicles. The *foraminal zone* is located between the medial and lateral pedicle borders. The *extraforaminal zone* is located beyond the lateral pedicle border. This anatomic scheme is applicable to lumbar spinal stenosis syndromes and lumbar disc problems.

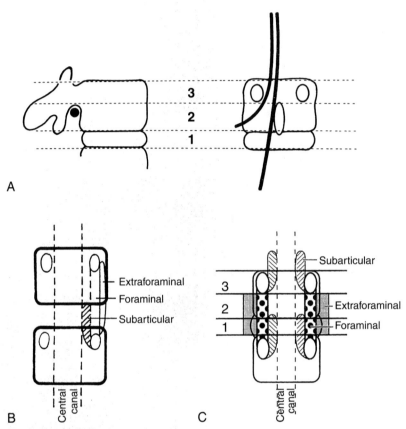

Figure 49-2. Localizing the lumbar disc herniation. **A,** Identify the herniation in relation to the three stories of the spinal canal (story 1, disc space level; story 2, foraminal level; and story 3, pedicle level). **B,** Determine if the pathology lies within the central spinal canal or the lateral zone. **C,** Identify the pathology on the anatomic grid for the involved spinal segment and determine the surgical plan. (From McCullough JA. Microdiscectomy: the gold standard for minimally invasive disc surgery. Spine State Art Rev 1997;11:373–396, with permission.)

11. How does the location of a disc herniation along the circumference of the annulus of the disc determine the pattern of nerve root compression?

Discs herniations are described by their relationship along the circumference of the annulus fibrosus as *central* (midline), *posterolateral* (most common), *foraminal*, or *extraforaminal*. The location of the disc herniation determines the pattern of nerve root compression. The nerve roots of the lumbar spine exit the spinal canal beneath the pedicle of the corresponding numbered vertebra and above the caudad intervertebral disc. A posterolateral L4–L5 disc herniation compresses the L5 nerve root (the traversing nerve root of the L4–L5 motion segment). An L4–L5 foraminal or extraforaminal disc herniation compresses the L4 nerve root (the exiting nerve root of the L4–L5 motion segment). A central disc herniation compresses one or more of the caudal nerve roots.

12. What initial treatment is advised for patients with a suspected acute lumbar disc herniation?

Initial treatment options include a short period of bedrest (not to exceed 3 days), oral medications (nonsteroidal antiinflammatory drugs [NSAIDs], aspirin, mild opioids), progressive ambulation, return to activity, and patient reassurance. Epidural injections can be considered. As acute pain subsides, physical therapy and aerobic conditioning are advised. If a patient fails to improve with 4 to 6 weeks of nonsurgical care, further evaluation is indicated. The optimal time for nonsurgical treatment ranges from a minimum of 4 weeks to a maximum of 6 months.

13. What are the indications for surgical treatment for a lumbar disc herniation?

Occasionally an acute massive disc herniation can result in cauda equina syndrome, which is best managed by emergent surgical treatment. However, most patients undergo elective surgical treatment due to failure of radicular pain to improve with nonsurgical treatment. Surgical treatment is directed at improving the patient's leg pain. When the predominant symptom is back pain, symptom relief is unpredictable, and discectomy is not advised. Appropriate criteria for surgical intervention include:

- Functionally incapacitating leg pain extending below the knee within a nerve root distribution
- Nerve root tension signs with or without neurologic deficit
- Failure to improve with 4 to 8 weeks of nonsurgical treatment
- Confirmatory imaging study (preferably MRI), which correlates with the patient's physical findings and pain distribution

14. How does surgery compare with nonoperative treatment for a symptomatic lumbar disc herniation?

Surgery has been shown to lead to a more rapid and greater degree of improvement compared with nonoperative treatment. Operative treatment is associated with a low rate of complication. However, patients who prefer nonoperative treatment and are able to tolerate their symptoms often improve and achieve an acceptable level of pain and function.

15. What surgical procedure is recommended for treatment of a symptomatic lumbar disc herniation?

Open lumbar discectomy using microsurgical technique remains the gold standard for the treatment of a symptomatic lumbar disc herniation (Fig. 49-3). Important technical points include use of a small incision, limited muscle and bone dissection, and limited removal of displaced or loose disc material. A surgical microscope or headlight and loupe magnification is used to enhance intraoperative visualization. Uncomplicated patients typically go home within 24 hours of surgery and are able to return to work in 1 month. The success rate for relief of leg pain exceeds 90% in appropriately selected patients.

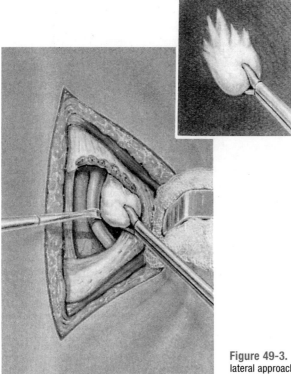

Figure 49-3. Lumbar disc fragment excision. (From McCullough JA. The lateral approach to the lumbar spine. Oper Tech Orthop 1991;1:27, 55, with permission.)

16. How does the location of a disc herniation influence selection of the appropriate surgical approach?

Disc herniations located within the central spinal canal are treated through an **interlaminar** surgical approach. Disc herniations located in the extraforaminal zone are treated through an **intertransverse** surgical approach (except at L5–S1 where an interlaminar approach is preferred). The surgical approach for disc herniations located in the foraminal zone is determined by a combination of factors, including the level and size of the disc herniation (Fig. 49-4).

17. What are the surgical alternatives to microsurgical lumbar discectomy?

A variety of alternative procedures have been proposed. However, no procedure has demonstrated superior surgical outcomes compared with microsurgical lumbar discectomy. Alternative procedures include chymopapain injection, percutaneous automated discectomy, laser discectomy, and a variety of endoscopic surgical techniques.

18. What complications have been reported in association with microsurgical lumbar discectomy?

Fortunately complications are rare but may include:

- Vascular injury
- Nerve root injury
- Dural tear
- Infection
- Increased back pain

- Recurrent disc herniation
- Cauda equina syndrome
- Medical complications (e.g. thrombophlebitis, urinary tract infection)

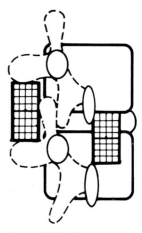

Figure 49-4. The two windows of opportunity into the spinal canal: interlaminar *(right)* and intertransverse *(left)*. (From McCullough JA. The lateral approach to the lumbar spine. Oper Tech Orthop 1991;1:27, 55, with permission.)

19. What is the most common cause of surgical failure after lumbar disc excision?

Poor patient selection is the most common cause of treatment failure following lumbar discectomy. Other factors that may contribute to a poor surgical outcome include prolonged symptoms (> 6 to 12 months), abnormal pain behavior, workman's compensation situation, litigation, and tobacco use.

20. What is the incidence of recurrent disc herniation after microsurgical lumbar discectomy?

The incidence of recurrent disc herniation following microsurgical lumbar discectomy is 5% to 10%. Higher rates of recurrence (up to 26%) have been reported in patients in whom large annular defects were present at conclusion of discectomy. If symptoms are predominantly radicular in nature, repeat lumbar discectomy may be beneficial. If symptoms include a combination of radiculopathy and low back pain, discectomy combined with fusion may be considered in select patients with recurrent lumbar disc herniations.

Key Points

1. The majority of patients with a lumbar disc herniation improve with nonoperative treatment.
2. Relief of leg pain is the primary goal of lumbar discectomy.

Websites

Epidural steroid injection compared with discectomy: http://www.jbjs.org/Comments/pdf/JBJA086040670.pdf
Disc pathology: http://www.nlm.nih.gov/medlineplus/herniateddisk.html#cat3

BIBLIOGRAPHY

1. Atlas SJ, Keller RB, Wu YA, et al. Long-term outcomes of surgical and nonsurgical management of sciatica secondary to a lumbar disc herniation: 10 year results from the Maine Lumbar Spine Study. Spine 2005;30:927–35.
2. Carragee EJ, Han MY, Suen PW, et al. Clinical outcomes after lumbar discectomy for sciatica: the effects of fragment type and anular competence. J Bone Joint Surg 2003;85A:102–8.
3. McCulloch JA, Young PA. Essentials of Spinal Microsurgery. Philadelphia: Lippincott-Raven; 1998.
4. Moschetti W, Pearson AM, Abdu WA. Treatment of lumbar disc herniation: an evidence-based review. Semin Spine Surg 2009;21:223–9.
5. Weber H. Lumbar disc herniation: a controlled prospective study with ten years of observation Spine 1983;8:131–140.
6. Weinstein JN, Lurie JD, Tosteson TD, et al. Surgical versus nonoperative treatment for lumbar disc herniation: four-year results for the Spine Patient Outcomes Research Trial (SPORT). Spine 2008;33:2789–2800.

DISCOGENIC LOW BACK PAIN

Eeric Truumees, MD

CHAPTER 50

1. Define lumbar disc degeneration.
Lumbar disc degeneration has been defined by the North American Spine Society Consensus Committee on Nomenclature in terms of morphologic changes involving the anatomic components of the lumbar disc. These changes may include:
- Desiccation, fibrosis, vacuum changes, or cleft formation in the *nucleus*
- Fissuring, mucinous degeneration, or calcification in the *annulus*
- Defects and sclerosis of the *vertebral endplates*
- Osteophytes at the *vertebral apophysis*

2. What is lumbar degenerative disc disease?
Although disc degeneration is virtually universal in the aging spine, disc degeneration is inconsistently and only occasionally associated with pain and functional limitation. *Degenerative disc disease (DDD)* is broadly defined as a clinical syndrome characterized by manifestations of disc degeneration and symptoms attributed to these changes. Causal connections between degenerative changes and clinical symptoms are often difficult clinical distinctions. No evidence-based consensus exists for differentiating pathologic degenerative disc changes from disc changes associated with normal aging.

3. How is the clinical syndrome of lumbar DDD characterized?
Lumbar DDD refers to a continuum of nonradicular pain disorders of degenerative origin. Specifically excluded are symptoms related to disc impingement on neural elements, facet-mediated back pain, and spinal deformities secondary to lumbar DDD (e.g. spondylolisthesis, degenerative scoliosis).

Presenting symptom is primarily low back pain, which may radiate to the sacroiliac and/or buttock region. Common physical examination findings include tenderness with palpation over the lumbar region and limited lumbar range of motion. Low back pain is often more severe with flexion and less severe with extension in the absence of associated facet joint degeneration.

Radiographic findings in lumbar DDD include disc height loss, decreased lumbar lordosis, vacuum phenomena, osteophytes, and endplate sclerosis. Similar degenerative changes are frequently noted in asymptomatic patients. A change in radiographic alignment from supine to standing or from flexion to extension may occur.

Magnetic resonance imaging (MRI) findings include disc desiccation, annular fissures, high-intensity zones (HIZ), loss of disc space height, and changes in vertebral endplate morphology. No pathognomonic findings have been identified that permit distinction of asymptomatic age-related changes from symptomatic lumbar DDD.

Lumbar discography is utilized as a provocative test to assess patients with DDD. Although controversial, this test attempts to directly identify a cause and effect relationship between MRI findings of DDD and clinical symptoms. Findings that support a diagnosis of discogenic pain include concordant pain on injection of a specific disc level with absent or minimal pain on injection of adjacent control levels. Additional criteria for diagnosis include pain reproduction with a low pressure/low volume injection and presence of abnormal disc morphology. Discography remains a controversial test in patients with abnormal psychometric profiles, chronic pain illness, worker's compensation claims, and secondary gain issues.

4. What is a high-intensity zone (HIZ)?
An HIZ is an area of increased signal intensity in the posterior annular region of the disc present on T2-weighted MRI. Initial reports suggested that an HIZ was a marker for symptomatic internal disc disruption and concordant pain reproduction with discography. However, additional studies have demonstrated that an HIZ is not a specific marker for symptomatic disc disruption as this finding is present in many asymptomatic individuals.

5. What is the significance of endplate changes on lumbar MRI?
Changes in vertebral endplate morphology adjacent to degenerating discs are frequently observed on MRI. These changes have been classified by Modic into three types:
- **Type I** changes reflect acute disruption and fissuring of vertebral endplates, which leads to growth of vascularized fibrous tissue into the adjacent vertebral body marrow. This tissue exhibits a diminished T1 and increased T2 signal pattern

- **Type II** changes develop in the context of chronic degeneration as the hematopoietic (red) peridiscal marrow undergoes fatty degeneration. A type II pattern exhibits increased T1 signal and an isointense or slightly hyperintense T2 signal
- **Type III** changes reflect extrinsic bone sclerosis as seen on plain radiographs. Dense bone in the vertebral endplates yields a hypointense signal on both T1 and T2 images

   The clinical significance of endplate changes in patients with degenerative disc changes is unclear. Just as the pathologic changes of disc degeneration are likely a normal part of aging, the MRI findings associated with those changes frequently do not correlate with low back pain.

6. What is the cause of the pain associated with lumbar degenerative disc disease?

The answer to this question remains elusive. The outer layers of the annulus fibrosis are innervated by sympathetic pain fibers via the sinuvertebral nerve. Theories that have evolved to explain the painful symptoms associated with disc degeneration include:

- **Chemical:** The disc releases inflammatory mediators, which irritate the annular nerve fibers
- **Disc nocioception:** Motion and loading of a degenerated disc becomes painful following nerve fiber ingrowth into the outer annular region
- **Instability:** The degenerative process leads to excessive and abnormal painful motion of the degenerative lumbar segment
- **Neutral zone:** The *neutral zone* is conceptualized as a region of intervertebral motion around the neutral posture where little or no resistance to motion exists due to the passive structures of the spinal motion segment. Although the overall flexion-extension arc of motion may decrease with DDD, the types of motion and force required to produce motion may change. In early DDD, disc dehydration and nuclear resorption cause the peripheral annulus to become lax. This laxity increases translatory motion in the motion segment's *neutral zone.* Abnormal motion or laxity may cause pain by abnormally loading the annulus or by inducing lumbar extensor muscle spasticity in an effort to control abnormal motion.
- ***Stone in the shoe* hypothesis:** Focal abnormal loads (the *stone in the shoe*) cause areas of focal endplate overloading resulting in pain

7. Are there easily defined subtypes of DDD?

A variety of terms have been applied to patients with nonradicular lumbar pain disorders of a degenerative origin including discogenic pain syndrome, annular tear syndrome, *dark disc disease,* internal disc disruption (IDD), isolated disc resorption, and lumbar spondylosis (LS). Currently there is no level I evidence to support subsegregation of DDD, and no universally accepted classification exists. Patients with chronic low back pain of discogenic origin with tall discs and normal radiographs (IDD) are often contrasted with patients with marked disc collapse, osteophyte formation, and vacuum disc changes (LS). These disease subgroups may be associated with varied responses to operative and nonoperative interventions. For example, stand-alone anterior fusion procedures may fail at a higher rate in IDD. LS patients may not respond as well to lumbar disc replacement. Ongoing research is directed at clarification of such issues.

8. How much is known about the natural history of DDD?

Understanding of the natural history of DDD is limited. The available natural history data yield the following conclusions:

- The pathophysiology of lumbar DDD is not well understood
- The natural history of lumbar DDD is, for the most part, benign
- There are more elements at work than mechanical factors alone
- Patients with fewer radiographic abnormalities may have more pain and functional limitation than ones with much "worse" radiographic change
- Similarly, a patient's pain may worsen without concomitant change on imaging or may improve despite radiographic progression
- The subjective nature of these pain complaints makes objective grading of disease state severity impossible

9. Discuss common nonsurgical treatment options for chronic low back pain due to lumbar DDD.

Nonsurgical treatment options for chronic low back pain due to lumbar DDD include:

- **Observation:** For patients with limited symptoms, reasonable function, and good core strength, observation is an appropriate treatment
- **Medication:** Nonsteroidal antiinflammatory medications are effective for short-term relief of symptoms. Muscle relaxants (benzodiazepine and non-benzodiazepine) and anticonvulsant medications are considered second-line medication options. Tricyclic antidepressants are a useful adjunct. Tramadol, a synthetic analgesic, has been shown to significantly reduce pain and improve physical function in chronic low back pain patients. Long-term use of opioids is controversial due to decreasing efficacy over time and high rates of substance abuse. Corticosteroids do not have a clearly defined role in treatment of lumbar DDD
- **Physical therapy:** Exercise therapy with emphasis on core muscle strengthening (abdominal wall muscles, lumbar muscles), stretching, and endurance training have shown benefit
- **Epidural injections:** Epidural injections may provide short-term relief of symptoms
- **Miscellaneous:** A myriad of traditional (e.g. chiropractic, orthoses, traction, laser, transcutaneous electrical nerve stimulation) and nontraditional (e.g. acupuncture, massage, herbs, meditation) treatments have been advocated based on varying levels of supportive medical evidence

10. What is the most important component of an exercise program for the treatment of low back pain due to lumbar DDD?

The most important component of a low back exercise program is to address fear-avoidance behavior of the patient by reassuring the patient that it is safe to exercise despite the chronic pain he or she may experience. The appropriate exercise program is a supervised active physical therapy program that uses progressive, non–pain contingent exercise (i.e. the patient is encouraged to exercise despite their pain) to increase strength and endurance. Successful outcomes may be achieved with a variety of exercise programs including core strengthening, McKenzie therapy, Pilates, and aerobic conditioning. It is counterproductive to tell patients, "Let pain be your guide." Patients with lumbar DDD must be reassured that they will not do any damage to their spine, even if exercise is painful.

Table 50-1. Popular Treatment Options for Lumbar Degenerative Disc Disease

TYPE OF MANAGEMENT	ADVANTAGES	DISADVANTAGES	COMMENTS
Nonoperative Management	• Least costly • Least morbid	• Some patients will fail	• Trial of nonoperative treatment for all patients
Decompression Procedures (e.g. laser, nucleoplasty)	• Low initial morbidity • Motion preserving	• High rates of failure in patients with mechanical back pain	• Lack of evidence to support efficacy
Posterior Motion-Preserving Implants (e.g. CoFlex)	• Less invasive • May be revised to fusion	• Success rates unknown	• Theoretical advantages remain unproven
Posterolateral Fusion (PLF)	• Decreases axial pain • Breakdown unlikely after successful healing	• Increased surgical morbidity • Adjacent segment degeneration (ASD) • Painful micromotion may persist due to unfused anterior column	• Appropriate for many patients
Noninstrumented PLF	• Less morbidity and cost than instrumented fusion	• High pseudarthrosis risk	• Appropriate in select cases
Instrumented PLF	• Higher fusion rates • No brace required • Sagittal alignment may be improved	• Increased morbidity and costs • May further increase ASD risk • Fails in osteoporotic bone • Screw misplacement may injure nerves	• Used in most cases • Increased fusion rates may not be associated with improved outcomes
Anterior Lumbar Interbody Fusion (ALIF)	• Direct removal of pain generator • Avoids disruption of posterior extensor muscles • Avoids manipulation of neural structures	• Access surgeon available • Difficult if prior abdominal surgery • More difficult at L4–L5 • Exposure-related complications	• Stand-alone ALIF controversial due to complications, especially in multilevel cases
Circumferential Fusion (Anterior + Posterior)	• Higher fusion rate and superior functional outcomes compared with posterior fusion	• Exposure-related complications due to anterior approach • ASD risk	• Recent studies show better outcomes and less cost to society compared with posterior fusion
PLIF/TLIF Techniques	• Allow circumferential fusion via single incision • Provide advantages of ALIF and PLF	• ASD risk • Autologous bone graft frequently utilized	• Many different techniques • Outcome is more technique-dependent compared with circumferential fusion
Artificial Disc Replacement	• Motion preservation • Removal of pain generator	• Difficult to revise • Long-term stability unknown • Strict indications	• Potentially useful for select patients in absence of facet joint arthropathy

11. What surgical options are available for treatment of lumbar DDD?

A wide range of surgical procedures has been advocated (Table 50-1).
- **Interbody fusion procedures** are favored by many surgeons as they directly address the pain generator (lumbar disc). Interbody fusion can be performed through various approaches:

  Anterior approach (anterior lumbar interbody fusion, ALIF)

  Posterior approach (posterior lumbar interbody fusion, PLIF; transforaminal lumbar interbody fusion, TLIF)

  Lateral approach (direct lateral approach, DLIF; extreme lateral interbody fusion, XLIF—not indicated at the L5–S1 level)

  Combined circumferential approaches

  A variety of implants can be used to promote interbody fusion including autograft, allograft, or fusion cages used in combination with autograft, allograft, synthetic graft material, or bone morphogenetic protein. Posterior spinal instrumentation is commonly performed in conjunction with interbody fusion. A posterolateral fusion may be combined with an interbody fusion. Minimally invasive approaches have been popularized in an attempt to decrease exposure-related surgical morbidity.
- **Artificial disc replacement** is an alternative to fusion. However, candidates for artificial disc replacement represent a much narrower group of patients than those considered for fusion. For example, patients with facet joint arthrosis or severe disc space narrowing (<4 mm) are not candidates for artificial disc replacement (Fig. 50-1).

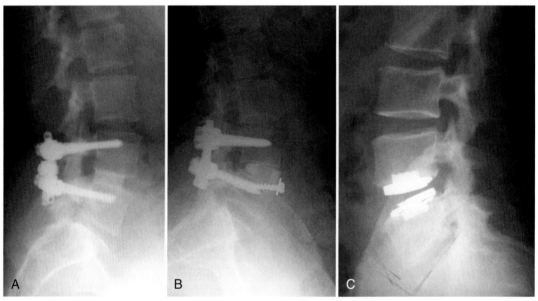

Figure 50-1. Surgical options for lumbar degenerative disc disease. **A,** Interbody fusion through a posterior approach using cortical allograft combined with posterior spinal instrumentation and fusion. **B,** Interbody fusion through an anterior approach using femoral allograft combined with posterior spinal instrumentation and fusion. **C,** Artificial disc replacement with the ProDisc-L implant. (**A** from Herkowitz HN, Garfin SR, Eismont FJ, et al., editors. Rothman Simeone The Spine. 5th ed. Philadelphia: Saunders; 2006. Fig. 91-10, p 1531; **B** from Vincent J. Devlin, MD; **C** from Yue JJ, Bertagnoli R, McAfee PC, et al., editors. Motion Preservation Surgery of the Spine. Philadelphia: Saunders; 2008. Fig. 39-2A, p 321.)

12. How does surgical treatment compare with nonoperative treatment for patients with discogenic low back pain?

Data from randomized controlled trials permit comparison of nonoperative and operative treatment for patients with discogenic low back pain. Conclusions drawn include:
- Spinal fusion is superior to nonstructured nonoperative treatment
- Spinal fusion outcomes are similar to outcomes obtained with a structured nonoperative treatment program consisting of intensive outpatient physical rehabilitation
- Outcomes of artificial disc replacement are similar or slightly better than outcomes of spinal fusion

13. Which patients are the most appropriate candidates for surgical treatment for lumbar DDD?

It is challenging to successfully select surgical candidates who will benefit from lumbar fusion procedures for discogenic back pain. Lumbar fusion may be considered for treatment of low back pain of discogenic origin in patients who fail to improve after a minimum of 6 months of appropriate nonsurgical care. Many spine specialists use discography in an attempt to correlate the patient's symptoms and imaging studies. Appropriate surgical criteria include:

- Patients with pain and disability for more than 1 year
- Failure of aggressive physical conditioning and conservative treatment for more than 6 months
- Single-level degeneration on MRI with concordant pain response on discography
- Absence of psychiatric or secondary gain issues

 Patients with multilevel disc degeneration (greater than two levels) are considered to be poor candidates for lumbar surgery because procedures typically fail to provide significant benefit for such patients.

14. Which patients are less than ideal candidates for surgical treatment for lumbar DDD?

Surgical treatment is associated with poor outcomes in patients with unresolved secondary gain issues, worker's compensation claims, litigation, multiple emergency department visits, high levels of opioid usage, abnormal psychometrics, chronic pain illness, and exaggerated pain behaviors. Patients off work greater than 3 months tend to have worse results. To have any sense that surgery might benefit the patient, the surgeon must get to know the patient. Overreliance on MRI or discography data will lead to a high rate of clinical failures. Motivated patients without psychosocial overlay that fall within the narrow indications are likely to do well. Deviation from these strict criteria exposes the patient to significant operative risks with much less potential benefit.

Key Points

1. The pathophysiology of lumbar DDD and its relation to low back pain symptoms is poorly understood.
2. Mechanical, traumatic, chemical, psychosocial, and genetic factors may interact and play a role in the development of disc degeneration.
3. Evidence-based treatment options for symptomatic lumbar degenerative disc disease include a structured outpatient physical rehabilitation program, spinal fusion, and artificial disc replacement.

Websites

High-intensity zone of the lumbar disc: http://www.josonline.org/pdf/v17i2p190.pdf
Lumbar degenerative disc disease: http://radiology.rsna.org/content/245/1/43.full
North American Spine Society Consensus Committee on Nomenclature: http://www.spine.org/Documents/Nomenclature.pdf
Lumbar degenerative disc disease: http://emedicine.medscape.com/article/309767-overview
Degenerative disc disease condition center: http://www.spineuniverse.com/conditions/degenerative-disc/degenerative-disc-disease-condition-center

BIBLIOGRAPHY

1. Coe M, Mirza S, Sengupta D. The role of fusion for discogenic axial back pain without associated leg pain, spondylolisthesis or stenosis: an evidence-based review. Semin Spine Surg 2009;21:246-256.
2. Fardon DF, Herzog RJ, Mink JH, et al. Nomenclature and classification of lumbar disc disorders. In: Garfin SR, Vaccaro AR, editors. Orthopaedic Knowledge Update-Spine. Rosemont, IL: American Academy of Orthopaedic Surgeons; 1997. p. A3–A14.
3. Rainville J, Nguyen R, Suri P. Effective conservative treatment for chronic low back pain. Semin Spine Surg 2009;21:257–263.
4. Soegaard R, Bünger CE, Christiansen, et al. Circumferential fusion is dominant over posterolateral fusion in a long-term perspective. Spine 2007;32:2405–2414.
5. Truumees E, Fischgrund J, editors. Axial low back pain. Semin Spine Surg 2008;20:73–160.
6. Zdeblick TA. Discogenic back pain. In: Herkowitz HN, Garfin SR, Balderston RA, et al., editors. The Spine. Philadelphia: Saunders; 1999. p. 749–66.

LUMBAR SPINAL STENOSIS

Vincent J. Devlin, MD

1. What is lumbar spinal stenosis?

Lumbar spinal stenosis is defined as any type of narrowing of the spinal canal, nerve root canals, or intervertebral foramen. This narrowing can be caused by soft tissue, bone, or a combination of both. The resultant nerve root compression leads to nerve root ischemia and a clinical syndrome associated with variable degrees of low back, buttock, and leg pain.

2. What are the two main types of spinal stenosis?

The two main types of spinal stenosis are (1) congenital-developmental and (2) acquired spinal stenosis. In the most widely accepted classification, spinal stenosis is subdivided into two congenital-developmental subtypes and six acquired subtypes.

CONGENITAL-DEVELOPMENTAL STENOSIS
- Idiopathic
- Achondroplastic

ACQUIRED STENOSIS
- Degenerative
- Combined congenital and degenerative stenosis
- Spondylolytic or spondylolisthetic
- Iatrogenic (e.g. following laminectomy or spinal fusion)
- Post-traumatic
- Metabolic (e.g. Paget's disease, fluorosis)

3. What is the most common type of spinal stenosis?

The acquired degenerative type of spinal stenosis is the most common type.

4. How does degenerative spinal stenosis develop?

Pathologic changes in the lumbar disc and facet joints are responsible for the development of spinal stenosis. With the passage of time, biochemical and mechanical changes in the intervertebral disc decrease its ability to withstand cyclic loading. These changes predispose to anular tears, loss of disc height, annular bulging, and osteophyte formation. A degenerative sequence also occurs posteriorly in the facet joint complex. Disc space narrowing increases loading on posterior facet and capsular structures leading to joint erosion, loss of cartilage, and capsular laxity. Ultimately, facet hypertrophy and osteophyte formation occur.

Osteophytes on the inferior articular process encroach medially resulting in **central spinal canal stenosis.** Ligamentum flavum hypertrophy and annular bulging further contribute to stenosis involving the central spinal canal.

Osteophytes on the superior articular process enlarge resulting in **lateral zone stenosis.** Osteophytes may also form circumferentially at the vertebral margins at the attachment of the anulus in an attempt to autostabilize the motion segment. Portions of these osteophytes, termed uncinate spurs, may protrude from the subjacent vertebral endplate or disc margin into the lateral nerve root canal above and provide an additional source of lateral nerve root entrapment. Loss of disc space height can also decreases the cross-sectional area of the neural foramen and lead to symptomatic lateral zone stenosis.

Spinal instability may develop as a result of the degenerative process and lead to the development of degenerative spondylolisthesis, lateral listhesis, scoliosis, and complex spinal deformities.

5. What is the epidemiology of spinal stenosis?

Spinal stenosis may present at any age (e.g. congenital type). However, the acquired degenerative type of spinal stenosis typically becomes symptomatic in the sixth and seventh decades of life. The most common levels of involvement in the lumbar region are L3–L4 and L4–L5. Up to 15% of patients with degenerative lumbar spinal stenosis have coexistent cervical spinal stenosis (tandem stenosis).

6. Describe the typical history reported by a patient with acquired degenerative spinal stenosis.

The typical patient reports the gradual onset of low back, buttock, thigh, and calf pain. Patients may report numbness, burning, heaviness, or weakness in the lower extremities. The lower extremity symptoms may be unilateral or bilateral. Symptoms are exacerbated by activities that promote spinal extension such as prolonged standing or walking (neurogenic claudication). Maneuvers that permit spinal flexion such as sitting, lying down or leaning forward on a shopping cart tend to relieve symptoms as these positions increase spinal canal diameter. Changes in urinary function or impotence due to lumbar spinal stenosis are rare but occasionally noted.

7. **What common conditions should be considered in the differential diagnosis of spinal stenosis?**
Common conditions that should be ruled out during assessment include:
- Degenerative arthritis involving the hip joints
- Peripheral neuropathy
- Vascular insufficiency
- Metastatic tumor

8. **Compare and contrast the presentation of neurogenic claudication and vascular claudication.**
Patients with **neurogenic claudication** report tiredness, heaviness, and discomfort in the lower extremities with ambulation. The distance walked until symptoms begin and the maximum distance that the patient can walk without stopping varies from day to day and even during the same walk. Patients report that leaning forward relieves symptoms. These patients may not experience symptoms during activities performed in a flexed posture such as riding a bicycle or walking uphill. In contrast, activities performed in extension such as walking downhill tend to worsen symptoms. Patients with **vascular claudication** describe cramping or tightness in the calf associated with ambulation. The distance they are able to walk before symptoms occur is constant. Their symptoms are not affected by posture. They are unable to tolerate walking uphill, walking downhill, or cycling.

9. **What findings are typically noted on physical examination of the patient with spinal stenosis?**
Although most patients with lumbar spinal stenosis have significant subjective complaints, physical examination generally reveals few objective findings. The most frequent physical findings include reproduction of pain with lumbar extension, weakness of the extensor hallucis longus muscle, and sensory deficits over the lower extremities. Neurologic findings not otherwise detectable are sometimes demonstrated by performing a stress test (walking until symptoms occur and repeating the neurologic examination).

10. **Contrast the role of radiographs, magnetic resonance imaging (MRI), computed tomography (CT), and CT-myelography in the assessment of spinal stenosis.**
- **Radiographs:** Useful to diagnose spinal deformities (scoliosis, spondylolisthesis, lateral listhesis). Flexion-extension radiographs are useful to diagnose spinal instabilities. Radiographs can also exclude pathologic processes such as neoplasm, infection, or hip osteoarthritis.
- **MRI:** The best initial study for the diagnosis of spinal stenosis. In many cases it provides sufficient diagnostic information to eliminate the need for further diagnostic studies.
- **CT:** Its strength is assessment of osseous anatomy in relation to spinal stenosis syndromes. It does not provide optimal soft tissue detail and does not optimally visualize the neural structures.
- **CT-myelography:** An excellent test that is generally limited to the presurgical patient due to its invasive nature. It can visualize posturally dependent stenosis of the lumbar spinal canal, which is not visible with any other imaging modality.

11. **What are the options for nonsurgical management of lumbar spinal stenosis?**
The nonsurgical treatment options for lumbar spinal stenosis include:
- Medication (nonsteroidal antiinflammatory drugs [NSAIDs], opioid analgesics, third-generation anticonvulsants)
- Physical therapy (flexion exercises, functional stabilization exercises)
- General fitness and conditioning (cycling, pool exercise)
- Injections (epidurals, selective nerve root blocks)
- Manual therapy

12. **What are the indications for surgical treatment for patients with spinal stenosis?**
Surgical treatment is indicated for patients with severe spinal stenosis accompanied by intractable pain or significant neurogenic claudication or patients who fail to improve with appropriate nonsurgical treatment. Surgical treatment for spinal stenosis is elective in nature except in the presence of bowel or bladder dysfunction (cauda equina syndrome).

13. **What are the surgical treatment options for lumbar spinal stenosis?**
The basic surgical treatment for spinal stenosis is spinal **decompression** to remove those structures (lamina, ligamentum flavum, hypertrophied portions of facet joints, uncinate spurs) that are responsible for compression of the dural sac and nerve roots. Decompression of the neural elements may be achieved by **laminectomy** (complete removal of the lamina) or **laminotomy** (partial removal of the lamina). In certain specific situations (e.g. spondylolisthesis) a spinal fusion should be performed in conjunction with spinal decompression. Insertion of an **interspinous process spacer** to provide indirect decompression of the spinal canal is a recently developed alternative to laminectomy in select patients with lumbar spinal stenosis.

14. **Explain the basic steps involved in a laminectomy procedure performed to treat central spinal stenosis between L4 and S1.**
A skin incision is made between L3 and S1. The paraspinal muscles are elevated from the lamina between L3 and S1. The L4 and L5 spinous processes are resected. The pars interarticularis is identified at each level to ensure that bone

removal does not compromise its integrity. The hypertrophic lamina of L4 and L5 are thinned with a motorized burr to facilitate removal with angled Kerrison rongeurs. Adhesions between the dural sac and surrounding tissue are released with a Penfield elevator. Starting from the L5–S1 interspace, lamina and hypertrophic ligamentum flavum are resected between L4 and S1. The midline decompression is widened to permit visualization of the lateral border of the dural sac as well as the medial border of the pedicle at each level to ensure adequate decompression (Fig. 51-1).

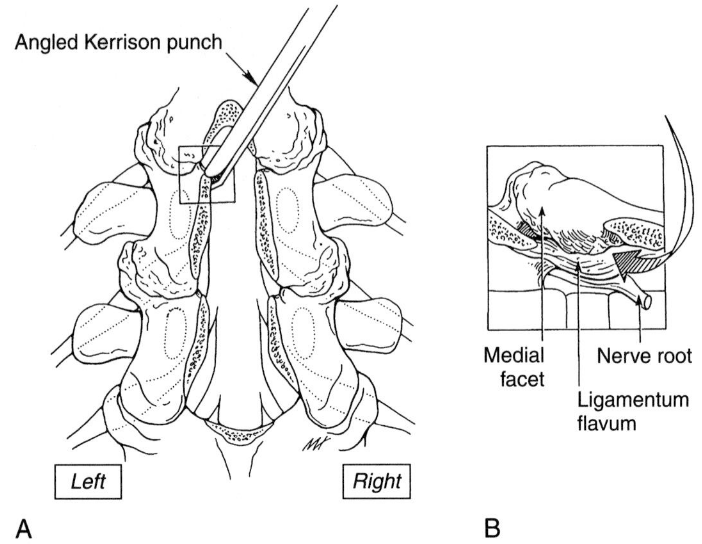

Angled Kerrison punch

Figure 51-1. Decompression for central spinal stenosis. **A,** Midline bilateral laminectomy provides decompression of the cauda equina. **B,** Removal of the medial aspect of hypertrophic facet joints and infolded ligamentum flavum is necessary. (From Stambough JL. Technique for lumbar decompression of spinal stenosis. Oper Tech Orthop 1997;7:36–43, with permission.)

Medial facet

Nerve root

Ligamentum flavum

Left   Right

A

B

15. Explain the basic steps involved in decompression of lateral zone stenosis.

Clinical evaluation and preoperative imaging studies are reviewed to determine the extent of lateral zone stenosis. Potential sources of neural compression include:

- **Zone 1** (also called the subarticular zone, entrance zone, or lateral recess). Osteophytes from the superior articular process may compress the exiting nerve root in this zone
- **Zone 2** (also called the foraminal zone, midzone, pedicle zone, or hidden zone). A variety of pathology may cause nerve root impingement including facet and ligamentum flavum hypertrophy, disc bulges, and uncinate spurs
- **Zone 3** (also called the extraforaminal zone, exit zone or far-lateral zone). Nerve root compression may result from disc protrusion, uncinate spurs, facet subluxation, and ligamentous structures

   After the midline decompression is completed, each nerve root in the surgical field must be inspected and decompressed. Each nerve root is identified along the medial border of its respective pedicle. Medial facet overgrowth and ligamentum flavum hypertrophy are resected with a Kerrison rongeur. The goal is to undercut the facet joint without sacrificing its integrity. The intervertebral disc is palpated or visualized to ensure the disc is not causing significant nerve root compression. Resection of disc and/or uncinate spurs is performed as needed to enlarge the foramen. Adequacy of decompression is checked by assessing the ability to retract the nerve root 1 cm medially and laterally without tension at the entrance zone. In addition, it should be possible to pass a blunt probe dorsal and volar to the nerve root out through the neural foramen (zone 3) without resistance (Fig. 51-2).

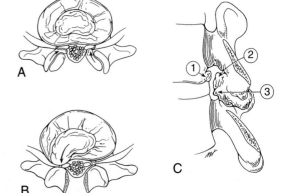

Figure 51-2. Decompression for lateral zone stenosis. **A,** Zone 1—stenosis due to hypertrophy of the superior articular process. **B,** Zone 2—stenosis due to lateral disc bulging and uncinate spurs. **C,** Zone 3—stenosis due to uncinate spur (1) and superior articular process hypertrophy (2,3). (From Stambough JL. Technique for lumbar decompression of spinal stenosis. Oper Tech Orthop 1997;7:36–43, with permission.)

A

B

C

16. **What complications may occur with lumbar decompression procedures for spinal stenosis?**

Some commonly encountered complications include:
- Dural tear
- Arachnoiditis
- Infection
- Nerve root injury
- Spinal instability
- Inadequate decompression
- Persistent symptoms
- Recurrent stenosis

17. **Compare and contrast laminectomy and laminotomy for treatment of lumbar spinal stenosis.**

Laminectomy is the traditional procedure for surgical decompression for lumbar stenosis. It involves removal of the midline osseous and ligamentous structures including the lamina, spinous processes, interspinous ligaments, and portions of the facet joints. It provides excellent visualization of neural structures and facilitates complete decompression of involved neural structures. However, spinal instability is not uncommon following laminectomy and often requires treatment with spinal instrumentation and fusion. **Laminotomy** involves partial removal of the lamina and facet complex but preserves the midline structures including the spinous processes and interspinous ligaments. Preservation of the midline structures decreases the risk of developing spinal instability. The disadvantages of laminotomy include technical difficulty of the procedure and the risk of inadequate decompression due to limited exposure. An intermediate approach between laminectomy and laminoplasty is an **interlaminar decompression,** which enhances visualization of the neural elements for decompression but minimizes bone resection and is less destabilizing than laminectomy. Laminotomies are most appropriate for treatment of patients with spinal stenosis limited to the level of the facet joints and disc space. Laminectomies are most appropriate for patients with congenital stenosis and multilevel severe spinal stenosis. Regardless of which procedure is utilized, preservation of pars interarticularis and at least 50% of the facet joints bilaterally is recommended to prevent iatrogenic spinal instability.

18. **What are the indications for fusion in lumbar spinal stenosis procedures?**

The indications for fusion fall into two broad categories:

PREOPERATIVE STRUCTURAL PROBLEMS THAT PREDISPOSE TO INSTABILITY AFTER DECOMPRESSION
- Degenerative spondylolisthesis or lateral listhesis
- Progressive scoliosis or kyphosis
- Recurrent spinal stenosis requiring repeat decompression at the same level

INTRAOPERATIVE STRUCTURAL ALTERATIONS THAT WARRANT CONSIDERATION OF A FUSION
- Excess facet joint removal (>50%)
- Pars interarticularis fracture or removal
- Radical disc excision with resultant destabilization of the anterior spinal column

19. **What types of fusion procedures are performed for unstable spinal stenosis syndromes?**

The most common type of fusion procedure is a posterior fusion combined with posterior pedicle screw fixation. Interbody fusion may be added for patients with severe coronal and/or sagittal imbalance, rotatory subluxations, severe foraminal stenosis (to provide indirect decompression through restoration of foraminal height), deficient posterior facet joints, or biologic factors that negatively affect fusion success.

20. **How do interspinous process distraction devices improve spinal stenosis symptoms?**

A device is inserted between adjacent spinous processes to create segmental flexion at the operative level. This indirectly increases the cross-sectional area of the spinal canal and neural foramina. Appropriate candidates for this type of device are patients with mild to moderate spinal stenosis whose symptoms are relieved with sitting and flexion maneuvers. These devices are appealing to patients because the procedure for insertion is less invasive than a laminotomy or laminectomy procedure. Short-term data have shown that interspinous spacers are superior to nonoperative treatment and comparable to laminectomy in the short term. However, long-term data are not available and the durability of clinical improvement is unknown. An example of a contemporary interspinous implant is the X-STOP® IPD®implant. It is currently Food and Drug Administration (FDA) approved for implantation at one or two levels between L1 and L5 in patients with intermittent neurogenic claudication due to spinal stenosis.

Key Points

1. Lumbar spinal stenosis is defined as any type of narrowing of the spinal canal, nerve root canals, or intervertebral foramen.
2. Spinal stenosis symptoms are typically position dependent and exacerbated by activities that promote spinal extension such as prolonged standing or walking and relieved with spinal flexion maneuvers.
3. Surgical treatment options for lumbar spinal stenosis include insertion of an interspinous spacer, lumbar decompression (laminotomy or laminectomy), and lumbar decompression combined with spinal instrumentation and fusion.

Websites

Lumbar spinal stenosis: http://www.aafp.org/afp/980415ap/alvarez.html
Lumbar spinal stenosis: http://orthoinfo.aaos.org/topic.cfm?topic=A00329
Spinal stenosis: http://www.nlm.nih.gov/medlineplus/spinalstenosis.html

BIBLIOGRAPHY

1. Arnoldi CC, Brodsky AE, Cauchoix J, et al. Lumbar spinal stenosis and nerve root entrapment syndromes: definition and classification. Clin Orthop 1976;115:4–5.
2. Atlas SJ, Keller RB, Wu YA. Long-term outcomes of surgical and nonsurgical management of lumbar spinal stenosis: 8-10 year results from the Maine Lumbar Spine Study. Spine 2005;30:936–43.
3. Herkowitz HN, Sidhu KSD. Lumbar spine fusion in the treatment of degenerative conditions: current indications and recommendations. J Am Acad Orthop Surg 1995;3:123–35.
4. Katz JN, Lipson SJ, et al. Seven- to ten-year outcome of decompressive surgery for degenerative lumbar spinal stenosis. Spine 1996;21:92–8.
5. Kim DH, Anderson PA. Interspinous process distraction devices for spinal stenosis. Semin Spine Surg 2007;19:206–14.
6. O'Leary PF, McCance SE. Distraction laminoplasty for decompression of spinal stenosis. Clin Orth Rel Res 2001;384:26–34.
7. Weinstein JN, Toteson TD, Lurie JD, et al. Surgical versus nonsurgical therapy for lumbar spinal stenosis. N Engl J Med 2008;358:794–810.

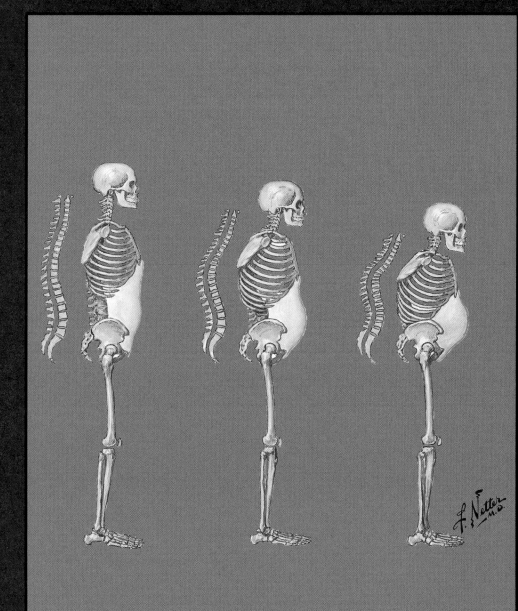

ADULT IDIOPATHIC AND DEGENERATIVE SCOLIOSIS

Brian A. O'Shaughnessy, MD, Charles H. Crawford, III, MD, and Keith H. Bridwell, MD

1. What are the two types of adult lumbar scoliosis?
- Idiopathic with superimposed degenerative changes
- De novo/degenerative scoliosis

2. Define degenerative or de novo scoliosis. How does it differ from adult idiopathic scoliosis?
De novo scoliosis begins at age 40 in patients with no preexisting deformity. The deformity occurs in conjunction with multilevel asymmetric disc degeneration. At various levels, the discs degenerate more on one side than the other, resulting in a lumbar deformity. By contrast, adult patients with idiopathic scoliosis presumably had some degree of deformity as a teenager. Although each patient is different, patients with idiopathic scoliosis tend to have more rotational deformity at each segment of their curve than do patients with de novo scoliosis.

3. What is the association of spinal stenosis with idiopathic scoliosis and superimposed degenerative changes?
It is uncommon to see a substantial amount of central spinal stenosis in patients who have preexisting idiopathic scoliosis with superimposed degenerative changes. It is more common to see either lateral recess stenosis or foraminal stenosis on the concavity of the distal segments.

4. Which levels are most commonly affected by spinal stenosis in patients with idiopathic scoliosis and superimposed degenerative changes in the lumbar spine?
L3–L4, L4–L5, and L5–S1. At L3–L4 stenosis may be somewhat related to the rotatory subluxation commonly found at this level. At L4–L5, lateral recess stenosis is most common; at L5–S1, foraminal stenosis is most common. The stenosis at L4–L5 and L5–S1 is usually on the concavity of the fractional curve below.

5. What is the most common curve pattern with lumbar degenerative scoliosis?
Usually one sees a double lumbar curve pattern in which one curve, most commonly left-sided, is from T12 to L3 and the second curve is right-sided from L3 to the sacrum. At L3–L4 there is usually a rotatory subluxation with lateral listhesis, which forms the transitional segment between the two curves.

6. With adult scoliosis and foraminal stenosis at L5–S1, what nerve root is most commonly affected?
The nerve root exiting between the L5 and S1 pedicle is the L5 root. Most commonly one sees a left-sided lumbar curve from T12 to L4 and then a fractional curve from L4 to the sacrum that swings the other way. In this situation, the concavity of the fractional curve is on the left side; the left L5 nerve root is the one most commonly affected.

7. What are the most common indications for surgical treatment of lumbar idiopathic scoliosis with subsequent degenerative changes?
- Progressive deformity
- Progressive pain
- Spinal claudication symptoms
- Neurologic deficit

8. What are the indications for surgical treatment in young adults with scoliosis who do not have substantial degenerative changes?
- A deformity over 50° by Cobb measurement that the patient perceives as either unacceptable or progressive
- Documented progression of the deformity
- Coronal or sagittal imbalance

9. Is significant back pain a common presentation in a young adult with scoliosis in the absence of substantial degenerative changes?
No. Patients with significant back pain without advanced degenerative changes should raise the suspicion of a tumor, arteriovenous malformation, or intrinsic abnormality of the spinal cord. Particular attention on the neurologic

examination should be paid to evaluation of gait, motor/sensory testing, and the presence of any upper motor neuron signs (e.g. clonus, Babinski reflex). In such patients, especially if the neurologic examination is abnormal, magnetic resonance imaging (MRI) or computed tomography myelography may be warranted.

10. **Define neutral sagittal balance.**
Sagittal balance is defined by a plumb dropped from the cervical spine. Some prefer to drop the plumb from C2, and others prefer to drop it from C7. The plumb on a standing lateral x-ray should fall through the lumbosacral disc. Falling through the lumbosacral disc is neutral balance. Falling behind it is negative sagittal balance, and falling in front of it is positive sagittal balance.

11. **What is the most common sagittal alignment associated with progressive lumbar scoliosis?**
Adults with progressive lumbar scoliosis usually have coexisting disc degeneration at all segments. The result is loss of anterior column height and thus segmental kyphosis. This results in positive sagittal imbalance.

12. **Does positive sagittal imbalance correlate with poor functional status in adult patients with scoliosis?**
Yes. In a study by Glassman and colleagues, positive sagittal balance was identified as the radiographic parameter most highly correlated with adverse health status outcomes. Moreover, although even mildly positive sagittal balance was found to be somewhat detrimental, the severity of symptoms increased in a linear fashion with progressive sagittal imbalance. Positive sagittal imbalance related to lumbar hypolordosis was most poorly tolerated.

13. **Name four common causes for flatback syndrome or fixed sagittal imbalance syndrome.**
1. Harrington instrumentation in the lumbar spine
2. Multisegment anterior compression instrumentation/fusion without structural grafting
3. Progressive postlaminectomy kyphosis
4. Junctional kyphosis above a multisegment lumbar fusion

14. **What are the three primary osteotomy techniques used in adult spinal deformity?**
1. Smith-Petersen osteotomy or Ponte osteotomy
2. Pedicle subtraction osteotomy
3. Vertebral column resection (VCR)

15. **What is the effect of a Smith-Petersen osteotomy in the anterior, middle, and posterior column?**
Smith-Petersen osteotomy opens up the anterior column, closes the middle column somewhat, and closes the posterior column (Fig. 52-1).

16. **What is the effect of a pedicle subtraction osteotomy (PSO) on the anterior, middle, and posterior column?**
A PSO hinges on the anterior column and closes the middle and posterior columns (Fig. 52-2).

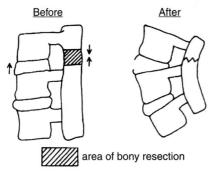

Figure 52-1. Smith-Petersen osteotomy. (From Booth KC, Bridwell KH, Lenke LG, et al. Complications and predictive factors for the successful treatment of flatback deformity (fixed sagittal imbalance). Spine 1999;24:1712–20.)

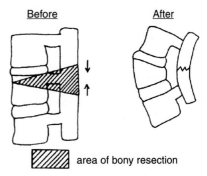

Figure 52-2. Three-column pedicle subtraction osteotomy. (From Booth KC, Bridwell KH, Lenke LG, et al. Complications and predictive factors for the successful treatment of flatback deformity (fixed sagittal imbalance). Spine 1999;24:1712–20.)

17. Name four acceptable forms of anterior structural grafting used with multisegment fusions in the lumbar spine.

1. Fresh frozen femoral rings packed with morselized bone graft
2. Titanium mesh cages packed with bone graft
3. Polyetheretherketone (PEEK) or carbon fiber cages packed with bone graft
4. Autogenous tricortical iliac bone graft. There is rarely enough bone stock, however, for more than two levels

18. What type of bone graft is most effective for achieving fusion when packed within these structural grafts or cages?

Either morselized autogenous graft from iliac crest harvest, local autogenous bone graft, or recombinant human bone morphogenetic protein-2 (rhBMP-2).

19. Name four surgical principles that should be accomplished to have a reasonable chance of getting a long fusion to the sacrum solid.

1. Segmental fixation of all segments of the lumbar spine without jumps or gaps
2. Structural grafting at L4–L5 and L5–S1
3. Neutral or slightly negative sagittal balance
4. Four-point fixation of the sacrum and pelvis

20. What are the principal indications for surgical treatment of degenerative/de novo scoliosis?

1. Progressive deformity that is unacceptable for the patient
2. Major coronal or sagittal imbalance
3. Spinal claudication symptoms

21. List options for spinal cord monitoring in the surgical treatment of adult scoliosis.

- Stagnara wake-up test
- Somatosensory evoked potentials
- Motor-evoked potentials
- Hoppenfeld clonus test

22. List complications of surgical treatment of adult scoliosis.

- Pseudarthrosis
- Superficial wound infection
- Deep wound infection
- Neurologic deficit
- Progressive coronal deformity
- Progressive sagittal deformity
- Fixed sagittal imbalance
- Increasing pain

23. How much sagittal correction is usually achieved with a lumbar pedicle subtraction osteotomy?

30° to 35°.

24. How does a pedicle subtraction osteotomy (PSO) differ from a vertebral column resection (VCR)?

Both a PSO and VCR can be performed in the thoracic and lumbar spine; however, most commonly for fixed deformity, a PSO is performed in the lumbar spine and a VCR is carried out in the thoracic spine. The most distinguishing feature that differentiates a PSO from VCR is correction mechanics. In a PSO, there is a fixed angle of closure determined by the size of the wedge resection. In a VCR, the spine is dissociated in two separate segments and the arc of correction falls anterior to the spinal column with no fixed closure angle. For this reason, VCR is often best suited for sharp, angular deformities that can be significantly corrected, provided the spinal cord can tolerate the configurational change the osteotomy affords.

25. Does thoracic scoliosis ever progress in adulthood?

Which curves do and do not progress into adulthood is highly variable. It is generally thought that a significant percentage of curves over 50° progress into adulthood. A relatively small percentage of curves between 30° and 50° progress, and progression of thoracic curves below 30° is unlikely.

26. Is lumbar degenerative scoliosis generally progressive or nonprogressive?

This question does not have a simple answer. It is generally thought that a high percentage of degenerative scoliosis cases progress in adulthood. Degenerative scoliosis may be more inclined to progress than long-standing preexisting idiopathic scoliosis. Multiple rotatory subluxations and a relative lack of osteophyte formation seem to be predisposing factors for progression.

27. Can an adult lumbar fusion for scoliosis be stopped at L4 even in the presence of disc degeneration at L4–L5 and L5–S1?

This issue is highly controversial. Some authors believe that the fusion can be stopped at L4 if the disc degeneration at L4–L5 and L5–S1 is not substantial. Others believe that if disc degeneration is present at these two segments, the fusion should automatically be carried to the sacrum. A middle-of-the-road philosophy is that stopping at L4 is possible and feasible only if there is no substantial deformity between L4 and the sacrum and if the disc degeneration at these two segments is *mild* (Fig. 52-3).

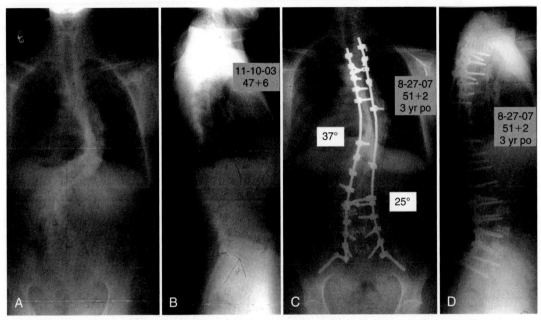

Figure 52-3. **A** and **B,** Adult idiopathic scoliosis. A 47-year-old female with progressive thoracic and lumbar curves and superimposed degenerative changes. Notice the rotatory subluxation at L3–L4, the fixed tilt at L4–L5, and disc space collapse at L5–S1. **C** and **D,** Three years after a long posterior fusion to the sacrum and anterior interbody grafting with titanium mesh cages, her Oswestry Disability Index has improved from 32 to 0.

28. List potential complications associated with an anterior approach that is performed from T12 to the sacrum.
- Sympathectomy effect in the ipsilateral leg
- Deep venous thrombosis in association with extensive mobilization of the venous structures from L4 to the sacrum
- Bulging or diastasis of the abdominal wall postoperatively
- Retroperitoneal fibrosis

29. Which anterior surgical approach accomplishes exposure anteriorly of all segments from T10 to the sacrum?
The thoracoabdominal approach, which usually involves entering the chest through the 10th rib and then taking down the diaphragm and the superficial and deep abdominal muscles.

30. For a left lumbar scoliosis, if exposure is desired from T10 to the sacrum, is it better to do the approach from the left side or the right side?
It is generally best to approach a curve on the convexity of the curve. In most left lumbar curve patterns, the major curve has an apex between T12 and L2 and extends from T10 or T11 to L4. From L4 to the sacrum, there is usually a fractional curve that extends the other way—to the right side. Generally exposure can be accomplished from the left side behind the aorta and vena cava from L4 to L5. Exposure at L5–S1 is variable from patient to patient. Sometimes it is possible to expose L5–S1 from the left side behind the bifurcation, and in other cases, it is necessary to expose the L5–S1 disc beneath the bifurcation. The same skin incision can be used for both exposures.

31. Are anterior approaches commonly performed today for the treatment of adult scoliosis?
As a result of the potential morbidity from an anterior approach and the fact that recent data suggest the same correction and similar fusion rates are achievable through a posterior-only approach, the enthusiasm for anterior fusions or combined anterior/posterior fusions for adult spinal deformity has declined over recent years. A *mini-open* anterior retroperitoneal approach is, however, still commonly performed to achieve anterior column structural interbody grafting at caudal segments of a long fusion to the sacrum.

32. What is the effect of thoracoplasty on pulmonary function in the adult population?
Few studies have addressed this issue. However, current literature suggests a substantial drop in pulmonary function in the first 3 months after surgery, which improves over the next 2 years. At 2 years postoperatively, pulmonary function is usually close to baseline, although frequently not entirely back to baseline. For this reason, a thoracoplasty in an adult patient who does not have exceptionally good pulmonary function may not be advisable.

33. What is the role for parenteral hyperalimentation in adults with scoliosis?
To date, no multicenter, randomized, prospective series has definitively answered this question. However, several articles suggest that parenteral nutrition seems to reduce complications somewhat in the adult population, particularly in patients having anterior and posterior surgery, either staged or continuous; patients with reduced protein stores preoperatively; and patients having fusions greater than 10 segments.

34. Do long scoliosis fusions reduce back pain in the adult population?
This question is difficult to answer definitively. Most current literature suggests that back pain is substantially improved for most patients. However, it is clear that not all patients have a reduction of pain. Furthermore, it is uncommon for back pain to be *cured* with scoliosis surgery. However, the most common outcome is substantial reduction in back pain.

35. Which is a greater problem in adult scoliosis—progression and pain with thoracic deformity or progression and pain with lumbar deformity?
One study has reported more progression with thoracic scoliosis than lumbar scoliosis in adulthood. However, most investigators have found that lumbar curves are more inclined to progress than thoracic curves. Each patient, however, is different, and one cannot always predict whether lumbar or thoracic curves will progress in adulthood.

36. For long fusions to the sacrum, which technique is currently considered the gold standard for posterior fixation at L4, L5, and the sacrum?
Currently pedicle fixation at L4, L5, and the sacrum is highly favored over hook fixation and sublaminar wire fixation. However, fixation of the sacrum is somewhat controversial. There is controversy over the best way of fixing the sacrum beyond simply the use of bicortical sacral screws.

37. With a long instrumentation to the sacrum in adults with scoliosis, if the S1 screws are inadvertently directed laterally toward the ala rather than medially toward the promontory and the screws perforate the anterior cortex, which nerve root is likely to be irritated?
The L5 root. The L5 root exits between the pedicle of L5 and S1 and then travels anterior to the sacral ala. If an S1 pedicle screw is directed medially toward the sacral promontory and protrudes beyond the anterior sacral cortex, the screw will be medial to the path of the L5 root. If an S1 pedicle screw is directed laterally and protrudes beyond the anterior sacral cortex, the screw may irritate the L5 root. This complication (L5 root irritation) is most likely to occur in a male patient with a narrow pelvis, in whom it is technically difficult to angle the S1 pedicle screws in a sufficiently medial direction. Irritation of the S1 nerve root may occur if the S1 pedicle screw were to perforate the medial cortex of the S1 pedicle and directly impinge upon the S1 nerve root.

Key Points

1. Scoliosis presenting in adulthood may represent *idiopathic scoliosis,* which initially developed in adolescence, or scoliosis, which developed in adulthood secondary to asymmetric disc degeneration and is termed *de novo* or *degenerative scoliosis.*
2. Surgical indications for adult scoliosis include progressive deformity, pain, and symptomatic neural compression.
3. The goals of surgical treatment include achievement of optimal sagittal and coronal plane balance, successful arthrodesis, and decompression of symptomatic neural compression.
4. Appropriate surgical treatment for adult scoliosis often requires anterior structural grafting, osteotomies, segmental pedicular fixation, use of osteobiologics, and iliac fixation.

Websites

North American Spine Society: http://www.spine.org/Pages/Default.aspx
Scoliosis Research Society: http://www.srs.org/
Spine Universe: http://www.spineuniverse.com/

BIBLIOGRAPHY

1. Bradford DS, Tay BK, Hu SS. Adult scoliosis: surgical indications, operative management, complications, and outcomes. Spine 1999;24:2617–2629.
2. Bridwell KH. Osteotomies for fixed deformities in the thoracic and lumbar spine. In: Bridwell KH, DeWald RL, editors. The Textbook of Spinal Surgery. 2nd ed. Philadelphia: Lippincott-Raven; 1997. p. 821–36.
3. Dickson JH, Mirkovic S, Noble PC, et al. Results of operative treatment of idiopathic scoliosis in adults. J Bone Joint Surg 1995;77A:513–23.
4. Glassman SD, Bridwell K, Dimar JR, et al. The impact of positive sagittal balance in adult spinal deformity. Spine 2005;30:2024–9.
5. Grubb SA, Lipscomb HJ, Conrad RW. Degenerative adult onset scoliosis. Spine 1988;13:241–5.
6. Kostuik JP. Adult scoliosis: the lumbar spine. In: Bridwell KH, DeWald RL, editors. The Textbook of Spinal Surgery. 2nd ed. Philadelphia: Lippincott-Raven; 1997. p. 733–75.
7. Weinstein SL, Ponseti IV. Curve progression in idiopathic scoliosis. J Bone Joint Surg 1983;65A:447–55.

SAGITTAL PLANE DEFORMITIES IN ADULTS

Munish C. Gupta, MD, and Vincent J. Devlin, MD

1. Describe the normal sagittal contour of the adult spine.

In the sagittal plane, the normal spine possesses four balanced curves (Fig. 53-1). The kyphotic thoracic and sacral regions are balanced by the lordotic cervical and lumbar regions. In the normal state, the sagittal vertical axis (determined by dropping plumb line from the center of the C7 vertebral body) passes anterior to the thoracic spine, through the center of the L1 vertebral body, posterior to the lumbar spine, and through the lumbosacral disc. A positive sagittal vertical axis (SVA) is present when this line passes in front of the anterior aspect of S1. Negative SVA is present when this line passes behind the posterior aspect of S1. Sagittal imbalance has been defined as an SVA passing more than 5 cm anterior to the posterior margin of the superior S1 endplate.

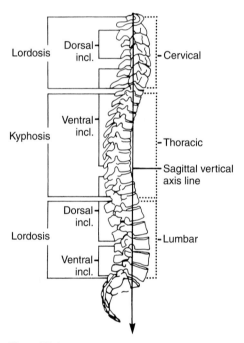

Figure 53-1. Normal sagittal alignment of the spinal column. Note the sagittal vertical axis line and the orientation of each individual vertebrae. (From DeWald RL. Revision surgery for spinal deformity. Instructional Course Lectures vol. 41. Park Ride, IL: American Academy of Orthopaedic Surgeons; 1992.)

2. What are normal values for thoracic kyphosis, lumbar lordosis, and sagittal vertical axis in adults?

There is a wide range of normal values in adults. Thoracic kyphosis (T2–T12) varies between 30° and 50°. Lumbar lordosis varies between 45° and 70°. The sagittal vertical axis passes within 2 cm of the posterior superior corner of S1. A correlation between increasing thoracic kyphosis and lumbar lordosis tends to maintain spinal balance. In general, lumbar lordosis exceeds thoracic kyphosis by 20° to 30° to maintain spinal balance and normal position of the sagittal vertical axis.

3. **How does normal sagittal alignment change with age?**
   Aging is associated with loss of anterior spinal column height secondary to degenerative disc changes and vertebral body compression, resulting in increased thoracic kyphosis and decreased lumbar lordosis. The C7 plumb line moves anterior relative to the sacrum as thoracic kyphosis (the angle between the upper end plate of T2 and the lower end plate of T12 on the lateral radiograph) increases and lumbar lordosis (from the top of L1 to the top of S1) decreases. Even asymptomatic people lean forward with age.

4. **List common causes of sagittal plane spinal deformity requiring surgical treatment in the adult population.**
   Degenerative spinal disorders, fractures, scoliosis, spondylolisthesis, ankylosing spondylitis, and iatrogenic spinal disorders are common causes of sagittal plane deformity requiring surgical treatment in the adult patient. Any adult spinal deformity of sufficient severity to warrant surgical intervention requires analysis of preoperative sagittal plane alignment.

5. **What radiographs are required for evaluation of sagittal plane alignment?**
   A lateral standing spine radiograph performed on a 36-inch cassette to permit evaluation of thoracic kyphosis, lumbar lordosis, sacral orientation, and the sagittal vertical axis. It is important that the patient stand with the hips and knees fully extended. The elbows should be flexed and the patient's hands should rest in the supraclavicular fossa. Lateral flexion-extension views and supine cross-table lateral hyperextension films performed over a radiolucent bolster may provide additional information about a specific spinal region.

6. **Why is it important to visualize the femoral heads on the lateral standing spine radiograph?**
   There is an interrelationship between the orientation of the distal lumbar spine, sacrum, and the pelvic unit, which influences sagittal alignment of the spine. Three pelvic parameters are measured: pelvic incidence (PI), sacral slope (SS), and pelvic tilt (PT). Pelvic incidence (PI) is a fixed anatomic parameter unique to the individual. Sacral slope (SS) and pelvic tilt (PT) are variable parameters. The relationship among the parameters determines the overall alignment of the sacropelvic unit according to the formula $PI = PT + SS$. Increased pelvic tilt is a compensatory mechanism for a positive shift in SVA and should be considered when planning reconstructive spinal surgery for sagittal imbalance. (See Chapter 10, Question 28.)

7. **Explain the biomechanical factors responsible for the development of kyphotic deformities.**
   The spine can be conceptualized as consisting of two columns, the anterior spinal column (vertebral bodies, intervertebral disc, and anterior and posterior longitudinal ligaments) and the posterior spinal column (facets, laminae, and associated ligaments). The anterior column resists compressive forces, whereas the posterior column resists tensile forces. Disruption of either column can lead to development of a kyphotic deformity.

8. **What descriptive terms are used in association with kyphotic deformities?**
   - **Short-radius kyphosis:** An acute angular kyphosis occurs over a few vertebral segments
   - **Long-radius kyphosis:** A uniform posterior curvature develops over many segments of the spine
   - **Flexible kyphosis:** Corrects within the normal range with hyperextension
   - **Rigid kyphosis:** Deformity resists correction with hyperextension
   - **Rotational kyphosis:** The vertebral bodies rotate out of the sagittal plane and a complex spinal deformity develops involving the sagittal, axial, and coronal planes

9. **What general concepts guide the surgical treatment of kyphotic deformities?**
   The goal of surgical treatment of kyphotic deformities is to restore the function of the compromised spinal columns. The anterior spinal column length and anterior column load sharing are maintained or restored. Integrity of the posterior spinal column is restored with spinal instrumentation. The length of the posterior spinal column is shortened by application of compression forces. Neural compression, if present, is relieved through either direct or indirect techniques. Lasting deformity correction is maintained by successful arthrodesis.

10. **Describe the principles of surgical treatment for Scheuermann's kyphosis.**
    Scheuermann's kyphosis is a long-radius kyphotic deformity that may be either flexible or rigid. Adult deformities of sufficient severity to require surgical treatment tend to be rigid.
    - **Traditional surgical treatment** consists of a first-stage anterior approach to release contracted anterior spinal column structures, including the anterior longitudinal ligament, annulus, and intervertebral disc. The disc spaces are filled with nonstructural bone graft. The deformity is corrected with second-stage procedure using posterior segmental spinal instrumentation placed above and below the apex of the kyphotic deformity.
    - **An alternative approach (Ponte technique)** that permits deformity correction through a single-stage posterior surgical approach has evolved. Multilevel interlaminar closing wedge resections are performed over the full length of the deformity and compression forces are applied to the spine via segmental fixation in order to shorten the posterior spinal column and achieve correction of the kyphotic deformity.

11. **Describe the principles of surgical treatment for posttraumatic kyphosis.**

Posttraumatic kyphosis is most commonly a short-radius kyphotic deformity that may be either flexible or rigid. Factors to consider in the surgical treatment of posttraumatic kyphosis include the magnitude of deformity, the number of involved levels, global sagittal balance, effects of prior surgical procedures, the presence or absence of neurologic deficit, and the stability of the anterior and posterior spinal columns. Isolated anterior surgical procedures are often insufficient because the posterior osteoligamentous structures impede adequate deformity correction and restoration of normal spinal biomechanics. Decision making regarding surgical treatment must be individualized. Valid treatment options for posttraumatic kyphotic deformities include pedicle subtraction osteotomies, Smith-Petersen osteotomies, and combined anterior and posterior procedures. See Figure 53-2.

12. **What factors are responsible for the development of kyphotic deformities in senior citizens?**

The most common etiologies responsible for the development of kyphotic deformities in senior citizens include loss of posterior muscular and ligamentous tone, compression fractures secondary to osteoporosis, and loss of disc height secondary to degenerative disc changes.

13. **How is sagittal plane alignment altered in ankylosing spondylitis?**

Patients with ankylosing spondylitis may develop fixed flexion deformities of the hips and spine. Patients with severe deformities are unable to look straight ahead and have extreme difficulties carrying out activities of daily living. Initial surgical treatment is most frequently directed at the hip joints. Total hip arthroplasty is an effective procedure in this population. Severe deformities require additional surgery with spinal osteotomy at the site of major deformity.

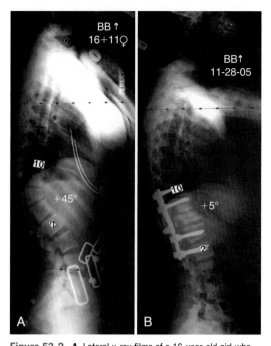

Figure 53-2. A, Lateral x-ray films of a 16-year-old girl who sustained a three-column flexion-distraction injury during a motor vehicle accident. She was treated with a posterior spinal fusion from T10 to L2 with a T12 pedicle subtraction osteotomy with correction of her deformity and restoration of normal sagittal balance as seen in **(B)** the postoperative lateral x-ray. (From Buchowski JM, Kuhns CA, Bridwell KH, et al. Surgical management of posttraumatic thoracolumbar kyphosis. Spine J 2008;8:666–77.)

14. **What is flatback deformity?**

Flatback deformity describes symptomatic loss of normal sagittal plane alignment resulting from loss of lumbar lordosis. This moves the C7 plumb line and head to an anterior position relative to the sacrum. This deformity was initially reported in association with Harrington instrumentation that corrected the coronal plane deformity of scoliosis through the application of posterior distraction forces. This approach had the unintended consequence of decreasing the normal lordotic alignment of the lumbar region creating an iatrogenic spinal deformity. Current terminology for this deformity includes *fixed sagittal imbalance, sagittal malalignment,* or *sagittal imbalance syndrome.*

15. **In addition to Harrington instrumentation, what are some other causes of sagittal imbalance syndrome?**

Sagittal imbalance syndrome may occur for many reasons in addition to Harrington instrumentation for scoliosis treatment. Sagittal plane malalignment may occur after lumbar fusion for degenerative spinal disorders when adequate lumbar lordosis is not restored during the initial surgery. Transition syndrome (breakdown of spinal segments above or below a solid spinal fusion) is another frequent cause of sagittal imbalance. Autofusion of the spine as a result of Forestier's disease (diffuse idiopathic skeletal hyperostosis, DISH) or ankylosing spondylitis may also lead to spinal imbalance. Osteoporotic compression fractures are a common cause of sagittal imbalance. Additional etiologies include spinal tumors, spinal trauma, spinal infections, and iatrogenic deformities following instrumented spinal fusion surgery.

16. **How does loss of lumbar lordosis increase muscle fatigue?**

Loss of lordosis causes anterior translation of the C7 plumb line and center of gravity, resulting in an increased flexion moment applied to the spine. The distance between the spine and the lumbar erector spinae muscles decreases, thus shortening the moment arm of the spinal extensors. The erector spinae muscles must work harder to balance the body; as a result, these muscles fatigue earlier.

17. List early and late compensatory mechanisms that attempt to accommodate for loss of lumbar lordosis.

Early compensatory mechanisms include hyperextension of adjacent mobile lumbar, thoracic, and cervical segments, as well as hip hyperextension. With further decompensation, knee flexion helps keep the head above the pelvis but results in quadriceps fatigue. Patients present with a *flexed-knee, flexed-hip* appearance.

18. What are the consequences of compensatory hyperextension of adjacent spinal motion segments?

Increased facet loads lead to facet and disc degeneration, as well as pain. Spondylolisthesis may develop secondary to facet degeneration and/or fracture through the pars interarticularis.

19. How does operative positioning affect lumbar lordosis?

Hip flexion significantly reduces lumbar lordosis. Although hip flexion can facilitate access to the spinal canal for surgical decompression, the reduction of lumbar lordosis must be taken into account if a fusion is performed during the same procedure. Lumbar instrumentation and fusion should be performed with the hips extended to maintain and restore maximal lumbar lordosis.

20. What are the surgical options for correction of sagittal deformity in the previously unfused spine?

Posterior fusion with segmental instrumentation using appropriately contoured spinal rods can improve sagittal alignment. More severe deformity may require a wide posterior release and transforaminal lumbar interbody fusion or anterior release and anterior interbody fusion to restore the intervertebral disc height and segmental lordosis.

21. What are the surgical options for correction of the sagittal plane deformity in the previously fused spine?

Smith-Petersen osteotomy (resection of a posterior column wedge to achieve correction through the disc space or through a prior anterior osteotomy) and **pedicle subtraction osteotomy** (resection of a three-column wedge hinging at the anterior longitudinal ligament) are powerful methods for correction sagittal deformity. Combined coronal and sagittal deformity may be corrected with a **vertebral column resection procedure.** See Figure 53-3.

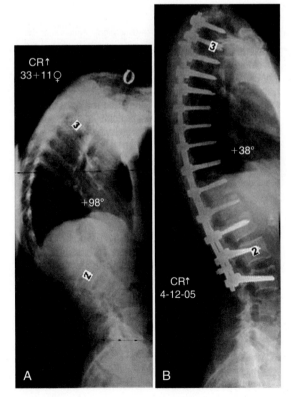

Figure 53-3. **A,** Preoperative lateral x-ray film of a 33-year-old woman who sustained T5 and T8 compression fractures and a T12 burst fracture when she was hit by a falling tree. The patient underwent posterior segment al spinal instrumentation from T2 to L1 with posterior spinal fusion from T11 to L1, where a year after the initial surgery, the instrumentation was removed. The patient presented approximately 6 years after the removal of instrumentation with increasing thoracic pain and hyperkyphosis. She was treated with multiple Smith-Petersen osteotomies from T5 to L1 and an instrumented posterior spinal fusion from T2 to L3 by using pedicle screws with restoration of normal sagittal contours and balance as seen in **(B)** the postoperative lateral x-ray films of the spine. (From Buchowski JM, Kuhns CA, Bridwell KH, et al. Surgical management of posttraumatic thoracolumbar kyphosis. Spine J 2008;8:666–77.)

Key Points

1. Any adult spinal deformity patient considered for surgical treatment involving multilevel spinal instrumentation and fusion requires detailed preoperative analysis of sagittal plane alignment.
2. Prevention of postoperative sagittal imbalance following spinal instrumentation and fusion begins with patient positioning on an operating table, which permits enhancement of lumbar lordosis.
3. Important techniques for achieving optimal sagittal alignment include appropriate sagittal rod contouring and restoration of segmental sagittal alignment using interbody fusion, wide posterior releases, and spinal osteotomies as needed.
4. Surgical options for treatment of sagittal imbalance in the previously fused spine include Smith-Petersen osteotomies, Ponte osteotomies, pedicle subtraction osteotomy, combined anterior and posterior osteotomy, and vertebral column resection.

Websites

Spinal osteotomies: http://www.coa-aco.org/coa-bulletin/issue-85/themes-complex-procedures-revision-surgeries-and-spinal-osteotomies.html
Vertebral column resection: http://www.spinal-deformity-surgeon.com/vcr-paper.html
Adult sagittal plane deformity: http://www.spineinstituteny.com/research/assets/Joseph_2009.pdf
Pedicle subtraction osteotomy: http://www.spineuniverse.com/professional/pathology/deformity/ankylosing-spondylitis-treated-pedicle-subtraction
Decisions and expectations with osteotomy surgery: http://www.spineuniverse.com/professional/technology/surgical/thoracic/decisions-expectations-osteotomy-surgery-fixed

BIBLIOGRAPHY

1. Bernhardt M, Bridwell KH. Segmental analysis of the sagittal plane alignment of the normal thoracic and lumbar spines and thoracolumbar junction. Spine 1989;14:717–21.
2. Bradford DS, Tribus CB. Vertebral column resection for the treatment of rigid coronal decompensation. Spine 1997;22:1590–9.
3. Bridwell KH. Decision making regarding Smith-Petersen vs. pedicle subtraction vs. vertebral column resection for spinal deformity. Spine 2006;31:S171–8.
4. Buchowski JM, Kuhns CA, Bridwell KH, et al. Surgical management of posttraumatic thoracolumbar kyphosis. Spine J 2008;8:666–77.
5. Joseph SA, Morena AP, Brandoff J, et al. Sagittal plane deformity in the adult patient. J Am Acad Orthop Surg 2009;17:378–88.
6. Lafage V, Schwab F, Patel A, et al. Pelvic tilt and truncal inclination: two key radiographic parameters in the setting of adults with spinal deformity. Spine 2009;34:E599–E606.
7. Legaye J, Duval-Beaupère G, Hecquet J, et al. Pelvic incidence: a fundamental pelvic parameter for three-dimensional regulation of spinal sagittal curves. Eur Spine J 1998;7:99–103.
8. Rinella AS, Bridwell KH. Iatrogenic fixed sagittal imbalance. In: Herkowitz HN, Garfin SR, Eismont FJ, Bell GR, Balderston RA, editors. Rothman and Simeone The Spine. 5th ed. Philadelphia: Saunders; 2006. p. 1564–78.

SPONDYLOLYSIS AND SPONDYLOLISTHESIS IN ADULTS

Vincent J. Devlin, MD

1. **Discuss similarities and differences between adult and pediatric patients with spondylolysis and spondylolisthesis in regard to classification, clinical presentation, radiographic workup, and treatment.**

CLASSIFICATION

Contemporary classifications (Wiltse, Marchetti, and Bartolozzi) do not distinguish between pediatric and adult patients with spondylolisthesis. However, the degenerative type of spondylolisthesis is seen only in adult patients. Degenerative spondylolisthesis is covered in this chapter while basic principles regarding spondylolisthesis with emphasis on isthmic spondylolisthesis are covered in detail in Chapter 38.

CLINICAL PRESENTATION

In pediatric patients, back pain is the most common presenting symptom. Pain is directly related to instability at the site of spondylolysis/spondylolisthesis. Symptoms of hamstring spasm are not uncommon. Occasionally, L5 radicular symptoms occur. In pediatric high-grade developmental spondylolisthesis patients, spinal stenosis symptoms may develop including cauda equina-related symptoms. In contrast, adult patients frequently present with both back and leg pain symptoms. In adult patients, symptoms may be related either to the level of spondylolisthesis or to degenerative pathology (disc protrusion, stenosis, discogenic pain) at adjacent spinal levels. It is critical to precisely localize the pain generator in adult patients with spondylolisthesis because pain may not be related to the spondylolisthesis.

DIAGNOSTIC WORKUP

Standing spinal radiographs are the initial radiographic study for assessment of spondylolisthesis in both pediatric and adult patients. The degree of slip (Meyerding classification) and the slip angle are important for decision making in both patient groups. The need for additional diagnostic imaging is more frequent in adults to assess the cause of leg pain and status of the lumbar discs. Magnetic resonance imaging (MRI) is the standard for evaluating neural compression in both pediatric and adult patients. Computed tomography (CT) is the method of choice for assessing osseous anatomy in both groups. Discography is occasionally used in adult patients to assess whether a particular disc is a pain generator but has little role in pediatric patients. Technetium bone scans are sometimes used in pediatric patients to assess osseous activity related to spondylolysis and assess healing of pars defects. In adult patients, bone scans are of little value for assessment of spondylolysis because pars defects are typically inactive in adults.

SURGICAL TREATMENT

In pediatric patients, options for treatment of spondylolysis include either direct pars repair or intertransverse fusion. In adults, surgical treatment of symptomatic spondylolysis requires a fusion because the disc at the level of the pars defect typically demonstrates degenerative changes demonstrates degenerative changes and the chronic pars defects have poor healing potential.

   With respect to treatment of low-grade isthmic spondylolisthesis (grade 1 and grade 2) in children, in situ posterolateral fusion with or without posterior spinal instrumentation is associated with a high success rate due to the excellent healing potential of pediatric patients. Adults with low-grade isthmic spondylolisthesis generally receive more complex surgery, but surgical decision making remains controversial. Adult patients are most commonly treated with posterior spinal fusion combined with pedicle fixation and direct neural decompression. The addition of an interbody fusion is advocated by many surgeons and may be performed through either an anterior or posterior approach. Some surgeons prefer to perform posterior fusion without direct neural decompression in the absence of severe neurologic deficits in order to preserve greater osseous surface area for posterior fusion. Other surgeons advocate posterior fusion without use of instrumentation for low-grade slips. The rationale for use of posterior spinal instrumentation is to decrease the risk of postoperative slip progression and enhance the success rate of posterior fusion.

With respect to treatment of high-grade spondylolisthesis (grade 3 and 4), circumferential fusion provides the most reliable rate of fusion in both pediatric and adult patients. Circumferential fusion may be performed with reduction (partial vs. complete) or without reduction of the spondylolisthesis. Direct decompression of central and foraminal stenosis is generally performed in conjunction with instrumentation and fusion.

ISTHMIC SPONDYLOLISTHESIS

2. Does isthmic spondylolisthesis progress after skeletal maturity?
Sometimes. When slip progression occurs in the adult patient with isthmic spondylolisthesis, the degree of slip is most likely to progress during the fourth and fifth decades of life. Progression of slippage is associated with the development of degenerative disc changes at the level of the pars defect. The ability of the intervertebral disc to resist shear forces at the level of the pars defect is compromised and progression of spondylolisthesis occurs. This explains how a pars defect that has been asymptomatic since childhood may become symptomatic in later life in the absence of precipitating trauma.

3. What nonoperative treatment options are available for adults with isthmic spondylolisthesis?
Nonoperative treatment options include nonsteroidal antiinflammatory drugs, physical therapy, epidural injections, and orthoses. Weight reduction is an appropriate recommendation for overweight patients. Smoking cessation is advised due to its association with back pain symptoms and its adverse effect on healing of spinal fusion in the event that future fusion surgery is considered.

4. When is surgery considered for an adult patient with isthmic spondylolisthesis?
Surgery is infrequently required for adult patients with spondylolisthesis. General indications to consider surgical intervention for adult isthmic spondylolisthesis include:
- Failure of nonsurgical treatment for disabling back and/or leg pain
- Patients with symptomatic and radiographically unstable isthmic spondylolisthesis
- Documented slip progression ($>$ grade 2 slippage)
- Symptomatic grade 3 or 4 spondylolisthesis or spondyloptosis
- Associated symptomatic spinal stenosis or progressive neurologic deficit
- Cauda equina syndrome related to spondylolisthesis

5. What pattern of neural compression is most commonly associated with L5–S1 isthmic spondylolisthesis?
L5 nerve root compression (exiting nerve root of the L5-S1 motion segment) is the type of neural compression most commonly associated with L5–S1 isthmic spondylolisthesis. L5 nerve root compression may occur secondary to:
- Hypertrophy of fibrocartilage at the site of the pars defect (zone 1)
- Compression in the foraminal zone (zone 2) as the L5 root is compressed between a disc protrusion or osteophyte and the inferior aspect of the L5 pedicle
- Compression between the inferior aspect of the L5 transverse process and the superior aspect of the sacral ala (zone 3)
- Increased tension within the L5 nerve root secondary to forward displacement of the L5 vertebra

The sacral nerve roots can become involved in high-grade isthmic spondylolisthesis as these nerves become stretched over the L5–S1 disc and posterior aspect of the sacrum.

6. What are the contemporary surgical treatment options for L5–S1 isthmic spondylolisthesis in adult patients?
- Decompression and in situ posterolateral fusion with or without posterior pedicle fixation
- Decompression, posterolateral fusion, and posterior pedicle fixation combined with interbody fusion and reduction (reduction may be partial vs. complete, interbody fusion may be performed through either an anterior or posterior approach)
- Decompression, posterolateral fusion, and posterior pedicle fixation combined with partial reduction and placement of a trans-sacral interbody graft (fibula strut or cage) and/or trans-sacral screws

7. List benefits associated with combining an interbody fusion with a posterior spinal instrumentation and fusion in isthmic spondylolisthesis (Fig. 54-1).
- Increase in the surface area available for fusion healing leading to an increased rate of successful arthrodesis
- Increase in neuroforaminal height, thereby providing for indirect nerve root decompression
- Reduction in slip angle and degree of slip
- Interbody support decreases stress on pedicle screws, thereby preventing screw and implant construct failure

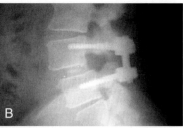

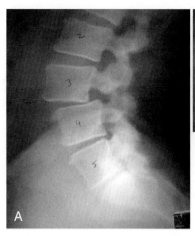

Figure 54-1. Low-grade adult isthmic spondylolisthesis. **A,** Standing lateral radiograph. **B,** Postoperative lateral radiograph following treatment with L3–L4 posterior fusion, posterior pedicle fixation, and transforaminal lumbar interbody fusion (TLIF) using a radiolucent interbody cage in combination with iliac autograft bone graft. (From Herkowitz H, Garfin S, Eismont F, et al. Rothman-Simeone The Spine. 5th ed. Philadelphia: Saunders; 2006. p. 366.)

8. **Is it necessary to achieve a complete reduction of a high-grade spondylolisthesis in order to obtain a successful clinical outcome following surgical treatment?**
   No. The factors associated with a successful outcome in high-grade spondylolisthesis surgery are maintenance or restoration of sagittal balance and achievement of a solid fusion. It has been demonstrated that reduction of the slip angle (lumbosacral kyphosis) is more important than complete reduction of the degree of slip for restoration of sagittal alignment. Complete reduction of a high-grade spondylolisthesis is associated with a high rate of L5 nerve root injury. Circumferential fusion is associated with the highest rate of successful arthrodesis, and surgical techniques have evolved to permit a circumferential fusion construct without the need to achieve complete reduction of spondylolisthesis. However, in extreme cases with severe deformity, complex procedures including complete reduction, sacral osteotomy, or L5 vertebrectomy remain valid treatment options.

9. **What is the rationale for trans-sacral interbody fusion and transvertebral screw fixation?**
   - *Secure implant fixation:* It is challenging to place L5 pedicle screws in a high-grade L5–S1 spondylolisthesis without reduction of listhesis. Secure fixation of L5 can be achieved by placing medially directed S1 screws across the anterior sacral cortex and across the L5–S1 disc and into the adjacent L5 vertebra
   - *Simplified technique for anterior column fusion:* Placement of a fibular graft or axial fusion cage can be achieved from either a posterior or anterior approach without the need for anatomic reduction of spondylolisthesis
   - *Potential for deformity correction:* Partial correction of the slip angle is feasible using this technique when indicated

DEGENERATIVE SPONDYLOLISTHESIS

10. **Define degenerative spondylolisthesis.**
    Degenerative spondylolisthesis is an anterior subluxation of one vertebra relative to the adjacent inferior vertebra in the presence of an intact posterior neural arch. The subluxation is a consequence of degenerative changes in the intervertebral disc and posterior facet joints.

11. **Who is most likely to develop degenerative spondylolisthesis?**
    Degenerative spondylolisthesis generally occurs in patients older than 40 years. It is most common in the sixth decade. Risk factors include female sex (female-to-male ratio: 4:1), diabetes, osteoporosis, and sacralization of the L5 vertebra.

12. **What level of the spine is most commonly involved in degenerative spondylolisthesis?**
    Ninety percent of cases of degenerative spondylolisthesis occur at L4–L5, and 10% of cases occur at L3–L4 or L5–S1.

13. **What are the common presenting symptoms of degenerative spondylolisthesis?**
    Symptoms include neurogenic claudication, low back pain, and radicular pain. Neurogenic claudication presents as buttock and thigh pain and cramping associated with prolonged standing or walking. Relief of these symptoms is achieved by sitting or flexion maneuvers. Patients may also report numbness, heaviness, or weakness in the lower extremities. Occasionally mild bowel or bladder dysfunction dysfunction may be reported.

14. **What nonspinal disorders must be ruled out during the examination of a patient with degenerative spondylolisthesis?**
    Degenerative arthritis of the hip joint and peripheral vascular disease. Hip joint arthrosis may cause buttock and thigh pain that mimics the symptoms of spinal stenosis. Assessment of hip joint range of motion can determine whether radiographs are necessary to evaluate the hip joints. If both hip arthritis and degenerative spondylolisthesis are present, injection of the hip

joint under fluoroscopic guidance can aid in sorting out which problem is more symptomatic. Peripheral vascular disease can also cause claudication. Assessment of lower extremity peripheral pulses is a routine part of assessment of patients with adult spinal disorders. Vascular claudication is associated with increased muscular exertion independent of trunk position. Symptoms due to vascular claudication typically occur in the distal calf and foot and are not associated with back pain.

15. What imaging studies should be obtained to assess a patient with symptoms suggestive of degenerative spondylolisthesis?

Initial studies include standing anteroposterior (AP) and lateral lumbar radiographs and lateral flexion-extension radiographs. A lumbar MRI is ordered to evaluate the spinal canal for neural compression. In patients who are unable to tolerate MRI (e.g. claustrophobia, pacemaker) and patients with associated scoliosis and spondylolisthesis, a CT-myelogram is obtained (Fig. 54-2).

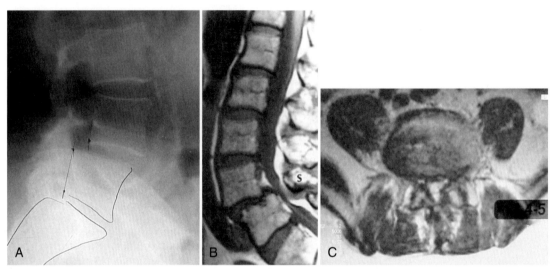

Figure 54-2. Imaging studies for degenerative spondylolisthesis. **A,** Standing lateral radiograph. **B,** Magnetic resonance imaging (MRI) sagittal view. **C,** MRI axial view. (B from Barckhausen RR, Math KR. Lumbar spine disease. In: Katz DS, Math KR, Groskin SA, editors. Radiology Secrets. Philadelphia: Hanley & Belfus; 1998.)

16. What MRI finding suggests the presence of lumbar degenerative spondylolisthesis despite normal spinal alignment on MRI?

Fluid in the facet joints. Degenerative spondylolisthesis is position dependent in many cases. Although standing radiographs will document spondylolisthesis, supine positioning for radiographs or MRI may result in spinal realignment and reduction of spondylolisthesis leading to a failure to diagnose the condition. Fluid in the facet joints is a marker that is helpful for diagnosis of a mobile spondylolisthesis (Fig. 54-3).

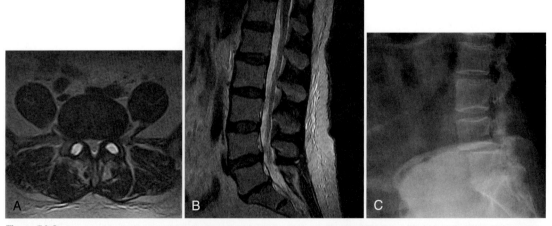

Figure 54-3. Dynamic degenerative spondylolisthesis. **A,** Axial magnetic resonance imaging (MRI) shows facet joint effusions, which suggest segmental instability. **B,** MRI sagittal view shows normal alignment at L4–L5 in the supine position. **C,** Standing lateral radiograph documents spinal instability with L4–L5 degenerative spondylolisthesis.

17. What pattern of neural compression is most commonly associated with L4–L5 degenerative spondylolisthesis?

Degenerative spondylolisthesis leads to central spinal stenosis at the level of subluxation combined with subarticular (zone 1) stenosis due to compromise of the traversing nerve root of the involved motion segment. The exiting nerve root is generally spared from compression unless there is severe loss of disc space height.

Degenerative spondylolisthesis at the L4–L5 level leads to central and subarticular stenosis with compromise of the L5 nerve root (traversing nerve root of the L4–L5 motion segment). The L4 nerve root (exiting nerve root of the L4–L5 motion segment) is spared from compression unless severe loss of disc space height results in foraminal narrowing.

18. What degree of subluxation can be associated with degenerative spondylolisthesis?

In a patient who has not undergone prior spine surgery, degenerative spondylolisthesis presents with subluxation less than 50% (grade 1 or 2 slips). Further slippage is limited by the intact neural arch.

19. What are the nonsurgical treatment options for degenerative spondylolisthesis?

Options include nonsteroidal antiinflammatory medication, physical therapy, and orthoses. Active physical therapy consisting of aerobic conditioning and lumbar flexion exercises is advised. Epidural injections are more likely to be effective for patients with significant lower extremity symptoms rather than for patients whose predominant symptom is back pain. Prescription of a walker may be helpful. Alternative treatments such as acupuncture may be considered.

20. When is surgery considered for degenerative spondylolisthesis?

- Persistent or recurrent symptoms despite adequate nonsurgical management
- Progressive neurologic deficit
- Significant reduction in quality of life
- Confirmatory imaging studies consistent with the diagnosis and symptoms

21. What are the surgical treatment options for degenerative spondylolisthesis?

- Decompression (laminotomies, interlaminar decompression, complete laminectomy)
- Decompression and posterior fusion without spinal instrumentation
- Decompression and posterior fusion and posterior spinal instrumentation
- Decompression and posterior fusion and posterior spinal instrumentation combined with interbody fusion (anterior or posterior approach)
- Innovative technologies: interspinous spacers, dynamic stabilization, minimally invasive approaches for decompression and fusion

22. What is the preferred surgical treatment for degenerative spondylolisthesis?

Outcome studies have shown that decompression combined with posterior fusion provides superior results compared with decompression without fusion. There remains lack of consensus regarding routine use of posterior spinal instrumentation, selection of the most appropriate option for bone graft (autogenous iliac graft, local bone graft, bone morphogenetic proteins) and the role of supplemental interbody fusion. Regarding use of posterior spinal instrumentation, short-term studies report a higher rate of successful fusion with spinal instrumentation but no difference in patient outcome. However, longer-term studies have shown that patients with successful fusion were significantly improved compared with those who developed pseudarthrosis. This finding has led many surgeons to recommend the use of posterior spinal instrumentation to increase the rate of successful posterior fusion and decrease the rate of slip progression.

23. Describe what is involved in a typical open decompression for L4–L5 degenerative spondylolisthesis. Does decompression without fusion ever have a role?

A typical open decompression for L4–L5 spondylolisthesis involves removal of the inferior one-half of the lamina of L4 and the superior one-half of the lamina of L5 to decompress the central spinal canal. Next the L5 nerve roots are decompressed by removing the medial one-half of the L4–L5 facet joints and accompanying ligamentum flavum. The decompression of the L5 nerve root is continued until the L5 nerve root is mobile and a probe passes easily through the neural foramen. The L4 nerve root and foramen should also be checked for potential compression.

Although a posterior fusion is generally recommended for treatment of patients with degenerative spondylolisthesis and spinal stenosis, in select situations decompression without fusion can achieve a good outcome. Potential candidates for this approach are usually low-demand elderly patients. Such patients generally have a narrow L4–L5 disc space (<2 mm) and exhibit no motion on flexion-extension radiographs. They may have anterior vertebral osteophytes, which provide additional stability to the L4–L5 motion segment. Decompression in these patients should preserve at least 50% of the L4–L5 facet joints bilaterally to prevent increased listhesis post-operatively. Minimally invasive or microsurgical limited foraminotomies have been advocated as a potentially less destabilizing option in this situation (Fig. 54-4).

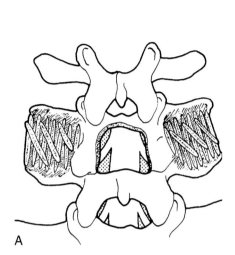
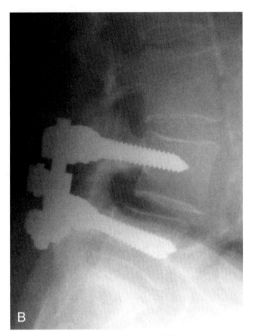

Figure 54-4. Posterolateral L4–L5 decompression and fusion. **A,** Without spinal instrumentation. **B,** With pedicle screw fixation. (A from Grobbler LJ, Wiltse LL. Classification, non-operative and operative treatment of spondylolisthesis. In: Frymoyer JW, editor. The Adult Spine: Principles and Practice. New York: Raven Press; 1991. p. 1696, with permission.)

24. Describe how a posterior fusion is performed for L4–L5 degenerative spondylolisthesis. What is the role of posterior spinal instrumentation?

After completion of the decompression, the transverse processes of L4 and L5 are carefully exposed and soft tissue is removed from the intertransverse membrane extending between the transverse processes. The transverse processes are decorticated with a curette or burr to expose their cancellous surface. Cancellous and corticocancellous bone graft from the patient's iliac crest is applied to the intertransverse region to complete the fusion procedure. If internal fixation is used, a facet fusion may also be performed. However, if no instrumentation is used, facet disruption may increase the risk of post-operative instability.

The addition of internal fixation in the form of pedicle fixation at the level of listhesis has many advantages. Pedicle fixation has been shown to increase the rate of successful fusion and decrease the risk of postoperative progressive slippage and recurrent stenosis. Use of pedicle fixation facilitates early patient mobilization following surgery, and its routine use is preferred by many surgeons. Some surgeons believe that use should be limited until there is unequivocal evidence that pedicle fixation positively improves patient outcome. Noninstrumented fusion is considered reasonable in the patient with mild degenerative spondylolisthesis (<5 mm) in whom there is no pathologic motion on flexion-extension radiographs. Most surgeons today agree that pedicle fixation should be used if greater than 5 mm of motion is noted on dynamic radiographs.

25. What are some situations in which addition of an interbody fusion is considered for treatment of L4–L5 degenerative spondylolisthesis?

- Degenerative spondylolisthesis in which the L4 and L5 vertebrae are in a position of kyphosis relative to one another
- Degenerative spondylolisthesis with severe disc space narrowing associated with L4 foraminal stenosis. In this situation, addition of an interbody fusion will increase the dimensions of the neural foramen between L4 and L5 resulting in decompression of the L4 nerve root.
- Degenerative spondylolisthesis in which the required decompression has compromised the amount of available posterior bone surface available for posterior fusion. For example, if the facet joints are completely removed and/or the pars interarticularis is violated, a posterior fusion alone is less likely to heal

Key Points

1. Radiculopathy most commonly involves exiting nerve root in isthmic spondylolisthesis while the traversing nerve root is most commonly involved in degenerative spondylolisthesis.
2. For degenerative spondylolisthesis, patient outcomes are improved when decompression is combined with posterior fusion compared with decompression without fusion.
3. Circumferential fusion performed in conjunction with posterior spinal instrumentation provides the highest likelihood of successful arthrodesis for adult patients with isthmic spondylolisthesis.

Websites

Spondylolysis and spondylolisthesis: http://emedicine.medscape.com/article/310235-overview
Evidence-based guidelines for degenerative lumbar spondylolisthesis: http://www.spine.org/Documents/spondylolisthesis_Clinical_Guideline.pdf
Cost effectiveness — surgical treatment of degenerative spondylolisthesis with and without degenerative spondylolisthesis: http://www.annals.org/content/149/12/845.full.pdf+html

BIBLIOGRAPHY

1. Berven SH, Herkowitz HN. Evidence-based medicine for the spine: Degenerative spondylolisthesis. Semin Spine Surg 2009;21:238–45.
2. DeWald CJ, Vartabedian JE, Rodts MF, et al. Evaluation and management of high-grade spondylolisthesis in adults. Spine 2005;30:S49–S59.
3. Floman Y. Progression of lumbosacral isthmic spondylolisthesis in adults. Spine 2000;25:342–7.
4. Kornblum MB, Fischgrund JS, Herkowitz HN, et al. Degenerative lumbar spondylolisthesis with spinal stenosis: A prospective long-term study comparing fusion and pseudarthrosis. Spine 2004;29:726–33.
5. Kwon BK, Albert TJ. Adult low-grade acquired spondylolytic spondylolisthesis—evaluation and management. Spine 2005;30:S35–S41.
6. Majid K, Fischgrund JS. Degenerative lumbar spondylolisthesis: Trends and management. J Amer Acad Ortho Surg 2008;16:208–15.
7. Smith J, Deviren V, Berven S, et al. Clinical outcome of trans-sacral interbody fusion after partial reduction for high-grade L5–S1 spondylolisthesis. Spine 2001;26:2227–34.
8. Swan J, Hurwitz E, Malek F, et al. Surgical treatment for unstable low-grade isthmic spondylolisthesis in adults: A prospective controlled study of posterior instrumented fusion compared with anterior-posterior fusion. Spine J 2006;6:606–14.
9. Weinstein JN, Lurie JD, Tosteson TD, et al. Surgical compared with nonoperative treatment for lumbar degenerative spondylolisthesis: Four-year results in the spine patient outcomes research trial (SPORT) randomized and observational cohorts. J Bone Joint Surg 2009;91A:1295–1304.

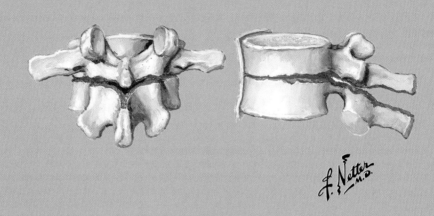

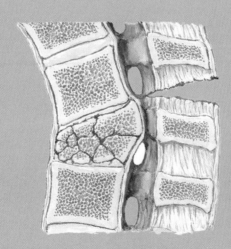

UPPER CERVICAL SPINE TRAUMA

Jens R. Chapman, MD, and Richard J. Bransford, MD

1. What are the major types of injuries involving the upper cervical (occiput–C2) region?

The major types of injuries can be classified according to location:

1. Occipitocervical articulation
   - Occipital condyle fractures
   - Atlanto-occipital dislocation
2. Atlas (C1)
   - Atlas fractures
   - Transverse ligament injuries
3. Axis (C2)
   - Odontoid fractures
   - Hangman's fractures

2. How are upper cervical spine injuries diagnosed?

Any patient with a suspected cervical spine injury requires a thorough evaluation. Frequently, no specific symptoms or findings on physical examination strongly point to the presence of a significant osseous or ligamentous injury involving the upper cervical region. Symptoms are notoriously vague and may include headaches or suboccipital pain. Not infrequently, the patient may be unconscious following trauma. A neurologic evaluation is performed, according to the American Spinal Injury Association (ASIA) guidelines. Assessment of the upper cervical spine should include evaluation of lower cranial nerve function. Most upper cervical spine injuries can be diagnosed on the lateral cervical spine radiograph. An open-mouth anteroposterior (AP) odontoid view and lateral skull radiograph should be obtained if radiographs are used for cervical spine clearance. Computed tomography (CT) with sagittal and coronal plane reformatted views is required to assess the full magnitude of injury and is considered the imaging modality of choice for initial workup in the trauma setting. Magnetic resonance imaging (MRI) is indicated for patients with cervical spinal cord injury and for evaluation of suspected ligament injuries that are not evident with other imaging modalities. Immobilization with a cervical collar (for stable injuries) or Gardner-Wells tong traction (for most unstable injuries) should be maintained in the emergency setting.

3. What is the role of flexion-extension radiographs in the assessment of acute upper cervical spine injuries?

Although flexion-extension radiographs can identify instability of the atlantoaxial motion segment, they are of limited value and even potentially dangerous in the acute trauma setting. Physician-supervised traction films are preferable to assess stability of the upper cervical spine.

4. How is a cervical traction test performed?

With the patient in the supine position, an image intensifier is used to obtain a baseline lateral radiographic image of the cervical spine. Traction weights are added in 5-lb increments (20-lb limit) using a head halter or skeletal traction device (halo, Gardner-Wells tongs) as the cervical region is monitored radiographically. If distraction of more than 3 mm between the occipital condyles and atlas or between the atlas and axis occurs, the test is considered positive and is discontinued.

5. Are upper cervical spine injuries common?

Because of the fragile nature of the bony and ligamentous components of the upper cervical spine, injuries are relatively common, especially in the setting of closed head trauma. Typical injury mechanisms include flexion, extension, or compressive forces applied to the head during motor vehicle accidents, falls from a height, or sporting injuries. Approximately 50% of fractures involving the atlas are accompanied by a second spine fracture. Fractures of the axis account for 27% of associated injuries; odontoid fractures account for 41%. The exact incidence of upper cervical ligamentous injuries is undetermined. Disruption of the craniocervical ligaments is reported to be the leading cause of fatal motor vehicle occupant trauma (Fig. 55-1).

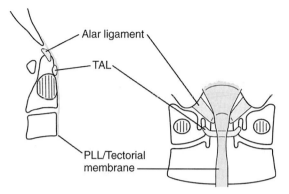

Figure 55-1. Craniocervical ligaments. The tectorial membrane is the uppermost extension of the posterior longitudinal ligament (PLL) and attaches to the occipital condyles providing for stability against cranial traction and flexion forces. The alar ligaments extend from the tip of the odontoid process and attach to the anterior aspect of the foramen magnum serving as checkreins against rotation and distraction. These ligaments run from the occiput to C2 without attaching directly to C-1, which serves as a bushing. The transverse atlantal ligament (TAL) restricts translation of C1 on C2. (© Jens R. Chapman.)

6. Are upper cervical spine injuries commonly associated with neurologic deficits?

Because of the relatively large size of the upper cervical spinal canal, neurologic deficits are relatively rare in association with upper cervical injuries. However, when upper cervical spinal cord injuries occur, they are often fatal because of injury to the respiratory and cardiac centers in the medulla and upper cervical cord. Incomplete spinal cord injuries in the upper cervical region may present as a cervicomedullary syndrome or cranial nerve injury.

OCCIPITOCERVICAL ARTICULATION

7. What is the mechanism for occipital condyle fractures and how are these injuries classified?

Occipital condyle fractures typically result from a direct blow to the head or from a rapid deceleration injury. These injuries are frequently associated with C1 fractures and cranial nerve injuries. CT is used to classify these injuries into three subtypes according to the classification developed by Anderson and Montessano:
- Type 1: a stable comminuted fracture resulting from an axial loading injury
- Type 2: a stable skull base fracture that extends into the occipital condyle
- Type 3: an avulsion fracture of the condyle at the attachment of the alar ligament. This fracture type is potentially unstable and may be associated with an atlanto-occipital dislocation.

8. How are occipital condyle fractures treated?

Unilateral Type 1 and 2 injuries are usually treated with a rigid cervical orthosis. Isolated Type 3 avulsion injuries are managed with a halo orthosis. Type 3 injuries associated with atlanto-occipital dislocation require posterior occipitocervical fusion.

9. What is an atlanto-occipital dislocation (AOD)?

High-speed deceleration injuries may result in disruption of important craniocervical ligaments (tectorial membrane, anterior occipito-atlantal membrane, alar ligaments) resulting in craniocervical junction instability. These injuries are frequently fatal. Survivors frequently present with a spinal cord injury above the C4 segment. Incomplete spinal cord injuries associated with AOD include respiratory impairment and cranial nerve injuries (cervicomedullary syndrome). Young children are the most commonly injured age group due to their relatively large head size, shallow atlanto-occipital joints, and ligamentous laxity compared with adults. In the pediatric age group, AOD may be the result of shaken baby syndrome, pedestrian versus car injuries, or deceleration injuries in a car crash with the child immobilized in a car seat.

10. How is atlanto-occipital dislocation identified?

The most effective initial screening test remains the lateral cervical spine radiograph. The most important radiographic parameters to assess include:
- **Soft tissue swelling** adjacent to the upper cervical vertebral bodies (> 6mm)
- **Diastasis or subluxation** of atlanto-occipital articulation (Fig. 55-2A)
- Disruption of **Harris' lines**—this is a combination of two measurements that have been termed the *rule of twelve* (Fig. 55-2C):
    - **Dens-basion interval (DBI):** The distance from the dens to the basion should be less than 12 mm
    - **Basion-atlantal interval (BAI):** A measurement from a perpendicular line extending along the posterior margin of the C2 vertebral body (posterior axis line [PAL-B]) should not be more than 4 mm anterior and should be less than 12 mm posterior to the basion

Additional measurements have been described but are less reliable than Harris's lines. These include **Wackenheim's line** and **Power's ratio** (Fig. 55-2B). A Power's ratio greater than 1 suggests an anterior dislocation of the atlanto-occipital joint. This ratio between the distance from the basion to the posterior arch of C1 and the distance from the opisthion to the anterior arch of C1 is usually less than 1.

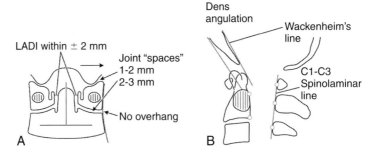

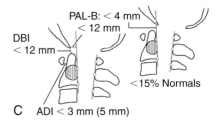

Figure 55-2. **A,** The lateral masses of the atlas should closely articulate with the superior articular processes of the atlas. The odontoid should be centered symmetrically between the lateral masses of the atlas (lateral atlantodens interval [LADI]). **B,** Additional screening lines include Wackenheim's line and the C1 to C3 spinolaminar line. **C,** The tip of the odontoid should remain in close proximity to the basion, as shown with the reference lines described by Harris. ADI, atlantodens interval; PAL-B, posterior axis line. (© Jens R. Chapman.)

The diagnosis of AOD is confirmed with a fine-cut CT scan and/or MRI. Occasionally, a cervical traction test is necessary to confirm the presence of an occult AOD.

11. How is an atlanto-occipital dislocation classified?

There are two major methods used to classify AODs. The initial classification of Traynelis assessed the direction of displacement of the head relative to the cervical spine and described anterior, vertical, posterior, and oblique dislocations. However, classification according to displacement in the presence of global ligamentous failure is somewhat arbitrary as displacement can be altered by patient positioning. In addition, such a classification does not grade injury severity or the potential for spontaneously reduced dislocations, which would be overlooked if the sole criterion for injury is displacement. It is important to distinguish incomplete injuries that retain partial meaningful craniocervical ligamentous integrity from occult injuries in which a rebound phenomenon led to partial or complete deformity reduction. Spontaneously reduced injuries are easily overlooked yet may have catastrophic consequences if left untreated.

An alternative classification, the Harborview classification, attempts to stratify injuries according to severity:

- Type I: These injuries are relatively stable and can be treated nonoperatively. MRI shows edema or hemorrhage at the craniocervical junction, but Harris' lines show normal cervical alignment. A traction test performed with 25 pounds of traction is normal and rules out a spontaneously reduced injury
- Type II: These injuries feature complete disruption of key ligaments of the cranio-cervical junction and are innately unstable, requiring surgical treatment. MRI shows edema or hemorrhage at the craniocervical junction, but Harris's lines show borderline screening measurement values. A spontaneous partial reduction of the cranium to its cervical location, through remaining residual ligamentous attachments, has occurred and is potentially misleading. Traction at weights less than 25 pounds shows sufficient distraction to meet craniocervical dissociation criteria, according to Harris's lines
- Type III: These injuries demonstrate obvious major cranio-cervical displacement on static plain radiographs

12. What is the treatment for an atlanto-occipital dislocation?

Stage I lesions are usually treated with 8 to 12 weeks of halo vest immobilization. Stage II and III AOD are potentially life-threatening injuries. Emergent reduction and external immobilization attempts can be made with a halo vest or head immobilization using a neck collar and sand bags. Definitive treatment of stage II and III lesions consists of posterior occipitocervical arthrodesis with rigid segmental spinal instrumentation. Attempts at occiput to C1 fusion are unwarranted because this treatment does not address the disrupted alar ligaments and tectorial membrane, which extend between C2 and the occiput. Significant ethical challenges, in terms of sustaining life-preserving support measures, may arise in cases of patients with associated anoxic or traumatic brain injury.

ATLAS FRACTURES AND TRANSVERSE ATLANTAL LIGAMENT (TAL) INJURIES

13. How are C1 fractures and TAL injuries diagnosed?

Radiographs should include an open-mouth odontoid view and a lateral C1–C2 view. On the lateral view, the atlantodens interval (ADI) should be less than 3 mm in adults and less than 5 mm in children. On the open-mouth view, the symmetry of the dens in relation to the adjacent lateral masses should be assessed. Any outward displacement of the lateral masses of C1 in relation to C2 should be noted. Atlantoaxial offset greater than 7 mm indicates C1–C2 instability and disruption of the TAL (Fig. 55-3), although TAL disruption may also be present if atlantoaxial offset is less than 7 mm. Definitive assessment is achieved with a fine-cut CT scan with reformatted images. Efforts at visualizing the TAL on MRI have remained unreliable. Isolated TAL injuries may occasionally require flexion-extension radiographs to assess for atlantoaxial instability.

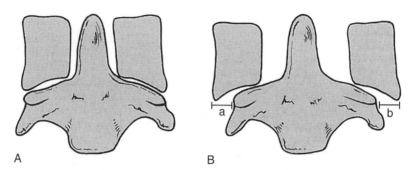

A   B

Figure 55-3. A, Lateral displacement of the C1 lateral masses of more than 7 mm indicates disruption of the transverse ligament. **B,** The sum of the displacements of the left and right sides (a + b) is used to determine the total displacement. (From Browner BD, Jupiter JB, Levine AM, editors. Skeletal Trauma. Philadelphia: Saunders; 1998.)

14. How are C1 fractures classified?

Five primary types of atlas fractures have been defined (Fig. 55-4):

- Type 1: Transverse process fracture
- Type 2: Posterior arch fracture
- Type 3: Lateral mass fracture
- Type 4: Anterior arch fracture
- Type 5: Burst fracture (Jefferson's fracture). Burst fractures may consist of three or four parts. This injury may occur as a ligamentous combination injury with associated TAL disruption.

Types 3, 4, and 5 fractures can be inherently stable or unstable, depending on fracture comminution, displacement, and concurrent ligamentous disruption. In general, Type 3 injuries with a sagittal fracture line and segmental anterior arch fractures are unstable.

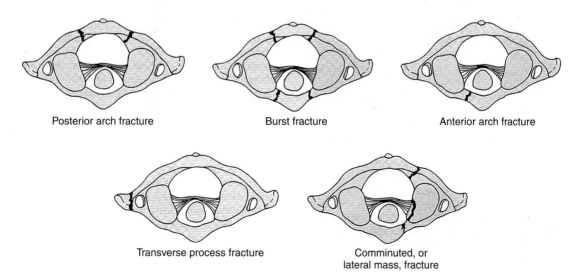

Posterior arch fracture   Burst fracture   Anterior arch fracture

Transverse process fracture   Comminuted, or
                                   lateral mass, fracture

Figure 55-4. Classification of atlas fractures. (From Browner BD, Jupiter JB, Levine AM, editors. Skeletal Trauma. Philadelphia: Saunders; 1998.)

15. How are atlas fractures treated?

Type 1 injuries are treated with a cervical collar.

Type 2 injuries are treated with a cervical collar if they occur as an isolated injury. However, there is a greater than 50% chance of an association injury (e.g. odontoid fracture), and the presence of additional injury alters the treatment plan.

Type 3 injuries require close follow-up for potential loss of reduction and secondary collapse. If subsidence of the occipital condyle through the lateral mass of the atlas occurs, treatment options consist of closed reduction with skeletal cranial traction over a period of several weeks, followed by halo immobilization or primary posterior atlantoaxial arthrodesis.

Type 4 fractures, in which the odontoid has displaced through the anterior ring of the atlas, are highly unstable. If atlantoaxial alignment is maintained, nonoperative treatment with a halo vest is considered. Closed reduction and atlantoaxial arthrodesis are usually required.

Type 5 (Jefferson-type) fractures are treated based on integrity of the TAL. Disruption of the TAL is suspected if the lateral masses of C1 overhang those of C2 by the sum of 7 mm or more on the AP open-mouth radiograph (Spence's rule). TAL disruption is also present if there is translational atlantoaxial displacement of 3 mm or more in any direction. Nonoperative treatment of type 5 atlas fractures consists of fracture reduction with traction and conversion to a halo vest after a period of days to weeks. Upon mobilization, maintenance of satisfactory alignment is checked with upright lateral and open mouth odontoid views. Surgical stabilization has been advocated based upon an unstable fracture configuration, for patients with purely ligamentous injury of the TAL, or if recumbent traction or halo treatment is unsuccessful or contraindicated.

Certain variants of C1 injuries can be treated with primary open reduction and internal fixation.

16. What are the different types of TAL injuries?

TAL injuries have been differentiated into:
- Type 1 injuries (bony avulsion)
- Type 2 injuries (purely ligamentous injuries)

17. How are TAL injuries treated?

Treatment options depend on the type of TAL injury.
- Type 1 injuries (bony avulsion) can be successfully treated with rigid immobilization in a significant number of patients
- Type 2 injuries (purely ligamentous injuries) are unlikely to heal with nonsurgical management and require reduction of the deformity and atlantoaxial arthrodesis

18. What surgical techniques are used for posterior stabilization of atlas fractures and TAL injuries?

Historically, fusion of the C1–C2 motion segment was performed utilizing **wire or cable fixation**. The Gallie technique places wires under the posterior arch of C1 and around the C2 spinous process. The Brooks technique places wires under the lamina of C1 and C2. However, in the presence of a fracture through the ring of C1, neither technique is applicable. Today, wiring techniques are rarely used as a stand-alone option due to advances in spinal instrumentation techniques.

Placement of **transarticular screws** has been described for types 3, 4, and 5 atlas fractures. This technique requires anatomic reduction of the atlas on the axis to ensure safe placement and optimal fixation of each transarticular screw. It is also limited by anatomic factors such as patient size and body habitus, as well as the location of the vertebral artery within the C2 segment. Alternatively, placement of lateral mass screws into the atlas and pedicle screws or laminar screws in the axis, linked to a cervical rod on each side, has gained popularity. Advantages of **C1–C2 screw-rod fixation (Harm's technique)** include flexibility to adapt fixation according to individual patient anatomy and provision for intraoperative fracture reduction by manipulation of independent screws in C1 and C2. **Occipitocervical instrumentation and fusion** have been utilized to stabilize severe C1 injuries by spanning the injured level. Some experts have advocated treatment of select C1 fractures with **osteosynthesis techniques** utilizing lateral mass screws placed from either a posterior or transoral approach to achieve direct fracture repair and avoid fusion across motion segments.

AXIS FRACTURES: ODONTOID FRACTURES AND HANGMAN'S FRACTURES

19. What is the usual mechanism of injury for an odontoid fracture?

Odontoid fractures typically occur secondary to forced extension or flexion of the head and neck during a fall or collision. Associated fractures of the atlas occur in 10% to 15% of cases. Odontoid fractures are the most common cervical fracture in patients younger than 8 years or older than 70 years.

20. How are odontoid fractures classified?

The Anderson and D'Alonzo classification (Fig. 55-5) is widely accepted and is based on the location of the fracture line:
- Type 1: Stable avulsion fracture occurring at the tip of the odontoid. This must be differentiated from an avulsion fracture associated with AOD or os odontoideum
- Type 2: Unstable transverse fracture involving the cortical bone of the waist of the odontoid

- Type 3: Unstable fracture extending into the cancellous portion of the C2 vertebral body
  Important fracture variables with potential therapeutic implications include segmental comminution, fracture displacement, and fracture obliquity. A more precise distinction between Type 2 and Type 3 fractures has been proposed. Type 2 fractures lack involvement of the superior articular facets of C2, whereas Type 3 fractures involve the superior articular facet.

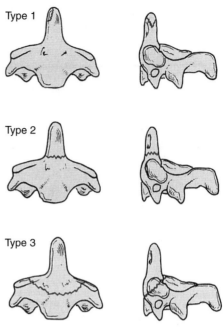

Figure 55-5. Anderson and D'Alonzo's classification of odontoid fractures. Type 1 fractures involve the tip of the odontoid process and are stable. Type 2 fractures penetrate the base of the odontoid. Type 3 fractures extend into the body of C2. (From Browner BD, Jupiter JB, Levine AM, editors. Skeletal Trauma. Philadelphia: Saunders; 1998.)

21. How are odontoid fractures treated?

Type 1 fractures are treated with a cervical collar. It is important to evaluate the craniocervical junction to rule out concomitant ligamentous injuries.

Type 2 fractures are associated with a high incidence of nonunion (15%–85%). Risk factors associated with nonunion include initial fracture displacement greater than 4 mm, patient age older than 50 years, posteriorly displaced fractures, angulation greater than 10°, and inappropriate initial treatment. Treatment of Type 2 fractures is determined by a variety of factors including initial fracture displacement, presence of associated cervical fractures, fracture comminution, fracture obliquity, and bone quality. Nondisplaced or minimally displaced fractures may be treated with a halo vest or rigid collar for 8 to 12 weeks. Maintenance of fracture reduction is checked with lateral cervical spine radiographs taken in both the recumbent and upright positions. Anterior screw fixation or posterior C1–C2 fusion is performed for displaced fractures and for patients who are unable to tolerate halo immobilization. Treatment with benign neglect consisting of a soft neck collar has been suggested for geriatric patients too feeble to tolerate attempts at definitive care.

Type 3 fractures are reduced with skeletal traction as needed and externally immobilized. Severely comminuted or unstable fracture patterns may require posterior fusion and screw-rod fixation.

22. What options exist for surgical stabilization of odontoid fractures?

1. **Anterior screw fixation:** Single- or double-screw fixation can be performed for patients with transverse or posterior oblique odontoid fractures (fracture line courses from anterior superior to posterior inferior). Prerequisites include a fracture that is less than 3 weeks old and a patient with reasonable bone quality. Certain factors, such as a large body habitus, may preclude this form of treatment. There is also controversy with respect to anterior screw fixation in the elderly, secondary to swallowing difficulties encountered postoperatively. Contraindications to anterior screw fixation include fractures that course from anterior inferior to posterior superior (parallel to screw trajectory) and fractures with significant comminution
2. **Posterior fusion with wires or cables:** For patients with an intact C1 ring, posterior wire or cable fixation can be successful. Substantial limitations to this technique include insufficient biomechanical stiffness in rotation and the possibility of undesirable C1 posterior translation. With modern day techniques, stand-alone wiring is rarely utilized
3. **Transarticular screw fixation:** Placement of a small fragment screw from the midpoint of the inferior articular processes of C2 across the pars of C2 into the lateral mass of C1 provides excellent biomechanical stiffness and leads to a very high rate of bony union. Risks associated with this technique include iatrogenic injury to the vertebral artery as it passes laterally to the vertebral body of C2. Preoperative planning including CT evaluation to assess screw trajectory in relation to the vertebral artery and meticulous surgical technique are important for successful execution of this procedure
4. **Posterior C1–C2 screw-rod fixation:** This technique utilizes lateral mass screws for C1 fixation and pedicle screws for C2 fixation. Alternatively, C2 screw fixation can engage the laminae on either side. The screws are connected by rods along each side of the spine. Biomechanically, these segmental fixation constructs have similar biomechanical fixation strength compared with transarticular screw constructs

23. What is the usual mechanism of injury for a hangman's fracture?

The term *hangman's fracture* was originally used to describe the C2 fracture dislocation that occurred when criminals were treated by judicial hanging. A radiographically similar injury to the second cervical vertebra occurs as a result of motor vehicle trauma and is more appropriately termed *traumatic spondylolisthesis of the axis*. This fracture results in disruption of the bony bridge between the inferior and superior articular processes of the C2 segment. The fracture may be accompanied by injury to the C2–C3 disc, as well as disruption of the posterior ligaments between C2 and C3. Concurrent soft tissue injuries heavily influence fracture stability and treatment.

24. How is traumatic spondylolisthesis of the axis classified?

The Effendi classification, as modified by Levine and Edwards, is widely accepted (Fig. 55-6):

- Type I injuries consist of a fracture through the neural arch with no angulation and up to 3 mm of displacement
- Type II fractures have both significant angulation and fracture displacement (>3 mm)
- Type IIA injuries show minimal displacement but are associated with severe angulation as a result of a flexion-distraction injury mechanism. This injury may not be recognized until a radiograph is obtained in traction
- Type III injuries combine severe angulation and displacement with a unilateral or bilateral facet dislocation between C2 and C3

There is a low incidence of spinal cord injury with type I, II, and IIA injuries but a high incidence of spinal cord injury with type III injuries.

Eismont and Starr have described an atypical type of hangman's fracture (subsequently classified as type IA) in which on one side there is the typical location of fracture but the line of the fracture then cuts obliquely across the body in a similar pattern to a type III odontoid fracture. This injury type has a higher than usual rate of spinal cord injury. In the typical traumatic spondylolisthesis fracture patterns, the vertebral body displaces anteriorly and the corresponding posterior elements displace posteriorly, resulting in increased space for the spinal cord. In the atypical type IA variant, the circumference of the spinal canal is unchanged and bone or hematoma may result in cord compression and neurologic injury.

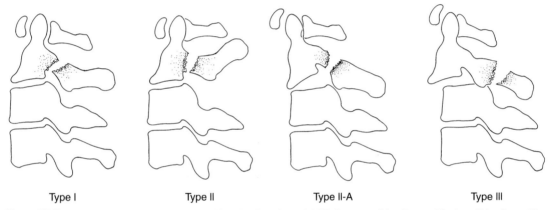

| Type I | Type II | Type II-A | Type III |

Figure 55-6. Types of traumatic spondylolisthesis of the axis. (From Leventhal MR. Fractures, dislocations and fracture-dislocations of the spine. In: Crenshaw AH, editor. Campbell's Operative Orthopaedics. 8th ed. St. Louis: Mosby-Year Book; 1992.)

25. How is traumatic spondylolisthesis of the axis treated?

Treatment is based on the fracture type:

- Type I injuries can be treated in a rigid neck collar
- Type II injuries are usually treated with traction, followed by immobilization in a halo or a rigid collar. If significant disruption of the C2–C3 disc exists, surgical stabilization may be considered to avoid morbidity associated with prolonged traction and halo immobilization
- Type IIA injuries are usually treated by closed reduction by positioning in extension, followed by halo immobilization. If significant disruption of the C2–C3 disc exists, surgical stabilization is considered
- Type III injuries require surgical treatment for reduction of the facet dislocation and surgical stabilization

26. What are the surgical treatment options for unstable traumatic spondylolisthesis of the axis?

Unstable type II and IIA fractures not amenable to treatment with nonoperative means can be surgically stabilized by placement of C2 transpedicular screws or anterior C2–C3 plating. Type III fractures require open reduction of the facet dislocation and stabilization of the dislocation with lateral mass fixation to C3 and either C2 pedicle screws or fixation to C1. The fracture of the neural arch can be treated by placement of C2 transpedicular screws.

Key Points

1. The craniocervical junction consists of the osseous, ligamentous, and neurovascular structures that extend from the skull base to C2.
2. Injuries to the craniocervical junction are associated with a significant likelihood of death.
3. Nonoperative treatment options include recumbent skeletal traction, cervical orthoses, and halo immobilization.
4. Direct fracture osteosynthesis is an option for surgical treatment of select type 2 odontoid fractures and C2 pars interarticularis fractures.
5. Open reduction and stable internal fixation is indicated for unstable craniocervical injury patterns.

Websites

Internal decapitation: survival after head to neck dissociation injuries: http://www.medscape.com/viewarticle/577910_3
Measurement techniques for upper cervical spine injuries: http://www.medscape.com/viewarticle/555355
Upper cervical trauma: http://fhs.mcmaster.ca/surgery/documents/upper_cervical.pdf

BIBLIOGRAPHY

1. Anderson LD, D'Alonzo RT. Fractures of the odontoid process of the axis. J Bone Joint Surg 1974;56A:1663–74.
2. Bellabarba C, Mirza SK, West GA, et al. Diagnosis and treatment of craniocervical dislocation in a series of 17 consecutive survivors during an 8-year period. J Neurosurgery Spine 2006;4:429–40.
3. Bellabarba C, Mirza SK, Chapman JR. Injuries to the craniocervical junction. In: Bucholz RW, Heckman JD, Court-Brown CM, editors. Rockwood & Green's Fractures in Adults. 6th ed. Philadelphia: Lippincott Williams & Wilkins; 2006.
4. Chutkan NB, King AG, Harris MB. Odontoid fractures: Evaluation and management. J Am Acad Orthop Surg 1997;5:199–204.
5. Dickman CA, Greene KA, Sonntag VK. Injuries involving the transverse atlantal ligament: Classification and treatment guidelines based upon experience with 39 injuries. Neurosurgery 1996;38:44–50.
6. Dvorak MF, Johnson MG, Boyd M, et al. Long-term health-related quality of life outcomes following Jefferson-type burst fractures of the atlas. J Neurosurg Spine 2005;2:411–17.
7. Grauer JN, Shafi B, Hilibrand AS, et al. Proposal of a modified treatment-oriented classification of odontoid fractures. Spine J 2005; 5:123–9.
8. Greene KA, Dickman CA, Marciano FF, et al. Acute axis fractures: Analysis of management and outcome in 340 consecutive cases. Spine 1997;22:1843–52.
9. Levine AM, Edwards CC. Fractures of the Atlas. J Bone Joint Surg 1991;73A:680–91.
10. Levine AM, Edwards CC. The management of traumatic spondylolisthesis of the axis. J Bone Joint Surg Am 1985;67(2):217–26.

LOWER CERVICAL SPINE INJURIES

Vincent J. Devlin, MD, John C. Steinmann, DO, and Paul A. Anderson, MD

INITIAL MANAGEMENT

1. **Describe the initial evaluation of a trauma patient with respect to potential lower cervical spine injury.**
   - The cervical spine is immobilized in the blunt trauma patient until the spine has been cleared
   - Initial evaluation and management is carried out according to the elements of the Advanced Trauma Life Support (ATLS) protocol
   - The posterior cervical region is palpated for tenderness, and the patient is log rolled to permit inspection and palpation of all spinal regions
   - Neurologic examination is performed according to American Spinal Injury Association (ASIA) criteria

2. **Describe an evidence-based approach to clearance of the cervical spine.**
   Following initial clinical examination, the cervical clearance process is initiated by assigning the patient to one of four groups:
   - **Asymptomatic** (i.e. alert, oriented, absent cervical pain/tenderness, normal neurologic examination, no intoxication, no distracting injuries). These patients may be cleared based on clinical assessment without obtaining imaging studies (NEXUS criteria, Canadian C-Spine Rule)
   - **Asymptomatic, Temporarily Unable to Assess** (i.e. presence of intoxication or distracting injuries that impair clinical examination and that are expected to improve over a 24-hour period). These patients are initially immobilized in a cervical collar. Reevaluation at 24 to 48 hours may permit patient clearance based on clinical criteria if the patient is assessable and asymptomatic. If the patient cannot be assessed clinically, the patient is evaluated according to the protocol for an obtunded patient
   - **Symptomatic** (i.e. presence of pain, tenderness, neurologic symptoms). Imaging studies are required. Options include plain radiography (limited ability to visualize occipitocervical and cervicothoracic junctions), multidetector computed tomography (CT) scan (increased sensitivity for osseous injury but may miss ligamentous injury), and magnetic resonance imaging (MRI) (important for unexplained neurologic deficits, ligamentous injury, potential disc herniations associated with facet injuries). CT has become the study of choice for initial evaluation
   - **Obtunded** No consensus exists regarding an optimal clearance protocol. Options include a multidetector CT scan or a combination of CT and MRI

3. **When is emergent closed reduction of a cervical spine injury indicated?**
   Emergent closed reduction is considered in patients with cervical canal compromise and a neurologic deficit, especially spinal cord injuries. Common fractures requiring immediate reduction include burst fractures and facet dislocations. If the patient is alert and neurologic status can be assessed clinically, traction reduction can commence without MRI. If the patient is obtunded or uncooperative, MRI is obtained prior to proceeding with closed reduction. Contraindications to closed reduction using skull traction include patients with skull fractures, distraction injuries (e.g. atlanto-axial dislocations), and concomitant subaxial and upper cervical injuries (e.g. odontoid fracture).

4. **In a patient with a traumatic spinal cord injury, what medical treatments have proven beneficial?**
   Initial resuscitation to raise and maintain blood pressure to a mean arterial blood pressure between 80 and 85 mm Hg is beneficial to the injured spinal cord. In an acute spinal cord injured patient, this usually requires the addition of pressor agents. Hypoxemia must be avoided. Supplemental oxygen is routinely administered, and ventilatory support is utilized as indicated. The use of neuroprotective agents such as methylprednisolone is controversial. Each institution should determine a protocol for use of methylprednisolone because it has been shown to have limited efficacy and is associated with serious complications including mortality.

5. **What is the optimal timing of surgical decompression in spinal cord injured patients?**
   Recent multicenter studies have shown that early surgery (within 24 hours) is safe and may lead to better neurologic outcomes than delayed surgery. In addition, those patients treated within 12 hours of initial injury may have even better outcomes. Before undergoing early cervical surgery, patients should be fully resuscitated, have a mean arterial blood pressure of 80 to 85 mm Hg, and be well oxygenated.

INJURY CLASSIFICATION

6. What factors serve as the basis for classification of subaxial cervical spine injuries?

Classification systems for subaxial cervical spine injuries have evolved based on various factors including mechanism of injury, anatomic site of injury, radiologic description of injury morphology, the presence/absence of neurologic deficit, and injury severity. Classification based on mechanism of injury has been criticized due to lack of reliability and validity.

7. How are subaxial cervical spine injuries classified on the basis of injury morphology?

Description of subaxial cervical spine injuries according to injury morphology and location is valuable to allow communication and categorization. An injury may be **isolated** (bony or ligamentous involvement of a single column) or **complex** (both bony and ligamentous involvement of single column or involvement of multiple columns) (Table 56-1).

Table 56-1. Subaxial Cervical Spine Fracture Morphology

A. INJURIES INVOLVING THE ANTERIOR COLUMN	
Isolated	Compression fracture
	Transverse process fracture
	Traumatic disc disruption
Complex	Burst fracture
	Disc distraction injury ± anterior avulsion fracture
	Flexion axial load fracture
B. INJURIES INVOLVING THE POSTERIOR COLUMN	
Isolated	Spinous process fractures
	Lamina fractures
Complex	Posterior ligamentous disruption ± fracture
C. INJURIES INVOLVING THE LATERAL COLUMN	
Isolated	Superior facet fracture
	Inferior facet fracture
Complex	Fracture separation of the lateral mass
	Unilateral facet dislocations with or without fractures
	Bilateral facet dislocations with or without fractures

(Adapted from Moore TA, Vaccaro AR, Anderson PA: Classification of Lower Cervical Spine Injuries. Spine 31: 11S, 537-543, 2006.)

8. How is neurologic function classified?

Neurologic function is classified using guidelines created by the American Spinal Injury Association (ASIA). Cranial nerve function, upper and lower extremity sensory and motor function, and perineal function are evaluated. Neurologic injury may involve the spinal cord, conus medullaris, cauda equina or isolated nerve root(s). Spinal cord injuries are classified as complete or incomplete. In **complete cord injuries**, sensory and motor function is absent below the level of injury including S4 and S5 sacral nerve root function. In **incomplete cord injuries**, partial preservation of sensory or motor function is present and these injuries are associated with a better prognosis for recovery than for complete injuries. The **motor level** is the lowest functioning root level with grade 3 or better strength.

9. How are subaxial cervical injuries classified according to injury severity?

Two new classification systems based on injury severity have been developed to aid in decision making:
- Cervical Spine Injury Severity Score (CSISS)
- Subaxial Cervical Spine Injury Classification (SLIC)

10. Explain how to use the Cervical Spine Injury Severity Score (CSISS) for classification of a subaxial cervical spine injury.

The cervical spine is conceptualized in terms of **four columns** (anterior, posterior, and right and left lateral columns). Each column is scored from 0 to 5 using an analog scale based on degree of osseous displacement and ligamentous injury (Fig. 56-1). The resulting injury severity score ranges from 0 (no injury) to 20 (most severe injury). Scores of 7 or more generally require surgery and scores less than 5 are generally treated nonoperatively.

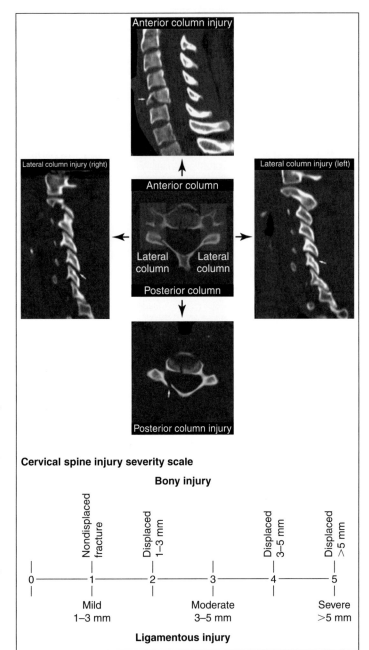

Figure 56-1. The Cervical Spine Injury Severity Score. The algorithm is used to quantify the mechanical instability of the injury with the intention of guiding treatment. The cervical spine is divided into four columns: anterior column (anterior and posterior longitudinal ligaments, vertebral body, disc, uncinate processes, and transverse processes), right and left lateral columns (pedicle, superior and inferior facet joints, facet joint capsules, and lateral mass), and posterior column (lamina, spinous processes, ligamentum flavum, and the posterior ligament complex). The severity of the bony or ligamentous injury to each column is assigned a number according to the analog scale, with 0 being uninjured and 5 being the most severely injured. The sum of the scores for each of the four columns represents the Cervical Spine Injury Severity Score. Scores greater than 7 indicate sufficient instability to warrant surgical stabilization. (From Kwon BK, Anderson PA. Injuries to the lower cervical spine. In: Browner BD, Jupiter JB, Levine AM, et al, editors. Browner Skeletal Trauma. 4th ed. Philadelphia: Saunders; 2009.)

11. Explain how to use the Subaxial Injury Classification (SLIC) scoring system.
The SLIC classification system analyzes three injury characteristics:
- **Injury morphology:** Assess the injured vertebra and its relationship with adjacent vertebral bodies
- **Disco-ligamentous complex integrity:** Assess the status of the disc, annulus, anterior and posterior longitudinal ligaments, facet capsules, and posterior ligaments
- **Neurologic status:** Neurologic injury, if present, may involve the nerve roots or spinal cord (complete vs. incomplete injury). Incomplete neurologic injury in the setting of persistent neural compression is most likely to benefit from surgical intervention and is associated with the highest score
See Table 56-2.

Table 56-2. Subaxial Cervical Spine Injury Classification (SLIC)

1	FRACTURE MORPHOLOGY	SCORE
	No injury	0
	Compression	1
	Burst	2
	Distraction	3
	Rotation/ Translation	4
2	**Disco-ligamentous complex**	
	None	0
	Indeterminate	1
	Disrupted	2
3	**Neurologic function**	
	Intact	0
	Root injury	1
	Complete cord injury	2
	Incomplete cord injury	3
	Ongoing compression with deficit	+1
	Total*	

*Total score ≤ 3 nonoperative treatment is recommended, a score = 4 either surgery or nonoperative treatment is indicated, and a score ≥ 5 surgery is recommended.
(From Vaccaro AR, Hulbert RJ, Patel AA, et al. The subaxial cervical injury classification system: A novel approach to recognize the importance of morphology, neurology and integrity of the disco-ligamentous complex. Spine 2007;32:2365–74.)

ANTERIOR COLUMN INJURIES

12. What are the characteristic features of compression fractures?

Compression fractures result from axial loading forces with or without associated hyperflexion. Anterior vertebral body wedging and superior endplate fractures occur. If injury is associated with a hyperflexion component, the posterior ligamentous complex may be disrupted.

13. What are the characteristic features of burst fractures?

Burst fractures result from axial loading of the cervical spine. Loss of anterior and posterior vertebral height is noted (Fig. 56-2). Posterior displacement of a portion of the posterior vertebral body wall may occur and lead to spinal canal compromise with neurologic injury. Disruption of the posterior osteoligamentous structures may occur. Burst fractures are most common in the lower cervical spine (C6 and C7).

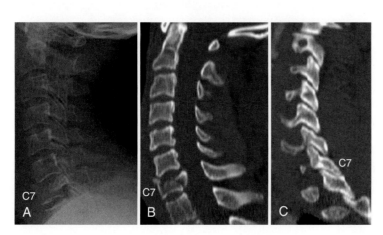

Figure 56-2. C7 burst fracture. This 32-year-old cyclist suffered an isolated C7 burst fracture when hit by a car. On plain radiograph **(A)** and sagittal computed tomographic reconstruction **(B)**, the C7 injury has the classic burst fracture appearance, with superior endplate rupture and retropulsion of the posterior vertebral body into the spinal canal. Sagittal alignment is well maintained and no interspinous widening is present. **C,** The facet joints are intact.

Continued

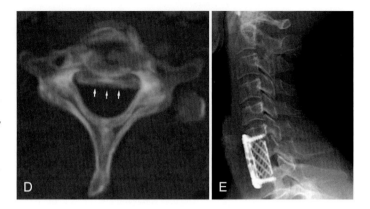

Figure 56-2, cont'd. **D,** The axial computed tomography demonstrates the retropulsed posterior body of C7 *(arrows)*, which narrow the spinal canal. **E,** The patient underwent a C7 corpectomy with titanium cage reconstruction and anterior cervical plating. (From Kwon BK, Anderson PA. Injuries to the lower cervical spine. In: Browner BD, Jupiter JB, Levine AM, et al, editors. Browner Skeletal Trauma. 4th ed. Philadelphia: Saunders, 2009.)

14. What are the characteristic features of flexion-axial loading fractures?

Flexion-axial loading fractures (also termed *flexion tear-drop fractures*) represent a spectrum of injuries resulting from combined anterior column compression and posterior column distraction. Compression of the anterior superior aspect of the vertebral body is associated with a fracture line extending vertically from the anterior vertebral cortex to the inferior vertebral endplate. In severe injuries, the spine is cleaved into an anterior inferior segment (tear-drop segment) while the remaining portion of the vertebral body displaces posteriorly toward the spinal cord (Fig. 56-3). Associated injuries include lamina fractures, spinous process fractures, and posterior ligament complex disruption. This fracture type has the highest rate of neurologic injury of all cervical fractures.

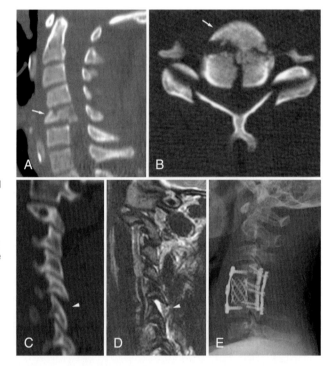

Figure 56-3. Flexion-axial loading fracture. This patient presented with a severe C5 flexion-axial loading fracture and complete quadriplegia. Notice on the sagittal **(A)** and axial **(B)** images the large anterior fragment of the C5 vertebral body *(arrow)*. There is a sagittal split in the C5 vertebral body, bilaminar fractures, and facet disruption *(arrowheads)* as seen on sagittal computed tomography **(C)** and confirmed on T2-weighted magnetic resonance imaging **(D)**. Due to the severe instability, a circumferential stabilization was performed **(E)**. The autogenous bone from the C5 corpectomy was used to fill a titanium reconstruction cage, followed by anterior plating and posterior lateral mass fixation from C4 to C6. (From Kwon BK, Anderson PA. Injuries to the lower cervical spine. In Browner BD, Jupiter JB, Levine AM, et al, editors. Browner Skeletal Trauma. 4th ed. Philadelphia: Saunders, 2009.)

15. Provide an overview of the treatment options for anterior column subaxial spine injuries.

The injuries are classified to determine the Cervical Spine Injury Severity Score (CSISS) and Subaxial Cervical Spine Injury Classification (SLIC) scores.

- *Compression fractures* are associated with low CSISS and SLIC scores, and nonsurgical treatment with a cervical collar or cervicothoracic orthosis is indicated. For the rare case of a compression fracture associated with disruption of the posterior ligamentous complex, treatment with posterior screw-rod fixation and posterior fusion is recommended
- *Burst fractures* and *flexion-axial loading fractures* in neurologically intact patients with low CSISS and SLIC scores can be considered for nonsurgical management with a halo vest. More commonly, these injuries are initially reduced with traction and treated surgically. Preferred treatment is an anterior procedure with corpectomy, placement of a

strut graft or fusion cage, and anterior plate fixation. Combined anterior and posterior instrumentation and fusion is indicated in the presence of concomitant severe posterior column disruption

POSTERIOR COLUMN INJURIES

16. What are the different types of posterior column injuries?
Posterior column injuries may be *isolated* (spinous process fracture, lamina fractures, posterior ligament injury without facet joint disruption) or *complex* (fractures in an ankylosed spine, traumatic spondylolisthesis).

17. How are posterior column injuries managed?
Isolated spinous process or lamina fractures are effective treated with immobilization in a cervical collar. Treatment of isolated posterior ligament injuries without obvious facet joint disruption is more unpredictable. The degree of ligament injury can be difficult to determine initially even with MRI. Initial treatment with a cervical collar or cervicothoracic orthosis is reasonable unless there is radiographic evidence of increasing deformity or excessive motion. In severe cases, surgical stabilization is indicated. MRI should be performed prior to surgical intervention to rule out an associated disc disruption and to guide the selection of the appropriate surgical approach.

LATERAL COLUMN INJURIES

18. What are the different types of unilateral facet injuries?
A wide spectrum of injuries may occur:
- *Unilateral ligamentous facet injuries:* These are soft tissue injuries without an associated fracture. The facet joints may be subluxed, perched (tip to tip), or dislocated
- *Unilateral facet fracture without facet subluxation or dislocation*
- *Facet fractures with associated facet subluxations or dislocations*

19. What treatment is indicated for an isolated facet fracture without associated subluxation or dislocation?
Initial treatment is immobilization in a cervical collar. Erect radiographs in the collar are necessary to assess for displacement, subluxation, or the development of segmental kyphosis. Careful clinical and radiographic follow-up is critical because it can be difficult to predict which injuries will develop signs of instability and require surgical intervention. Treatment options for unstable injuries include single-segment anterior cervical discectomy and fusion with plate fixation or posterior screw-rod fixation and posterior fusion.

20. What is the significance of a fracture separation of the lateral mass?
An ipsilateral lamina and pedicle fracture functionally separates the injured lateral mass from the facet above and below the fracture and is called a **fracture separation of the lateral mass** (Fig. 56-4). This injury creates potential instability at two adjacent motion segments with the possibility of anterior subluxation at both the cranial and caudal levels. Nondisplaced injuries are treated with immobilization in a cervical collar, cervicothoracic orthosis, or halo vest. Surgical treatment is indicated for injuries associated with displacement. Surgical treatment options include posterior and anterior approaches. Surgical treatment is anterior or posterior instrumentation and fusion over two motion segments. Single-level anterior discectomy and fusion can be considered if subluxation is present at a single level (usually the lower level) but is associated with risk of late subluxation at the untreated level.

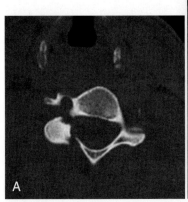 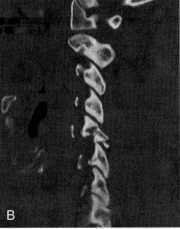

Figure 56-4. Fracture separation of the lateral mass. **A,** Axial computed tomography (CT) shows ipsilateral pedicle and lamina fractures, which create a free-floating lateral mass. **B,** Sagittal CT image shows rotational deformity of the fractured lateral mass.

Continued

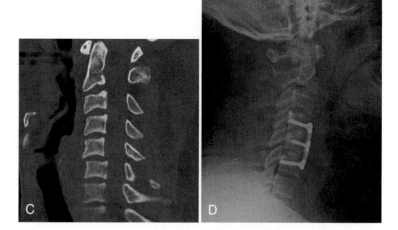

Figure 56-4, cont'd. C, CT image shows associated anterolisthesis at C5–C6. **D,** Treatment consisted of anterior reduction and two-level discectomy and fusion combined with anterior plate fixation.

21. What are the characteristic features of traumatic cervical spondylolisthesis?

This injury pattern typically occurs at the C7 or T1 levels. Spondylolisthesis develops following bilateral fractures involving the pars interarticularis and/or pedicles. Due to separation of the anterior and posterior spinal columns, the spinal canal is widened. As a result, neurologic function may remain intact despite the presence of vertebral body translation at the injured level. Required treatment is posterior open reduction and posterior spinal instrumentation and fusion with screw-rod fixation.

22. What are the characteristic features of a unilateral facet dislocation?

Unilateral facet dislocations typically result from a high-energy injury involving combined distractive flexion and rotational forces (Fig. 56-5). Patients present with neck pain that may be accompanied by a mild torticollis. The injury may be overlooked on initial radiographs. Careful inspection shows less than 25% anterolisthesis, rotational asymmetry of adjacent spinous processes, interspinous widening, and the "bow-tie sign" (due to displacement of adjacent facet joints). CT scan will clearly identify the facet dislocation and any associated facet fractures. MRI will identify injury of the posterior ligaments and facet capsules, as well as disc disruption or herniation if present. Associated nerve root injury is more common than spinal cord injury.

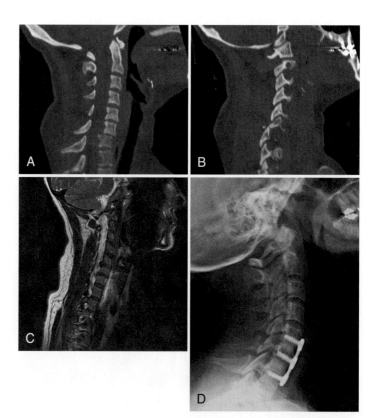

Figure 56-5. Unilateral facet dislocation. Middle-aged female driver involved in motor vehicle accident presented with neck pain and unilateral arm weakness. **A,** Sagittal computed tomography shows mild C6–C7 anterolisthesis and unilateral C6–C7 facet dislocation. **B** and **C,** Sagittal magnetic resonance imaging shows concomitant disc herniation above the level of listhesis (C5–C6). **D,** Treatment was anterior cervical discectomy, fusion, and plate fixation C5 to C7.

23. What are the characteristic features of bilateral facet dislocations?

Bilateral facet dislocations or fracture dislocations are high-energy injuries resulting from hyperflexion with or without associated rotational injury (Fig. 56-6). The lateral radiographs demonstrate greater than 50% subluxation. MRI findings include disruption of facet capsules, posterior ligaments, and intervertebral disc, and in many cases an associated disc herniation is present. CT is important for accurate assessment of posterior and lateral column osseous injuries. Associated neurologic injury is common and may be incomplete or complete.

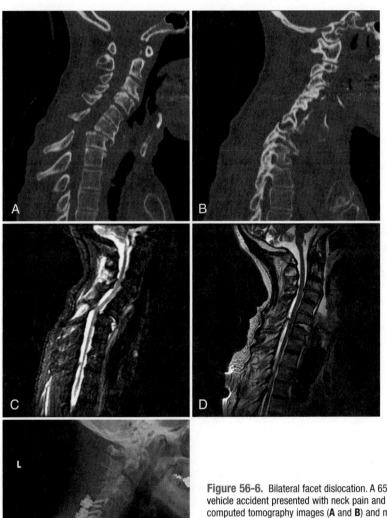

Figure 56-6. Bilateral facet dislocation. A 65-year-old man involved in a motor vehicle accident presented with neck pain and an incomplete spinal cord injury. Sagittal computed tomography images (**A** and **B**) and magnetic resonance imaging (MRI) **(C)** show anterolisthesis at C6–C7 with bilateral facet dislocations. Note the anterior osteophyte formation that suggests the injury occurred through a spinal segment stiffened by chronic spondylosis. Awake closed reduction with cervical tong traction was performed. **D,** Postreduction MRI shows restoration of alignment and facet reduction. Note the distracted disc space at C6–C7. **E,** Treatment consisted of posterior spinal instrumentation and fusion followed by anterior grafting and plate fixation.

24. What controversy is associated with closed reduction of facet dislocations?

When neurologic impairment exists, emergent reduction is desirable to reestablish spinal canal alignment and provide neural decompression in order to maximize chances for neural recovery. Controversy surrounds the need to image the intervertebral disc with MRI at the level of injury prior to reduction. A significant number of facet dislocations are associated with disc disruption and disc herniation. If the disc fragment is associated with the superiorly translated vertebra, reduction has the potential to displace disc material into the spinal canal and cause a catastrophic neural deficit. In the neurologically intact patient who is awake and cooperative, some surgeons recommend a prereduction MRI to rule out a potentially dangerous disc herniation. If a disc herniation is present, anterior discectomy is recommended prior to reduction. However, multiple studies have shown that immediate traction and reduction can be performed safely in the alert, awake, and cooperative patient whose neurologic status can be clinically monitored. Closed reduction should not be attempted in an unconscious patient or in a patient in whom a reliable neurologic examination is not possible. An MRI should be obtained prior to attempting reduction in uncooperative or unconscious patients to guide the selection of the appropriate treatment approach. In all patients, a cervical MRI should be obtained following closed reduction and prior to operative intervention.

25. How is emergent closed reduction of a cervical facet-dislocation accomplished?
Reduction is accomplished in a setting that allows constant monitoring, cervical traction, and frequent radiographs or fluoroscopy. Use of intravenous analgesics, muscle relaxants, and nasal oxygen is recommended. Gardner Wells tongs (preferably stainless steel) are safe, easily applied, and allow traction in excess of 70% of the patient's body weight (weights up to 140 lb have been used). Pin sites are prepped with Betadine and anesthetized with lidocaine. Tongs are applied by inserting pins into the skull above and in line with the external auditory meatus. An initial weight of 5 to 10 lb is applied. Neurologic examination and radiographic assessment are performed. This process is repeated as weight is added in 5- to 10-lb increments until reduction is achieved. The patient requires careful clinical examination to detect any sign of deterioration in neurologic function. Serial radiographs are monitored for signs of excessive disc space distraction (disc height > 1.5 times the height of adjacent disc spaces). When reduction occurs, the head is slightly extended and weight is decreased to 20 lb. MRI-compatible tongs are substituted for stainless steel tongs while maintaining alignment with manual in-line traction and the patient is transported for a cervical MRI study.

26. Discuss surgical treatment decision making for unilateral and bilateral facet dislocations.
MRI following attempted closed reduction of unilateral and bilateral facet dislocations is required to plan surgical treatment. If an acute disc herniation is suspected on the postreduction MRI, an anterior approach with anterior discectomy, fusion, and anterior plate fixation is indicated. In patients with reduced facet dislocations without associated disc herniation, either an anterior or posterior approach may be utilized. Combined anterior and posterior procedures are indicated for dislocations not completely reducible from an anterior approach and for highly unstable injury patterns. Open reduction is required for injuries that fail closed reduction, and techniques for reduction have been described using both anterior and posterior approaches.

INJURIES IN SPECIAL CIRCUMSTANCES

27. What unique features are associated with cervical spine injuries in patients with ankylosing spondylitis (AS) and diffuse idiopathic skeletal hyperostosis (DISH)?
AS and DISH patients who present for evaluation following trauma require special consideration:
- Diagnosis may be difficult, especially with nondisplaced fractures in patients with osteopenia and spinal deformity. AS and DISH patients complaining of neck pain are presumed to have a cervical fracture until ruled out with advanced imaging studies
- Fracture patterns are frequently three-column spinal injuries and are highly unstable due to the long rigid lever arms created by fused spinal segments proximal and distal to the level of injury
- Multiple noncontiguous spine fractures or *skip fractures* may be present
- Neurologic injury is common and may result from initial fracture displacement, from subsequent fracture displacement during transport or hospitalization, or from associated epidural hematoma (surgical emergency)
- When such a fracture is recognized, immobilization of the cervical spine in its preinjury position is necessary. In the patient with preexisting kyphotic deformity, this requires placing bolsters underneath the occiput to maintain prefracture alignment
- Surgical treatment consists of expedient multilevel posterior instrumentation (three levels above and below the injury if possible). Fusion of the fracture site may not be necessary due to the bony proliferative disease in these patients. Supplemental anterior fusion and plate fixation is indicated in the presence of a significant anterior column osseous defect

28. What incomplete spinal cord injury syndrome is commonly associated with a hyperextension injury mechanism in patients with preexistent cervical spondylosis?
Central cord syndrome is the incomplete spinal cord injury syndrome most commonly associated with a hyperextension injury mechanism in older patients with cervical spondylosis and a narrow spinal canal. A spectrum of neurologic deficits ranging from weakness limited to the hands to complete quadriparesis may occur. More severe neurologic involvement is noted in the upper extremities compared with the lower extremities. Initial surgical treatment is indicated for patients with associated fractures, spinal instability, or deterioration in neurologic status. Data to support indications and timing of surgery to optimize neurologic recovery in patients with stable spines and static or improving neurologic status are limited, although there is a current trend toward earlier decompression.

Key Points

1. Initial evaluation and management of a patient with a subaxial cervical spine injury is carried out according to the ATLS protocol.
2. The objective of cervical spine clearance is to exclude a significant cervical spine injury.
3. Appropriate management of subaxial cervical spine injuries is dependent on neurologic status, injury morphology, and spinal stability.

Websites

Lower cervical spine fractures and dislocations: http://emedicine.medscape.com/article/1264065-overview
Subaxial Cervical Spine Injury Classification: http://jdc.jefferson.edu/cgi/viewcontent.cgi?article=1013&context=orthofp

BIBLIOGRAPHY

1. Anderson PA, Gugala Z, Lindsey RW, et al. Clearing the cervical spine in the blunt trauma patient. J Am Acad Orthop Surg 2010;18:149–59.
2. Anderson PA, Moore TA, Davis KW, et al. Cervical spine injury severity score: Assessment of reliability. J Bone Joint Surg 2007;89A:1057–65.
3. Bellabarba C, Anderson PA. Injuries of the lower cervical spine. In: Herkowitz HN, Garfin SR, Eismont FJ, Bell GR, Balderston RA, editors. Rothman-Simeone The Spine. 5th ed. Philadelphia: Saunders; 2006. p. 1100–31.
4. Brandenstein D, Molinari RW, Rubery PT, et al. Unstable subaxial cervical spine injury with normal computed tomography and magnetic resonance initial studies: A report of four cases and review of the literature. Spine 2009;34:E743–E750.
5. Dvorak MF, Fisher CG, Fehlings MG, et al. The surgical approach to subaxial cervical spine injuries: An evidence-based algorithm based on the SLIC classification system. Spine 2007;32:2620–9.
6. Kwon BK, Anderson PA. Injuries of the lower cervical spine. In: Browner BD, Jupiter JB, Levine AM, Trafton PG, Krettek C, editors. Browner Skeletal Trauma. 4th ed. Philadelphia: Saunders; 2009.
7. Kwon BK, Vaccaro AR, Grauer JN, et al. Subaxial cervical spine trauma. J Am Acad Orthop Surg 2006;14:78–89.
8. Moore TA, Vaccaro AR, Anderson PA. Classification of lower cervical spine injuries. Spine 2006;31:S37–S43.
9. Nowak DD, Lee JK, Gelb DE, et al. Central cord syndrome. J Am Acad Ortho Surg 2009;17:756–65.
10. Vaccaro AR, Hulbert RJ, Patel AA, et al. The subaxial cervical injury classification system: A novel approach to recognize the importance of morphology, neurology and integrity of the disco-ligamentous complex. Spine 2007;32:2365–74.

57 CHAPTER THORACIC AND LUMBAR SPINE FRACTURES

Edward A. Smirnov, MD, D. Greg Anderson, MD, Todd J. Albert, MD, and Vincent J. Devlin, MD

1. Why is it important to assess radiographically the entire spinal axis when a significant spine fracture is identified in one region of the spine?

There is a 5% to 20% chance that a patient has a second fracture in a different region of the spine. Factors that increase the risk of missed spine fractures on initial evaluation include head injuries, intoxication, drug use, and polytrauma.

2. What factors increase the risk of neurologic injury with thoracic and lumbar spine fractures?

1. High-energy injuries, especially burst fractures and fracture dislocations
2. Fractures located above the L2 level. The conus medullaris and spinal cord occupy the spinal canal in this location, and these neural elements are more prone to neurologic injury than the nerve roots of the cauda equina

3. Are plain radiographs sufficient to distinguish the common types of thoracic and lumbar spine fractures?

No! Although anteroposterior (AP) and lateral radiographs are the best first imaging test to assess a spine fracture, a computed tomography (CT) scan must be obtained when radiographs suggest a significant thoracic or lumbar fracture. Failure to obtain a CT scan may lead to inappropriate diagnosis and treatment. Magnetic resonance imaging (MRI) plays a complementary role and is useful in the assessment of patients with neurologic deficit and for evaluation of the posterior ligamentous complex (PLC).

4. What parameters are important to assess on radiographs of thoracic and lumbar fractures? (Fig. 57-1)

- **Percentage of vertebral body compression:** The anterior vertebral height (B) is divided by the posterior vertebral height (A) or the height of an adjacent non-fractured vertebra and multiplied by 100.
- **Local kyphotic deformity:** The angle (C) between the vertebral endplates above and below the injured level is determined (Cobb method). This value (kyphosis angle) is compared with the normal sagittal alignment for the specific levels of the spine under evaluation.
- **Integrity of the posterior spinal column:** Findings that suggest disruption of the posterior spinal column include widening or splaying of the spinous processes or a localized kyphotic deformity of a thoracolumbar spinal segment.
- **Signs of major spinal column disruption:** Relative distraction, translation, or rotational displacement of adjacent vertebrae implies a severe injury with disruption of all three spinal columns.

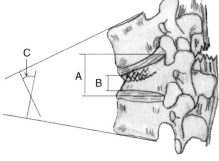

Figure 57-1. Useful radiographic parameters for assessing thoracic and lumbar fractures: (1) percentage of vertebral body compression, (2) local kyphotic deformity, and (3) disruption of the posterior spinal column. Percentage of vertebral body compression is determined by dividing the anterior vertebral height (B) by the posterior vertebral height (A). The local kyphotic deformity is determined by measuring the angle (C) between the vertebral endplates above and below the injured level.

5. Define the three-column model of the spine as described by Denis (Fig. 57-2).

- The **anterior column** is composed of the anterior longitudinal ligament, anterior half of the vertebral body, and anterior half of the disc
- The **middle column** is composed of the posterior half of the vertebral body, the posterior half of the disc, and the posterior longitudinal ligament
- The **posterior column** includes the pedicles, facet joints, lamina, and posterior ligament complex

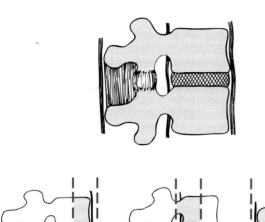

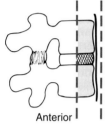
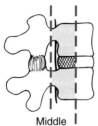
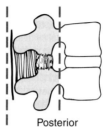

Anterior | Middle | Posterior

Figure 57-2. Denis' three-column model of the spine. The middle column is made up of the posterior longitudinal ligament, the posterior annulus fibrosis, and the posterior aspects of the vertebral body and disc. (Lee YP, Templin C, Eismont F, et al. Thoracic and upper lumbar trauma. In: Browner BD, Jupiter JB, Levine AM, et al., editors. Skeletal Trauma, 4th ed. Philadelphia: Saunders; 2008.)

6. What are the six most common patterns of thoracolumbar fractures described by McAfee?

McAfee expanded Denis's concepts and classified thoracic and lumbar spine fractures into six patterns based on CT scan analysis. Injury patterns were determined based on the forces (compression, axial distraction or translation) that disrupt the middle spinal column (Fig. 57-3) (Table 57-1).

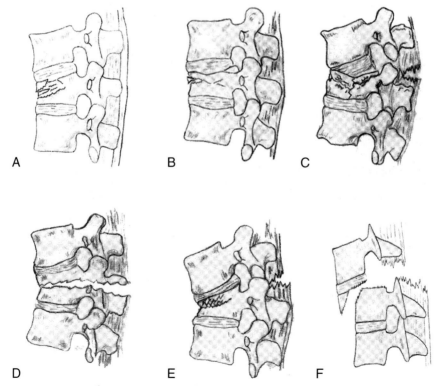

Figure 57-3. McAfee classification of thoracic and lumbar fractures. **A,** Compression fracture. **B,** Stable burst fracture. **C,** Unstable burst fracture. **D,** Chance fracture. **E,** Flexion-distraction injury. **F,** Fracture-dislocation or translational injury.

Table 57-1. The McAfee Classification of Thoracic and Lumbar Fractures

| FRACTURE TYPE | MODE OF SPINAL COLUMN FAILURE | | | INJURY MECHANISM |
	ANTERIOR	MIDDLE	POSTERIOR	
Compression	Compression	Intact	Intact	Axial load, flexion
Stable Burst	Compression	Compression	Intact	Compression
Unstable Burst	Compression	Compression	Compression, lateral flexion, or rotation	Compression, lateral flexion, rotation
Flexion-Distraction	Compression	Tension	Tension	Flexion-distraction
Chance	Tension	Tension	Tension	Tension
Translational (Fracture-Dislocation)	Shear, Rotation	Shear, Rotation	Shear, Rotation	Shear, rotation

7. **Discuss limitations regarding classification systems for thoracic and lumbar spine fractures.**

A wide variety of classification schemes have been proposed including the AO/Magerl classification, the Denis classification, the McAfee classification, and the Load-Sharing classification.

- The **AO/Magerl classification** identifies three primary injury patterns: *compression, distraction,* and *torsion.* However, these injuries are subdivided into more than 50 distinct injury patterns, which makes application of this classification challenging in clinical practice.
- Similarly, the **Denis classification** proposed four main fracture types—*compression, seat-belt, burst,* and *fracture-dislocations*—but described more than 16 injury subtypes. Its complexity and the discovery that the middle spinal column plays a secondary role in determining spinal instability have stimulated additional research.
- The **McAfee classification** provides sufficient detail to place injuries into six distinct categories and facilitates communication with the multidisciplinary team involved in trauma care.
- The **Load-Sharing classification** provides valuable guidance in determining an appropriate surgical approach for thoracolumbar fracture repair.

However, the previous classifications do not stratify neurologic injury, do not define spinal instability, fail to incorporate MRI data, and lack guidelines for nonoperative versus operative treatment. Such limitations have led to ongoing research to develop a comprehensive, valid, user-friendly classification to guide treatment. The Thoracolumbar Injury Classification and Severity Score (TLICS) has recently been introduced to address these issues. This score is based on three factors:

- Injury mechanism
- Neurologic status
- Integrity of the posterior ligamentous complex (PLC)

A score of 3 or less suggests nonoperative treatment; a score of 4 suggests nonoperative or operative treatment; and a score of 5 or greater suggests operative treatment. Point values are assigned to each factor as follows:

- **Injury mechanism:** compression fracture (1), burst fracture (2), translational-rotational injury (3), distraction injury (4)
- **Neurologic status:** Intact (0), nerve root injury (2), incomplete cord/conus injury (3), complete cord/conus injury (2), cauda equina injury (3)
- **PLC status:** Intact (0), indeterminate (2), disrupted (3)

COMPRESSION FRACTURES

8. **Describe the mechanism, injury pattern, and treatment of a thoracic or lumbar compression fracture.**

Compression fractures represent an isolated failure of the anterior spinal column due to a combination of flexion and axial compression loading (Fig. 57-4). Because the structural stability of the spine is not compromised by this single-column injury, treatment consists of early patient mobilization. Typically the patient is treated with an orthosis (e.g. Jewett brace, thoracolumbosacral orthosis [TLSO]) until back pain resolves. Radiographic and clinical follow-up is generally carried out on a monthly basis for the first 3 months after injury.

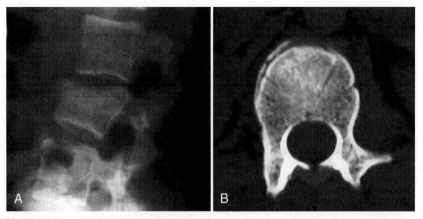

Figure 57-4. Compression fracture. **A,** Lateral radiograph. **B,** Axial computed tomography scan. A compression fracture represents an injury of the anterior spinal column. Note the loss of anterior vertebral height. Treatment with an orthosis led to complete resolution of symptoms within 2 months.

9. **What radiographic features are considered worrisome when assessing compression fractures?**
   - Loss of vertebral height exceeding 50% (suggests possible posterior ligamentous injury)
   - Segmental kyphosis exceeding 20° (suggests possible posterior ligamentous injury)
   - Multiple adjacent compression fractures (may require surgical treatment if significant kyphotic deformity occurs)
   - Loss of the pedicle shadow on the anteroposterior (AP) radiograph or presence of a soft tissue mass on MRI (suggests possibility of a pathologic fracture secondary to tumor or infection)

10. **Why is a compression fracture with greater than 40% to 50% loss of anterior vertebral body height considered *unstable*?**
    Because it is highly likely that an associated posterior ligament complex disruption is present. The posterior ligament complex experiences about one third of the tensile load transmitted to the vertebral body to cause fracture. In young persons with good bone quality, the magnitude of the load required to create a compression fracture may result in tensile failure of the posterior ligamentous complex.

11. **Outline the treatment of compression fractures secondary to osteoporosis.**
    Osteoporotic compression fractures are usually due to low-energy trauma in patients with weakened bone. They are common in the elderly, as well as patients on chronic steroid therapy. Multiple fractures may occur and may lead to significant spinal deformities and/or pain. It is important to rule out pathologic fracture due to tumor (e.g. multiple myeloma, metastatic disease) or metabolic bone disease (e.g. osteomalacia). Fracture treatment depends on severity and location of injury. Most fractures can be managed with an orthosis. It is important to diagnose and treat the underlying osteoporosis in addition to treating the fracture. Baseline bone density studies of the spine and hip should be performed. Osteoporosis treatment options include exercise, hormone replacement therapy, bisphosphonate therapy, calcitonin, or teriparatide. Open surgical treatment with spinal canal decompression combined with stabilization and fusion is generally reserved for fractures associated with neurologic deficit. Minimally invasive surgical procedures such as vertebroplasty and kyphoplasty have been popularized for the treatment of select acute and subacute compression fractures. These procedures attempt to relieve pain by supplementing the structural integrity of the collapsed vertebral body via the injection of polymethylmethacrylate (PMMA) bone cement.

STABLE BURST FRACTURES

12. **Describe the mechanism and injury pattern associated with a stable burst fracture.**
    Key features that identify a stable burst fracture (Fig. 57-5) include:
    - Fracture involves the anterior and middle spinal columns
    - Height loss of the vertebral body is present
    - Posterior vertebral body cortex is disrupted
    - Facet joints and lamina do not demonstrate any displaced fractures
    - Preservation of posterior spinal column integrity (absence of widening between the spinous processes at the fracture level when compared with adjacent spinal levels)
    - The patient has intact neurologic status

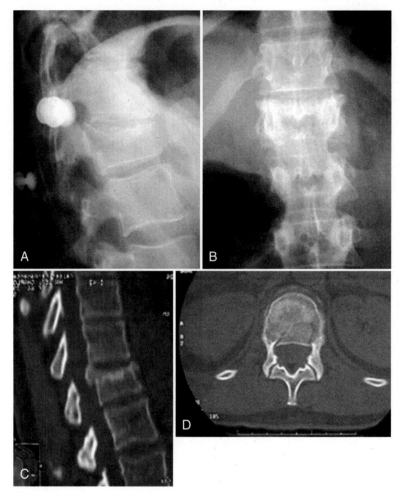

Figure 57-5. Stable L1 burst fracture. This fracture involves the anterior and middle spinal columns. Note the disruption of the posterior vertebral body cortex. The posterior spinal column is not disrupted. **A,** Lateral radiograph. **B,** Anteroposterior radiograph. **C,** Sagittal computed tomography (CT). **D,** Axial CT. Treatment with a thoracolumbosacral orthosis led to resolution of symptoms.

Although bone may be retropulsed into the spinal canal, the resultant compromise of the spinal canal is less than 50%. Loss of anterior column vertebral height is less than 50%. The local kyphotic deformity is generally less than 15° to 25°. Despite the possible presence of a nondisplaced vertical fracture in the lamina, the facet joints and the posterior ligament complex remain intact.

13. **What are the treatment options for a stable burst fracture?**
    Stable burst fractures are usually treated by nonoperative techniques. An excellent method is closed reduction and body-cast immobilization. Immobilization in a TLSO is the most common method used currently. A cervical extension is added for fractures above T7, and a thigh cuff is considered for low lumbar fractures (L4, L5). The cast or brace is generally worn for 3 months.

14. **What percent of burst fractures is misdiagnosed as compression fractures on plain radiographs?**
    Approximately 25% of burst fractures are misdiagnosed as compression fractures if radiographs alone are evaluated. For this reason, it is important to evaluate significant thoracic and lumbar spine fractures with a CT scan.

15. **What radiographic criteria help to distinguish a burst fracture from a compression fracture?**
    Loss of posterior vertebral body height (compared with the vertebrae above and below), any break in the posterior aspect of the vertebral body, or interpedicular widening on the AP view are signs of a burst fracture. The posterior vertebral body angle may aid diagnosis. This angle is formed by a line drawn along the vertebral endplate and the posterior vertebral body margin. If this angle is greater than 100°, a burst fracture is likely present.

UNSTABLE BURST FRACTURES

16. Describe the mechanism and injury pattern of an unstable burst fracture.

Unstable burst fractures result from axial compression forces that disrupt all three columns of the spine. The anterior and middle columns fail in compression with loss of vertebral body height and retropulsion of the posterior vertebral body wall into the spinal canal. The AP radiograph shows a widening of the distance between the pedicles at the level of fracture. Unlike a stable burst fracture, the posterior ligamentous complex (PLC) is disrupted. Posterior spinal column disruption permits development of a kyphotic deformity. CT scans are used to determine the percentage of spinal canal compromise and the presence or absence of an associated laminar fracture.

17. What is the major concern about a burst fracture associated with a laminar fracture?

Possible incarceration of the dura or neural elements in the fracture site with associated cerebrospinal (CSF) leakage may be present. One study demonstrated incarceration of the dural sac in the fracture site in more than one third of burst fractures associated with a laminar fracture.

18. What nonspinal injuries are commonly associated with burst fractures?

Calcaneus fractures, long bone fractures, and closed head injuries.

19. What are the major criteria for recommending nonsurgical treatment for burst fractures?

Burst fractures without neurologic deficit, with canal compromise less than 50%, and with less than 30° of initial kyphosis may be considered for nonsurgical treatment. Such patients require close clinical and radiographic monitoring for the potential development of neurologic deficit and progressive kyphotic deformity.

20. What are the major criteria for recommending surgical treatment for burst fractures?

Indications for surgical treatment of burst fractures are controversial and include:
- Progressive neurologic deficit
- CT evidence of spinal canal compromise associated with incomplete neurologic deficit
- Burst fracture associated with significant disruption of the posterior column—for example, facet subluxation, significant disruption of the posterior ligamentous complex
- Greater than 50% loss of vertebral body height
- Kyphosis greater than 25° to 30° at the level of fracture
- Inability to immobilize the patient with a brace due to associated injuries or body habitus

See Figure 57-6.

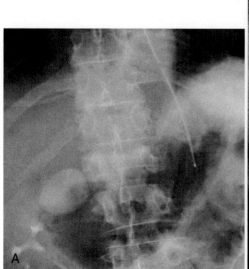
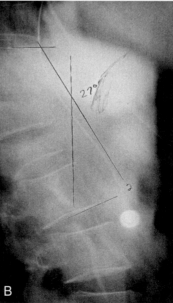
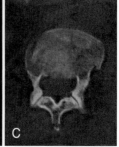

Figure 57-6. Unstable burst fracture. Treatment with long segment fixation. A 43-year-old man sustained a T12 burst fracture when a mobile home roof fell on him during a storm. The patient was neurologically intact. **A,** A preoperative anteroposterior (AP) radiograph shows approximately 50 percent loss of height at T12 and L1. **B,** A preoperative lateral view shows local kyphosis measuring 27°. **C,** Axial computed tomography shows a minimal burst component at L1.

Continued

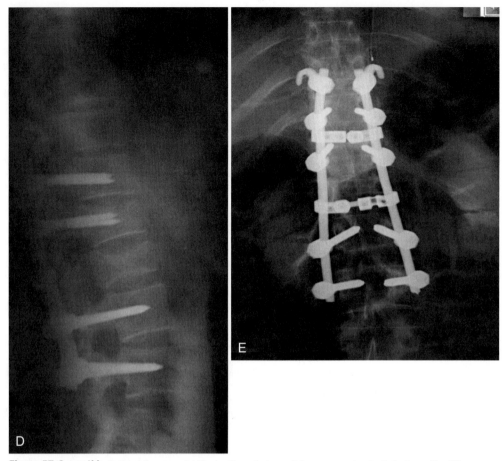

Figure 57-6, cont'd. **D,** This injury was stabilized with posterior pedicle screws and rods. **E,** Postoperative AP radiograph showing two cross-connectors used for additional stability. (Lee YP, Templin C, Eismont F, et al. Thoracic and upper lumbar trauma. In: Browner BD, Jupiter JB, Levine AM, et al, editors. Skeletal Trauma. 4th ed. Philadelphia: Saunders; 2008.)

21. What are the surgical goals in treating unstable burst fractures?
- **Decompression:** Spinal canal decompression is generally indicated for patients with neurologic deficits, especially incomplete deficits. Neurologic assessment should include lower extremity sensory and motor function, as well as bowel and bladder function
- **Realignment:** Spinal realignment is achieved through use of spinal instrumentation with correction of kyphotic deformity
- **Stabilization:** The combination of spinal instrumentation and spinal fusion can restore long-term stability to injured spinal segments

22. What are three options for decompression of spinal canal stenosis resulting from a burst fracture in a patient with a neurologic deficit?
- **Indirect decompression:** Distraction applied to the fracture through the use of posterior spinal instrumentation has the potential to reduce the fracture fragments and decompress the spinal canal through *ligamentotaxis.* This technique is most likely to be successful if performed within the first 72 hours after the fracture occurs
- **Direct posterolateral decompression:** The fragments impinging on the neural elements are pushed away anteriorly to decompress the dural sac after exposure of the spinal canal is achieved through a laminectomy or transpedicular approach. This procedure is performed in conjunction with posterior spinal instrumentation and fusion
- **Direct anterior decompression:** The fracture may be exposed directly through an anterior approach, and the entire vertebral body may be removed (corpectomy) to decompress the spinal canal. A bone graft or cage is used to reconstruct the anterior spinal column. Spinal stability is restored by placement of anterior spinal instrumentation, posterior spinal instrumentation, or a combination of both anterior and posterior spinal implants

See Figure 57-7.

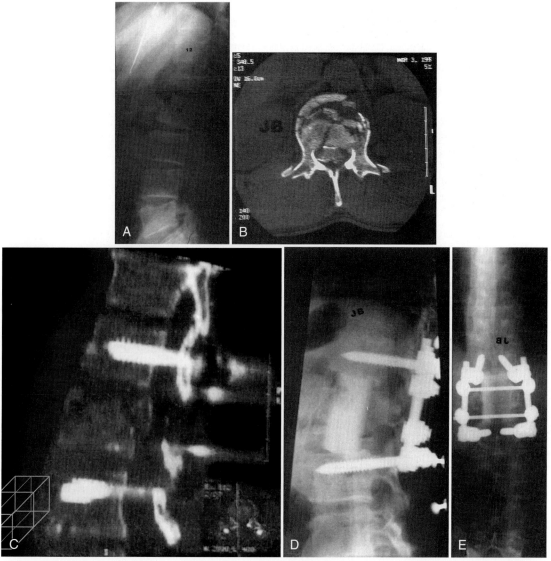

Figure 57-7. Unstable burst fracture. L1 burst fracture treated with posterior pedicle screw fixation followed by anterior decompression and reconstruction using structural allograft. The preoperative lateral radiograph **(A)** and computed tomography (CT) scan **(B)** demonstrate 60% loss of vertebral body height and 90% spinal canal occlusion. **C,** CT following urgently performed posterior decompression and short segment fixation demonstrate approximately 50% residual canal compromise. The lateral **(D)** and anteroposterior **(E)** radiographs demonstrate tibial allograft placement after anterior decompression. This second surgery was performed 10 days after the posterior procedure. The patient sustained multiple injuries following a high-speed motorcycle accident. (From Chapman JR, Mirza SK. Anterior treatment of thoracolumbar fractures. Spine State Art Rev 1998;12:647–61.)

23. What are the advantages and disadvantages of using pedicle screws for treatment of thoracolumbar burst fractures?
Advantages:
- Emergent decompression and short-segment instrumentation and fusion can be expeditiously performed and permits early patient mobilization.
- Fewer spine segments require instrumentation and fusion when pedicle screws are used, compared with when rod and hook constructs are utilized.
- Pedicle screws can be used with contoured rods to maintain and restore normal sagittal alignment.
Disadvantages:
- Second-stage anterior corpectomy and fusion may be required in fractures with extensive vertebral body comminution because pedicle screw constructs without anterior column structural support are prone to screw breakage
- Patients with residual cord/root compression in the setting of persistent neurologic deficit will require delayed anterior decompression and fusion

24. What are the common indications for use of an anterior approach and anterior instrumentation in a thoracolumbar burst fracture?

Indications include fractures from T11 to L3, especially when an incomplete neurologic lesion with compromise of the spinal canal would benefit from direct decompression of the spinal canal. Significant kyphotic deformities in which anterior column structural grafting is indicated also respond well to an anterior approach (Fig. 57-8).

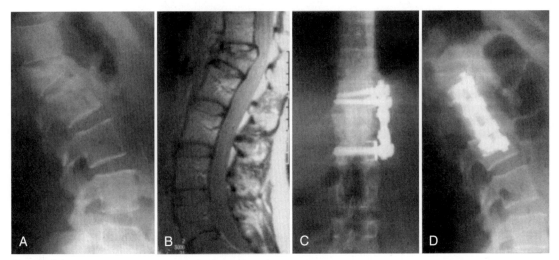

Figure 57-8. Unstable burst fracture. L1 burst fracture treated with corpectomy, anterior femoral allograft, and anterior rod-screw construct (Kaneda instrumentation). **A,** Preoperative lateral radiograph. **B,** Preoperative sagittal MRI. Postoperative **C,** anteroposterior and **D,** lateral radiographs. (From Devlin VJ, Pitt DD. The evolution of surgery of the anterior spinal column. Spine State Art Rev 1998; 12:493–527.)

25. Discuss the major limitations of an anterior approach to thoracolumbar burst fractures.

Fractures below L3 are difficult to treat with anterior instrumentation because of local anatomic constraints due to the proximity of the aorta, vena cava, and iliac vessels. Anterior corpectomy for acute fractures is frequently accompanied by significant bleeding from the fractured vertebra. There is limited ability to realign the spine from an anterior approach in the presence of posttraumatic translational or scoliotic deformities, and such injuries are more effectively treated with initial posterior instrumentation. It is not possible to explore lamina fractures noted on CT scan for potential incarceration of the dura with associated CSF leak from the anterior approach. Care must be taken in cases with significant disruption of the posterior column, and patients with osteoporotic bone as the anterior screw fixation may not provide adequate stability in these cases. Noncompliant/combative patients represent additional contraindications to anterior-only approaches. These patients require the added stability of posterior instrumentation because they will be noncompliant with postoperative brace wear.

CHANCE FRACTURES

26. Describe the mechanism and injury pattern of a Chance fracture.

Chance fractures generally result from a flexion injury mechanism in a lap-belt-restrained car passenger. Radiographs show three spinal columns injured transversely due to failure of the spinal segment in tension. The axis of rotation for this injury is anterior to the vertebral body. The disruption of the spine may progress through bone (vertebral body, pedicle, and spinous process), soft tissue (disc, facet joint, and interspinous ligament), or a combination of bone and soft tissue structures.

27. What nonspinal injuries are commonly associated with Chance fractures?

A high incidence of intraabdominal (bowel) injury (45%) is associated with Chance fractures.

28. What are the treatment options for a Chance fracture?

In general, patients with Chance fractures are treated with posterior spinal instrumentation and fusion (Fig. 57-9). A short-segment posterior instrumentation construct, which applies compression forces across the fracture, is appropriate. The pattern of injury determines the minimum number of levels requiring instrumentation. If the injury to the middle column involves the posterior disc, MRI is indicated to identify a disc herniation that may require excision prior to application of posterior compression forces. Uncommonly, patients who sustain injuries entirely through bone and do not have concomitant abdominal or neurologic injuries may be treated with extension casting.

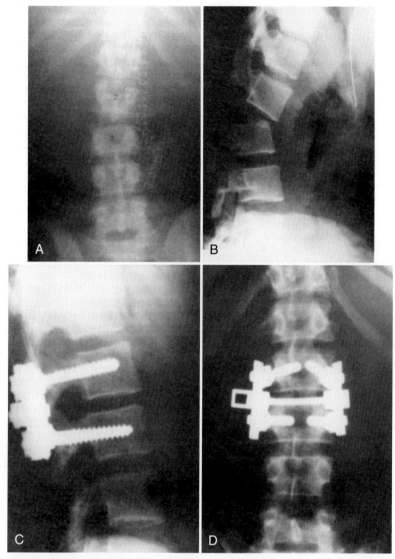

Figure 57-9. Chance fracture. **A,** Anteroposterior radiograph. **B,** Lateral radiograph. **C,** Postoperative lateral radiograph. **D,** Postoperative anteroposterior radiograph. (From Puno RM, Bhojraj SY, Glassman SD, et al. Flexion distraction injuries of the thoracolumbar and lumbar spine in the adult and pediatric patient. Spine State Art Rev 1993;7:223–48.)

FLEXION-DISTRACTION INJURIES

29. Describe the mechanism and injury pattern of a flexion-distraction injury.

Common injury mechanisms for flexion-distraction injuries include motor vehicle accidents and falls from a height. Such injuries result in tensile failure of the posterior spinal column and compressive failure of the anterior column and possibly the middle column. Posterior column injuries include separation of the spinous processes and facet joints. The vertebral body is wedged anteriorly (see Fig. 57-10). Bony fragments from the middle column may be retropulsed into the spinal canal. The axis of rotation for a flexion-distraction injury is within the vertebral body, in contrast to a Chance fracture where the axis of rotation is located anterior to the vertebral body. A flexion-distraction injury may be misdiagnosed initially as a compression fracture if the disruption of the posterior spinal column is unrecognized.

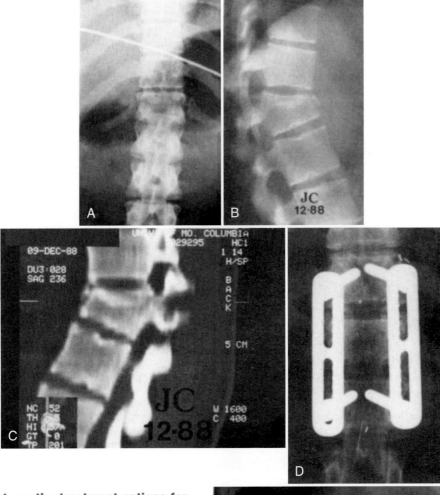

30. What are the treatment options for a flexion-distraction injury?

These unstable injuries are treated with posterior spinal instrumentation and posterior fusion (see Fig. 57-10).

Figure 57-10. Flexion-distraction injury. **A,** Preoperative anteroposterior (AP) radiograph. **B,** Preoperative lateral radiograph. **C,** Preoperative computed tomography scan. **D,** Postoperative AP radiograph. **E,** Postoperative lateral radiograph. (From Holt BT, McCormack T, Gaines RW Jr. Short-segment fusion: Anterior or posterior approach? Spine State Art Rev 1993;7:277–86.)

TRANSLATIONAL INJURIES (FRACTURE-DISLOCATIONS)

31. Describe the mechanism and injury pattern of a translational injury (fracture-dislocation).

Fracture-dislocations result from high-energy injuries and are the most unstable type of spine fractures. The structural integrity of all three spinal columns is completely disrupted with resultant displacement of the spine in one or more planes (Fig. 57-11). Severe neurologic deficits generally accompany this injury pattern.

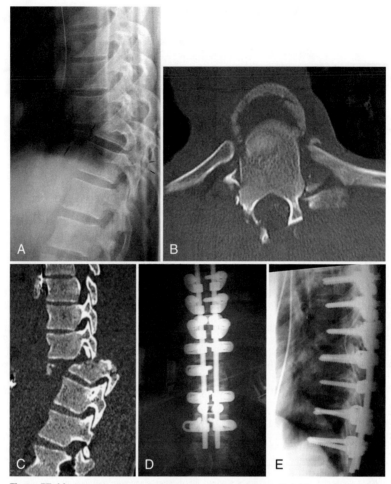

Figure 57-11. Translational injury. **A,** Preoperative lateral radiograph. **B,** Axial computed tomography (CT) image. **C,** Sagittal CT image. **D,** Postoperative anteroposterior radiograph. **E,** Postoperative lateral radiographs.

32. What are the treatment options for a translational injury (fracture-dislocation)?
These injuries require surgical stabilization regardless of the patient's neurologic status. These injuries are best treated initially from a posterior approach to realign the spine and restore spinal stability by fixation two or three levels above and below the injury. Anterior column reconstruction may be indicated if there is severe comminution precluding achievement construct stability with isolated posterior instrumentation or if spinal canal decompression is required (especially for patients with incomplete neurologic deficits) (see Fig. 57-11).

GUNSHOT INJURIES TO THE SPINE

33. How does the treatment of thoracolumbar injuries due to gunshot wounds differ from other mechanisms of injury?
Gunshot injuries generally spare the spinal ligaments, and thus most gunshot injuries are *mechanically stable*. However, many patients may have a neurologic deficit resulting from the blast wound to the neurologic elements. Most patients can be treated nonoperatively and mobilized in a TLSO. Tetanus prophylaxis should be considered. Broad-spectrum antibiotics should be administered for 48 to 72 hours. Transcolonic gunshots to the spine are treated with antibiotics for 7 to 14 days. Steroid use does not improve neurologic outcome, and use of steroids is associated with an increased rate of complications. Evidence of acute lead intoxication, an intracanal copper bullet, or new-onset neurologic deficit are potential indications for surgical decompression and bullet removal. Literature does not support bullet removal for intracanal cervical and thoracic gunshots but does support intracanal bullet removal for the T12 to L5 levels.

Key Points

1. Computed tomography (CT) is an integral part of the initial assessment of thoracic and lumbar spine fractures.
2. Comprehensive assessment of a thoracic or lumbar fracture includes a description of the injury mechanism, neurologic status, and integrity of the posterior ligamentous complex (PLC).
3. Abdominal visceral injuries are frequently associated with a flexion-distraction spinal injury mechanism.

Websites

Decision making in thoracolumbar fractures: http://www.neurologyindia.com/text.asp?2005/53/4/534/22626
Orthopaedic Trauma Association Spine Lectures: http://www.ota.org/res_slide/Spine_INDEX.ppt
Surgical treatment of thoracolumbar spine fractures: http://www.coluna.com.br/revistacoluna/volume5/vol_5_%5B2%5Dpg_84-89.pdf
Thoracic spine fractures and dislocations: http://emedicine.medscape.com/article/1267029-overview
Thoracolumbar injury classification and severity scale (TLICSS): http://www.orthopaedia.com/display/Main/Thoracolumbar+Injury+Classification+and+Severity+Scale+%28TLICSS%29

BIBLIOGRAPHY

1. Bono CM, Heary RF. Gunshot wounds to the spine. Spine J 2004;4:230–40.
2. Cammisa FP, Eismont FJ, Green BA. Dural lacerations occurring with burst fractures and associated laminar fractures. J Bone Joint Surg 1989;71A:1044.
3. Denis F. The three-column spine and its significance in the classification of acute thoracolumbar spinal injuries. Spine 1983;8:817–31.
4. Kim DH, Ludwig SC, Vaccaro AR, et al, editors. Atlas of Spine Trauma: Adult and Pediatric. Philadelphia: Saunders; 2008.
5. Magerl F, Aebi M, Gertzbein SD, et al. A comprehensive classification of thoracic and lumbar injuries. Eur Spine J 1994;3:184–201.
6. McAfee PC, Yuan HA, Frederickson BE, et al. The value of computed tomography in thoracolumbar fractures. J Bone Joint Surg 1983;65A:461–73.
7. Mirza SK, Mirza AJ, Chapman JR, et al. Classifications of thoracic and lumbar fractures: Rationale and supporting data. J Am Acad Orthop Surg 2002;10:364–77.
8. Oner FC, vanGils APG, Faber JAJ, et al. Some complications of common treatment schemes of thoracolumbar spine fractures can be predicted with magnetic resonance imaging. Spine 2002;27:629–36.
9. Parker JW, Lane JR, Karaikovic EE, et al. Successful short-segment instrumentation and fusion for thoracolumbar spine fractures. Spine 2000;25:1157–70.
10. Reitman CR, editor. Management of thoracolumbar fractures. Monograph Series, American Academy of Orthopaedic Surgeons, Rosemont, IL; 2004.
11. Vaccaro AR, Baron EM, Sanfilippo J, et al. Reliability of a novel classification system for thoracolumbar injuries: The Thoracolumbar Injury Severity Score. Spine 2006;31:S62–S69.

SACRAL FRACTURES

Jens R. Chapman, MD, Thomas A. Schildhauer, MD, and Carlo Bellabarba, MD

CHAPTER 58

1. What is the role of the sacrum?
The sacrum connects the lumbar spine and the left- and right-sided iliac wings by means of well-developed ligaments with little inherent bony stability. The sacrum is kyphotically aligned in the sagittal plane in a variable dimension ranging from 0° to over 90°. The sacrum distributes the torso load from the lumbar spine mainly through its S1 segment into the sacroiliac joints and distally to the hip joints.

2. Who is affected by sacral fractures?
Basically two distinct patient groups are affected by sacral fractures:
1. *High-energy injury mechanisms:* These patients require assessment and treatment as polytrauma victims (e.g. motor vehicle accidents, falls from a height, crush injuries)
2. *Low-impact insufficiency fractures:* These patients require comprehensive metabolic and neoplasia workup (osteoporosis, previously undiagnosed neoplastic disorder)

3. How are sacrum fractures diagnosed?
Subjective symptoms of patients with sacrum fractures are notoriously vague and usually consist of back pain aggravated by sitting, standing, and walking. A detailed patient history including mechanism of injury and associated injuries is critical. Physical examination is important and consists of inspection and palpation of the patient's back side and thorough examination of neurologic function. Specific imaging and electrodiagnostic tests are critical.

4. Describe the components of the neurologic examination for patients with a sacral fracture.
Regardless of the patient's cognitive status, an evaluation consistent with the *Guidelines of the American Spinal Injury Association* is performed. A detailed rectal examination is performed. Components of this evaluation include assessment for blood in the rectal vault, as well as presence of the prostate in the expected position. From a neurologic perspective, rectal assessment should include *four components*:
1. Presence of spontaneous anal sphincter tone
2. Maximum voluntary anal sphincter contractility
3. Perianal sensation to light touch and pinprick
4. Presence of anal wink and bulbocavernosus reflex

Postvoid residuals (PVR) can be used as a follow-up test for patients with neurogenic bladder to assess for reinnervation. In female patients, examination of the vaginal vault is also important.

5. What imaging tests are helpful in assessing sacral fractures?
The basic radiographic assessment starts with an *anteroposterior (AP) pelvis radiograph.* Due to the inclined nature of the sacrum, visualization of the sacrum is limited. Attention to subtle details, such as disruption of the foraminal lines, is important in screening for sacral fractures. If a fracture is suspected, further radiographs should be ordered, including *pelvic inlet and outlet views* and a *lateral sacral radiograph.* If a pelvic ring fracture is suspected, a *pelvic computed tomography (CT)* is ordered to assess the three-dimensional complexities of the fracture. If a significant sacral fracture is diagnosed, a *sacral CT* including sagittal and coronal reformatted images is required. *Magnetic resonance imaging (MRI)* is not routinely necessary but is helpful for diagnosis of insufficiency or stress fractures and to evaluate unclear neurologic injuries. *MRI neurography* is useful to localize known root or plexus injury. *Technetium bone scans with single-photon emission computed tomography (SPECT) images* are helpful in identifying insufficiency fractures of the sacrum.

6. What electrodiagnostic tests are helpful in assessing patients with sacral fractures and neurologic injuries?
- Electromyogram (EMG) of L5 and S1 innervated muscles
- Anal sphincter EMG
- Somatosensory-evoked potentials (SSEPs) of tibial and peroneal nerves
- Pudendal sensory-evoked potentials (pudendal SEPs)
- Cystomyography (CMG)

Pudendal SEPs are helpful for patients with impaired cognitive status or unclear physical examination findings and suspected lumbosacral root injury. Pudendal SEPs are useful in the assessment of the acutely injured patient. In contrast, conventional EMG is limited to assessment of the L5 and S1 roots and usually has a delay time of 3 weeks before injury-related changes are detectable. Anal sphincter EMG and CMG can diagnose lower sacral root damage but are not useful in the immediate postinjury period. CMG has been used as a follow-up study for patients with neurogenic bladder and may demonstrate bladder reinnervation.

7. Why is the diagnosis of sacral fractures frequently overlooked or delayed?

The diagnosis of sacral fractures is overlooked or delayed in up to half of cases. Causes for missed injuries range from vague physical symptoms and findings to difficulties in interpreting an AP pelvis radiograph for sacral abnormalities. This can be especially challenging in obese patients and in the presence of an osteopenia or osteophytes. In multiply-injured patients, a challenging resuscitation setting can distract diagnostic attention from the posterior pelvic ring. A high index of suspicion is important to avoid potential secondary damage from a missed sacral fracture.

8. What are possible consequences of a missed sacral fracture?

- Chronic pain with weightbearing
- Sacral or posterior pelvic malunion
- Secondary neurologic deficits from progressive fracture displacement and/or neural element impingement
- Posterior soft tissue breakdown from progressive sacral kyphosis

9. How are sacral fractures classified?

The wide range of sacral fracture patterns and their frequent association with pelvic fractures has led to development of many different fracture classification systems. The **Denis classification** is the most helpful general classification of sacral fractures because of its significant implications regarding incidence and type of associated neurologic injury. It uses the *most medial fracture extension* to distinguish three types of fractures (Fig. 58-1):

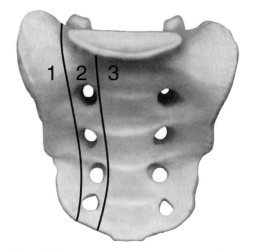

- **Zone 1 fractures** remain lateral to the sacral foramina. This is the most frequent fracture type and is associated with the lowest rate of neurologic injury (5%). Neurologic injury in Zone 1 fractures is limited to the L5 root or sciatic nerve
- **Zone 2 fractures** extend through the sacral foramina. These are the second most frequent fracture type. Associated lumbo-sacral root injuries occur in one quarter of patients
- **Zone 3 fractures** involve the central sacral spinal canal. These are the least common injury type but have the highest rate of neurologic injuries (>50%) ranging from sacral root deficits to cauda equina transection with associated bowel and bladder control deficits

Figure 58-1. Three-zone system of Denis: zone I injuries remain lateral to the neuroforamina; zone II fractures involve the neuroforamina but do not involve the central spinal canal; zone III injuries extend into the central spinal canal.

The Denis classification, however, does not specifically address *zone 3 transverse fractures.* The **Roy-Camille classification** provides a helpful subclassification system (Fig. 58-2) to address these injuries. It differentiates simple kyphotic fractures (type 1), kyphotically and partially translated fractures (type 2), fully displaced fractures (type 3), and segmentally comminuted fractures (type 4, as described by Strange-Vognsen).

L5–S1 facet joint disruption may occur in association with sacral fractures and can compromise pelvic ring stability and influence treatment. The **Isler classification** distinguishes three injury types: type 1 (lateral to the facet joint), type 2 (fracture line passes through the L5–S1 facet joint), and type 3 (fracture line passes medial to the L5–S1 facet joint). Type 1 fractures are least likely to disrupt lumbosacral stability.

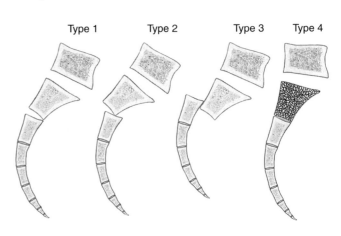

Figure 58-2. Subclassification of Denis zone III fractures as suggested by Roy-Camille. Type 1 injuries are angulated but not translated, whereas type 2 injuries are angulated and translated. Type 3 injuries show complete translational displacement of upper and lower sacrum, whereas type 4 injuries are segmentally comminuted due to axial impaction (as suggested by Strange-Vognsen). (From Chapman JR, Mirza SK. Sacral fractures. In: Fardon D, Garfin S, et al, editors. Orthopaedic Knowledge Update: Spine 2. Rosemont, IL: American Academy of Orthopaedic Surgeons, 2002.)

Sacral fractures associated with pelvic ring injuries require additional classification. Standard pelvic injury classifications (e.g. Tile classification, Young Burgess classification) are utilized to assess stability, injury mechanism, and associated injuries.

10. What factors influence selection of treatment options for sacral fractures?
Decision making regarding management of patients with sacral fractures is multifactorial. Variables include presence/absence of multiple injuries, open vs. closed fracture, associated soft tissue compromise, neurologic injury, and injury mechanism. There are no simple treatment algorithms.

11. What are the nonoperative treatment options for sacral fractures?
Criteria for nonoperative management include (1) stable, nondisplaced, closed, single-system injury; (2) no associated pelvic ring injury or L5–S1 facet joint disruption; and (3) intact neurologic status. Nonoperative management options include:
- Early, protected weightbearing
- Immobilization with a thoracolumbosacral orthosis (TLSO) with a unilateral or bilateral thigh extension or pantaloon spica cast
- Prolonged bed rest with recumbent skeletal traction

12. What surgical treatment options exist for sacral fractures?
Surgical interventions can be classified as decompression procedures and procedures that provide fracture reduction and stabilization.

13. When is a surgical decompression indicated after a sacral fracture?
In presence of lumbosacral or sacral nerve deficits or sacral radicular pain, surgical decompression within 2 weeks of injury has been associated with improved outcome compared with nonsurgical management. Decompression can be accomplished with direct decompression through a dorsal midline laminotomy and foraminotomy or with indirect decompression via fracture disimpaction or fracture reduction and stabilization.

14. What drawbacks are associated with surgical decompression of sacral fractures?
Surgical decompression may be ineffective in presence of traumatic sacral neural transsection. Approximately 35% of displaced transverse sacral fractures are associated with transected sacral roots based on autopsy study. Unfortunately, no imaging or electrophysiologic studies can conclusively establish the presence of transected sacral roots. Other risks associated with decompression surgery for sacral fractures include wound healing problems, persistent cerebrospinal fluid leakage, and additional fracture destabilization.

15. When is surgical stabilization of a sacral fracture indicated?
There are few strict guidelines for surgical sacral fracture stabilization. Typically, fracture displacement of 1 cm or more is considered to be consistent with fracture instability. Injuries that disrupt significant ligamentous lumbopelvic support structures usually have a poor prognosis for healing. Most patients who require surgical decompression of lumbosacral neural elements should also be considered for surgical stabilization to prevent further fracture displacement and enhance chances of neural recovery.

16. What are the options for surgical stabilization of sacral fractures (Table 58-1)?
All sacral fractures should be evaluated in the context of their effect on posterior pelvic ring and spinopelvic junction stability. Anterior pelvic ring stabilization has a supplemental role in sacral fracture stabilization, which can be achieved with anterior external fixation or symphyseal plating. Posterior pelvic ring fixation has undergone considerable evolution. Percutaneous sacroiliac screw placement has been reported to have a high success rate in the treatment of noncomplex sacral fractures. This technique allows effective indirect fracture reduction and stabilization when applied within 2 to 3 days from injury and has a relatively low incidence of reported complications. It is, however, limited in its biomechanical stability, especially for vertically displaced fractures and high-grade Denis zone 3 injuries. The most stable sacral fracture stabilization consists of lumbopelvic stabilization using lumbar pedicle and iliac screw fixation. This technique allows comprehensive stabilization of the sacrum through a posterior midline exposure.

Table 58-1. Options for Surgical Stabilization of Sacral Fractures

ANTERIOR (INDIRECT METHODS)	POSTERIOR
Symphyseal plating	Sacroiliac screw fixation (open or closed)
Anterior external fixation	Posterior tension band plating
Retrograde superior ramus screw fixation	Sacral alar plating (Roy-Camille technique)
	Lumbopelvic instrumentation
	Combined procedures

17. What is the optimal time for surgical intervention for a sacral fracture?

Optimal timing of surgical intervention for sacral fractures is multifactorial. Posterior exposures usually require a posterior midline approach with the patient in the prone position. Truly emergent open surgical decompression and stabilization of sacral fractures are rarely indicated. Because of the risk of significant blood loss, emergent surgical intervention using the open approach in the prone position is frequently postponed in favor of a delayed postprimary procedure within the first 2 weeks after injury. Additional factors to consider are presence of soft tissue deglovement (Morel-Lavalle lesion), open sacral fractures, and posterior soft tissue compromise caused by prominent bony fragments.

18. How are percutaneous sacroiliac screws placed?

Intricate knowledge of pelvic anatomy and high-quality intraoperative C-arm is prerequisite. Satisfactory closed reduction is achieved by skeletal traction or percutaneous manipulation. Radiographic anatomy should be reviewed to rule out the presence of congenital sacroiliac bony anomalies. Typically, a 7.0-mm large fragment cannulated screw system is used for unilateral or bilateral fixation. With the patient positioned supine on a fluoroscopy table, appropriate percutaneous starting points and guide-pin trajectories are determined using sacral lateral, as well as inlet and outlet projections on C-arm. Intraoperative screw placement under computed tomography (CT) guidance can be used as an imaging alternative. However, this approach is not feasible for polytraumatized patients or if intraoperative fracture manipulation is required. Screws are usually advanced over guidewires into the vertebral body of the S1 segment. Compression screws can be used in the presence of noncomminuted fractures. Fully threaded screws are preferred for patients with comminuted zone 2 fractures.

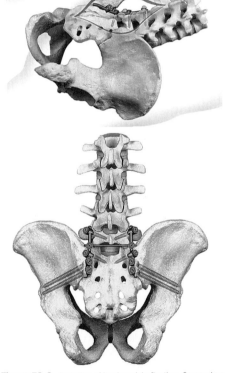

19. How is lumbopelvic instrumentation accomplished?

The ideal instrumentation system for lumbopelvic fixation is low profile and biomechanically stable, possesses a simple screw-linkage mechanism, and is adaptable to individual needs (Fig. 58-3). The instrumentation technique for lumbopelvic fixation differs significantly among various implant makers. Using side-loading implants, such as the Universal Spine System (Synthes), bilateral L5 pedicle fixation is obtained. If the S1 segment is intact, additional pedicle screws are placed into this segment. After decompression of the sacrum from the L5 segment downward, reduction of the sacral segments and the iliac wings can be accomplished with temporary threaded pins. Rods are then contoured to connect from the L5 and S1 screws to the region of the posterior iliac crest overhang and the posterior sacral ala. Using the outer iliac table as an inclination guide, one or two drill holes are then placed just lateral to the rod under lateral C-arm visualization. A starting point is selected approximately 2 cm inferior to the posterior superior iliac spine and aiming toward the anterior inferior iliac spine. The thickened portion of the ilium within 2 to 3 cm above the sciatic notch offers the most predictable passageway for such pelvic anchoring devices. Screws of up to 130 mm in length and 8 mm in diameter have been shown to be safely anchored in the iliac wing using this technique.

Figure 58-3. Insertion of lumbopelvic fixation. Comprehensive stabilization of the sacrum and complete decompression of the sacrum can be achieved with the insertion of long iliac screws that are attached to conventional, caudally extended lumbosacral rods.

20. What is triangular osteosynthesis?

The term *triangular osteosynthesis* is used to denote implant constructs that combine longitudinal vertebropelvic fixation (i.e. pedicle screw-rod fixation between the lower lumbar pedicles and iliac column or sacral ala) with horizontal fixation using an iliosacral screw. Triangular osteosynthesis provides greater stability than isolated iliosacral screw constructs. It is intended to facilitate early progressive weight-bearing for patients with vertically unstable sacral fractures.

Key Points

1. A high index of clinical suspicion, targeted physical examination, and appropriate imaging studies are required for timely diagnosis of sacral fractures.
2. Sacral fractures may result in posterior pelvic ring instability, spinopelvic instability, or combined instabilities.
3. Surgical treatment is indicated for sacral fractures associated with neurologic deficit, instability, or deformity.

Websites

Sacral fractures: Current strategies in diagnosis and management: http://www.orthosupersite.com/view.asp?rID=44034
Sacral insufficiency fracture: http://rheumatology.oxfordjournals.org/cgi/content/full/40/9/1065
Sacrum and sacral fractures: http://www.wheelessonline.com/ortho/sacrum_and_sacral_fractures

BIBLIOGRAPHY

1. Denis F, Davis S, Comfort T. Sacral fractures: An important problem: retrospective analysis of 236 cases. Clin Orthop 1988;227:67–81.
2. Nork S, Jones CB, Harding SP, et al. Percutaneous stabilization of U-shaped sacral fractures using iliosacral screws: Technique and early results. J Orthop Trauma 2001;15:1236–44.
3. Schildhauer TA, Bellabarba C, Nork SE, et al. Decompression and lumbopelvic fixation for sacral fracture-dislocations with spino-pelvic dissociation. J Orthop Trauma 2006;20:447–57.
4. Schildhauer TA, Josten C, Muhr G. Triangular osteosynthesis of vertically unstable sacrum fractures: A new concept allowing early weight-bearing. J Orthop Trauma 2006;20:S44–S51.
5. Schildhauer TA, McCullough P, Chapman JR, et al. Anatomic and radiographic considerations for placement of transiliac screws in lumbopelvic fixations. J Spinal Disord Tech 2002;15(3):199–205.

SPINAL CORD INJURY

Thomas N. Bryce, MD

1. Which of the following terms are currently favored to describe impairment or loss of motor and/or sensory function due to damage of neural elements within the spinal canal: (1) tetraplegia, (2) paraplegia, (3) quadriplegia, (4) quadriparesis, and/or (5) paraparesis?

Tetraplegia refers to the impairments resulting from damage to neural elements within the cervical spinal canal, whereas *paraplegia* refers to the impairments resulting from damage to neural elements within the thoracic, lumbar, or sacral spinal canal. As *tetra*, *para*, and *plegia* are of Greek origin and *quadri* is of Latin origin, to maintain uniformity in word root origins, tetraplegia is preferred over quadriplegia. Because the American Spinal Injury Association (ASIA) Impairment Scale (AIS) (see Question 7) more precisely defines incomplete tetraplegia and paraplegia than the terms quadriparesis and paraparesis, their use is discouraged.

2. What is the difference between a skeletal level and a neurologic level of injury in assessing a person with a traumatic spinal cord injury (SCI)?

The **skeletal level of injury** is defined as the level in the spine where the greatest vertebral damage is found on radiographic examination.

The **neurologic level of injury** is defined as the most caudal segment of the spinal cord with normal sensory and motor function bilaterally.

3. How are the sensory and motor components assessed in the determination of a neurologic level of spinal cord injury?

Sensory and motor functions are assessed according to the *International Standards for Neurological Classification of Spinal Cord Injury*:

- **Sensory component:** Light touch and pinprick sensation are tested for each dermatome and graded on a three-point scale:

  0 = Absent

  1 = Impaired (partial or altered appreciation, including hyperesthesia)

  2 = Normal

The **sensory level** is the most caudal dermatome where both light touch and pinprick are normal and where all rostral dermatomes are also normal.

- **Motor component:** A key muscle is tested from each myotome in a rostral-caudal sequence by manual muscle test and graded on a six-point scale:

  0 = Total paralysis, no palpable or visible contraction

  1 = Palpable or visible contraction

  2 = Active movement, full range of motion (ROM) with gravity eliminated

  3 = Active movement, full ROM against gravity only

  4 = Active movement, full ROM against resistance

  5 = Normal

The **motor level** is the most caudal muscle having grade 3 or better strength where all muscles above are graded 5. If the level of injury is at a site for which there is no key muscle (e.g. C2–C4, T2–L1, S2–S4/5), the motor level is defined by the sensory level.

4. Identify the key muscles that are tested in determining the motor level.

C5 = Elbow flexors (biceps, brachialis)

C6 = Wrist extensors (extensor carpi radialis longus and brevis)

C7 = Elbow extensors (triceps)

C8 = Finger flexors (flexor digitorum profundus) to the middle finger

T1 = Small finger abductors (abductor digiti minimi)

L2 = Hip flexors (iliopsoas)

L3 = Knee extensors (quadriceps)

L4 = Ankle dorsiflexors (tibialis anterior)

L5 = Long toe extensors (extensor hallucis longus)

S1 = Ankle plantar flexors (gastrocnemius, soleus)

5. **Identify the key point for each sensory dermatome that is tested in determining the sensory level.**

C2 = Occipital protuberance
C3 = Supraclavicular fossa
C4 = Top of acromioclavicular joint
C5 = Lateral side of antecubital fossa
C6 = Thumb
C7 = Middle finger
C8 = Little finger
T1 = Medial (ulnar) side of antecubital fossa
T2 = Apex of the axilla
T3 = Third intercostal space (IS)
T4 = Fourth IS (nipple line)
T5 = Fifth IS (midway between T4 and T6)
T6 = Sixth IS (level of xiphisternum)
T7 = Seventh IS (midway between T6 and T8)

T8 = Eighth IS (midway between T6 and T10)
T9 = Ninth IS (midway between T8 and T10)
T10 = Tenth IS (umbilicus)
T11 = Eleventh IS (midway between T10 and T12)
T12 = Inguinal ligament at mid-point
L1 = Half the distance between T12 and L2
L2 = Mid-anterior thigh
L3 = Medial femoral condyle
L4 = Medial malleolus
L5 = Dorsum of the foot at the third metatarsal phalangeal joint
S1 = Lateral heel
S2 = Popliteal fossa in the midline
S3 = Ischial tuberosity
S4–S5 = Perianal area (taken as one level)

6. **What is the difference between a complete and an incomplete SCI?**
   - **Complete spinal cord injury** is defined by the total absence of sensory and motor function below the anatomic level of injury in the absence of spinal shock. Recovery from spinal shock typically occurs within 48 hours following an acute spine injury
   - **Incomplete spinal cord injury** is present when residual spinal cord and/or nerve root function exists below the anatomic level of injury. Incomplete neurologic injuries are broadly classified by pattern of neurologic deficit into one of several syndromes, which is helpful in determining prognosis

7. **How is the severity of a spinal cord injury classified?**
   The AIS, a component of the International Standards for Neurological Classification of Spinal Cord Injury, is a 5-point scale (A, B, C, D, E) used to specify the severity of injury. It includes definitions of complete and incomplete injuries.
   - A = Complete: No sensory or motor function is preserved in the sacral segments S4–S5
   - B = Incomplete: Sensory but not motor function is preserved below the neurologic level and includes the sacral segments S4–S5
   - C = Incomplete: Motor function is preserved below the neurologic level, and more than half of key muscles below the neurologic level have a muscle grade less than 3
   - D = Incomplete: Motor function is preserved below the neurologic level, and at least half of key muscles below the neurologic level have a muscle grade 3 or greater
   - E = Normal: Sensory and motor function are normal

8. **Identify and describe six different patterns of incomplete neurologic injury which may be present following a traumatic spinal injury.**
   - **Cruciate paralysis:** damage to the anterior spinal cord at the C2 level (level of corticospinal tract decussation) with greater loss of motor function in upper extremities compared with the lower extremities, variable sensory loss, and variable cranial nerve deficits.
   - **Central cord syndrome:** damage to the central spinal cord below the C2 level with greater loss of motor function in upper extremities (especially in the hands) compared with the lower extremities with variable sensory loss, at least partial sacral sparing, and variable bowel and bladder involvement
   - **Anterior cord syndrome:** damage to the anterior spinal cord with relative preservation of proprioception and variable loss of pain sensation, temperature sensation, and motor function.
   - **Brown-Séquard syndrome:** damage to the lateral half of the spinal cord with relative ipsilateral proprioception and motor function loss and contralateral pain and temperature sensation loss.
   - **Conus medullaris syndrome:** damage to the sacral segments of the spinal cord located in the conus medullaris, which typically results in an areflexic bowel and bladder, lower extremity sensory loss, and incomplete paraplegia.
   - **Cauda equina syndrome:** damage to lumbosacral nerve roots within the neural canal results in variable lower extremity motor and sensory function, bowel and bladder dysfunction, and saddle anesthesia.

9. **What is the rationale for administering medications, such as methylprednisolone, following an acute spinal cord injury?**
   The pathophysiology of acute spinal cord injury involves both primary and secondary injury mechanisms.
   - **Primary injury** to the spinal cord results from mechanical forces applied to the spinal column at the time of injury and is not correctable.
   - **Secondary injury** to uninvolved neurologic tissue in the vicinity of the primary injury may occur due to a variety of mechanisms and potentially can be modified via pharmacotherapy.
   Methylprednisolone has been advocated based on its antioxidant and cell membrane stabilizing properties. A loading dose of 30 mg/kg is followed by 5.4 mg/kg for 23 hours if administered within 3 hours of injury or for 48 hours if administered between 3 and 8 hours after injury. Use of methylprednisolone remains controversial due to complications,

such as infection, gastrointestinal bleeding, pulmonary and endocrine problems, and an adverse effect on healing of spinal fusions. Research regarding alternative pharmacologic agents is currently under way.

10. Identify six complications of SCI that may manifest within the first 2 days after injury.
Hypotension, bradycardia, hypothermia, hypoventilation, gastrointestinal bleeding, and ileus.

11. What causes hypotension, bradycardia, and hypothermia?
Acute cervical or upper thoracic spinal cord injuries are associated with a functional total sympathectomy with resultant loss of vasoconstrictor tone in the trunk and extremities and loss of beta-adrenergic cardiostimulation, leading to a clinical picture of hypotension with paradoxical bradycardia. The loss of sympathetic tone also leads to an inability to regulate body temperature. After it is clearly established that no visceral or extremity injury is causing occult hemorrhage and blood loss, hypotension is best treated with sympathomimetic agents.

12. What causes hypoventilation?
The innervation to the diaphragm, the major muscle responsible for inspiration, is C3 to C5 ("3, 4, 5 keeps you alive"). The innervation to the internal intercostals and the abdominal muscles, the major muscles responsible for forced expiration (e.g. cough), are local thoracic and abdominal segmental nerves. Thus, a cervical or thoracic spinal cord injury can affect inspiration, cough, or both, depending on the level of injury. Patients with a C1–C2 complete SCI have no volitional diaphragmatic function and require mechanical ventilation or placement of a diaphragm/phrenic pacer. Patients with a C3–C4 complete SCI have severe diaphragmatic weakness and commonly require mechanical ventilation, at least temporarily. Patients with C5 to T1 complete SCI are usually able to maintain independent breathing but remain at high risk for pulmonary complications due to loss of innervation to the intercostal and abdominal muscles.
  Pneumonia is the most common cause of early death for persons with tetraplegia and is often related to aspiration of stomach or oropharyngeal contents, commonly occurring at or shortly after the initial injury. Atelectasis may result from hypoexpansion of the chest due to either pain or muscle weakness or to inadequate cough predisposing to inadequate clearing of secretions. Respiratory failure may develop immediately after SCI or over several days. Close monitoring of respiratory function is warranted in persons with cervical SCI during the first week after injury. See Table 59-1.

Table 59-1. Respiratory Function and Spinal Injury

INJURY LEVEL	RESPIRATORY SYSTEM CHANGES	MECHANICAL VENTILATION
Occiput–C2	(−) Diaphragm, (−) intercostals	Always needed
C3–C4	(+/−) Diaphragm, (−) intercostals	Often needed acutely
C5–T1	(+) Diaphragm, (−) intercostals	Only needed if there are associated pulmonary complications
T2–T12	(+) Diaphragm, (+/−) intercostals	Usually not needed

13. What causes gastrointestinal bleeding?
Risk is increased with any physical or psychologic trauma and is exacerbated by the standard high-dose steroid protocols used after SCI.

14. What causes ileus?
Adynamic (paralytic) ileus occurs after acute SCI in 8% of cases. After its resolution, usually within 2 to 3 days, a bowel routine of stool softeners, stimulant laxatives, and bowel evacuants is initiated to facilitate regularly timed evacuations of the bowel.

15. When should anticoagulant prophylaxis against venous thromboembolus (VTE) be started after SCI?
VTE is found in one half to three quarters of persons with traumatic SCI who are not receiving anticoagulant prophylaxis. The highest risk is within the first week after SCI. Therefore, anticoagulant prophylaxis should be started as soon as hemostasis has been achieved, unless there is a contraindication. Randomized controlled studies have shown a low risk of major bleeding when either low-molecular-weight heparin (LMWH) or unfractionated heparin prophylaxis is started within 72 hours of injury. LMWH has been shown to be more effective than unfractionated heparin in preventing pulmonary embolus. Mechanical compression devices have been shown to decrease the risk of VTE when used in conjunction with anticoagulant prophylaxis.

16. When should an inferior vena cava (IVC) filter be placed?
An IVC filter should only be placed in those in whom active bleeding is anticipated to last more than 72 hours or in those in whom adequate anticoagulant prophylaxis cannot be started. If an IVC filter is used, a temporary one should be chosen, and it should be removed within 8 to 12 weeks if no VTE develops. Historically, one third of those who receive permanent IVC filters ultimately develop VTE.

17. How can incontinence of stool be prevented after SCI?

A neurogenic bowel after SCI affects mainly the colon and rectum distal to the splenic flexure and can be classified as an upper motor neuron (UMN) type if sacral reflexes are present (e.g. bulbocavernosus or anocutaneous) or lower motor neuron (LMN) type if these reflexes are absent. Institution of a bowel routine or daily timed evacuation of the colon can prevent incontinence by allowing predictable evacuations in nearly everyone with SCI.

During a UMN-type bowel routine, digital stimulation of the rectum triggers reflex evacuation of stool. This can be further facilitated by inserting an irritant suppository or mini-enema into the rectum and performing this routinely after a meal to take advantage of the gastrocolic reflex.

During a LMN-type bowel routine, digital evacuation of the rectum empties the rectum of stool. Stool-bulking agents or fiber are useful in maintaining an optimal consistency of stool, because water absorption is usually impaired within an areflexic colon. Oral irritant or osmotic laxatives given 8 to 12 hours before the routine may be necessary to help propel the stool through the colon to the distal portion where it can be evacuated.

18. How should a neurogenic bladder be initially managed after an SCI?

An indwelling transurethral catheter (or suprapubic tube if indicated) should be placed as soon as feasible and should remain in place until the patient's fluid status has stabilized.

19. Identify five interventions that can help prevent the development of pressure ulcers after acute SCI.

1. The length of time spent on a spine board should be minimized, and pressure relief should be provided every 30 minutes if the time on the board exceeds 2 hours.
2. Patients in spinal traction should be immobilized on rotating kinetic beds.
3. Patients must be turned from side to side (30°–45° from supine) every 2 hours around the clock while in bed to prevent prolonged pressure over bony prominences.
4. Bowel and bladder incontinence should be managed with timed bowel evacuations and catheter drainage of the bladder.
5. Shear pressure on the skin can be avoided by lifting rather than dragging immobile patients.

20. Identify six reasons for transferring a person with tetraplegia to a specialized SCI center.

- Overall survival rates increase
- Complication rates (e.g. incidence of new pressure ulcers) decrease
- Length of hospital stay decreases
- Functional gains during rehabilitation are greater
- Home discharge is more likely
- Rehospitalization rates are lower

21. What is the prognosis for neurologic recovery of a patient with a complete tetraplegia?

Only **2% to 3%** of persons who have an initial **Asia Impairment Scale (AIS) score of A** convert to AIS D by 1 year. However, 30% to 80% of persons with motor complete tetraplegia recover a single motor level (gaining functional motor strength at that level) within 1 year of injury.

A muscle with grade 1 or 2 strength at 1 month has a 90% chance of reaching grade 3 by 1 year, whereas a muscle with grade 0 strength has only a 25% chance to reach grade 3 or better by 1 year. The chance of functional recovery of a muscle two levels below the motor level of injury, when the first muscle below the motor level is grade 0, is exceedingly rare.

22. What is the prognosis for neurologic recovery of someone who has an incomplete tetraplegia?

Among **sensory incomplete patients,** the type of sensation preserved below the level of injury is prognostically important. Persons with preservation of perianal pinprick sensation have a greater than 70% chance of regaining ambulatory ability, whereas persons who have spared light touch sensation only in the same region are unlikely to regain ambulatory ability.

Among persons with **motor incomplete SCI,** age and initial motor strength seem to be major determinants of ambulation. In one study of 105 persons with incomplete motor tetraplegia, in which age 50 was arbitrarily chosen as a cutoff, 91% of all persons younger than 50 years, either AIS C or D, ambulated at 1 year; all persons older than 50 years and AIS D ambulated; while only 40% of persons older than 50 years and AIS C ambulated.

23. What is the prognosis for neurologic recovery for someone who has paraplegia?

Among persons with **complete paraplegia,** 75% retain the same neurologic level of injury (NLI) at 1 year that they had at 1-month postinjury, 20% gain a single level, and 5% gain two neurologic levels. Persons with T1 to T8 complete paraplegia do not recover lower limb voluntary movement. Fifteen percent of persons with T9 to T11 complete paraplegia recover some lower limb function, while 55% of persons with T12 or below complete paraplegia recover some lower limb function.

Persons with **incomplete paraplegia** have the best prognosis for ambulation among all the groups of persons with traumatic SCI. Eighty percent of individuals with incomplete paraplegia regain functional hip flexion and knee extension within 1 year of injury, making both indoor and community-based ambulation possible.

24. What typical lower extremity motor function is required for community ambulation?
Typically, community ambulation requires bilateral grade 3 hip flexor strength and at least one knee with grade 3 knee extensor strength.

25. Compare the expected patterns of muscular weakness and the expected functional outcomes for eating, bed/wheelchair transfers, and wheelchair propulsion for persons with C1 to C3, C4, and C5 neurologic levels.
See Table 59-2.

Table 59-2. Functional Outcomes for C1 to C5 Spinal Cord Injuries

	C1–C3	C4	C5
Patterns of Muscular Weakness	Total paralysis of trunk, upper extremities, lower extremities, dependent on ventilator	Paralysis of trunk, upper extremities, lower extremities; inability to cough, endurance and respiratory reserve low secondary to paralysis of intercostals	Absence of elbow extension, pronation, all wrist and hand movement, total paralysis of trunk and lower extremities
Eating	Total assist	Total assist	Total assist for setup, then independent eating with equipment
Bed/Wheelchair Transfers	Total assist	Total assist	Total assist
Wheelchair Propulsion	Manual: total assist Power: independent with equipment	Manual: total assist Power: independent with equipment (sip and puff control or head array)	Manual: independent to some assist indoors on noncarpet, level surface; some to total assist outdoors Power: independent

26. Compare the expected patterns of muscular weakness and the expected functional outcomes for wheelchair propulsion and ambulation for persons with C6, C7–C8, T1 to T9, and T10 to L1 neurologic levels.
See Table 59-3.

Table 59-3. Functional Outcomes for C6 to L1 Spinal Cord Injuries

	C6	C7–C8	T1–T9	T10–L1
Patterns of Muscular Weakness	Absence of wrist flexion, elbow extension, hand movement; total paralysis of trunk and lower extremities	Paralysis of trunk and lower extremities; limited grasp release and dexterity secondary to partial intrinsic muscles of hand	Lower trunk paralysis; total paralysis of lower extremities	Paralysis of lower extremities
Wheelchair Propulsion	Manual: independent indoors; some to total assist outdoors Power: independent with standard arm drive on all surfaces	Manual: independent all indoor surfaces and level outdoor terrain; some assist with uneven terrain	Independent	Independent
Ambulation	Standing: total assist Ambulation: not indicated	Standing: independent to some assist in standing frame Ambulation: not indicated	Standing: independent in standing frame Ambulation: typically not functional	Standing: independent with equipment Ambulation: functional, some assist to independent with knee, ankle, foot orthosis and forearm crutches or walker

27. What is spasticity and what peripheral factors can cause an exacerbation of spasticity?

Spasticity is a motor disorder characterized by a velocity-dependent increase in tonic stretch reflexes (muscle tone) with exaggerated tendon jerks, resulting from hyperexcitability of the stretch reflex as one component of the upper motor neuron syndrome. Peripheral factors that may exacerbate spasticity include heterotopic ossification, urolithiasis, urinary tract infections, stool impaction, pressure ulcers, fracture/dislocations, and ingrown toenails.

28. Name six pathologic changes associated with late neurologic deterioration after SCI.
1. Posttraumatic cysts
2. Delayed spinal deformity
3. Residual cord compression
4. Tethering
5. Fibrosis
6. Subarachnoid cysts

29. A tetraplegic patient develops an L2–L3 destructive spinal lesion 10 years after a C5–C6 fracture-dislocation. Workup reveals no evidence of a spinal tumor or infection. What is the most likely cause of this lesion?

Neuropathic spinal arthropathy (Charcot spine). Destructive spinal lesions can develop in spinal cord–injured patients due to repetitive loads placed on the denervated spine in the course of daily activities. The most common clinical presentation is a spinal deformity. Patients may present with audible clicking or crepitus due to spinal instability, loss of sitting balance, cauda equina syndrome, nerve root compression, or obstructive uropathy. Surgical treatment is challenging and associated with a high complication rate.

30. What are the three most common causes of death after SCI?
1. Diseases of the respiratory system
2. Other heart disease
3. Infective and parasitic diseases

Key Points

1. Perform baseline and serial neurologic assessments using the International Standards for Neurological Classification of Spinal Cord Injury to detect neurologic changes, as well as to define the severity of injury.
2. Patients with spinal cord injury should be initially managed in an intensive care unit setting due to the high risk of respiratory complications and hypotension.
3. Early surgical stabilization allows earlier mobilization, enables more intensive rehabilitation, and results in a shorter hospital stay.
4. Persons with preserved perianal pinprick sensation, with or without motor function, have a good prognosis for functional motor recovery and ambulation.

Websites

Clinical practice guidelines, developed by the Consortium for Spinal Cord Medicine, are available for download at www.pva.org
   Bladder Management for Adults with Spinal Cord Injury
   Preservation of Upper Limb Function Following Spinal Cord Injury
   Respiratory Management Following Spinal Cord Injury
   Depression Following Spinal Cord Injury
   Neurogenic Bowel Management in Adults with Spinal Cord Injury
   Outcomes Following Traumatic Spinal Cord Injury
   Acute Management of Autonomic Dysreflexia
   Pressure Ulcer Prevention and Treatment Following Spinal Cord Injury
   Prevention of Thromboembolism in Spinal Cord Injury

BIBLIOGRAPHY

1. Bryce TN, Ragnarsson KT, Stein AS. Spinal cord injury. In: Braddom RL, editor. Physical Medicine and Rehabilitation. 3rd ed. Philadelphia: Saunders; 2007. p. 1285–1349.
2. Capagnolo DI, Heary RF. Acute medical and surgical management of spinal cord injury. In Kirshblum S, Capagnolo DI, DeLisa JA, editors. Spinal Cord Medicine. Philadelphia: Lippincott, Williams and Wilkins; 2002. p. 96–107.
3. Consortium for Spinal Cord Medicine. Early acute management in adults with spinal cord injury: A clinical practice guideline for health-care professionals. J Spinal Cord Med 2008:31(4):403–79.
4. Consortium for Spinal Cord Medicine. Neurogenic bowel management in adults with spinal cord injury. J Spinal Cord Med 1998;21(3):248–93.
5. Consortium for Spinal Cord Medicine. Outcomes following traumatic spinal cord injury: Clinical pratice guidelines for health-care professionals. J Spinal Cord Med 2000;23(4):289–316.
6. Marino RJ, Barros T, Biering-Sorensen, et al. International standards for neurological classification of spinal cord injury. J Spinal Cord Med 2003;26(Suppl 1):S50–6.
7. National Spinal Cord Injury Statistical Center, University of Alabama at Birmingham, 2006 annual statistical report, July 2006, University of Alabama, Birmingham. https://www.nscisc.uab.edu/public_content/pdf/NSCIC%20Annual%2006.pdf .
8. Piepmeier J. Late sequelae of spinal cord injury. In: Narayan R, Wilberger J, Povlishock J, editors. Neurotrauma. New York: McGraw-Hill; 1996. p. 1237–44.
9. Reference manual for the International Standards for Neurological Classification of Spinal Cord Injury. Chicago: American Spinal Injury Association; 2003. p. 21–45.
10. Yarkony G, Formal C, Cawley M. Spinal cord injury rehabilitation: Assessment and management during acute care. Arch Phys Med Rehabil 1997;78:S48–S52.

CERVICAL SPINE INJURIES IN ATHLETES

CHAPTER 60

Robert G. Watkins, IV, MD, and Robert G. Watkins, III, MD

1. What sports are associated with the highest risk for head and neck injuries?

The organized sports with the highest risk for head and neck injuries are football, gymnastics, wrestling, and ice hockey. Football is the sport associated with the highest risk of such injuries. Head and neck injuries also occur in a variety of nonorganized sports activities including diving, skiing, surfing, and trampoline use.

2. What types of cervical injuries must be considered in an athlete injured in a sporting event?

Sports-related cervical injuries can involve the muscles, ligaments, intervertebral discs, osseous structures, and the neural structures they protect. Injuries to consider include muscular strains, intervertebral disc injuries, major/minor cervical spine fractures, stinger/burner injuries, and transient quadriplegia. In addition, preexisting cervical conditions predispose an athlete to neurologic injury and may be discovered during subsequent evaluation. These include congenital cervical stenosis, Klippel-Feil syndrome, and os odontoideum.

3. If a player suffers a traumatic neck injury on the athletic field, should the headgear be removed?

It is important to engage in spinal precautions and leave the headgear in place until the cervical spine can be completely evaluated. The team personnel should have a means available for removal of the facemask so that the airway is readily accessible. Immediate removal of the helmet should not be performed until the proper medical personnel are prepared for an emergency situation. If circumstances require helmet removal, the shoulder pads should be removed at the same time because removal of only one piece of equipment can lead to a significant change in spinal alignment. When lifting a player with a suspected cervical injury, the physician should stabilize the head and neck to the torso by placing his or her hands under the scapulas and stabilizing the head between his or her forearms. Details of the methods and techniques for on-the-field management and transportation of the spine injured athlete are available at http://www.spine.org/Documents/NATA_Prehospital_Care.pdf

4. What is the most common sports-related injury of the cervical spine?

The most common sports-related injury of the cervical spine is a muscle strain. Direct trauma to the head or neck leads to eccentric contraction and muscle stretch injury. Sprains of the facet joint capsular ligaments may also occur. Patients report neck pain, muscle spasm, and limited cervical motion. Initial radiographs are obtained to rule out significant injury. The neck is immobilized, and symptoms are treated with nonsteroidal antiinflammatory drugs (NSAIDs), analgesics, and immobilization. In patients with persistent symptoms, magnetic resonance imaging (MRI) is performed to rule out a traumatic disc herniation or major ligamentous injury.

5. What is a "hidden flexion injury" of the cervical spine?

This term refers to a purely ligamentous injury associated with three-column disruption of the spine, including injury to the posterior longitudinal ligament, facet capsule, ligamentum flavum, and interspinous ligament in the absence of osseous injury. Such injuries can be missed on plain radiographs. Persistent posterior cervical tenderness following an acute injury should raise concern about this injury pattern. The lateral cervical radiograph should be carefully evaluated for subtle increase in the distance between adjacent spinous processes. Cervical MRI is useful to evaluate for posterior cervical ligamentous disruption. Physician-supervised flexion-extension lateral radiographs are considered only for alert, cooperative, and neurologically intact patients and are not advised or considered useful in the immediate postinjury period. Commonly used criteria for defining instability between motion segments in the subaxial cervical region are 11° greater angulation than an adjacent segment or 3.5-mm translation relative to an adjacent vertebra (Fig. 60-1).

6. What is the clinical presentation of a traumatic cervical disc herniation?

The clinical presentation of a traumatic cervical disc herniation is variable. Patients may present with isolated neck pain, radiculopathy, or an anterior cord syndrome with paralysis of the upper and lower extremities. In contrast to adults, immature athletes most commonly develop disc herniations at C3–C4 and C4–C5. Disc injury is associated with axial loading and hyperflexion during activities such as wrestling, diving, and football.

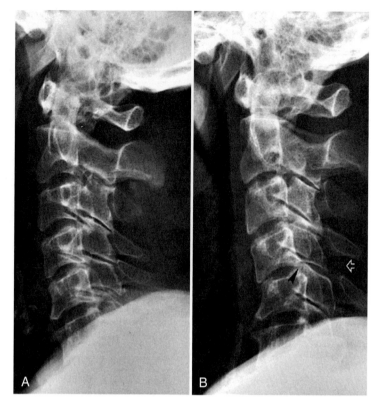

Figure 60-1. Hyperflexion ligament injury not apparent on neutral lateral cervical radiograph. **A,** Neutral position lateral radiograph of a trauma patient with cervical spine tenderness is unremarkable. **B,** Repeat view shows C4–C5 injury *(arrowhead)* with mild flaring of the spinous processes *(open arrow)* and facet joint widening. (From Mirvis SE. Spinal imaging. In: Browner BD, Jupiter JB, Levine AM, et al. Skeletal Trauma. 4th ed. Philadelphia: Saunders; 2008.)

7. What biomechanical force is the primary cause of fracture dislocations involving the cervical spine during football?

The National Football Head and Neck Injury Registry demonstrated that most cervical fracture dislocations occurred with axial loading of the cervical spine during headfirst contact. However, the full spectrum of major and minor spinal injuries has been reported in association with football injuries.

8. What is spear tackler's spine?

Spearing refers to contact at the crown of the head while the neck is maintained in a flexed posture. In this posture, the normal cervical lordosis is no longer present, and the cervical spine is predisposed to injury. Injuries due to this mechanism have been described in football, diving, and hockey. Spear tackler's spine was defined by analysis of football players with spearing injuries and is considered to be a contraindication to participation in contact sports. Criteria for diagnosis include:
- Developmental narrowing of the cervical spinal canal
- Persistent straightening or reversal of cervical lordosis on erect lateral cervical radiographs
- Posttraumatic radiographic changes on cervical radiographs
- History of use of spear tackling techniques during athletics

9. What is the most common neurologic injury in an athlete following impact to the head, neck, or shoulder?

Stingers or burners are the most common athletic cervical neurologic injuries in this setting. Symptoms result from injury to the brachial plexus or cervical nerve roots. Stingers have been reported to occur in up to 50% of athletes involved in contact or collision sports.

10. What is a stinger or burner?

A stinger or burner (burner syndrome) is a peripheral nerve injury associated with burning arm pain and paresthesias. A stinger presents with unilateral dysesthetic pain that often follows a dermatomal distribution. It may be accompanied by weakness, most often in the muscle groups supplied by the C5 and C6 nerve roots (deltoid, biceps, supraspinatus, infraspinatus) on the affected side. Although pain frequently resolves spontaneously in 10 to 15 minutes, it is not uncommon to have trace abnormal neurologic findings for several months. Normal, painless motion of the cervical spine is generally present and is crucial in distinguishing a stinger from other types of cervical pathology, such as disc herniation, foraminal stenosis, or fracture. Bilateral symptoms suggest a different etiology, such as a neurapraxic injury of the spinal cord.

11. What injury mechanisms are responsible for a stinger or burner?

Three different mechanisms have been described:
1. Hyperextension, compression, and rotation toward the involved arm, thereby closing the neural foramen and causing a nerve root contusion. This mechanism is essentially a replication of Spurling's maneuver
2. Lateral neck flexion associated with a shoulder depression injury, resulting in brachial plexus stretch
3. Direct blow to the brachial plexus with resultant injury

12. Describe a rational treatment protocol for an athlete with a stinger.

Most stingers resolve within minutes. For an athlete's first episode, with only brief transitory symptoms, treatment is conservative and no special testing is required. The athlete is permitted to return to unrestricted activity after complete resolution of symptoms if a normal neurologic examination, negative head compression test, and pain-free and unrestricted cervical range of motion are present. The athlete should not be allowed to return to sports until symptoms completely subside. Further workup is directed at patients with persistent symptoms or recurrent episodes to assess for other cervical problems, such as fracture, stenosis, disc herniation, or instability. Workup includes cervical radiographs with physician-supervised flexion-extension views, single-photon emission computed tomography (SPECT) bone scan, MRI, and electromyography (EMG).

13. What is the role of EMG in assessing the athlete who experiences a stinger?

If the symptoms have not resolved by 3 weeks, it is reasonable to obtain an EMG. This test can help define the specific nerve root involved and determine the degree of injury. Results of this test may lag behind an athlete's recovery, however. Players who demonstrate clinical weakness and moderate fibrillation potentials on EMG are withdrawn from play. When sequential EMG studies reveal spontaneous, mild, or scattered positive waves with end-motor recruitment (findings consistent with reinnervation), the athlete may return to sports provided painless and unrestricted cervical range of motion and full muscle strength are present.

14. What types of cervical stenosis affect athletes?

The same types of cervical stenosis affect athletes and the general population:
1. Developmental or congenital stenosis (typified by short pedicles and decreased sagittal diameter of the spinal canal)
2. Acquired stenosis (associated with osteophytes and degeneration at the level of the disc space)

15. What is cervical cord neurapraxia?

Cervical cord neurapraxia with transient quadriparesis and quadriparesthesia is characterized clinically by an acute transient episode of bilateral sensory and motor abnormalities. Sensory changes may include numbness, burning, tingling, or anesthesia. Motor changes may include paresis or paralysis of the arms, legs, or both. Neck pain is generally not present. An episode of cervical cord neurapraxia generally resolves in less than 10 to 15 minutes. The most commonly described mechanism of injury is axial compression with a component of either hyperflexion or hyperextension. This syndrome has been reported in association with cervical spinal stenosis, kyphosis, congenital fusions (Klippel-Feil syndrome), cervical instability (traumatic or developmental), and intervertebral disc herniation.

16. Is transient cervical cord neurapraxia associated with permanent neurologic injury?

A single event of uncomplicated transient cervical cord neurapraxia is not associated with permanent neurologic injury. However, two or more events increase the risk of permanent neurologic injury.

17. What is the risk of reoccurrence of transient cervical cord neurapraxia after the athlete returns to contact sports?

Studies have shown that 56% of athletes returning to contact sports experienced a recurrent episode of transient cervical cord neurapraxia. This number was higher when an athlete returned to football as compared with other sports.

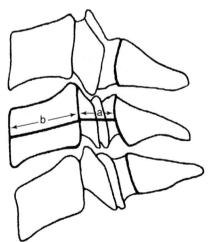

18. Define the Torg ratio.

The Torg ratio is determined on a lateral cervical radiograph as the sagittal diameter of the spinal canal (a) divided by the anteroposterior vertebral body diameter (b) (Fig. 60-2). The sagittal diameter of the spinal canal is determined by measuring the distance between the middle of the posterior surface of the vertebral body and the nearest point on the spinolaminar line. This ratio method avoids the potential for error secondary to radiographic magnification when absolute numbers are used to determine the sagittal diameter of the cervical canal.

Figure 60-2. The ratio of the spinal canal to the vertebral body is the distance from the midpoint of the posterior aspect of the vertebral body to the nearest point on the corresponding spinolaminar line (distance a) divided by the anteroposterior width of the vertebral body (distance b). (From Torg JS, Pavlov H, Genuario SE, et al. Neurapraxia of the cervical spine cord with transient quadriplegia. J Bone Joint Surg 1986;68A:1354–70.)

19. What is the significance of the Torg ratio?

A ratio less than 0.8 suggests the presence of cervical spinal stenosis. The Torg ratio is a highly sensitive method of determining cervical stenosis (93% sensitivity) but has an extremely low positive predictive value for determining future injury (0.2%). It is not a useful screening method for determining athletic participation in contact sports and should not be used as the sole criterion for the diagnosis of cervical stenosis in an athlete. Although an athlete may have the same size spinal canal as a nonathlete, the athlete's vertebral body may be larger, thus falsely lowering the Torg ratio and implying stenosis. In addition, the Torg ratio has not been correlated with the development of permanent quadriparesis in athletes. The Torg ratio should not be used as the sole criterion in making a return-to-play decision after an episode of transient quadriplegia.

20. What is the most reliable way to identify cervical spinal stenosis?

MRI or computed tomography (CT)-myelography is the most reliable way to identify cervical spinal stenosis. Cross-sectional imaging with these modalities permits the relationship between the osseous spinal canal and spinal cord diameter to be determined. The most important parameter is the presence of an adequate protective cushion (functional reserve) of cerebrospinal fluid (CSF) around the spinal cord.

21. Describe a rational treatment protocol after an episode of transient quadriparesis.

Immediately following an episode of transient quadriparesis, the athlete should be prohibited from continuing to participate in the sport for that particular event, even if a full recovery occurs soon after the episode. A thorough history of all events leading up to and following the episode should be carefully documented. A complete onsite physical examination should be performed. Even if symptoms are momentary or resolve, a radiographic examination should be performed on a timely basis. The athlete should be considered to have a fracture until proven otherwise, especially if the patient complains of persistent or significant neck stiffness or pain. If a neurologic deficit is present at the time of evaluation, then a cervical orthosis should be applied and the patient should be transported for medical treatment and appropriate imaging studies.

22. What factors should be considered in making a return-to-play decision for an athlete after the first episode of transient quadriplegia?

Return to play guidelines following a single episode of transient quadriplegia have been proposed by Cantu and permit return to contact sports if there is complete resolution of symptoms, unrestricted cervical range of motion, normal cervical alignment, lack of spinal instability, and absence of stenosis on cervical MRI or CT-myelography. Contraindications to return to sports include instability, deformity, and loss of CSF functional reserve.

23. When should an athlete be allowed to return to play following cervical injury?

There are no universally accepted guidelines for determining when an athlete may return to play after a cervical injury. Basic principles guiding decision making include:
- The athlete should be symptom free with respect to neck pain
- Unrestricted and pain-free cervical motion should be present
- Neurologic evaluation should be normal
- Full muscle strength should be present
- There should be no evidence of radiographic instability, abnormal spinal alignment, or other spinal abnormalities on advanced imaging studies

General guidelines for return to play following cervical injury have been defined and are modified appropriately according to individual clinical factors. It is helpful to divide athletes into three general groups:
1. No contraindication to return to play
2. Relative contraindication to return to play
3. Absolute contraindication to return to play

24. Summarize guidelines for return to contact sports *without contraindication* for commonly encountered cervical spinal conditions.

The following conditions are considered to permit return to contact sports without restriction after comprehensive patient assessment:

POSTTRAUMATIC
- Healed, stable C1 or C2 fracture (treated nonoperatively) with normal cervical range of motion
- Healed stable subaxial spine fracture without sagittal plane kyphotic deformity
- Asymptomatic clay shoveler's fracture (C7 spinous process fracture)

CONGENITAL
- Single-level Klippel-Feil deformity (excluding the occipital–C1 articulation) without evidence of instability or stenosis noted on MRI
- Spinal bifida occulta

DEGENERATIVE
- History of cervical degenerative disc disease that has been treated successfully in the clinical setting of occasional cervical neck stiffness with no change in baseline strength profile

POSTSURGICAL
- After anterior single-level cervical fusion (below C3–C4), with or without instrumentation, that has healed
- After single- or multiple-level posterior cervical microlaminoforaminotomy

OTHER
- Prior history of two stingers within the same or multiple seasons. The stingers should last less than 24 hours, and the athlete should have full range of cervical motion without any evidence of neurologic deficit

25. **Explain what is meant by a *relative contraindication* to return to contact sports.**
A relative contraindication to return to contact sports is defined as a condition associated with a possibility for recurrent injury, despite the absence of any absolute contraindication. The athlete, family, and coach must be counseled that recurrent injury is a possibility and that the degree of risk is uncertain.

26. **List commonly encountered cervical conditions that are relative contraindications to return to play.**
- Previous history of transient quadriplegia or quadriparesthesia. The athlete must have full return to baseline strength and cervical range of motion with no increase in baseline cervical neck discomfort and imaging evidence of mild-to-moderate spinal stenosis
- Three or more stingers in the same season
- A prolonged stinger lasting more than 24 hours
- A healed single-level posterior fusion with lateral mass segmental fixation
- A healed single-level anterior fusion at C2–C3 or C3–C4 (sports that require head contact increase the risk of future injury)
- A healed, stable, two-level anterior or posterior cervical fusion with or without instrumentation (below C3–4) (sports that require head contact increase the risk of future injury)
- A healed cervical laminoplasty (sports that require head contact increase the risk of future injury)
- Cervical radiculopathy secondary to foraminal stenosis

27. **List *absolute contraindications* to return to contact sports.**
PREVIOUS TRANSIENT QUADRIPARESIS
- More than two previous episodes of transient quadriplegia or quadriparesthesia
- Clinical history or physical findings of cervical myelopathy
- Continued cervical neck discomfort or any evidence of a neurologic deficit or decreased range of motion from baseline after a cervical spine injury

POSTSURGICAL
- History of C1–C2 cervical fusion
- Three-level spine fusion
- Status post cervical laminectomy

SOFT TISSUE INJURY OR DEFICIENCIES
- Asymptomatic ligamentous laxity (i.e. greater than 11° of kyphotic deformity compared with the cephalad or caudal vertebral level)
- Radiographic evidence of C1–C2 hypermobility with an anterior dens interval of 4 mm or greater
- Radiographic evidence of a distraction-extension cervical spine injury
- Symptomatic cervical disc herniation

OTHER RADIOGRAPHIC FINDINGS
1. Plain radiography
- Evidence of a spear-tackler's spine on radiographic analysis
- A multiple-level Klippel-Feil deformity
- Clinical or radiographic evidence of rheumatoid arthritis
- Radiographic evidence of ankylosing spondylitis or diffuse idiopathic skeletal hyperostosis
- A healed subaxial spine fracture with evidence of a kyphotic sagittal plane or coronal plane abnormality
2. Magnetic resonance imaging
- Presence of cervical spinal cord abnormality noted on MRI
- MRI evidence of basilar invagination
- MRI evidence of Arnold-Chiari malformation
- MRI evidence of significant residual cord encroachment after a healed stable subaxial spine fracture
3. Computed tomography
- C1–C2 rotatory fixation
- Occipital–C1 assimilation

Key Points

1. During on-field evaluation of the injured athlete, a significant cervical spinal injury should be suspected until proved otherwise.
2. In the absence of special circumstances, such as respiratory distress combined with inability to access the patient's airway, the helmet should not be removed during the prehospital care of the injured athlete with potential head or neck injury. However, the facemask should be removed at the injury scene to permit airway access.
3. A stinger or burner represents a neuropraxia of cervical nerve roots or brachial plexus and typically presents with unilateral symptoms.
4. Cervical cord neuropraxia is characterized by an acute transient episode of bilateral sensory and/or motor abnormalities involving the arms, legs, or both.

Websites

Brachial plexus injury: http://emedicine.medscape.com/article/91988-overview
Cervical spine injuries in sports:
 http://emedicine.medscape.com/article/1264627-overview
Prehospital care of the spine-injured athlete: http://www.spine.org/Documents/NATA_Prehospital_Care.pdf

BIBLIOGRAPHY

1. Cantu RV, Cantu RC. Current thinking: return to play and transient quadriplegia. Curr Sports Med Rep 2005;4:27–32.
2. Clancy WG Jr, Brand RL, Bergfield JA. Upper trunk brachial plexus injuries in contact sports. Am J Sports Med 1977;5:209–15.
3. Levitz CL, Reilly PJ, Torg JS. The pathomechanics of chronic, recurrent cervical nerve root neurapraxia: The chronic burner syndrome. Am J Sports Med 1997;25:73–6.
4. Torg JS, Corcoran TA, Thibault LE, et al. Cervical cord neurapraxia: classification, pathomechanics, morbidity, and management guidelines. J Neurosurg 1997;87:843–50.
5. Torg JS, Pavlov H, Genuario SE, et al. Neurapraxia of the cervical spinal cord with transient quadriplegia. J Bone Joint Surg Am 1986;68A:1354–70.
6. Torg JS, Sennett B, Pavlov H, et al. Spear tackler's spine: An entity precluding participation in tackle football and collision activities that expose the cervical spine to axial energy inputs. Am J Sports Med 1993;21:640–9.
7. Vaccaro AR, Klein GR, Cicotti M, et al. Return to play criteria for the athlete with cervical spine injuries resulting in stinger and transient quadriplegia/paresis. Spine J 2002;2:351–6.
8. Vaccaro AR, Watkins RG, Albert TJ, et al. Cervical spine injuries in athletes: Return to play criteria. Orthopedics 2001;24:699–705.
9. Watkins RG. Spine in sports—criteria for return to athletic play after a cervical spine injury. Spine Line 2001;2(4):14–16.
10. Weinstein SM. Assessment and rehabilitation of an athlete with a stinger: A model for the management of noncatastrophic athletic cervical spine injury. Clin Sports Med 1998;17:127–35.

LUMBAR SPINE INJURIES IN ATHLETES

Robert G. Watkins, IV, MD, and Robert G. Watkins, III, MD

CHAPTER 61

1. **What is the differential diagnosis for an athlete who presents with symptoms of low back pain with or without radiculopathy?**
   - Muscle strain/ligament sprain
   - Lumbar disc injury (annular tear, discogenic pain syndrome, disc herniation)
   - Ring apophyseal injury (adolescents)
   - Overuse syndrome
   - Stress fracture (e.g. spondylolysis, sacral stress fracture)
   - Spondylolysis/spondylolisthesis
   - Minor lumbar fracture (e.g. transverse process fracture)
   - Major lumbar fracture
   - Degenerative disc disease
   - Lumbar spinal stenosis
   - Serious underlying spinal condition (discitis/osteomyelitis, neoplasm)
   - Nonspinal conditions that mimic spinal pathology (e.g. renal disease, sacroiliac pathology, intrapelvic pathology, gynecologic disorders, aortic aneurysm)

2. **Are the causes of back pain different in adolescent athletes and adult athletes?**
   In adolescent athletes, the most common causes of back pain are lumbar strain, spondylolysis/spondylolisthesis, lumbar disc injuries, and overuse syndrome. In adult athletes, the most common causes of back pain are lumbar strain, degenerative disc problems, disc herniations, and spinal stenosis.

3. **Are certain lumbar spinal injuries associated with specific sports activities?**
   Certain lumbar disorders have been associated with specific sports activities, and this information may be helpful in evaluation of the injured athlete. Some common associations include:
   - Spondylolysis—football, gymnastics, diving, wrestling, weightlifting
   - Lumbar disc herniation—weightlifting
   - Vertebral ring apophyseal injury—wrestling, ice hockey
   - Sacral stress fracture—running
   - Lumbar disc degeneration—gymnastics

4. **Describe the workup for an athlete with symptoms of low back pain with or without radiculopathy.**
   An accurate history and physical examination are essential.
   Key points to glean from the history are:
   - The time of day when the pain is worse. Is the patient awakened at night by pain?
   - A comparison of pain levels during activities (walking, sitting, standing)
   - The type of injury and duration of low back symptoms
   - The effect of a Valsalva maneuver, coughing, and sneezing on pain
   - The percentage of back versus leg pain (axial vs. radicular pain)
   - The presence of any bowel or bladder dysfunction
   Key points to assess during the physical examination are:
   - The presence of sciatic nerve tension signs
   - The presence of any neurologic deficit
   - Back and lower extremity stiffness or loss of range of motion
   - The exact location of tenderness and radiation of pain or paresthesias
   - Maneuvers that reproduce the pain, especially flexion versus extension with or without rotation
   Diagnostic workup must first rule out the possibility of tumor, infection, and impending neurologic crisis.
   - If the main complaint is **leg pain**, plain x-rays and magnetic resonance imaging (MRI) of the lumbar spine are performed to diagnose nerve root compression from disc or bony structures. Electromyography (EMG) and nerve conduction velocity (NCV) studies can help differentiate a peripheral nerve lesion from a radiculopathy. A computed tomography (CT) myelogram can be added if the etiology of pain remains unclear

- If **back pain** is the predominant symptom, workup is initiated with plain x-rays. In the adolescent and young adult athlete, single-photon emission computed tomography (SPECT) bone scan is a vital part of the diagnostic armamentarium. If the SPECT scan is positive and thus suspicious for a pars fracture, a CT scan with thin cuts is ordered to evaluate the abnormal area. If the SPECT scan is negative, MRI is indicated. In senior athletes, low back pain is rarely due to acute spondylolysis and more commonly due to muscle strain/ligament sprain, lumbar degenerative disorders, or idiopathic causes. If radiographs do not show a significant osseous injury, treatment is initiated for acute low back pain according to adult protocols and further imaging studies are deferred pending the outcome of standard treatment algorithms

5. **Describe the clinical presentation, workup, and treatment of a sacral stress fracture.**
A sacral stress fracture typically presents with the gradual onset of unilateral buttock or low back pain without a specific episode of inciting trauma. This injury develops in running athletes (e.g. marathon runners) and is more common in females. Tenderness is present over the sacroiliac region. Provocative maneuvers that stress the sacroiliac region may be painful. One-legged stance on the affected side is typically painful. Plain x-rays are usually negative. Diagnosis is possible with a SPECT scan, MRI, or CT scan. Treatment is activity restriction including a period of protected weight-bearing or non-weight-bearing, followed by a rehabilitation program. This injury has a good prognosis with athletes returning to sports after 8 weeks.

6. **Define spondylolysis, pars stress reaction, and spondylolisthesis.**
   - **Spondylolysis** is a defect in the pars interarticularis. It may be unilateral or bilateral
   - **Pars stress reaction** is an impending spondylolysis (microfracture) without a true pars defect. Bony healing can occur at this stage and prevent development of spondylolysis
   - **Spondylolisthesis** is the forward slippage of one vertebra in relation to another. Isthmic spondylolisthesis refers to forward slippage in the presence of bilateral pars defects

7. **What is the single leg extension test?**
The patient is asked to stand on one leg while simultaneously extending the lumbar spine. Increased lumbar pain on the supported side suggests a diagnosis of unilateral spondylolysis.

8. **What factors are related to the development of isthmic spondylolisthesis?**
Isthmic spondylolisthesis is not a true congenital disorder but does have a hereditary predisposition. An important contributing factor in athletes is repetitive microtrauma resulting in stress concentration in the region of the pars interarticularis. Repetitive hyperextension is the mechanism of injury reported in gymnasts, divers, wrestlers, weightlifters, and football linemen. Repetitive flexion and rotational injuries are also contributing factors.

9. **At what lumbar spinal level is isthmic spondylolisthesis most common?**
L5 is the most common location. The L5–S1 level is the region where maximum stress concentration and maximum lordosis occur.

10. **How prevalent is spondylolysis in athletes compared with the general population?**
The prevalence is 5% to 7% in the general population. Studies have documented higher rates in Olympic divers (43%), wrestlers (30%), weightlifters (23%), and gymnasts (16%). Many studies have shown increased rates in football interior linemen (15%–50%). Thus, clinical suspicion in athletes should be high, especially in athletes with persistent low-grade back pain that has been unresponsive or aggravated by physical therapy or other local modalities.

11. **What is the risk for progression of spondylolysis?**
Only about 10% of people with spondylolysis develop spondylolisthesis. This progression most commonly occurs during the adolescent growth spurt and is more common in girls. Children and younger adolescents with spina bifida occulta and a dome-shaped S1 endplate have a higher propensity for slip progression.

12. **How does one evaluate and treat an athlete with spondylolysis?**
Spondylolysis is evaluated with standing lumbar radiographs, SPECT bone scan, CT, and possibly MRI. The treatment plan starts with rest or restriction of enough activity to relieve or improve the symptoms. This plan may require merely stopping the sport or immobilization in a lumbosacral corset. No specific immobilization method has been proven scientifically to heal an athlete's spondylolysis. A neutral-position trunk stabilization program is initiated after a period of activity restriction or immobilization. A skilled therapist or trainer is important. Starting flexion, extension, or rotation exercises exacerbate the symptoms, whereas neutral isometric core stabilization exercises are less likely to increase symptoms. Healing can occur in an early lesion and not in a late lesion. In patients with persistent low-back pain symptoms despite a proper core stabilization program, surgery may be considered for repair of the pars interarticularis defect or in situ fusion (Table 61-1).

Table 61-1. Evaluation and Treatment of Spondylolysis

X-RAY STUDY	BONE SCAN	TREATMENT	LIKELIHOOD OF PARS HEALING	LENGTH OF IMMOBILIZATION	TIME OFF ATHLETICS
Negative	Unilateral pars uptake	Off athletics Trunk stabilization Wear corset	Nearly 100%	Until bone scan shows significant healing	Until bone scan shows significant healing Up to 6 months
Possible unilateral pars fracture	Bilateral pars uptake	Off athletics Trunk stabilization Wear corset	Nearly 100%	Until bone scan shows significant healing	Until bone scan shows significant healing Up to 6–9 months
Possible bilateral pars fracture	Bilateral pars uptake	Off athletics Trunk stabilization Wear corset	Fair	Until x-rays and bone scans show pars healing, or it is clear that healing will not take place	Until x-rays and bone scans show pars healing, or it is clear that healing will not take place
Definite bilateral pars fracture, appears acute	Still very "hot"	Off athletics Trunk stabilization Wear corset	Poor	Until x-rays and bone scans show pars healing, or it is clear that healing will not take place	Until x-rays and bone scans show pars healing, or it is clear that healing will not take place
Chronic pars fractures	Negative or only mildly positive	Treat symptomatically, posterior fusion, or pars repair	Poor, nearly nonexistent	May choose not to use a corset	Only until symptoms allow return

13. **Can athletes with spondylolysis and low-grade isthmic spondylolisthesis continue playing their sport?**
Yes. There is a high incidence of spondylolysis and low-grade spondylolisthesis (grades 1 and 2) in athletes. Semon and Spengler reported that 21% of football players presenting with back pain had spondylolysis. In these symptomatic football players, there was no difference in time lost from sports between athletes with spondylolysis and athletes with back pain and negative findings on radiographs.
A recent study by Brophy showed that spondylolisthesis did not significantly reduce the chance of playing in the NFL for any position, while a history of acute spondylolysis did have a significant effect for running backs. Patients with high-grade spondylolisthesis (grades 3 and 4) are not likely to participate in high-level sporting activity.

14. **What is the common mechanism producing vertebral endplate injury?**
Axial compression.

15. **What is the common mechanism producing intervertebral disc injury?**
Rotation is the most common mechanism causing intervertebral disc injury.

16. **What is an annular tear?**
The annulus fibrosus is a tough, multilayered ligamentous structure configured as concentric rings. Annular fibers are arranged in various orientations surrounding the central nucleus pulposus and connect adjacent vertebrae. Injury may cause concentric or radial tears in the annulus. Resultant inflammation from the tear may result in symptoms of spasm, back pain, and buttock and lower extremity pain. The outer annular layers are richly innervated, as is the granulation tissue that grows into the tear. This inflammatory membrane is believed to be a pain generator.

17. **What nerve innervates the posterior annulus?**
The sinuvertebral nerve with anastomosis through the spinal nerve and the posterior primary ramus.

18. **What are the options for treatment of an annular tear?**
Annular injuries are treated much like other ligamentous injuries. The first step is to control the inflammation with judicious use of antiinflammatory medications, oral steroids, steroid injections, and ice packs. A trunk-stabilization program is started as soon as possible after pain and inflammation decrease. This program concentrates on trunk strength, balance, coordination, flexibility, and aerobic conditioning. The vast majority of patients improve with nonoperative care. For patients with annular tears unresponsive to nonoperative care artificial disc replacement or fusion, surgery is a potential option.

19. What is the treatment of choice for athletes with herniated discs unresponsive to nonoperative treatment?

The surgical gold standard is microscopic lumbar discectomy from a posterior approach. This procedure involves making a 2-cm skin incision, extending caudally from the midportion of the disc space. The fascia is incised, the interlaminar area is exposed by gently elevating the muscle, and a retractor is placed. A small laminotomy is often necessary, depending on the size of the interlaminar area and the cephalad/caudal location of the herniation. Just enough ligamentum flavum is removed to gain access to the epidural space, protect the nerve, and remove the herniation.

Other potential surgical options include posterior endoscopic discectomy and selective endoscopic discectomy by a posterolateral/foraminal approach. Regardless of the approach, the goal in athletes, as in any patient, is to cause as little damage to the muscle and fascia as possible.

20. What percentage of athletes return to their sport after microscopic lumbar discectomy?

In a study by Watkins of professional and Olympic athletes, 88% returned to their sport after microscopic lumbar discectomy.

21. What are some general recommendations for returning to sports after lumbar spinal decompression procedures?

General recommendations include restoration of normal back strength, endurance, power, and pain-free activity. A minimum of 6 to 12 weeks is allowed for healing of the annulus fibrosus to prevent recurrent disc herniation.

22. What are some general recommendations for returning to sports after lumbar and thoracolumbar spinal fusion procedures?

Limited data assist with decision making for return to play after spinal fusions. According to a survey of North American Spine Society members about sports participation after spinal fusions, 80% returned to high school sports, 62% returned to collegiate sports, and only 18% returned to professional sports. Some of the criteria used to determine return to play included a solid fusion based on clinical assessment and imaging studies and full recovery as determined by near normal range of motion and normal muscular strength. Return-to-play decisions must be made on a case-by-case basis, and various factors, such as the number of levels fused, must be taken into account. For example, after a multilevel fusion, as for scoliosis or kyphosis, return to gymnastics or contact sports would not be advised by some experts because of the risk of injury due to increased stress at levels adjacent to the fusion. In contrast, after a limited fusion for spondylolysis or spondylolisthesis, return to contact sports may be a consideration after the fusion has healed and a comprehensive rehabilitation program has been completed.

23. What type of rehabilitation is recommended for athletes after spinal surgery?

A neutral-position, isometric coordinated core stabilization program is initiated shortly after surgery. The key to the core stabilization program is to use balance and coordination exercises to train the core muscles to dynamically protect the spine while performing the functions necessary to the sports activity. This program helps decrease future spine injury. The stabilization program has five levels of proficiency based on the ability of the athlete to perform the exercises.

24. Should the rehabilitation program start with flexion or extension exercises?

Neither. The authors advise starting with neutral isometric control exercises as part of the trunk stabilization program.

25. What type of aerobic activity can the athlete perform after spinal surgery?

It depends. Aerobic exercise is a vital part of the trunk-stabilization rehabilitation program. The key is to diversify the aerobic conditioning to methods that are best tolerated.

26. Can the recovering athlete lift weights while recovering from spinal surgery?

Yes, after establishing good core strength and trunk stability.

27. What objective factors can guide an athlete's return to play after spinal surgery?

Return-to-play decisions are complex and must be individualized on a case-by-case basis. Factors such as patient age, type of surgery (fusion vs. decompression), radiographic factors, and type of sport activity enter into decision making. Objective factors that can guide the physician in determining that an athlete may be ready to be considered for full return to play are as follows:

- Completion of an appropriate level in the trunk stabilization program (professional athletes Level 5, recreational golfers Level 3)
- Completion of a course of sport-specific exercises
- Attainment of an appropriate level of aerobic conditioning for the sport
- Practicing the sport fully
- Successful slow return to the sport with some limit on minutes played
- Commitment to continue to do the stabilization exercises after return to play

Key Points

1. In adolescent athletes, the most common causes of low back pain are lumbar strain, spondylolysis/spondylolisthesis, lumbar disc injuries, and overuse syndrome.
2. In adult athletes, the most common causes of low back pain are lumbar strain, degenerative disc disorders, disc herniations, and spinal stenosis.
3. Patients with lumbar strain, lumbar disc herniation, and spondylolysis can anticipate successful return to sports activities if they are able to successfully complete an appropriate trunk-stabilization rehabilitation program.
4. Limited data exist to assist with decision making for return to play after lumbar spinal fusions, and return-to-play decisions are determined on a case-by-case basis.

Websites

Lumbar disc problems in the athlete:
    http://emedicine.medscape.com/article/93419-overview
Lumbar spine injuries in athletes: http://www.medscape.com/viewarticle/553959
Trunk and pelvic stabilization program: http://pbats.com/index.php?page=trunk

BIBLIOGRAPHY

1. Bono CM. Low-back pain in athletes. J Bone Joint Surg 2004;86A:382-96.
2. Brophy RH, Lyman S, Chehab EL, et al. Predictive value of prior injury on career in professional American football is affected by player position. Am J Sports Med 2009;37:768-75.
3. Brown GA, Wood KB, Garvey TA. Lumbar spine problems in athletes. In: Arendt EA, editor. Orthopaedic Knowledge Update 2-Sports Medicine. Rosemont, IL: American Academy of Orthopaedic Surgeons; 1999. p. 417–27.
4. Hambly MF, Wiltse LL, Peek RD. Spondylolisthesis. In: Watkins RG, editor. The Spine in Sports. St. Louis: Mosby; 1996. p. 157–63.
5. Rossi F, Dragoni S. Lumbar spondylolysis: Occurrence in competitive athletes. J Sports Med 1990;30:450-2.
6. Rubery PT, Bradford DS. Athletic activity after spine surgery in children and adolescents. Spine 2002;27:423-7.
7. Semen RL, Spengler D. Significance of lumbar spondylolysis in college football players. Spine 1981;6:172-4.
8. Watkins RG, Williams LA. Lumbar spine injuries in athletes. In: Fu FH, Stone DA, editors. Sports Injuries. 2nd ed. Philadelphia: Lippincott Williams & Wilkins; 2001. p. 988–1014.
9. Watkins RG, Williams LA, Lin PM, editors. The Spine in Sports. St. Louis: Mosby; 1996.
10. Wright A, Ferree B, Tromanhauser S. Spinal fusion in the athlete. Clin Sports Med 1993;12:599–602.

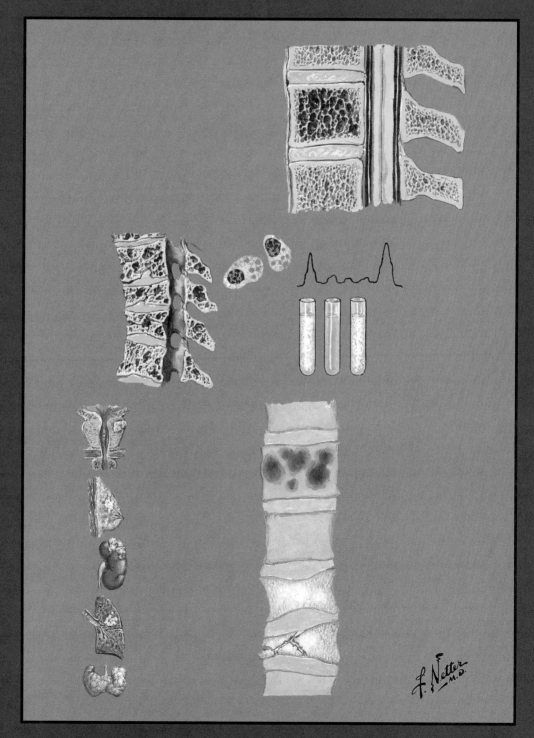

DISORDERS OF THE SPINAL CORD AND RELATED STRUCTURES

Darren L. Jacobs, DO, and Vincent J. Devlin, MD

SPINAL CORD TUMORS

1. **How does one describe the anatomic location of a spine tumor?**

   Spine tumors are localized according to the anatomic compartment in which they occur (Fig. 62-1): *extradural, intradural-extramedullary,* or *intramedullary.* Certain tumors may invade multiple anatomic planes.

   - **Extradural tumors** may be *primary* spinal tumors (benign or malignant) or *secondary* tumors (due to metastatic disease). Primary tumors most commonly develop from osseous structures. Metastatic disease involving the spine occurs most commonly secondary to breast, lung, prostate, thyroid, and renal malignancies

   - **Intradural-extramedullary tumors** arise within the dura but outside the spinal cord. These tumors displace the spinal cord toward the contralateral side of the thecal sac. The most common tumors arise from the sheath cells covering the spinal nerve root (schwannoma, neurofibroma) or from the meningeal cells along the spinal cord surface (meningioma). If the tumor arises as the nerve root leaves the dural sac, it may possess both an intradural and extradural component (dumbbell-shaped tumor)

   - **Intramedullary tumors** originate from the parenchyma of the spinal cord. The characteristic pattern on magnetic resonance imaging (MRI) is widening of the spinal cord and narrowing of the cerebrospinal fluid (CSF) space over several vertebral levels. These tumors are centrally located within the spinal cord and typically enhance with administration of gadolinium. Syringomyelia and perilesional cysts are frequently associated with these lesions

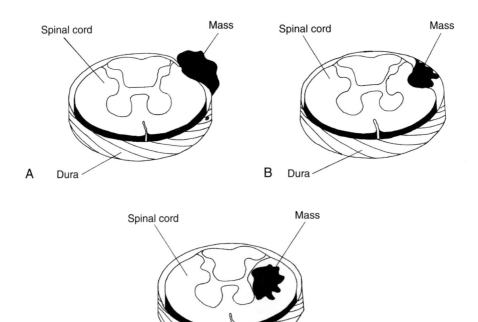

Figure 62-1. Location of spinal tumors. **A,** Extradural. **B,** Intradural-extramedullary. **C,** Intramedullary. (From Rolak LA. Neurology Secrets. 4th ed. Philadelphia: Mosby; 2005.)

2. What are the most common types of extradural spinal tumors?

Extradural tumors (Fig. 62-2) may be primary tumors originating from the vertebra and adjacent soft tissues or develop secondary to metastatic disease. The most common extradural spinal tumor is a metastatic tumor. The most common primary bone tumor is multiple myeloma. The differential diagnosis of an extradural spinal tumor is listed in Table 62-1.

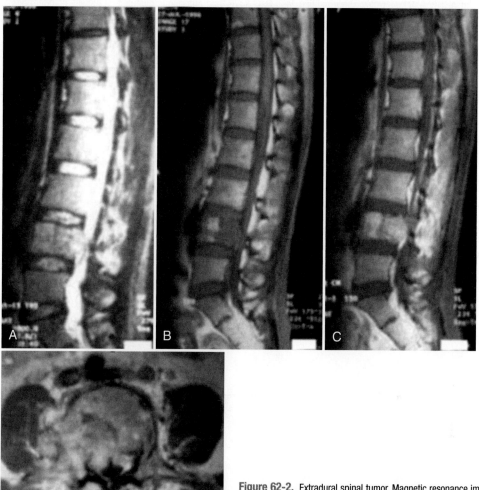

Figure 62-2. Extradural spinal tumor. Magnetic resonance imaging (MRI) of primary osteosarcoma in lumbar spine. **A,** Low to intermediate signal change is seen at L4 vertebral body on T2-weighted MRI. **B,** Low signal change on T1-weighted MRI. **C,** With gadolinium, a moderate enhancement pattern is shown. **D,** On axial view, soft tissue mass is accompanied with intraosseous mass through cortical breakage. (From Kim DH, Chan UK, Kim SH, et al. Tumors of the Spine. Philadelphia: Saunders; 2008.)

Table 62-1. Extradural Spine Tumors

PRIMARY SPINE TUMORS		METASTATIC SPINE TUMORS
BENIGN	**MALIGNANT**	
Osteoid osteoma	Myeloma/plasmacytoma	Breast
Osteoblastoma	Lymphoma	Prostate
Osteochondroma	Osteosarcoma	Lung
Giant cell tumor	Ewing's sarcoma	Thyroid
Aneurysmal bone cyst	Chondrosarcoma	Renal
Eosinophilic granuloma	Chordoma	Melanoma
Hemangioma		Gastrointestinal

3. What symptoms may be associated with an intradural spinal tumor?

Because of the slow-growing nature of many tumors, symptoms tend to precede diagnosis by an average of 2 years. Pain is often the earliest symptom and is typically reported as occurring at night. The clinical signs and symptoms associated with an intradural spinal tumor are related to the *level of the lesion* along the spinal column (cervical, thoracic, lumbar, sacral) as well as *tumor location* within the dura and spinal cord (extramedullary, intramedullary). Motor dysfunction, sensory dysfunction, reflex abnormalities, long tract signs, and autonomic dysfunction (bowel, bladder and/ or sexual dysfunction) may occur. *Extramedullary tumors* frequently cause unilateral symptoms due to their eccentric location (i.e. unilateral radicular pain, unilateral spastic weakness, Brown-Sequard syndrome). *Intramedullary tumors* typically cause dissociated sensory loss (loss of pain and temperature sensation without loss of position and vibration sensation). Intramedullary tumors typically develop in the central region of the spinal cord and disrupt the spinothalamic tracts but spare the dorsal columns, which are relatively resistant to tumor infiltration. Pain is described as burning, poorly localized, and involving large areas of the body. Intradural tumors may present with acute neurologic deterioration secondary to subarachnoid or epidural hemorrhage.

4. What are the most common types of intradural-extramedullary spinal cord tumors?

Eighty percent of the tumors in the intradural-extramedullary space are schwannomas, neurofibromas, or meningiomas (Fig. 62-3). Tumors of the intradural-extramedullary space account for 60% of all intradural spinal tumors in adults but are less common in children. Nerve sheath tumors (schwannomas, neurofibromas) arise from sheath cells covering the spinal nerve roots while meningiomas arise from meningeal cells localized at the spinal cord surface. *Neurofibromas* occur commonly in patients with neurofibromatosis type 1 (NF1), may present with multiple lesions, and occasionally may undergo malignant degeneration. *Schwannomas* are more common than neurofibromas and usually occur as solitary lesions. *Meningiomas* are typically isolated lesions most commonly located in the thoracic region. Other tumor types may occur in the intradural-extramedullary space but are less common (Table 62-2).

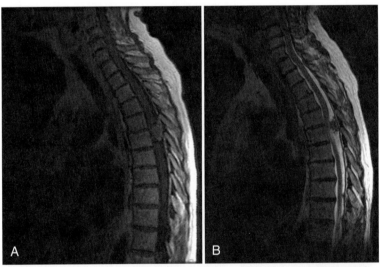

Figure 62-3. Intradural-extramedullary spinal cord tumor. Meningioma. **A,** Sagittal T1-weighted MRI with contrast material reveals a dura-based lesion with homogeneous enhancement, which is consistent with meningioma. **B,** Sagittal T2-weighted magnetic resonance imaging (MRI) reveals an isointense lesion in the posterior intradural compartment, which causes anterior displacement of the cord and cord compression at T6. Strong signal within the cord itself can be seen adjacent to the lesion (From Schapira AHV. Neurology and Clinical Neuroscience. 1st ed. Philadelphia: Mosby; 2007.)

Table 62-2. Intradural–Extramedullary Spinal Tumors	
Schwannoma	Ependymoma
Neurofibroma	Paraganglioma
Meningioma	Epidermoid and dermoid cysts
Hemangiopericytoma	Subarachnoid seeding of metastatic disease
Lipoma	

5. What are the most common types of intramedullary spinal cord tumors?

The most common types of intramedullary tumors (Table 62-3, Fig. 62-4) are ependymomas, astrocytomas, and hemangioblastomas. In children, astrocytomas are the most common tumor type, while in adults, ependymomas are most common. *Ependymomas* arise from the cuboidal ependymal cells that surround the ventricular system and central canal of the spinal cord. As the tumor enlarges in the central canal, the flow of CSF is obstructed and cystic cavities frequently develop above and below the lesion. *Astrocytomas* result from malignant transformation of astrocyte cells, which are glial cells that provide nutritional support to neurons and axons. The majority of tumors are low grade, but more aggressive and infiltrating types occur. These are typically categorized as high-grade or malignant neoplasms. *Hemangioblastomas* are the most common intramedullary spinal cord tumor of nonglial origin. Hemangioblastomas are tumors that are more commonly seen in patients with von Hippel-Lindau disease.

Table 62-3. Intramedullary Spinal Tumors	
Ependymoma	Neuroblastoma
Astrocytoma	Gliomas (malignant oligodendroglioma, ganglioglioma)
Hemangioblastoma	Epidermoid and dermoid cysts
Lipoma	Spinal cord metastasis

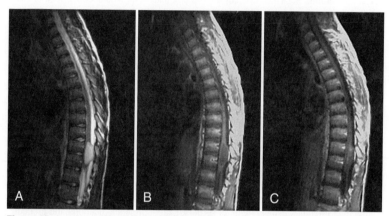

Figure 62-4. Intramedullary spinal cord tumor. Astrocytoma. **A,** Sagittal T2-weighted magnetic resonance imaging (MRI) reveals an expansile mass in the thoracic spinal cord, representing a World Health Organization grade II astrocytoma. Sagittal T1-weighted MRI before **(B)** and after **(C)** gadolinium administration demonstrates heterogeneous enhancement. (From Schapira AHV. Neurology and Clinical Neuroscience. 1st ed. Philadelphia: Mosby; 2007.)

6. What is the differential diagnosis of tumors of the cauda equina?

The most common tumors presenting in the region of the cauda equina include ependymoma, schwannoma, meningioma, lipoma, and metastasis.

7. Discuss and contrast the general approach to treatment of intradural-extramedullary spinal cord tumors versus intramedullary spinal cord tumors

Intradural-extramedullary spinal cord tumors tend to be histopathologically benign and can be successfully resected in the majority of patients, most commonly through a posterior surgical approach. Tumors in an anterior location and dumbbell-shaped tumors are more challenging to treat surgically. Radiotherapy or chemotherapy is generally reserved for tumors with malignant histologic characteristics and for recurrent tumors.

Intramedullary spinal cord tumors are typically treated with open surgical resection. Surgical advances that have transformed the surgical treatment of these lesions include MRI, microscopic surgical techniques, improved surgical instrumentation, intraoperative ultrasound, the ultrasonic aspirator, and intraoperative neurophysiologic monitoring. The aggressiveness of surgical resection is dependent on the histologic diagnosis based on intraoperative frozen section and the ability to locate and maintain a surgical plane. Well-circumscribed tumors such as ependymoma and hemangioblastoma are typically amenable to complete resection. Well-differentiated astrocytomas are amenable to resection, but infiltrative and high-grade types are impossible to completely resect and their treatment remains controversial. Radiotherapy is reserved for malignant lesions and for lesions that are not surgically resectable.

SYRINGOHYDROMYELIA AND CHIARI MALFORMATION

8. **What is syringohydromyelia?**

A **syrinx** is a cystic dilatation or cavitation that develops within the substance of the spinal cord. **Hydromyelia** refers to a dilatation of the central canal with an ependymal-cell lining. **Syringomyelia** is an eccentric cavitation that is not lined by ependyma. A syrinx extending into the brainstem is called **syringobulbia**. Current terminology groups these lesions as **syringohydromyelia**. A cavity greater than 5 cm with or without edema is more likely to cause symptoms.

9. **What are some causes of syringohydromyelia?**

Syringohydromyelia may be idiopathic or arise as the result of spinal cord trauma, tumor, spinal cord infarction, post radiotherapy, hemorrhage, or developmental anomalies (e.g. Chiari malformation, basilar invagination).

10. **Describe classic clinical features associated with syringohydromyelia.**

- **Dissociated sensory loss:** A centrally located syrinx disrupts the decussating spinothalamic tracts (loss of pain and temperature sensation) while dorsal column function remains intact (position and vibration sensation is preserved). The pattern of sensory loss involves the shoulders and upper trunk and is described as a "capelike" pattern
- **Dysesthetic pain:** Severe pain may develop and most commonly involves the trunk and upper extremities
- **Lower motor neuron lesions:** Involvement of the anterior horn cells leads to atrophy, weakness, and absent reflexes below the level of the lesion. Lesions that involve the cervical cord lead to muscle atrophy, which begins distally in the hands and progresses to involve more proximal musculature
- **Bulbar lesions:** Syringobulbia can manifest as tongue fasciculations, hoarseness, facial anesthesia, dysphagia
- **Autonomic system involvement:** Horner's syndrome, impaired bowel or bladder function
- **Musculoskeletal problems:** Scoliosis, Charcot arthropathy (classically the shoulder joint is involved), basilar invagination, Klippel-Feil anomaly

11. **What are the treatment options for a symptomatic syrinx?**

Syringohydromyelia has been classified into two main types:
- Communicating (associated with Chiari malformation, basilar arachnoiditis)
- Noncommunicating (associated with cord trauma, cord tumor, or arachnoiditis)

Surgical treatment of communicating syringohydromyelia initially involves suboccipital decompression. Placement of a ventriculoperitoneal shunt may also be indicated if hydrocephalus is present. Surgical treatment options for noncommunicating hydrocephalus vary and include syringostomy, shunting, and expansile duraplasty (to create a path for CSF flow around the lesion).

12. **What is the Chiari malformation?**

The spectrum of Chiari malformations consists of four hindbrain abnormalities that share a common entity of impaired CSF flow around the brainstem and through the foramen magnum. These disorders may be congenital or acquired. The tonsillar herniation is usually greater than 5 mm, but this is not essential or diagnostic of the disorder. Treatment of symptomatic Chiari malformations usually requires surgery. Exact surgical indications and procedures remain controversial.

13. **What are the types of Chiari malformations and their respective features?**

TYPE I

- Caudal descent of the cerebellar tonsils into the cervical spine, rarely below C2, results in crowding of the subarachnoid space at the craniocervical junction
- Usually adults or adolescents without myelomeningocele
- May be associated with scoliosis, hand weakness, craniovertebral osseous anomalies, Klippel-Feil anomaly, syringomyelia (50%–75%), hydrocephalus (10%)

TYPE II

- Caudal descent of the cerebellar vermis and medulla into the cervical spine, commonly below C2 (Fig. 62-5)
- Occurs almost exclusively in children with myelomeningoceles
- Associated with hydrocephalus (90%), syringomyelia (20%–95%), kinking of medulla, Klippel-Feil, atlantoaxial abnormalities

TYPE III

- Dorsal protrusion of a craniocervical sac containing posterior fossa contents (cerebellum, brainstem), seen externally, may be confused with occipital encephalocele
- Rare, frequently fatal during infancy

TYPE IV

- Crowded posterior fossa associated with hypoplastic cerebellum and brainstem without hindbrain herniation
- Rare, some authors have removed this from the Chiari classification

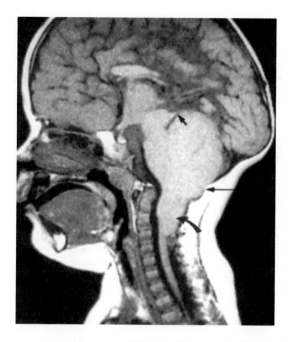

Figure 62-5. MRI image of a patient with Chiari II malformation. Note the upward herniation of the cerebellum as indicated by the *short arrow*. The *curved arrow* indicates downward herniation of the brainstem through the foramen magnum. The *thin long arrow* marks the foramen magnum. (From Fleisher LA (ed): Fleisher: Anesthesia and Uncommon Diseases. 5th ed., Philadelphia: Saunders; 2005.)

14. What are the indications for surgical decompression in Chiari malformations?
Indications remain controversial, but most authors agree that any Chiari malformation with an associated syrinx would portend surgery. Additionally, any signs of brainstem compression or cerebellar dysfunction are indications for surgical intervention. In Chiari II malformation patients with associated hydrocephalus, it is critical to ensure that the patient's ventriculoperitoneal shunt is functional prior to considering any additional surgical intervention. Controversy exists regarding the exact surgical procedure required to decompress the cervicomedullary junction and restore CSF circulation across the foramen magnum.

SPINAL DYSRAPHISM

15. Define spinal dysraphism.
Spinal dysraphism refers to a spectrum of congenital spinal anomalies due to failure of fusion of midline structures. The anomalies may involve the osseous vertebral elements, spinal cord, nerve roots, bladder, rectum, and genitalia.

16. What is spina bifida?
The neural tube usually closes between days 24 and 28 following conception during a process called *neurulation.* Spina bifida is a descriptive term applied to a group of neural tube defects associated disruption of neurulation leading to failure of posterior fusion of vertebral osseous elements (Fig. 62-6). Spina bifida is classified into two main types:
*   **Spina bifida occulta:** Intact skin overlies the underlying anomaly, which ranges from an osseous defect involving the posterior lamina without associated structural or neurologic significance to clinically significant involvement of

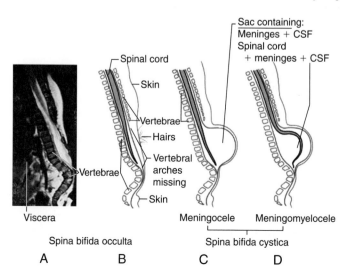

Figure 62-6. Sagittal views of spina bifida malformations. Magnetic resonance image and corresponding views showing **A** and **B**, Spina bifida occulta. **C**, Spina bifida cystica. **D**, Meningocele and meningomyelocele). CSF, cerebrospinal fluid. (From Haines DE. Fundamental Neuroscience for Basic and Clinical Applications. 3rd ed. Philadelphia: Churchill Livingstone; 2006.)

neural and meningeal structures with significant neurologic sequelae (e.g., diastematomyelia, lipomyelomeningocele, anterior sacral meningocele, tethered filum terminale)

- **Spina bifida cystica:** A mass extrudes through the defect and overlying skin. The mass may contain meninges and CSF (meningocele) or meninges, CSF, and spinal neural tissue (myelomeningocele). The spectrum of conditions may be detectable with prenatal imaging, is visible at birth and may be associated with severe neurologic sequelae. These sequelae may include hydrocephalus, neurogenic bowel and bladder dysfunction, and varying degrees of lower extremity paralysis.

17. Describe the clinical features of spina bifida occulta.

In spina bifida occulta the underlying spinal and/or neural defect is covered by intact skin and thus may not be grossly evident on examination. External signs may include a lumbosacral hair tuft (*faun's tail*), skin-covered lipoma, cutaneous hemangioma, or a lumbosacral skin dimple. If the defect is limited to failure of fusion of the vertebral arch, the finding has little clinical significance. However, more complex types are associated with neurologic, urologic, and/or orthopaedic abnormalities. The majority of more complex cases will require surgical intervention to prevent progression of neurologic deficits.

Associated neurologic findings may include lower extremity atrophy, weakness, radicular pain, or numbness. Urologic signs may include an abnormal voiding pattern in an infant, new incontinence after toilet training, or a urinary tract infection in a child of any age. Orthopaedic findings may include cavovarus foot deformities, clawtoes, leg-length discrepancy, and scoliosis. Diagnosis is often delayed until adolescence or adulthood, due to absent initial neurologic or urologic findings. Early identification is paramount because prophylactic surgery is usually indicated to preserve neurologic function.

18. What is diastematomyelia?

Diastematomyelia is a congenital spinal anomaly in which splitting of the spinal cord is identified. Two separate *hemicords* divided by a septum are present. Variations exist including two separate hemicords separated by a septum (osseous or cartilaginous) and contained in separate dural coverings or two separate hemicords (fibrous septum) in one dural covering. There is a female predominance and the condition most commonly presents in the lower thoracic or upper lumbar spine. Patients present with a tethered cord syndrome. Spinal deformities are commonly associated with diastematomyelia. Surgical intervention is indicated for patients with progressive neurologic deficits. If surgical correction of spinal deformity is planned, surgery to detether the spinal cord by removal of the septum should be performed prior to surgical procedures to correct spinal deformity.

19. What is the tethered cord syndrome?

Tethered cord syndrome presents with signs and symptoms that result from excessive tension on the spinal cord. At birth, the conus is usually located at the L2–L3 level and ascends to the L1–L2 level by 3 months of age. Spinal dysraphism is responsible for the majority of cases. A constellation of signs and symptoms is associated with this syndrome including neurologic deficits, back pain, cutaneous abnormalities, spinal deformities, bowel and bladder dysfunction, gait abnormalities, and orthopaedic deformities. MRI including dynamic imaging is the primary modality for confirmation of diagnosis. Surgical intervention is directed toward release of tethering structures to relieve chronic tension in the spinal cord.

20. What is a lipomyelomeningocele?

A **lipomyelomeningocele** is a common congenital spinal anomaly in which herniation of a lipoma into the conus medullaris or the dorsal spinal cord occurs through an osseous defect and communicates with an adjacent subcutaneous fatty mass. It is a common cause of tethered cord syndrome. Symptoms may include constipation, urinary urgency, dyspareunia, lumbar pain, or cephalgia (headache) with defecation. The term lipomyelomeningocele is actually a misnomer, because abnormal neural tissue does not extend outside of the spinal canal. Surgical treatment of this anomaly is extremely challenging and should be referred to a regional center with extensive treatment of these lesions.

21. Describe the presentation of an anterior sacral meningocele.

An **anterior sacral meningocele** is a rare congenital spinal anomaly in which herniation of dura mater and/or neural elements through a defect in the ventral spine is identified. The anomaly contains CSF and may contain neural elements. Unlike the myelomeningocele, this anomaly is not associated with hydrocephalus or Chiari malformation. Associated findings include the triad of sacral bony anomalies, a presacral mass, and anorectal anomalies (Currarino syndrome). Symptoms may include constipation, urinary urgency, dyspareunia, lumbar pain, or cephalgia (headache) with defecation. Examination findings include a smooth pelvic mass, palpable on pelvic or rectal examination. This entity is most commonly found at the sacral level and is more common in females.

22. Define myelomeningocele and describe the pertinent clinical findings.

Myelomeningocele is a neural tube defect in which the dorsal neural structures are open through the skin due to failure of the neural tube closure. This is the most common significant spinal birth defect. The incidence of this defect varies based on geography (worldwide: 1/1000 live births; United States: 0.6/1000 live births; Ireland: 4/1000 live births). Prevalence has diminished since the 1980s due to the utilization of perinatal folate and elective termination of the pregnancies upon identification by in utero imaging with ultrasound or MRI.

23. What is the etiology of myelomeningocele?

Embryologically, the defect occurs around day 28 following conception when the posterior neuropore fails to close or reopens due to distention of the central canal from CSF. This event has been associated with multiple factors including genetic factors, maternal nutritional factors (folic acid deficiency), season of conception, and environmental factors (socioeconomic status, degree of urbanization).

24. How is myelomeningocele diagnosed in the prenatal period?

Fetal diagnosis can be made prenatally by amniocentesis (increased alpha-fetoprotein and acetylcholinesterase levels) and ultrasound, with 90% accuracy. MRI imaging may be safely performed to further characterize the location of the lesion and to determine associated hydrocephalus or Chiari II malformation. This can allow for prenatal counseling and prognosis, including the options of termination of pregnancy, fetal closure, or elective cesarean section. Patients require careful evaluation for associated cardiac and renal defects. When the condition is identified prenatally, Caesarian section birth is usually recommended.

25. What is the management for a newborn patient with myelomeningocele?

Upon birth, the baby should be placed prone and the lesion covered with moist nonadherent dressing (Telfa). Trendelenburg position may prevent CSF accumulation at the lesion site. If the lesion is open and CSF leakage is noted, prophylactic antibiotics to prevent meningitis are administered. Careful neurologic examination is documented prior to surgery. Surgical closure should be performed within 48 to 72 hours of birth but may be delayed a week to allow for parental discussion regarding prognosis based on the spinal level of involvement (Fig. 62-7). The surgical procedure for closure of the defect involves resection of the *zona epitheliosa* and recapitulation of the *neural placode* into a tube. The dura and fascia are then closed over the closed placode in a water-tight fashion. The skin is then carefully closed over the repair. A rotational flap or a *Z-plasty* may be required to adequately cover the repair without tension. In utero repair of these lesions may be considered, and studies regarding the safety, efficacy, and success of this procedure are ongoing (Management of Myelomeningocele Study [MOMS], National Institute of Child Health and Human Development).

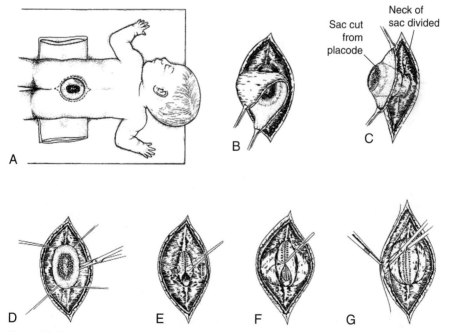

Figure 62-7. Technique for closure of a myelomeningocele. **A,** The infant is placed prone with towel rolls under the hips. An elliptical incision is outlined just outside the zona epithelioserosa, which may be oriented on a vertical or horizontal axis. **B,** The incision is to the level of the lumbodorsal fascia. The apices of the island of skin within the incision are grasped with clamps, and the skin is undermined medially until the dural sac is seen to funnel through the fascial defect. **C,** The dural sac is first incised at its base. The skin is then excised from the placode and discarded, allowing the placode to fall into the spinal canal. **D,** The everted dura is undermined and reflected medially to envelop the placode. The placode itself may be folded medially and sewn into a tube at this point. **E,** The dural layer is closed with nonabsorbable suture, using a running stitch. **F,** The fascia is incised to the muscle, undermined, and reflected medially to create a second layer of closure. **G,** The skin is undermined using blunt techniques to permit closure. (From Sutton LN, Schwartz DM. Congenital anomalies of the spinal cord. In: Herkowitz HN, Garfin SR, Eismont FJ, et al, editors. Rothman-Simeone The Spine. 5th ed. Philadelphia: Saunders; 2006.)

26. What are the clinical sequelae of myelomeningocele?

The clinical sequelae involve multiple body systems and include:
- **Neurologic:** 90% of patients develop clinically significant hydrocephalus, requiring CSF diversion procedures (e.g. ventriculoperitoneal shunt). Children will frequently have some degree of lower extremity motor, sensory, and/or autonomic dysfunction correlating to the level of the lesion. Cognitive deficits are common.
- **Urologic:** Nearly all patients have abnormalities in urologic function
- **Gastrointestinal:** Neurogenic bowel dysfunction is present in a high percentage of patients
- **Musculoskeletal deformities:** Spinal deformities are common and include scoliosis, kyphosis, and deformities associated with congenital osseous anomalies. A spectrum of lower extremity deformities may develop depending on the level of the lesion and may include hip dislocation, hip and knee contractures, and foot deformities.

MISCELLANEOUS DISORDERS INVOLVING THE SPINAL CORD

27. Define the terms myelopathy and myelitis.

Myelopathy and myelitis are disorders of the spinal cord that have numerous potential etiologies. **Myelopathy** usually indicates a compressive, toxic, or metabolic etiology. **Myelitis** usually indicates an inflammatory process due to infectious or autoimmune causes.

28. Describe the clinical picture of a patient presenting with a transverse myelopathy/myelitis.

- Chief complaint is usually lower extremity weakness and ambulatory dysfunction
- If the cervical cord is involved, upper extremity symptoms are also present
- Lhermitte's phenomenon (lightning-like electric shock pain radiating into the extremities and down the spine with neck flexion) may be present
- Sphincter incontinence, sexual dysfunction may be present
- Hoffmann's sign and Babinski's sign may be present
- Loss of abdominal and cremasteric reflexes is common
- Signs of spinal shock (flaccid paralysis with hypotension and bradycardia) may be present
- Treatment with steroids is common, but response is highly variable
- Most common type is idiopathic transverse myelitis

29. What is the differential diagnosis of a transverse myelopathy?

A. Idiopathic transverse myelitis
B. Demyelinating disease (multiple sclerosis, Devic syndrome)
C. Postvaccination
D. Infectious myelopathies
 1. Viral (HIV, HTLV-1, varicella-zoster virus [VZV], cytomegalovirus [CMV], Epstein-Barr virus [EBV], enteroviruses)
 2. Bacterial (syphilis, tuberculosis)
 3. Fungal
 4. Parasitic
E. Connective tissue diseases
 1. Rheumatoid arthritis
 2. Sjögren's disease
 3. Systemic lupus erythematosus
 4. Antiphospholipid antibody syndrome
F. Sarcoidosis
G. Nutritional (B_{12})

H. Paraneoplastic syndromes
 1. Small cell carcinoma of the lung
 2. Radiation myelopathy
 3. Intrathecal methotrexate
 4. Hodgkin's/lymphomas
I. Toxins
 1. Spinal anesthesia–epidural or intrathecal
 2. Spinal angiography
 3. Intrathecal steroids
J. Electrical injury (high-tension current, lightning, electroshock therapy)
K. Barotrauma (caisson work, scuba diving, flying)
L. Familial disorders (hereditary spastic paraplegia, Friedreich's ataxia)
M. Spinal cord compression (tumor, infection, trauma, cervical spondylosis)
N. Vascular disorders involving the spinal cord

30. What is multiple sclerosis?

Multiple sclerosis is a common disorder in which the myelin sheath within the central nervous system is destroyed by a poorly understood inflammatory process. Genetic and environmental factors have been implicated as triggers for the disease. Diagnosis is challenging and requires documentation of damage in at least two separate areas of the central nervous system and ruling out other possible diagnoses through careful medical history, neurologic examination, MRI, visual evoked potentials and CSF analysis. Symptoms associated with multiple sclerosis are variable and wide-ranging. These may include numbness, fatigue, gait problems, ataxia, bowel/bladder dysfunction, cognitive dysfunction, and spasticity. No cure is available, but a variety of medications are used in an attempt to limit disease activity and progression.

31. What is amyotrophic lateral sclerosis (ALS)?

Amyotrophic lateral sclerosis (ALS) is a progressive degenerative disorder of motor neurons in the spinal cord, brainstem, and motor cortex manifested clinically by muscular weakness, atrophy, and corticospinal tract involvement.

Clinical presentation typically includes atrophic weakness of hands and forearms, slight spasticity of the legs, and generalized hyperreflexia. Other findings may include hand and finger stiffness, cramping, fasciculations, and atrophy and weakness of tongue, pharyngeal, and laryngeal muscles. There is no sensory loss. The disease is characterized by middle life presentation and death is usually within 2 to 6 years. Diagnosis is made on the basis of history and neurologic examination and electromyography (EMG)/nerve conduction studies. Riluzole is a medication to treat ALS and may improve the neurologic function and survival. Its mechanism is not well understood. Physical therapy, occupational therapy, and speech therapy are necessary treatments. Symptomatic treatment for depression, secretion control, pain, fatigue, muscle spasms, and constipation are supportive measures. The disease is also called *Lou Gehrig's disease,* named for the New York Yankee's baseball player who died from this disorder.

Key Points

1. The differential diagnosis of a spinal cord tumor is determined by the anatomic compartment in which it occurs (i.e. extradural, intradural-extramedullary, or intramedullary).
2. Syringohydromyelia is an abnormal fluid cavity within the spinal cord, which may cause progressive neurologic dysfunction.
3. Spinal dysraphism is broadly classified into two forms: spina bifida occulta and spina bifida cystica.
4. Myelomeningocele is the most common significant spinal birth defect and results from disruption of the process of neurulation between days 24 and 28 following conception.

Websites

Chiari malformation: http://emedicine.medscape.com/article/1483583-overview
Intramedullary spinal cord tumors: http://emedicine.medscape.com/article/251133-overview
Neural tube defects: http://emedicine.medscape.com/article/1177162-overview
Spinal cord disorders: http://neuromuscular.wustl.edu/spinal.html
Spinal dysraphism and myelomeningocele: http://emedicine.medscape.com/article/413899-overview
Syringomyelia: http://emedicine.medscape.com/article/1151685-overview

BIBLIOGRAPHY

1. Batjer HH, Loftus C, editors. Textbook of Neurological Surgery: Principles and Practice. Philadelphia: Lippincott Williams and Wilkins; 2002.
2. Gebauer GP, Farjoodi P, Sciubba DM, et al. Magnetic resonance imaging of spine tumors: Classification, differential diagnosis, and spectrum of disease. J Bone Joint Surg 2008;90A:146-62.
3. Lew SM, Kothbauer KF. Tethered cord syndrome: an updated review. Pediatr Neurosurg 2007;43:236-48.
4. Sutton LN, Schwartz DM. Congenital anomalies of the spinal cord. In: Herkowitz HN, Garfin SR, Eismont FJ, Bell GR, Balderston RA, editors. Rothman-Simeone The Spine. 5th ed. Philadelphia: Saunders; 2006. p. 675–707.

PRIMARY SPINE TUMORS

William O. Shaffer, MD

1. **What types of tumors arise in the spine?**
   Primary tumors and secondary tumors.

2. **What is the difference between primary and secondary tumors of the spine?**
   Primary tumors of the spine arise de novo in the bone, cartilage, neural, or ligamentous structures of the spine. They may be classified as extradural or intradural. **Secondary tumors** are either metastatic to the spine from distant origins or grow into the spine from adjacent structures, such as a Pancoast tumor from the upper lobe of the lung. Primary spine tumors are extremely rare. Metastatic lesions involving the spine are the most common type of spinal tumor and account for 95% of all spinal tumors. Primary bone tumors of the spine are the emphasis of this chapter.

3. **What are the subtypes of primary bone tumors of the spine?**
   - Benign
   - Intermediate
   - Malignant
   - Tumor-like lesions

4. **What is a benign primary spine tumor?**
   Benign primary tumors of the spine are nonaggressive tumors, which may cause pain, local symptoms, and tissue destruction; however, they do not aggressively invade adjacent structures nor do they metastasize. Examples include:
   - Osteoid osteoma
   - Osteoblastoma
   - Chondroma
   - Chondroblastoma
   - Chondromyxoid fibroma
   - Giant-cell tumor
   - Hemangioma
   - Lymphangioma
   - Lipoma

5. **What is an intermediate primary spinal tumor?**
   An **intermediate tumor** is one that is locally invasive but rarely metastasizes. Examples include:
   - Aggressive osteoblastoma
   - Hemangiopericytoma
   - Hemangioendothelioma
   - Chordoma
   - Neurofibroma
   - Neurilemmoma

6. **What is a malignant primary spinal tumor?**
   A **malignant tumor** is locally invasive and metastasizes to other organs. It is a life-threatening tumor by its fundamental nature. Examples include:
   - Osteosarcoma
   - Chondrosarcoma
   - Ewing's sarcoma
   - Neuroectodermal tumor of bone
   - Malignant lymphoma
   - Myeloma
   - Malignant hemangiopericytoma
   - Angiosarcoma
   - Fibrosarcoma
   - Liposarcoma

7. **What are tumor-like lesions?**
   A **tumor-like lesion** arises in bone but is not neoplastic in its cell of origin. Such lesions can cause local vertebral collapse and secondary neural injury. Examples include:
   - Aneurysmal bone cyst
   - Eosinophilic granuloma
   - Brown tumor of hyperparathyroidism
   - Giant-cell (reparative) granuloma
   See Table 63-1

Table 63-1. World Health Organization Classification of Bone Tumors and Tumor-like Lesions

I. Bone-Forming Tumors	VI. Other Connective Tissue Tumors

1. Benign
  • Osteoma
  • Osteoid osteoma and osteoblastoma
2. Intermediate
  • Aggressive (malignant) osteoblastoma
3. Malignant (osteosarcoma)
  • Central (medullary): conventional central, telangiectatic, intraosseous well-differentiated (low-grade), round-cell
  • Surface (peripheral): parosteal, periosteal, high-grade surface
	1. Benign
	  • Benign fibrous histiocytoma
	  • Lipoma
	2. Intermediate
	  • Desmoplastic fibroma
	3. Malignant
	  • Fibrosarcoma
	  • Malignant fibrous histiocytoma
	  • Liposarcoma
	  • Malignant mesenchymoma
	  • Leiomyosarcoma
	  • Undifferentiated sarcoma

II. Cartilage-Forming Tumors	**VII. Other Tumors**

1. Benign
  • Chondroma: enchondroma, periosteal (juxtacortical)
  • Osteochondroma (osteocartilaginous exostosis): solitary, multiple hereditary
  • Chondroblastoma (epiphyseal chondroblastoma)
  • Chondromyxoid fibroma
2. Malignant
  • Chondrosarcoma
  • Juxtacortical (periosteal) chondrosarcoma
  • Mesenchymal chondrosarcoma
  • Dedifferentiated chondrosarcoma
  • Clear-cell chondrosarcoma
  • Malignant chondroblastoma
	1. Chordoma
	2. Adamantinoma of long bones
	3. Neurilemmoma
	4. Neurofibroma

	VIII. Unclassified Tumors
III. Giant-Cell Tumor (Osteoclastoma)	**IX. Tumor-Like Lesions**
IV. Marrow Tumors (Round-Cell Tumors)	1. Solitary bone cyst (simple or unicameral bone cyst) 2. Aneurysmal bone cyst 3. Juxta-articular bone cyst (intraosseous ganglion) 4. Metaphyseal fibrous defect (nonossifying fibroma) 5. Eosinophilic granuloma (histiocytosis X, Langerhans cell granulomatosis) 6. Fibrous dysplasia and osteofibrous dysplasia 7. Myositis ossificans (heterotopic ossification) 8. Brown tumor of hyperparathyroidism 9. Intraosseous epidermoid cyst 10. Giant-cell (reparative) granuloma
1. Ewing sarcoma of bone 2. Neuroectodermal tumor of bone 3. Malignant lymphoma of bone 4. Myeloma	
V. Vascular Tumors	

1. Benign
  • Hemangioma
  • Lymphangioma
  • Glomus tumor (glomangioma)
2. Intermediate or indeterminate
  • Hemangioendothelioma (epithelioid hemangioendothelioma, histiocytoid hemangioma)
  • Hemangiopericytoma
3. Malignant
  • Angiosarcoma (malignant hemangioendothelioma, hemangiosarcoma, hemangioendotheliosarcoma)
  • Malignant (hemangiopericytoma)	

From Schajowicz F, McDonald DJ. Classification of tumors and tumor lesions of the spine. Spine State Arts Rev 1998;10:1–11, with permission.

8. What is the most common primary tumor found in the spine?

Dreghorn found 55 cases of primary axial skeleton tumors in 1,950 cases in the Leeds Tumor Registry. Chordoma was the most common tumor of the spine, and osteosarcoma was the second most common. Multiple myeloma was considered a systemic disease, and only plasmacytoma was classified as a primary bone tumor in this study. Multiple myeloma has been shown to be the most frequent tumor arising in the spine by other studies.

9. Explain the relationship among age, location, and whether a spine tumor is benign or malignant?

There is a relationship between **age at diagnosis** and whether a tumor is benign. In patients younger than 18 years, 68% of all tumors are benign. If age at presentation is older than 18 years, more than 80% of all tumors are malignant. There is also a relationship between **tumor location** and whether a tumor is benign. Benign lesions tend to occur more frequently in the posterior elements (e.g. osteoblastoma, osteoid osteoma), whereas malignant lesions tend to involve the vertebral body.

10. **What are the common spine tumors according to patient age?**
    - **10 to 30 years:** Osteoid osteoma, osteoblastoma, osteochondroma, osteosarcoma, Ewing sarcoma, eosinophilic granuloma, giant cell tumor, aneurysmal bone cyst
    - **30 to 50 years:** Chordoma, chondrosarcoma, hemangioma
    - **Older than 50 years:** metastatic tumors, myeloma

11. **What are the most common spine tumors according to location in the spine?**
    - **Posterior spinal elements:** Osteoid osteoma, osteoblastoma, osteochondroma, aneurysmal bone cyst
    - **Vertebral body:** Chordoma, giant cell tumor, multiple myeloma, hemangioma, eosinophilic granuloma, aneurysmal bone cyst, metastatic disease
    - **Involvement of adjacent vertebra:** Aneurysmal bone cyst, chondrosarcoma, chordoma

12. **Why do primary spine tumors require classification according to an oncologic staging system?**
    Primary spine tumors are treated in accordance with principles of orthopaedic oncology, which require assessment of tumor biology, the relation of the tumor to surrounding structures, the risk of local tumor recurrence and metastasis, and the role of adjuvant therapies (e.g. embolization, radiation therapy).

13. **What oncologic staging system is used to classify primary benign and malignant bone tumors?**
    The Enneking staging system is used to classify primary bone tumors.
    - **Benign tumors** are classified using *arabic numerals* into three stages:
      - Stage 1: Latent lesions, which are generally asymptomatic and surrounded by a well-defined margin
      - Stage 2: Active lesions, which grow slowly and are bordered by a thin capsule
      - Stage 3: Aggressive lesions, which grow rapidly to invade surrounding structures
    - **Malignant tumors** are classified using *roman numerals* into three stages:
      - Stage I: Low-grade tumors
      - Stage II: High-grade tumors
      - Stage III: Tumor of any grade with regional or distant metastases
    - Malignant tumors are further subdivided depending on whether the tumor is **intracompartmental (A)** or **extracompartmental (B)**

14. **How does oncologic staging guide surgical tumor treatment?**
    The oncologic stage of a tumor determines the surgical margin required for treatment of a specific tumor, as well as the type of spine procedure required. The **four types of surgical margins** are:
    - **Intracapsular:** The plane of dissection is within the lesion (intracapsular) and may leave tumor at the margin of the lesion
    - **Marginal:** The plane of dissection is within the reactive zone surrounding the tumor (extracapsular) and may leave satellite lesions beyond the reactive zone
    - **Wide:** The plane of dissection is through normal tissue beyond the reactive zone (pseudocapsule surrounding the tumor). However, "skip" lesions may persist beyond a wide surgical margin
    - **Radical:** The plane of dissection includes removal of the tumor and the entire compartment of tumor origin. A radical margin cannot be achieved for spine tumors even if the spinal cord is sectioned above and below the lesion because the epidural space forms a continuous compartment from the skull to the sacrum
    In practice, surgical procedures performed for primary spine tumors can be considered as either *curettage* or *en bloc excision*.
    - **Curettage** refers to the piecemeal removal of tumor and is always an intracapsular (intralesional) procedure. This type of procedure is appropriate for stage 1 and 2 benign tumors
    - **En bloc excision** refers to an attempt to remove the entire tumor in a single piece, together with a surrounding cuff of normal healthy tissue. The surgical specimen requires gross and microscopic assessment to determine whether the surgical margin achieved was intracapsular, marginal, or wide. This type of procedure is appropriate for some stage 3 benign tumors and stage I and II malignant tumors

15. **What are the most common presenting symptoms of spinal tumors?**
    Pain is the most common presenting symptom. Pain is frequently described as persistent, progressive, and not typically associated with activity. Pain at night is a characteristic symptom. Subjective weakness, radiculopathy, objective neurologic deficit, and bladder or bowel dysfunction may develop over time. Other presenting symptoms include a palpable mass or painful spinal deformities. Pelvic girdle malignancies, including chordoma, osteosarcoma, chondrosarcoma, and malignant fibrous histiocytomas, may present with back pain and sciatica. Always remember to evaluate the pelvis if the spine appears normal or the degenerative lesion does not fit the patient's degree of pain or neurologic involvement.

16. **Are plain radiographs of value in the diagnosis of primary bone tumors of the spine?**
    Yes. Plain radiographs of the spine show a very high percentage of primary spinal tumors. The winking owl sign is a classic finding on the anteroposterior (AP) radiograph and reflects tumor destruction of the pedicle. However, a tumor may not be visible until more than 30% of trabecular bone is involved.

17. What workup is required to stage a spinal lesion?

Lab studies, plain radiography of the spine and chest, magnetic resonance imaging (MRI) of the spine, computed tomography (CT) (chest, abdomen, and pelvis, as well as CT of the lesion), technetium bone scan, and biopsy. Bone scans may be negative in the presence of myeloma, and a skeletal survey or positron emission tomography (PET) scan is preferred. CT myelography is an alternative for evaluation of the spine for patients who are unable to undergo MRI.

18. Should biopsy be performed at the same time as the CT scan?

No. A full metastatic workup, including renal ultrasound and/or intravenous pyelogram (IVP), is necessary to ensure that a renal cell tumor is not present. If a renal cell tumor is present, embolization of the spinal lesion should precede biopsy. If a renal cell tumor has been excluded prior to the CT scan, needle biopsy at the time of the CT scan is permissible. Other options for biopsy include percutaneous core needle biopsy or open biopsy (incisional vs. excisional). The selection of the appropriate technique depends on a variety of factors, including tumor location and suspected diagnosis. Oncologic principles require that biopsy technique must minimize local contamination and permit excision of the biopsy tract if a definitive surgical resection is required.

19. What lesions require selective arteriography and embolization?

- Highly vascular lesions
- Aneurysmal bone cyst
- Angiosarcoma
- Arterial vascular malformations
- Renal cell carcinoma metastasis
- Schwannomas or other neural-based tumors when resection requires sacrifice of the vertebral artery

20. Outline a recommended approach to assessment of primary spinal tumors.

Primary spine tumors benefit from an algorithmic approach, especially when a malignant primary tumor is suspected (Fig. 63-1).

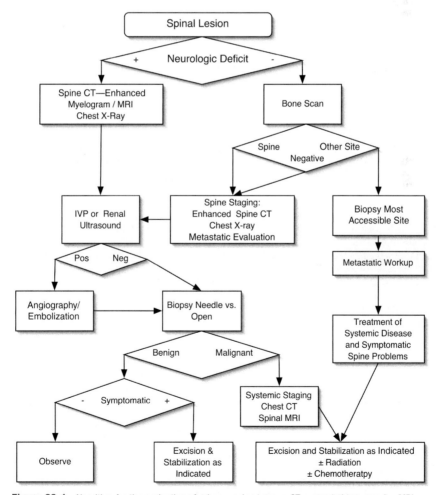

Figure 63-1. Algorithm for the evaluation of primary spine tumors. CT, computed tomography; MRI, magnetic resonance imaging. (From Weinstein JN, McLain RF. Primary tumor of the spine. Spine 1987;12:843–51, with permission.)

21. What results are expected when benign primary spine tumors are treated surgically?

Most benign primary spine tumors (e.g. osteoid osteoma, osteochondroma, Langerhans cell histiocytosis) can be adequately treated by curettage. A subset of benign lesions has either a high rate of local recurrence or causes severe local destruction (e.g. aggressive osteoblastoma, giant-cell tumor, aneurysmal bone cyst) and requires more extensive treatment. In such cases, an en bloc excision or intralesional surgery with the use of adjuvants (polymethylmethacrylate, embolization, radiation therapy) to extend the margin of the resection is considered. Overall reported success rates for surgical treatment of benign tumors range from 86% to 100%. In the Iowa study, there were no deaths and 86% of patients were alive after 5 years.

22. What results are expected when malignant primary spine tumors are treated surgically?

Surgical outcomes for malignant primary spine tumors depend on the type of surgical procedure performed and the surgical margin obtained. The 5-year survival rate for curettage of primary malignant spine tumors is 0%. The Iowa study showed a 5-year survival rate of 75% with complete resection. Incomplete resection of a malignant lesion had an 18% 5-year survival rate in this study.

23. Does the presence of neurologic structures within or adjacent to a primary malignant tumor influence the choice of surgical treatment?

No. The treatment of choice is complete resection of the tumor according to oncologic surgical principles, even if nerve roots that course through the tumor must be sacrificed. Of course, nerve roots not directly in contact with the tumor should be preserved.

24. Explain the Weinstein tumor zone system.

This zone system was developed to guide the selection of the most appropriate approach to the spine for excision and stabilization of primary bone tumors (Fig. 63-2). Four zones (I–IV) are identified and tumor extension is denoted as:
A. Intraosseous
B. Extraosseous
C. Distant tumor spread

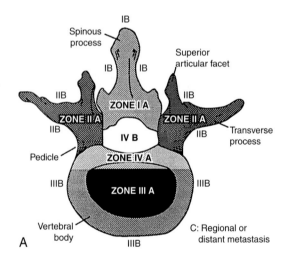

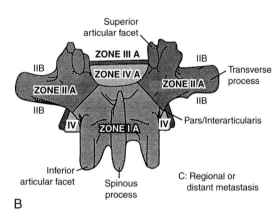

Figure 63-2. Weinstein's zones. **A,** Axial view. Zone I is composed of the spinous process, inferior articular process, and the lamina. Zone II is composed of the superior articular process, pedicle, and transverse process. Zone III is the anterior column. Zone IV is composed of the middle column and neural canal. **B,** Posterior view. **C,** Lateral view. (From Weinstein JN. Differential diagnosis and surgical treatment of primary benign and malignant neoplasms. In Frymoyer JW, editor. The Adult Spine: Principles and Practice. New York: Raven Press; 1991. p. 829–60, with permission.)

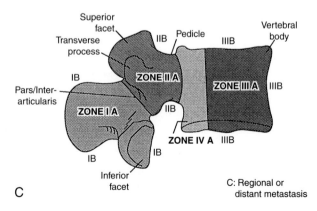

Surgical outcome depends on the zones involved, the extent of local or distant tumor spread, tumor type, and tumor grade. The appropriate surgical procedure must permit appropriate resection, adequate neural decompression, and spinal stabilization.

25. What approach is required for a tumor involving the spinous process?

An isolated tumor in the spinous process (zone IA or IB) can be adequately excised through a posterior approach with traditional laminectomy. However, a IB malignant tumor with invasion of the spinal canal becomes IV B and may be unresectable.

26. What extent of resection is required for a tumor involving the transverse process?

For a benign or intermediate tumor involving the transverse process, resection of the transverse process (for IIA tumor) or transverse process and surrounding musculature (for IIB tumor) is appropriate. If the pedicle is involved, the tumor is classified as IIA and requires removal of the pedicle for benign and intermediate tumor. A malignancy of stage IIA or IIB requires the complete removal of the transverse process, facet, and pedicle to achieve an adequate resection. If the canal is involved, the tumor becomes IVB and may not be resectable.

27. What extent of resection is required for a vertebral body tumor?

A tumor arising in the center of the body can be resected by performing an anterior vertebrectomy, frequently en bloc, in zone IIIA. If the tumor involves the cortical rim of the body, adjacent soft tissue requires resection in malignant tumors. If the back wall of the vertebral body is involved, the tumor becomes a zone IVA or IVB tumor, which may not be resectable. Zone IV tumors requiring en bloc excision are managed with combined anterior and posterior surgical approaches.

28. What is the WBB (Weinstein, Boriani, Biagini) surgical staging system for spinal tumors?

The WBB surgical staging system for spinal tumors attempts to correlate principles of oncologic surgery with the unique anatomy of the spine and to provide a guide for treatment. The vertebra is divided into 12 radiating zones in clockwise order. The spine is also divided into five tissue layers extending from the paravertebral extraosseous area to the dura:

A. Extraosseous soft tissue
B. Intraosseous superficial
C. Intraosseous deep
D. Extraosseous extradural
E. Extraosseous intradural

Based on this classification, three methods for performing en bloc tumor excisions are defined for the thoracic and lumbar lesions: *vertebrectomy*, *sagittal resection*, and *resection of the posterior arch* (Fig. 63-3).

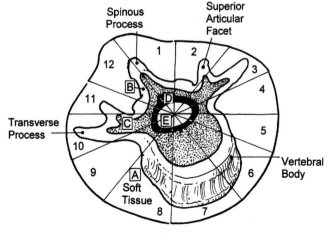

A. Extraosseous B. Intraosseous C. Intraosseous
   Soft Tissue   (Superficial)   (Deep)
D. Extraosseous E. Extraosseous
   (Extradural)   (Intradural)

Figure 63-3. WBB (Weinstein, Boriani, Biagini) surgical staging system for primary spine tumors. Tumor extent is described by dividing the involved vertebra into 12 sections in a clock-face arrangement. Five tissue layers are defined, moving from the superficial paraspinal soft tissue (layer A) to the dural compartment (layer E). The longitudinal extent of the tumor is recorded according to the levels involved. (From Hart RA, Weinstein JN. Primary benign and malignant musculoskeletal tumors. Semin Spine Surg 1995;7:288–303, with permission.)

29. When is a vertebrectomy indicated according to the WBB staging system?

Marginal or wide en bloc excision of the vertebral body can be performed if the tumor is confined to zones 4 to 8 or 5 to 9 (Fig. 63-4). In this situation, the tumor is located centrally and at least one pedicle is free from tumor. The posterior elements are removed first without entering the tumor. Subsequently the vertebral body is removed. Spinal reconstruction following tumor excision consists of an anterior allograft or structural spacer (fusion cage) combined with posterior spinal instrumentation. If the vertebral body is removed from an anterior surgical approach, anterior spinal instrumentation is typically used as well.

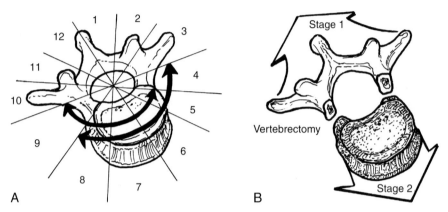

Figure 63-4. Vertebrectomy. **A,** En bloc excision with oncologically appropriate margin for a tumor located in the vertebral body is possible if at least one pedicle is uninvolved by tumor. **B,** A posterior approach is performed to remove the posterior spinal structures (spinous process, lamina, pedicles), transect the posterior longitudinal ligament, and separate the anterior surface of the dura from the posterior vertebral margin. An anterior approach is essential to maintain an oncologically appropriate margin if the tumor extends outside the vertebra.

30. When is a sagittal resection indicated according to the WBB staging system?

Sagittal resection to achieve a marginal or wide en bloc excision is indicated if tumor is confined to zones 3 to 5 or 8 to 11 (Fig. 63-5). In this situation, the tumor is located eccentrically in the vertebral body, pedicle, or transverse process. As in vertebrectomy, the first step is removal of the uninvolved posterior spinal structures. Then, with the patient in a lateral position, a combined anterior and posterior exposure permits the vertebra to be cut with a chisel remote from the tumor to permit en bloc excision. Spinal reconstruction is performed in a similar fashion to reconstruction following vertebrectomy.

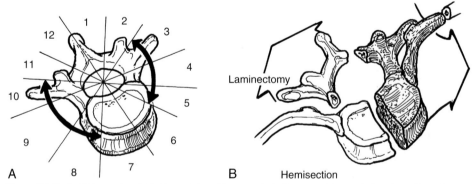

Figure 63-5. Sagittal resection. **A,** En bloc excision with an oncologically appropriate margin for a tumor located eccentrically in the body, pedicle, or transverse process is possible when the tumor is confined to zones 3 to 5 or 8 to 11. **B,** A posterior approach is performed to excise the posterior spinal structures uninvolved by tumor. A combined posterior and anterior approach is required to complete the en bloc excision safely with an oncologically appropriate margin.

31. When is resection of the posterior arch indicated according to the WBB staging system?
When a tumor is localized between zones 3 and 10, an en bloc excision can be achieved from a posterior approach (Fig. 63-6). A laminectomy is performed to expose the dural sac at the levels above and below the tumor. The pedicles are sectioned at the level of the tumor and the posterior arch is removed en bloc. The stability of the spine is restored with posterior spinal instrumentation and fusion.

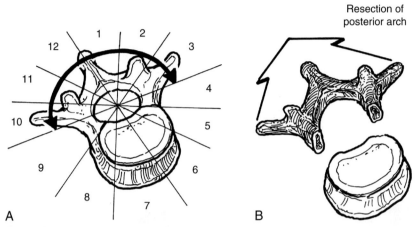

Resection of posterior arch

A   B

Figure 63-6. Resection of the posterior arch. **A,** The en bloc excision of a tumor to achieve an oncologically appropriate surgical margin is possible if tumor extent is limited between zones 3 and 10. The pedicles must be uninvolved by tumor. **B,** Surgery is performed through a posterior approach.

32. What primary tumors of the spine are amenable to kyphoplasty or vertebroplasty?
Marrow-based tumors, such as multiple myeloma and plasmacytoma, and hemangiomas.

33. How is the appropriate surgical approach selected for treatment of sacral tumors?
The appropriate surgical approach for treatment of sacral tumors depends on the amount of sacral involvement. Tumors that involve only the distal portion of the sacrum (S3 and below) can be treated with a single procedure from a posterior surgical approach. Tumors that involve the S1 and S2 segments or those that involve the entire sacrum require a combined anterior and posterior resection.

34. What is the relationship between the level of nerve root preservation and continence following sacral resection procedures?
If all sacral nerve roots can be preserved unilaterally, the patient will have near-normal bowel, bladder, and sexual function. If nerve root resection is required bilaterally, preservation of the S2 roots may preserve partial urinary and fecal continence in some patients. Preservation of at least one S3 nerve root is required for preservation of bowel and bladder function in most patients.

35. What vascular structures require control during the anterior approach for a complete sacrectomy?
The posterior divisions of the internal iliac vessels and the middle and lateral sacral vessels should be tied off during the anterior preparation for a complete sacrectomy. As the posterior resection is completed, the pelvis will hinge on the symphysis pubis. If the internal iliac vessels are not controlled, a tear of these vessels may lead to catastrophic bleeding.

36. In a complete sacrectomy, what other considerations must be taken into account during the anterior resection?
The patient is left incontinent by such a resection. Therefore, a diverting colostomy and ureterostomy should be performed during the anterior preparation. Staging the anterior preparation separately from the posterior resection should be considered. A myocutaneous vascularized flap is frequently used for posterior wound coverage. Success of this complex surgical procedure requires the support of a multidisciplinary team.

37. How does one stabilize the spine to the pelvis after complete sacrectomy?
Spinopelvic fixation is required in this setting. Interconnection of anchors in the ilium is utilized to form a foundation that allows stabilization of the ilium to the spine and opposite ilium. See Fig. 63-7.

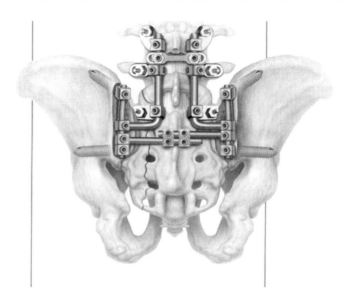

Figure 63-7. Spinopelvic fixation. (Courtesy of DePuy Spine, Raynham, MA.)

Key Points

1. Biopsy for primary spine tumors may lead to an adverse outcome unless performed according to strict oncologic principles.
2. En bloc resection with tumor-free surgical margins provides the best possible local control for malignant primary tumors of the spinal column and is the procedure of choice when technically feasible.

Websites

Comprehensive bone tumor information: http://www.bonetumor.org/navigation/pages/tumorInformation.htm
Spinal tumors: http://emedicine.medscape.com/article/1267223-overview
En bloc vertebrectomy: http://www.medscape.com/viewarticle/465369
Diagnostic tumor imaging: http://radiographics.rsna.org/content/28/4/1019.full.pdf+html?sid=990c6b4e-ef8b-4c8c-8c69-f93b103ee72d

BIBLIOGRAPHY

1. Anderson ME, McClain RF. Tumors of the spine. In: Herkowitz HN, Garfin SR, Eismont FJ, et al, editors. Rothman-Simeone The Spine. 5th ed. Philadelphia: Saunders; 2006. p. 1235–64.
2. Boriani S, Weinstein JN, Biagini R. Spine update: Primary bone tumors of the spine: Terminology and surgical staging. Spine 1997;22:1036-44.
3. Boriani S, Biagini R, De Iuri F. Primary bone tumors of the spine: A survey of the evaluation and treatment at the Istituto Orthpedico Rizzoli. Orthopedics 1995;18:993-1000.
4. Dickman CA, Fehlings MG, Gokaslan ZL, editors. Spinal Cord and Spinal Column Tumors: Principles and Practice. New York: Thieme; 2006.
5. Donthineni RD, Ofluoglu O, editors. Spine oncology. Orthop Clin North Am 2009;40:1-173.
6. Dreghorn CR, Newman RJ, Hardy GJ, et al. Primary tumors of the axial skeleton: Experience of the Leeds Regional Bone Tumor Registry. Spine 1990;15:137-40.
7. Enneking WF. A system of staging of musculoskeletal neoplasms. Clin Orthop Rel Res 1986;204:9-24.
8. Kim DH, Chang UK, Kim SH, et al, editors. Tumors of the Spine. 1st ed. Philadelphia: Saunders; 2008.
9. Scott DL, Pedlow FX, Hecht AC, et al. Tumors. In: Frymoyer JW, Wiesel SW, editors. The Adult and Pediatric Spine. 3rd ed. Philadelphia: Lippincott; 2004. p. 191–299.
10. Sundaresan N, Boriani S, Okuno S. State of the art management in spine oncology. Spine 2009;34:S7-S20.
11. Weinstein JN, McLain RF. Primary tumor of the spine. Spine 1987;12:843–51.

METASTATIC SPINE TUMORS

CHAPTER 64

Scott C. McGovern, MD, Winston Fong, MD, and Jeffrey C. Wang, MD

1. What is the most common tumor of the spine?
Metastatic lesions are the most common tumors of the spine. Metastatic lesions account for over 90% of all spine lesions. Spine metastases are the most common type of skeletal metastases.

2. What percentage of spinal metastases result in spinal cord compression?
Spinal cord compression occurs in 20% of patients who develop spinal metastases.

3. Which malignances most commonly metastasize to the spine?
In descending order of frequency: breast (21%), lung (14%), prostate (7.5%), renal (5%), gastrointestinal (GI) (5%), and thyroid (2.5%).
    A useful mnemonic to aid recall of common malignances that metastasize to the spine is P T Barnum Loves Kids (prostate, thyroid, breast, lung, kidney).

4. Where are metastatic spinal lesions most commonly located?
- **Within the vertebra**, metastatic lesions first involve the vertebral body, followed by subsequent invasion of the pedicles and surrounding tissues. The disc space remains relatively uninvolved by metastatic tumor
- **Within the spinal column**, metastatic lesions are found most commonly in the lumbar region, less commonly in the thoracic region, and least commonly in the cervical region
- **With respect to tumor type**, breast and lung tumors most commonly metastasize to the thoracic spine. Prostate tumors tend to metastasize to the lumbar spine, pelvis, and sacrum

5. What are the pathways by which metastatic disease spreads to the spine?
Potential pathways for spread of metastatic disease to the spinal column include:
1. Hematogenous spread (venous or arterial route)
2. Direct tumor extension
3. Lymphatic spread
    The most common pathway for spread of metastatic disease is the hematogenous route. Batson's plexus, a thin-walled system of veins that extend along the entire spinal column, provides a connection with the major organ systems and is a common pathway for tumor embolization.

6. What is the most common presenting complaint of a patient with a metastatic spinal tumor?
Progressive and unrelenting pain is the most common presenting complaint. The pain is often unrelieved with rest and is worse at night. Additional symptoms may include unintended weight loss, fatigue, and anorexia. Neurologic symptoms usually occur later in the disease process and may include weakness and radiculopathy. Occasionally patients may present with spinal deformity or a palpable mass.

7. What causes pain in patients with metastatic tumors of the spine?
Many causes of pain are possible: hyperemia and edema secondary to tumor, expansion of tumor into the periosteum of the vertebra and surrounding tissues, direct compression or invasion of nerve roots, spinal cord compression, and pathologic fractures with associated segmental spinal instability.

8. What radiographic signs are suggestive of a metastatic spinal lesion?
Radiographic signs suggestive of a metastatic lesion include an absent pedicle, vertebral cortical erosion/expansion, and loss of vertebral body height.

9. When are metastatic spinal tumors detectable on plain radiographs?
Most tumors of the spine are osteolytic. They are not demonstrated on plain films until more than 30% to 50% destruction of the vertebral body has occurred. An exception is prostate cancer, which tends to be blastic.

10. What is the "winking owl" sign?

This sign refers to the loss of one of the pedicle shadows on an anteroposterior (AP) spine radiograph. The cause for this radiographic finding is most frequently a metastatic vertebral lesion that has extended into the pedicle region and caused destruction of the pedicle.

11. What are the steps in evaluating a patient with a suspected metastatic spinal lesion?

Evaluation should occur in an organized and comprehensive fashion, as outlined below:

- **Patient history** should assess the pain pattern, sphincter control, neurologic symptoms, and pertinent factors such ambulatory status and ability to perform activities of daily living
- **Physical examination** should be comprehensive and include a full neurologic assessment, as well as examination of the breasts, thyroid, abdomen, prostate, and regional lymph nodes
- **Laboratory studies** should include routine tests such as complete blood count, erythrocyte sedimentation rate, electrolytes, calcium, phosphate, and liver function tests including alkaline phosphatase. Additional special tests such as prostate-specific antigen, serum and urine protein electrophoresis, thyroid function tests, and nutritional indices are obtained as indicated
- **Imaging studies** are critical for diagnosis and planning treatment. AP and lateral **spinal radiographs** are required to assess spinal anatomy and alignment. **Magnetic resonance imaging (MRI)** is the primary imaging study for defining the anatomic extent of metastatic spine tumors. Metastatic lesions generally demonstrate low signal intensity on T1 and high signal intensity on T2 and enhance when gadolinium contrast is administered. **Radioisotope studies** are valuable to survey the skeleton for metastatic lesions. Technetium total body bone scans are highly sensitive but nonspecific, and their ability to detect osseous metastases depends on tumor type. Osteoblastic metastases are readily detected on bone scan, whereas osteolytic lesions such as multiple myeloma and hypernephroma may not be detectable. Positron emission tomography (PET) is a newer radioisotope study that is highly sensitive and specific for cancer cells. Fluorine-18-labeled fluoro-deoxyglucose undergoes rapid uptake by tumor cells due to their increased metabolic activity. **Computed tomography (CT)** plays a role in the localization and quantification of bony vertebral destruction. If the primary tumor remains unknown, CT scans with intravenous and oral contrast should be obtained to assess the chest, abdomen, and pelvis in an attempt to locate the primary tumor. Women may require mammography
- **Biopsy** is performed if the diagnosis remains in question at this point. CT-guided biopsy is generally preferred. Thoracic and lumbar lesions are generally approached posterolaterally, cervical lesions are approached anterolaterally, and for sacral lesions a direct posterior approach is used. If there is a possibility of infection, cultures should be obtained at the time of biopsy. Bone marrow biopsy is performed if multiple myeloma is in the differential diagnosis

12. What is the goal for treatment of a metastatic spinal lesion?

The goal of treatment is generally palliation and not cure. Metastasis indicates that regional disease has progressed to a systemic illness that is generally incurable. Treatment is directed toward maximizing quality of life by providing pain relief and maintaining or restoring neurologic function. An exception is the patient with a solitary metastasis and potential for long-term survival with en bloc spondylectomy.

13. What are the options for treatment of a metastatic spinal lesion?

Potential treatment options include orthotic treatment, bisphosphonates, steroids, radiotherapy, chemotherapy, hormonal therapy, kyphoplasty and/or vertebroplasty, surgical decompression and stabilization, or a combination of these options.

14. What factors are important in determining a treatment plan for patients with a spinal metastatic lesion?

- Tumor type, grade, and location
- Tumor radiosensitivity
- Extent/pattern of spinal metastases
- Metastases to major internal organs
- Life expectancy
- Neurologic status
- Comorbid medical conditions
- Nutritional status
- Performance status and activity level
- Patient and family preferences

15. What classifications have been proposed to guide decision making for the patient with metastatic spinal disease?

Various classifications for patients with metastatic spinal disease have been proposed to:

- Guide treatment (Harrington classification)
- Determine prognosis and life expectancy (Tokuhashi classification)
- Determine the most appropriate surgical procedure (Tomita classification)

The Harrington classification stratified patients with spinal metastases into five groups based on *spinal stability* and *neurologic status*:
- Class 1: No significant neurologic dysfunction
- Class 2: Bone involvement without collapse or instability, minimal neurologic involvement
- Class 3: Major neurologic dysfunction without significant bone involvement or instability
- Class 4: Vertebral collapse or instability causing pain, no significant neurologic compromise
- Class 5: Vertebral collapse or instability with major neurologic impairment

As new treatment algorithms for metastatic spine disease evolve, alternative classification systems have been proposed. A decision framework (NOMS) based on neurologic (N), oncologic (O), mechanical instability (M), and systemic diseases and medical comorbidity (S) has been developed. An additional classification to identify neoplastic spinal instability and identify patients who could benefit from surgical consultation, the Spine Instability Neoplastic Score (SINS), has been proposed.

16. What is the role of bisphosphonates in treatment of metastatic spinal disease?
Bisphosphonates are useful for controlling bone pain due to metastatic tumor and also decrease the incidence of skeletal-related complications such as pathologic fracture and hypercalcemia of malignancy. Metastatic tumor cells secrete cellular modulators including parathyroid hormone-related protein receptor activator for nuclear factor κ B ligand (RANKL), and serine protease urokinase, which exert their effect through stimulation of osteoclasts. Bisphosphonates function by binding to bone matrix and lead to osteoclast dysfunction and apoptosis.

17. What is the role of steroid treatment for metastatic spinal lesions?
Steroids (usually dexamethasone) play a role in the initial treatment of edema associated with neural compression prior to definitive treatment. Complications associated with use of steroids include psychosis, diabetes, infection, avascular necrosis of the hip, and GI bleeding.

18. What are the indications for radiation therapy as the primary form of treatment for metastatic spinal lesions?
Radiation therapy plays a role in the treatment of malignancies by promoting reossification of the vertebral body and reducing tumor load. Pain relief has been reported in up to 80% of patients receiving radiation. Use of a spinal orthosis for 3 months following radiation therapy is recommended to prevent development of spinal fracture and instability. Tumors that are sensitive to radiation therapy include lung, breast, and prostate cancer, as well as lymphoma and myeloma. Radioresistant tumors include GI adenocarcinoma, metastatic melanoma, thyroid carcinoma, and renal cell carcinoma. Potential indications for radiation therapy as the primary form of treatment for metastatic spinal lesions include radiosensitive tumors with stable or slowly progressive neurologic symptoms, spinal canal compromise secondary to soft tissue tumor lesions, and patients who are not candidates for surgery due to medical comorbidities.

Radiation therapy is not indicated for patients with spinal canal compromise secondary to bone or for patients with spinal instability due to metastatic spinal disease. Patients with metastatic disease and epidural compression who are surgically treated with spinal cord decompression and reconstruction followed by radiation have been shown to have more favorable outcomes (improved neurologic function and pain relief) than patients treated with radiation alone.

19. What complications are associated with use of radiation therapy for metastatic spine lesions?
Complications associated with radiation therapy include bone marrow suppression, impaired wound healing, radiation myelopathy, neoplasia, and impaired healing of bone grafts. When appropriate, surgical decompression prior to radiation is preferred because this approach is associated with improved neurologic outcomes and decreased rates of postsurgical wound complications. In children, radiation therapy may lead to skeletal growth arrest, scoliosis, and neoplasia. The radiation sensitivity of the spinal cord and cauda equina limit the dose of radiation that can be safely administered with traditional external beam radiation therapy. New techniques such as intensity modulated radiation therapy (IMRT) and three-dimensional conformal radiation therapy (3D-CRT) have been developed to provide a higher radiation tumor dose without increasing damage to surrounding tissues.

20. What is the role of chemotherapy in the treatment of a metastatic spinal lesion?
Chemotherapy is used in patients with documented spinal metastases, patients at risk of developing spinal metastases, and patients with spinal lesions not amenable to surgical excision. The response to chemotherapy is determined by the tumor type. Tumors that are highly sensitive to chemotherapy include small-cell carcinoma of the lung, Ewing's sarcoma, thyroid carcinoma, breast carcinoma, lymphoma, germ cell tumors, and neuroblastoma. Tumors that are relatively resistant to chemotherapy include adenocarcinoma of the lung and GI tract, squamous cell carcinoma of the lung, metastatic melanoma, and renal cell carcinoma.

21. **What are the indications for surgical intervention for metastatic spinal lesions?**
Patients who are advised to undergo surgery for metastatic lesions of the spine should be predicted to survive the proposed procedure and must demonstrate adequate nutritional parameters to permit wound healing. The patient's expected lifespan should be greater than 3 months. Indications for surgical intervention in such patients include:
- Need for a definitive histologic diagnosis
- Impending pathologic fracture
- Spinal instability
- Pathologic fracture with bone in the spinal canal
- Increasing neurologic deficit despite steroid administration or during the course of radiation therapy
- Neurologic compromise at a previously irradiated level
- Radioresistant tumors

22. **What are the relative contraindications to surgical reconstruction for patients with metastatic spinal disease?**
- Widespread visceral or brain metastases
- Severe nutritional depletion
- Immunosuppression
- Significant metastases in all three spinal metastases regions
- Active infection
- Expected survival less than 3 months

23. **For patients with symptomatic spinal cord compression, what is the most important prognostic factor?**
The most important prognostic factor is the severity and latency of the neurologic deficit prior to treatment. Profound weakness lasting more than 48 hours generally fails to respond to radiation or surgical treatment. Epidural spinal cord compression is an oncologic emergency requiring prompt diagnosis and treatment.

24. **What is the role of embolization in the treatment of metastatic spinal disease?**
Embolization of spinal tumors can be used to reduce operative blood loss in hypervascular tumors such as renal cell carcinoma, thyroid carcinoma, and Ewing's sarcoma.

25. **What surgical approaches have been described for treating metastatic spinal lesions?**
Surgical approaches described for treatment of metastatic lesions include:
1. Posterior
2. Anterior
3. Combined anterior and posterior
4. Posterolateral
5. Minimally invasive (e.g. kyphoplasty, vertebroplasty)

26. **Why is laminectomy usually an inadequate procedure for treatment of a metastatic spinal lesion?**
In patients with neurologic deficit due to metastatic spinal lesions, 70% have anterior tumor compressing the dural sac, 20% have lateral compression of the dural sac, and only 10% have posterior neural compression by tumor mass. Inadequate decompression of the anterior spinal canal is obtained by a laminectomy. Furthermore, the destabilization of the spinal column created by a laminectomy increases the risk of postoperative spinal cord compression and paraplegia due to the development of postoperative kyphotic deformity and increased spinal instability. The primary indication for laminectomy as a stand-alone procedure is the relatively uncommon presentation of posterior epidural compression by metastatic tumor in a patient without anterior spinal column involvement by tumor.

27. **What factors determine the choice of surgical approach for metastatic spinal lesions?**
The approach to the spine depends on the location of the tumor, the presence/absence of spinal instability, and the presence/absence of neural compression/neural deficit. Because most metastases involve the vertebral body, reconstruction of the anterior and middle spinal columns is usually indicated. The anterior approach provides direct access to remove the affected vertebral body, decompress the dural sac, and reconstruct the anterior and middle spinal columns with an intracolumnar spacer and anterior spinal instrumentation. However, if two or more vertebral bodies require removal or if bone quality is poor, posterior spinal instrumentation is required. A single-stage posterolateral approach for decompression and stabilization is an alternative surgical option for patients with circumferential epidural spinal cord compression, patients who cannot tolerate an anterior approach due to medical comorbidities, and tumors located in the upper thoracic region that are difficult to approach through a thoracotomy.

28. **What are the options for reconstruction of the anterior and middle spinal columns after resection of a metastatic lesion involving the vertebral body?**
Options for reconstruction of the anterior and middle spinal columns include bone graft (autograft or allograft), methylmethacrylate, titanium mesh cages, and carbon fiber or polyether ether ketone (PEEK) cages. Expandable cages

have been popularized for use in this setting. All of these intracolumnar implants are used in combination with anterior spinal instrumentation (plate systems, rod systems) and/or posterior segmental spinal fixation.

29. **What is the role of kyphoplasty and vertebroplasty in the treatment of spinal metastatic disease?**

Kyphoplasty and vertebroplasty provide a minimally invasive approach for reduction of pain associated with pathologic spine fractures resulting from metastatic disease. The injected cement does not interfere with radiation therapy. The most common complication associated with these techniques is local cement extrusion.

Contraindications to these procedures include: vertebral body height loss exceeding 75%, posterior vertebral body cortex destruction, and significant spinal canal compromise due to epidural tumor.

30. **A 50-year-old woman with a history of breast cancer has been treated with a right mastectomy, radiation therapy, and chemotherapy. The patient presents with a several-week history of unrelenting back pain and increasing weakness in both lower extremities. The patient remains ambulatory and has intact bowel and bladder function. The patient has normal nutritional indices and has no other major medical problems. Plain radiographs (Fig. 64-1), axial MRI (Fig. 64-2), sagittal MRI (Fig. 64-3), and axial CT (Fig. 64-4) are shown below. What treatment should be advised?**

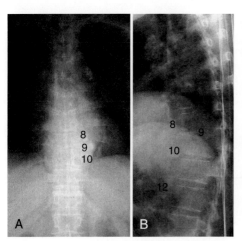

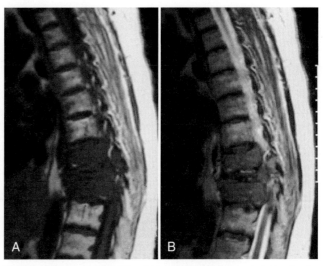

Figure 64-1. **A,** Anteroposterior and **B,** lateral radiographs show pathologic fractures involving the T9 and T10 vertebral bodies with associated loss of vertebral body height and kyphotic deformity.

Figure 64-3. **A,** T1- and **B,** T2-weighted sagittal MRI images depict two-level vertebral body destruction and severe spinal cord compression.

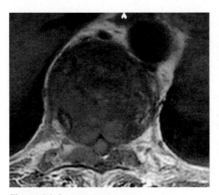

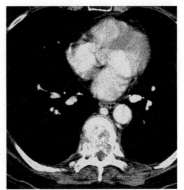

Figure 64-2. Axial MRI image shows tumor infiltration of all three spinal columns with tumor extension into the epidural space.

Figure 64-4. Axial CT image at the level of pathologic fracture shows infiltrative osseous destruction and narrowing of the spinal canal.

If the patient is willing to undergo surgery, this is the best treatment option. Two-level anterior thoracic spinal cord compression is most directly treated through a transthoracic anterior surgical approach. A kyphotic deformity due to multilevel tumor involvement and pathologic fracture is a classic indication for a combined approach with anterior and posterior spinal reconstruction. In this case, an initial anterior approach was used to decompress the spinal cord and place an expandable cage and bridging anterior plate. Subsequent posterior segmental spinal instrumentation was used to correct the kyphotic deformity and supplement the anterior spinal construct (Fig. 64-5). A single-stage posterior approach with posterolateral decompression and posterior placement of an expandable cage combined with posterior segmental spinal instrumentation is an alternative treatment option.

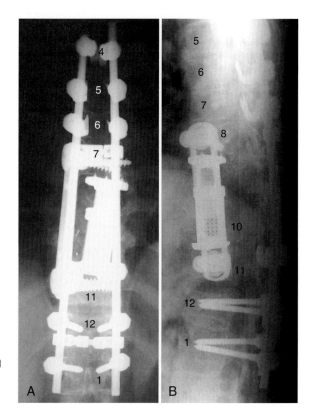

Figure 64-5. **A,** Anteroposterior and **B,** lateral radiographs following two-stage spinal reconstruction. In the first stage, an anterior transthoracic exposure was performed to permit T9 and T10 corpectomies and placement of an expandable cage and anterior plate. In the second stage, posterior segmental spinal instrumentation and posterior decompression were performed.

Key Points

1. Back pain is the most common presenting symptom in patients with metastatic spinal disease.
2. Treatment of metastatic spinal disease is directed toward maximizing quality of life by providing pain relief and maintaining or restoring neurologic function.
3. Treatment strategies for metastatic spine tumors include orthoses, bisphosphonates, steroids, radiotherapy, chemotherapy, hormonal therapy, vertebroplasty, kyphoplasty, surgical decompression and stabilization, or a combination of these options.

Websites

En bloc spondylectomy for spinal metastases: http://www.medscape.com/viewarticle/466858
Metastatic spine tumors: http://www.medscape.com/viewarticle/421498
Vertebroplasty and kyphoplasty for spinal metastases: http://www.orthonurse.org/portals/0/kyphoplasty%201.pdf

BIBLIOGRAPHY

1. Anderson MW, McLain RF. Tumors of the spine. In: Rothman RH, Simeone FA, editors. The Spine. 5th ed. Philadelphia: Saunders; 2006. p. 1235–64.
2. Bilsky MH, Azeem S. The NOMS framework for decision-making in metastatic cervical spine tumors. Curr Opinion in Ortho 2007;18:263–69.
3. Fisher CG, DiPaola CP, Ryken TC, et al. A novel classification system for spinal instability in neoplastic disease. An evidence-based consensus approach and expert consensus from the Spine Oncology Study Group. Spine 2010;35:E1221–E1229.
4. Hecht AC, Scott DL, Crichlow R, et al. Tumors: Metastatic disease. In: Frymoyer JW, Wiesel SW, Howard SA, et al, editors. The Adult and Pediatric Spine. 3rd ed. Philadelphia: Lippincott; 2004. p. 247–88.
5. Ibrahim A, Crockard A, Antonietti P, et al. Does spinal surgery improve the quality of life for those with extradural (spinal) osseous metastases? An international multicenter prospective observational study of 223 patients. J Neurosurg Spine 2008;8:271–8.
6. Patchell RA, Tibbs PA, Regine WF, et al. Direct decompressive surgical resection in the treatment of spinal cord compression caused by metastatic cancer: A randomized trial. Lancet 2005;366:643–8.
7. Tokuhashi Y, Matsuzaki H, Toriyama S, et al. Scoring system for the preoperative evaluation of metastatic spine tumor progression. Spine 1990;15:1110–3.
8. Tomita K, Kawahara N, Kobayashi T, et al. Surgical strategy for spinal metastases. Spine 2001;26:298–306.

METABOLIC BONE DISEASES OF THE SPINE

Edward D. Simmons, MD, MSc, FRCS(c), and Yinggang Zheng, MD

1. **What common metabolic bone diseases cause significant problems relating to the spinal column?**

   Osteoporosis, osteomalacia, Paget's disease, and renal osteodystrophy are common metabolic bone diseases associated with spinal pain and spinal deformity.

2. **What are two major functions of bone?**

   Two major bone functions are maintenance of calcium hemostasis and maintenance of skeletal integrity.

3. **Describe the two major types of bone tissue.**

   The skeleton is composed of two types of bone tissue: cortical (compact) bone (80%) and cancellous (trabecular) bone (20%). Cortical bone provides skeletal strength and rigidity, especially under torsional and bending loads. Cancellous bone serves two major functions: resistance to compressive loads and facilitation of bone remodeling by providing a high surface area for metabolic activity.

4. **Describe the composition of bone tissue.**

   Bone tissue is composed of cells and matrix. The cellular components of bone include osteoblasts, osteocytes, and osteoclasts. The matrix is composed of organic components (40%) and inorganic components (60%). The organic components include type 1 collagen, proteoglycans, noncollagenous matrix proteins (e.g. osteocalcin, osteonectin), and growth factors. The inorganic component, predominantly calcium hydroxyapatite $[Ca_{10} (PO_4)_6 (OH)_2]$, provides mineralization of the matrix and is responsible for the hardness and rigidity of bone tissue.

5. **Describe the cellular components of bone tissue.**
   - **Osteoclasts** develop from the hematopoietic stem cell line. These multinucleated giant cells are located in cavities along bone surfaces called Howship's lacunae and are responsible for bone resorption
   - **Osteoblasts** develop from the pluripotential mesenchymal stem cells of bone marrow and perform various functions, including synthesis of osteoid (unmineralized bone matrix), bone mineralization, and regulation of calcium and phosphate flux
   - **Osteocytes** arise from osteoblasts that have undergone terminal cell division and become surrounded by mineralized bone matrix. They possess extensive cell processes that communicate with other osteocytes and osteoblasts

6. **What factors are responsible for regulation of bone mineral balance?**

   Bone mineral balance is tightly regulated by the interaction of vitamin D metabolites (25-hydroxyvitamin D and 1,25-dihydroxyvitamin D), parathyroid hormone (PTH), and calcitonin. Calcium homeostasis depends on the interaction of these factors with various organ systems, including the liver, kidney, and gastrointestinal tract, as well as the thyroid and parathyroid glands.

7. **Distinguish among osteoporosis, osteomalacia, and osteopenia.**
   - **Osteoporosis** is a metabolic bone disease characterized by a decreased amount of normally mineralized bone per unit volume, resulting in skeletal fragility and increased risk of fracture
   - **Osteomalacia** is a metabolic bone disease characterized by delayed or impaired mineralization of bone matrix, resulting in bone fragility
   - **Osteopenia** is a descriptive and nonspecific term for decreased radiographic bone density
   See Figure 65-1.

8. **What are the different types of osteoporosis?**

   Osteoporosis has been classified into two major types: primary and secondary.
   - **Primary osteoporosis** is further subdivided into type 1 or postmenopausal osteoporosis and type 2 or senile osteoporosis
     - **Type 1** osteoporosis is due to estrogen deficiency and typically occurs in women 5 to 10 years after menopause. It predominantly affects trabecular bone and is associated with vertebral fractures, intertrochanteric hip fractures, and distal radius fractures

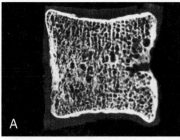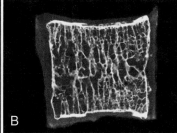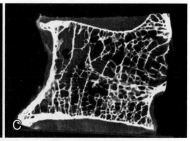

Figure 65-1. Specimen radiographs of 2-mm slices through the vertebral body of T2. **A,** The first specimen represents normal bone texture, density, and pattern. **B,** The second specimen shows a moderate degree of osteopenia, with accentuation of the vertical trabeculae and selective loss of the horizontal trabeculae. **C,** The third specimen shows severe osteoporosis, with irregular thin trabeculae and partial central collapse of the superior endplate. (From Bullough PG. Orthopaedic Pathology. 5th ed. Philadelphia: Mosby; 2010.)

○ **Type 2** osteoporosis occurs secondary to aging and calcium deficiency and is seen in both women and men after age 70 years. It affects both cortical and trabecular bone and is associated with vertebral fractures, femoral neck fractures, and pelvic fractures, as well as proximal tibia and humerus fractures
• **Secondary osteoporosis** occurs as a result of endocrinopathies or other disease states

9. What are the most common causes of secondary osteoporosis?
• **Endocrine disorders:** Cushing's disease, hypogonadism, hyperthyroidism, hyperparathyroidism, diabetes mellitus
• **Marrow disorders:** Lymphoma, multiple myeloma, metastatic disease, chronic alcohol use
• **Collagen disorders:** Osteogenesis imperfecta, Marfan's syndrome
• **Gastrointestinal disorders:** Malabsorption, malnutrition
• **Medications:** Thyroid replacement therapy, steroids, anticonvulsants, chemotherapy, aluminum-containing antacids

10. How can a physician determine the cause of osteoporosis?
Primary osteoporosis is a diagnosis of exclusion. The physician should perform a complete history and physical examination with attention to specific risk factors for secondary osteoporosis and osteomalacia. Laboratory tests, imaging tests, and transiliac bone biopsy may be indicated based on the history and physical examination. For example:
• *To rule out local bone tumor:* perform radiographs, magnetic resonance imaging (MRI), computed tomography (CT), and/or bone scan
• *To rule out bone marrow abnormality:* Perform complete blood count with differential, erythrocyte sedimentation rate, serum protein electrophoresis, and urinary protein electrophoresis
• *To rule out endocrinopathy:* Assess thyroid function tests, glucose, PTH, testosterone level
• *To rule out osteomalacia:* Assess serum calcium, phosphate, alkaline phosphatase, PTH, 25(OH) vitamin D, and 24-hour urine calcium level; consider a bone biopsy

11. What are the risk factors for osteoporotic fractures?
See Table 65-1.

Table 65-1. Risk Factors for Osteoporotic Fractures

Nonmodifiable Risk Factors	Potentially Modifiable Risk Factors
• Patient history of fracture during adulthood • History of fracture in a first-degree relative • Caucasian race • Advanced age • Female sex • Dementia • Poor health or frailty	• Smoking • Low body weight • Estrogen deficiency (menopause before age 45 years, bilateral ovariectomy, prolonged premenopausal amenorrhea >1 year) • Low calcium or vitamin D intake • Alcoholism • Impaired eyesight despite correction • Recurrent falls • Inadequate physical activity • Poor health or frailty

12. Summarize the major recommendations for physicians in relation to osteoporosis screening and treatment.
- Counsel all women about risk factors for osteoporosis, a silent disease process that is generally preventable and treatable
- Recommend bone mineral density (BMD) testing in accordance with current National Osteoporosis Clinical Practice Guidelines, which include:
  1. Women aged 65 years and older and men aged 70 years or older regardless of additional risk factors
  2. Postmenopausal women age 50 to 69 years with one or more additional risk factors for osteoporotic fracture
  3. Adults with diseases or using medications associated with low bone mass (e.g. rheumatoid arthritis, daily glucocorticoid use). http://www.nof.org/professionals/clinical-guidelines
- Advise all patients to maintain adequate dietary calcium and vitamin D intake
- Recommend a routine of weight-bearing and muscle-strengthening exercise to reduce the risk of falls and fractures
- Counsel patients to avoid smoking and limit alcohol intake
- Recommend pharmacologic therapy for osteoporosis prevention and treatment when appropriate

13. What is peak bone mass (PBM)?
Peak bone mass (PBM) is defined as the highest level of bone mass achieved as a result of normal growth. Bone mineral density (BMD) increases rapidly during adolescence until PBM is reached between 16 and 25 years of age. After age 30, men normally lose bone at a rate of 0.3% per year. After age 30, women normally lose bone at a rate of 0.5% per year until menopause, at which time the rate of bone loss accelerates to 2% to 3% per year over a 6- to 10-year period. The greater the PBM, the better the chance of avoiding osteoporosis later in life.

14. What are the daily recommended vitamin D and calcium requirements?
The daily adult requirement for vitamin D is 800 to 1000 units. The daily adult requirement for calcium (Ca) is 1200 mg for the 26-49 year age group. Recommendations regarding daily requirements are based on patient age and are frequently updated to reflect the current state of scientific knowledge See Table 65-2.

Table 65-2. Daily Calcium Requirements	
AGE GROUP	REQUIREMENT (MG OF ELEMENTAL CA/DAY)
1–10 years	800–1000
11–25 years	1200
26–49 years (premenopausal)	1200
>50 years (postmenopausal)	1500
Pregnancy	1500
Lactation	1500–2000

15. How is BMD measured?
The most widely accepted method of determining BMD is **dual-energy x-ray absorptiometry (DEXA)** at the hip. BMD is reported in terms of two absolute values: **T-score** (units of standard deviation compared with the bone density of a healthy 30-year-old) and **Z-score** (units of standard deviation compared with age- and sex-matched controls). The World Health Organization has defined osteoporosis in terms of the T-score. See Table 65-3.

The T-score can be used to predict fracture risk. A one-point decrease in standard deviation in T-score is associated with a 2.5 times increased risk of fracture. The Z-score is valuable in ruling out secondary causes of osteoporosis. Secondary causes of osteoporosis are unlikely in the presence of a normal Z-score.

Table 65-3. T-Score for Osteoporosis	
Normal	Between +1 and −1 standard deviation of peak
Osteopenia	Between −1 and −2.5 below peak
Osteoporosis	> −2.5 standard deviations below peak
Severe osteoporosis	> −2.5 standard deviations below peak plus fracture

16. What are the limitations of DEXA scans for predicting fracture risk?
DEXA scans do not convey all the necessary information to predict a specific patient's fracture risk. This is highlighted by the finding that up to half of all osteoporotic-related fractures occur in patients with BMD values classified as osteopenia. Thus, factors in addition to BMD require consideration in the assessment of fracture risk. The **FRAX® tool**

(http://www.sheffield.ac.uk/FRAX/) has been developed by the World Health Organization to integrate important clinical risk factors and bone density measurements to determine the 10-year probability of hip fracture and major osteoporotic fracture. These risk factors include age, body mass index, fracture history, family history of fracture, steroid use, rheumatoid arthritis, alcohol use, smoking, and secondary osteoporosis.

17. When is pharmacologic treatment advised for patients with osteopenia or osteoporosis?

Current indications for pharmacologic treatment in the United States include:

- Postmenopausal females or males age 50 or greater with a T-score of -2.5 or lower at the hip or spine or patients in this age range with a prior hip or spine fracture
- Patients with osteopenia (T-score -1 to -2.5) and a 10-year probability of hip fracture 3% or greater or a 10-year probability of any major osteoporosis-related fracture 20% or greater (fracture probabilities are determined by FRAX®).

18. What pharmacologic therapies are currently available for osteoporosis?

Food and Drug Administration (FDA)-approved medications for osteoporosis prevention and treatment include:

- **Oral bisphosphonates:** These antiresorptive agents are analogs of pyrophosphates and are absorbed onto the surface of hydroxyapatite crystals in bone. They alter bone remodeling by decreasing bone resorption
- **Intravenous bisphosphonates:** Provide an alternative medication for patients who are unable to tolerate an oral bisphosphonate
- **Estrogen/hormone replacement:** Estrogen replacement initiated after the onset of menopause is used to counteract the increased rate of bone loss noted during this period. Contraindications to estrogen use include a history of breast cancer, uterine cancer, or thromboembolism. Recent studies have raised controversy about the risks/benefits of estrogen use
- **Selective estrogen receptor modulators (SERMS):** This drug class was developed in an attempt to provide the beneficial effects of estrogen therapy in patients unable to take estrogen due to a history of breast or uterine cancer
- **Calcitonin:** This peptide hormone functions by reducing osteoclastic bone resorption. It is considered to be less effective than bisphosphonates or hormone replacement. It also provides an analgesic effect in patients with acute osteoporotic fractures. It may be administered by nasal spray or injection
- **Parathyroid hormone:** Teriparatide or PTH(1-34) is an anabolic agent that increases new bone formation and has demonstrated efficacy in the treatment of osteoporosis. It is administered by injection via a prefilled delivery device
- **Denosumab:** This monoclonal antibody binds to and inhibits RANK ligand (receptor activator of nuclear factor kappa B ligand [RANKL]). This action inhibits osteoclast formation, function, and survival.

19. Describe the typical clinical presentation of a patient with spinal osteoporosis.

The clinical presentation can be quite variable. In general, patients with osteoporosis are asymptomatic until a fracture occurs. However, not all patients with spinal fractures are symptomatic, and the initial presentation may be a significant loss of height associated with development of an exaggerated thoracic kyphosis (dowager's hump). Many patients present with acute severe pain after minimal trauma. Paravertebral muscle spasm is common, and tenderness can often be elicited at the fracture site with palpation. Neurologic signs and symptoms are uncommon but may occur (senile burst fracture). Complications associated with osteoporotic vertebral fractures include postural deformity, additional fractures, restrictive lung disease (following thoracic fractures), abdominal dysfunction (following lumbar fractures), chronic pain, disability, and an increased mortality rate.

20. What are the treatment options for painful vertebral compression fractures?

Treatment options for painful vertebral compression fractures include bedrest, narcotic analgesics, calcitonin, and spinal orthoses. Minimally invasive cement injection procedures (vertebroplasty, kyphoplasty) play a role in select patients. Major open surgical procedures are reserved for patients with severe spinal deformity or neurologic deficits because of the poor surgical outcomes noted in patients with osteopenic bone and advanced age.

21. What is the rationale for performing a vertebral bone biopsy in conjunction with a kyphoplasty procedure for cement augmentation of a vertebral body compression fracture?

Although the majority of vertebral body compression fractures are due to osteoporosis, other etiologies that may be responsible for compression fractures include osteomalacia, benign or malignant neoplasm, metastatic disease, and osteomyelitis. Vertebral bone biopsy during kyphoplasty does not add to the risk of the procedure and provides a potential means for diagnosis of such pathologic entities. However, it is critical to correlate the histologic findings with clinical and laboratory studies in order to arrive at an accurate diagnosis.

22. What are the causes of osteomalacia?

The causes of osteomalacia are varied. To arrive at the correct diagnosis, all of the causes must be considered in the course of an appropriate workup, including:

1. Nutritional deficiency
    - Vitamin D deficiency
    - Calcium deficiency due to dietary chelators (e.g. phytates, oxalates)
    - Phosphorus deficiency (e.g. secondary to aluminum-containing antacids)

2. Gastrointestinal malabsorption
   - Intestinal disease
   - Following intestinal surgery
3. Renal tubular acidosis
4. Renal tubular defects causing renal phosphate leak (e.g. vitamin-dependent rickets, type 1 and 2; Fanconi's syndrome)
5. Renal osteodystrophy
6. Miscellaneous causes
   - Anticonvulsants (induce hepatic P450 microsomal system, thereby increasing degradation of vitamin D metabolites)
   - Oncogenic
   - Heavy metal intoxication
   - Hypophosphatasia

23. **Compare and contrast important findings that aid in distinguishing osteomalacia and osteoporosis.**
    - **Symptoms:** Osteoporosis is generally asymptomatic until a fracture occurs. Osteomalacia is frequently associated with generalized bone pain and tenderness most commonly localized to the appendicular skeleton
    - **Radiographs:** Osteoporosis and osteomalacia have many similar features but axial involvement predominates in osteoporosis, and appendicular findings predominate in osteomalacia. Findings consistent with osteomalacia include pseudofractures, Looser's zones, and biconcave vertebra *(codfish vertebra)*
    - **Laboratory tests:** Laboratory tests are generally normal in osteoporosis. Osteomalacia is associated with decreased or normal serum calcium, low serum phosphate, increased serum alkaline phosphatase, and increased urine phosphate
    - **Bone biopsy:** In osteoporosis a biopsy reveals a decreased quantity of normally mineralized bone. The hallmark of osteomalacia is increased width and extent of osteoid seams

24. **What is Paget's disease?**
    Paget's disease is named after Sir James Paget, who described its clinical and pathologic aspects in 1876. Paget's disease is the second most common metabolic bone disease. It has been found in up to 5% of northern European adults older than 55 years. However, most affected individuals are asymptomatic. The cause is unknown, but viral infection and genetic factors are believed to be responsible. The disease causes focal enlargement and deformity of the skeleton. The pathologic lesion is abnormal bone remodeling. The disease progresses through three phases: lytic, lytic-blastic, and blastic. Radiographs are characteristic and show osteosclerosis with bone enlargement. Elevated alkaline phosphatase levels are typical. The wide spectrum of clinical presentation depends on the extent and site of skeletal involvement. Paget's disease commonly affects the skull, hip joints, pelvis, and spine. Back pain in the lumbar or sacral region is common. Neurologic deficits may occur due to the compression of spinal cord or nerve roots from enlarging vertebrae. Spinal stenosis is common when the lower lumbar spine is involved. Treatment options include medication to suppress osteoclastic activity (bisphosphonates, calcitonin, plicamycin), as well as surgical treatment for spinal stenosis, fracture, or degenerative joint disease. Approximately 1% of patients develop malignant degeneration within a focus of Paget's disease. This complication usually develops in the peripheral skeleton and rarely involves the spine. See Figure 65-2.

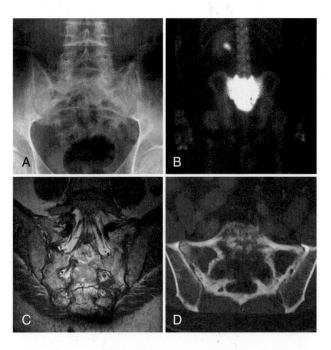

Figure 65-2. Radiographic abnormalities in Paget's disease: sacrum in a 76-year-old man. **A,** Radiograph shows few trabeculae, and the entire bone is osteopenic. The remaining trabecular pattern is coarsened, diagnostic of Paget's disease. **B,** Marked focal accumulation is seen throughout the entire sacrum, a pattern virtually diagnostic of Paget's disease. **C,** Oblique coronal T1-weighted (TR/TE, 500/20) spin echo MR image shows preservation of normal fatty marrow. The coarse trabeculae are not well appreciated. **D,** Axial CT scan viewed at a bone window demonstrates increased fatty marrow, with coarse trabeculae and thickened cortex. (From Resnick D, Kransdorf MJ, editors. Resnick: Bone and Joint Imaging. 3rd ed. Philadelphia: Saunders; 2005.)

Key Points

1. Osteoporosis is a metabolic bone disease characterized by a decreased amount of normally mineralized bone per unit volume.
2. Osteomalacia is a metabolic bone disease characterized by delayed or impaired mineralization of bone matrix.
3. Osteopenia is a descriptive and nonspecific term for decreased radiographic bone density.

Websites

Osteoporosis and bone physiology: http://courses.washington.edu/bonephys/index.html
Clinician's guide to prevention and treatment of osteoporosis (2010):
   http://www.nof.org/professionals/clinical-guidelines
The Paget foundation: http://www.paget.org/
World Health Organization Fracture Risk Assessment Tool (FRAX):
   http://www.sheffield.ac.uk/FRAX/

BIBLIOGRAPHY

1. Allen TR, Kum JB, Weidner N, et al. Biopsy of osteoporotic vertebral compression fractures during kyphoplasty: Unsuspected histologic findings of chronic osteitis without clinical evidence of osteomyelitis. Spine 2009;24:1486–91.
2. Dawson-Hughes B, Lindsay R, Khosla S, et al. Clinician's guide to prevention and treatment of osteoporosis. Washington, DC: National Osteoporosis Foundation; 2010.
3. Dell RM, Greene D, Anderson D, et al. Osteoporosis disease management: What every orthopaedic surgeon should know. J Bone Joint Surg 2009;91:S79–S86.
4. Garfin SR, Yuan HA, Reiley MA. New technologies in spine: Kyphoplasty and vertebroplasty for the treatment of painful osteoporotic compression fractures. Spine 2001;26:1511–15.
5. Lane JM, Sherman PJ, Madore GR. Metabolic bone disorders of the spine. In: Herkowitz HN, Garfin SR, Eismont FJ, Bell GR, Balderston RA, editors. Rothman–Simeone The Spine. 5th ed. Philadelphia: Saunders; 2006 p. 1317–40.

TREATMENT OPTIONS FOR OSTEOPOROTIC VERTEBRAL COMPRESSION FRACTURES

R. Carter Cassidy, MD, and Vincent J. Devlin, MD

1. What is the incidence of osteoporotic vertebral compression fractures?

Vertebral compression fractures are the most common fractures due to osteoporosis. Vertebral fractures are two to three times more prevalent than hip fractures or wrist fractures. The exact incidence of osteoporotic vertebral compression fractures is difficult to estimate but is quite high. In the United States alone, osteoporotic vertebral compression fractures are estimated to affect 200,000 to 700,000 persons per year. The difficulty estimating incidence arises because many people have a vertebral deformity due to an old fracture. This creates a problem when using radiographic parameters to determine incidence.

2. What is the economic impact of osteoporotic vertebral compression fractures on the health care system?

The estimated annual cost of treatment for vertebral compression fractures is estimated at 5 to 10 billion dollars in the United States. Hospital admissions for vertebral compression fractures exceed 150,000 admissions each year with an average cost of around $12,000 per admission.

3. Who is at greatest risk of developing an osteoporotic vertebral compression fracture?

The biggest risk factor for having a vertebral compression fracture is a prior osteoporotic fracture. A person who suffers a vertebral fracture is five times more likely to suffer an additional fracture, when compared with a control with no fracture. Because osteoporosis disproportionately affects older persons, age is a risk factor. In a large cohort of middle-aged individuals studied with serial radiographs over 2 decades, 24% of the women and 10% of the men sustained a vertebral fracture over the course of the study. Interestingly, although the rate of fracture of men and women older than 50 years is not significantly different, the prevalence of females with a fracture is higher due to longer life span.

Loss of bone mass is another risk factor. The relative risk of vertebral fracture is about 2.3 times the risk per standard deviation change in bone mineral density. Obesity is actually protective of bone loss and fracture.

The risk factors for vertebral compression fractures mirror the risk factors for osteoporosis and are classified as modifiable or nonmodifiable:

POTENTIALLY MODIFIABLE RISK FACTORS
- Smoking
- Low body weight
- Estrogen deficiency (menopause before age 45 years, bilateral ovariectomy, prolonged premenopausal amenorrhea > 1 year)
- Low calcium intake
- Alcoholism
- Impaired eyesight despite correction
- Recurrent falls
- Inadequate physical activity
- Poor health or frailty

NONMODIFIABLE RISK FACTORS
- Patient history of fracture during adulthood
- History of fracture in a first-degree relative
- Caucasian race
- Advanced age
- Female sex
- Dementia
- Poor health or frailty

4. What is the biomechanical explanation for the increased risk of additional osteoporotic vertebral body compression fractures following an initial fracture?

Following an initial compression fracture, the loss of vertebral body height leads to kyphotic deformity as the anterior spinal column load-bearing capacity is compromised. As the kyphosis at the fracture site increases, the posterior elements of the spine are unloaded, which further increases the load on the compromised anterior spinal column. A vicious cycle develops, which leads to progressive spinal deformity and additional fractures.

5. What is the effect, if any, of a vertebral compression fracture on patient mortality?

People who suffer a vertebral compression fracture appear to have an increased risk of death when compared with a control group. One study identified an age-adjusted relative risk of death of 1.6 in women with a compression deformity versus those without deformity. In a large review of a random Medicare population, patients with fracture had a statistically significant lower survival at various time periods up to 7 years following diagnosis than patients in a matched cohort.

6. In which part of the spine do osteoporotic vertebral compression fractures most commonly occur?

Osteoporotic vertebral compression fractures occur most commonly at the thoracolumbar junction and the midthoracic region but may occur at any location along the spinal column. Cervical osteoporotic fractures are much less prevalent than thoracic or lumbar fractures. Fractures above the T5 level are considered as suspicious for possible spinal tumor.

7. Describe key points to consider in the evaluation of a patient with a suspected osteoporotic compression fracture.

Vertebral compression fractures may present as *acute*, *subacute*, or *chronic* deformities. Statistics show that approximately 25% of radiographically detectable vertebral compression fractures are recognized clinically.

The diagnosis of a vertebral compression fracture can often be made by history and physical examination. Important elements of the **history** would include acuity of pain onset, history of antecedent trauma, and prior fractures. Query of medical conditions that affect bone mineral metabolism, such as renal failure, hypogonadism, or chronic steroid use, is important. The onset of symptoms may be insidious, with a specific inciting event reported only in 40% of patients. Pain is often described over the posterior spinal region near the level of the fracture. In some cases pain may radiate along the chest or abdominal wall or to proximal or distal spinal regions. Symptoms of back, flank, sacral, or abdominal pain in a patient with risk factors for osteoporosis should prompt consideration of a vertebral compression fracture.

On **physical examination**, the entire spine should be palpated to identify areas of tenderness because the level of the fracture often exhibits point tenderness with palpation or percussion over the posterior spinous process. Although usually normal, a thorough evaluation of motor strength, sensation, and reflexes in the upper and lower extremities should be documented.

Plain radiographs of the spine are obtained initially and display the characteristic loss of vertebral height associated with a fracture. Advanced imaging is helpful. **Magnetic resonance imaging (MRI)** or a **combination of a computed tomography (CT) and technetium-99m bone scan** are valuable when the acuity of the fracture is in question or when metastatic disease is a consideration (Fig. 66-1). **Dual-energy x-ray absorptiometry (DEXA)** scanning is a screening test for osteoporosis that uses x-ray to determine bone density. It is recommended for all Caucasian women older than 65 years, all postmenopausal women with at least one risk factor, and anyone who sustains a fragility fracture.

Laboratory tests play a role when infection, malignancy, or metabolic bone disease is suspected. Tests to order include a complete blood count, comprehensive metabolic panel, C-reactive protein level, erythrocyte sedimentation rate, serum and urine protein electrophoresis, and 25-hydroxy-vitamin D level.

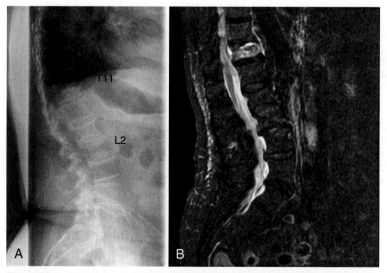

Figure 66-1. A, Lateral radiograph demonstrates fractures of T11 and L2 in an elderly woman with acute onset of thoracolumbar pain. **B,** T2 sequence magnetic resonance imaging (MRI) shows increased signal in T11, while the L2 body has no increased signal compared with the surrounding vertebral bodies. This signifies the T11 fracture as acute and the L2 fracture as chronic and healed.

8. **What are important features to assess on plain radiographs that demonstrate a compression fracture?**
   - **Loss of vertebral height** is assessed and described in terms of a percentage of normal height. Loss of height is described as mild (<25%), moderate (25%–40%) or severe (>40%). *Vertebrae plana* is a term used to describe extreme loss of vertebral body height that occurs when the vertebral body is reduced to a thin, flat shape.
   - **Kyphotic deformity** may be determined by measuring deformity at the level of the fractured vertebra or with reference to adjacent vertebrae: (1) **vertebral wedge angle** (angle between the superior and inferior endplates of the fractured vertebra); and (2) **local kyphotic deformity** (angle between the vertebral endplates above and below the level of fracture).
   - **Vertebral body fracture morphology** is described as a wedge (anterior height loss exceeds posterior height loss), crush (symmetric loss of height), or biconcave. Wedge fractures are more common in the thoracic spine while biconcave fractures are most common in the lumbar spine. Rarely, burst fractures may occur and result in retropulsion of bone into the spinal canal and may be associated with neurologic deficit.
   - **Discontinuity of the posterior vertebral body wall** is suspected in fractures with pedicle widening or loss of height exceeding 50%. CT and/or MRI are the best tests to assess integrity of the posterior vertebral body cortex.
   - **Dynamic mobility** is detected by comparing a supine cross-table lateral radiograph with a standing lateral radiograph centered at the level of fracture. Increased vertebral body height or decreased kyphotic deformity on a supine radiograph in comparison with findings on an upright radiograph suggest that vertebral height may be partially restored with a vertebral body augmentation procedure.
   - **Intravertebral clefts** (gas-filled cavities) within compression fractures may be present and represent fracture nonunions or ischemic necrosis of the vertebral body (Kümmell's disease) and imply dynamic mobility at the level of fracture.
   - **Fracture acuity** is difficult to determine from a single plain radiograph. Change in fracture configuration over time with loss of height supports the diagnosis of an acute or subacute fracture. Acute fractures are often defined as less than three months of age while chronic fractures are defined as greater than three months of age.

9. **What is the role of MRI in the diagnosis and treatment of osteoporotic vertebral compression fractures?**
   MRI is the single best imaging study for evaluating a vertebral body compression fracture. MRI is useful to distinguish between acute and chronic fractures when a patient presents with a spinal fracture on plain radiographs. An area of increased signal on T2 images or short-tau inversion recovery (STIR) sequences and low or iso-intensity on T1 sequences is indicative of an acute fracture. MRI is helpful in determining the integrity of the posterior vertebral body wall. MRI is also helpful in evaluating the patency of the spinal canal, especially if there is retropulsion associated with the fracture or in patients with preexisting spinal stenosis. MRI can also identify atypical cases where tumor or infection is the cause of the vertebral fracture.

10. **What is the role of a technetium bone scan in the diagnosis and treatment of compression fractures?**
    Increased vertebral body uptake on a bone scan occurs 48 to 72 hours following a vertebral fracture. However, bone scans can be positive for up to 18 months following a compression fracture, even if a vertebral fracture is healed and asymptomatic. Therefore, the role of bone scanning in an acute vertebral compression fracture is limited. It does play a role in evaluation of vertebral fractures in patients who are unable to undergo an MRI (e.g. due to a pacemaker).

11. **What are potential treatment options for osteoporotic compression fractures?**
    The goal of treatment is rapid return to baseline functional status, while limiting possible complications. Traditionally, osteoporotic compression fractures were treated nonoperatively except in unusual cases where the fracture was associated with neurologic compromise or extreme spinal instability. Rationale for this approach included the finding that a certain percentage of these fractures were associated with mild symptoms that improved over time. In addition, surgical treatment in this population is complicated by surgical morbidity due to associated medical comorbidities and implant complications due to poor fixation in osteoporotic bone using traditional surgical techniques. Over the past decade, studies have shown that, although some patients with compression fractures improve without intervention, up to two thirds may experience intense pain 1 year after their injury. This led to current treatment approaches that include analgesics, spinal orthoses, and medications (calcium, vitamin D, bisphosphonates) to prevent the next compression fracture by treating the underlying cause of osteoporosis. Administration of nasal calcitonin (200 IU [International Units]) for 4 weeks following an acute fracture has shown benefit in reducing pain. Minimally invasive vertebral augmentation provides an additional treatment option. Decision making is based on fracture-related factors (i.e. acuity, morphology) and patient-related factors including a medical comorbidities, pain level, ability to comply with treatment, and patient preference. Selection of a specific treatment option is tempered by realistic expectations and goals regarding the specific intervention in the context of the best available medical evidence regarding treatment effectiveness and outcomes (Table 66-1).

Table 66-1. Treatment Options for Osteoporotic Vertebral Body Compression Fractures

MEDICAL TREATMENT OPTIONS	SURGICAL TREATMENT OPTIONS
Analgesic Medication	Minimally Invasive Vertebral Body Augmentation • Vertebroplasty • Kyphoplasty

Spinal Orthoses	Traditional Maximally Invasive Spine Surgery
	• Anterior Approaches
	• Posterior Approaches
	• Combined Anterior and Posterior Approach
	  ○ Single Incision
	  ○ Separate Anterior and Posterior Incisions

Rehabilitation Approaches • Weight-bearing Exercise • Fall Prevention Program	Hybrid Approaches • Vertebral body augmentation combined with laminectomy • Vertebral body augmentation combined with laminectomy and posterior spinal instrumentation

Osteoporosis Medications
• Calcium
• Vitamin D
• Anticatabolics
  ○ Bisphosphonates
  ○ Hormone replacement
  ○ Selective estrogen modulators
  ○ Calcitonin
• Anabolics
  ○ Teriparatide
	Special Procedures
	• Pedicle subtraction osteotomy
	  ○ Burst fractures with canal compromise
	• Vertebral column resection
	  ○ Salvage revision for complex deformity

12. **What are potential complications associated with orthotic treatment of osteoporotic vertebral body compression fractures?**
    Orthotic treatment of osteoporotic spine fractures is challenging. Lack of compliance with treatment, due to the discomfort of a brace, frequently leads to persistent pain and unsatisfactory radiographic outcomes. If not monitored closely, skin breakdown can occur, especially in those of poor health and questionable mental status. The most common type of brace used is a limited contact orthosis such as a Jewett extension brace.

13. **What is vertebroplasty?**
    Vertebroplasty is the percutaneous injection of polymethylmethacrylate (PMMA) into a vertebral body to provide stabilization and relief of pain. The procedure was introduced in the 1980s, initially for treatment of vertebral hemangiomas. Currently, the procedure is most commonly used to treat acute and subacute osteoporotic vertebral body compression fractures. The procedure is performed with local anesthetic, with or without intravenous sedation, or with general anesthesia. The patient is placed prone on a radiolucent table and positioned to optimize fracture alignment. High-quality, high-resolution fluoroscopy is required and biplane fluoroscopy is preferable. Following placement of a needle into the vertebral body through either a pedicular or extrapedicular approach, bone cement mixed with barium contrast is introduced into the vertebral body with fluoroscopic monitoring. Multiple small syringes are commonly used to introduce the PMMA into the access needle. Alternatively, use of a remote cement delivery system permits the operator to stand away from the fluoroscope and needle to decrease radiation exposure to the operator. The typical amount of cement injected varies from 2 to 4 mL for thoracic vertebrae and 4 to 8 mL for lumbar vertebrae (Fig. 66-2).

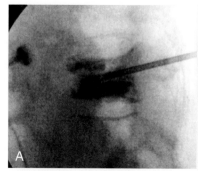 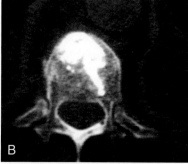

Figure 66-2. Vertebroplasty. **A,** Lateral fluoroscopic view during procedure. **B,** Postoperative computed tomography (CT) demonstrating cement placement. (From Resnick D, Kransdorf M. Bone and Joint Imaging. 3rd ed. Philadelphia: Saunders; 2005.)

14. What is kyphoplasty?

Kyphoplasty is a minimally invasive vertebral augmentation technique developed in the 1990s for treatment of painful vertebral body compression fractures. The procedure was intended to provide a method for achieving reduction of vertebral body compression fractures prior to injection of PMMA. It permits injection of high viscosity cement under low pressure, which is intended to minimize complications related to inadvertent cement leakage. The procedure is most commonly performed under general anesthesia. A Jamshidi needle is placed into the vertebral body through a pedicular or extrapedicular approach. A guidewire is used to place a working cannula into the vertebral body. If a biopsy is planned, it is performed at this time. Next a balloon tamp is placed and inflated with visible radiocontrast medium. Inflation of the balloon tamp reduces the fracture and creates a cavity for cement insertion. The balloon tamps are removed and cement is introduced under fluoroscopic visualization. Approximately 2 to 6 mL cement per side can be accepted at a single vertebral level (Fig. 66-3).

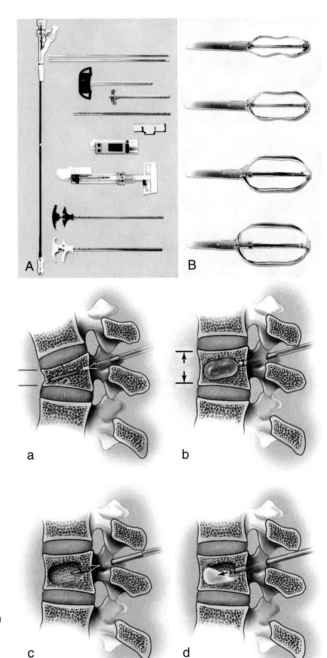

Figure 66-3. **A,** Instruments used in kyphoplasty, including large-bore trocars, drill, syringe for injecting cement with attached pressure monitor, cement delivery device, and bone tamp. **B,** Inflation of balloon tamp is demonstrated. **C,** Steps in the kyphoplasty procedure: **a,** Needle and cannula insertion. **b,** Placement of balloon tamp. **c,** Creation of cavity. **d,** Cement insertion. (**A, B,** from Majd ME, Farley S, Holt RT: Preliminary outcomes and efficacy of the first 360 consecutive kyphoplasties for the treatment of painful osteoporotic vertebral compression fractures. The Spine Journal 5:246, 2005. **C,** from Canale ST, Beaty JH: Campbell's Operative Orthopaedics, 11th ed., Philadelphia: Mosby; 2007.)

15. Compare and contrast the minimally invasive methods of vertebral augmentation, vertebroplasty and kyphoplasty.

Vertebroplasty and kyphoplasty are methods of stabilizing fractured vertebral bodies. Both techniques utilize a percutaneous approach to the vertebral body. A cannulated needle is inserted into the body, under fluoroscopy, through one or both pedicles.

- Vertebroplasty is performed by injecting liquid PMMA into the body. The cement fills the voids within the osseous trabeculae to stabilize the fractured vertebra. This is typically less viscous cement than is used in kyphoplasty, which theoretically is more likely to fill the trabecular bone but also more likely to leak out of the vertebral body. Fracture reduction occurs due to dynamic mobility at the fracture site and from patient positioning on the fluoroscopy table
- In kyphoplasty, a balloon is introduced into the body through the working cannula. The balloon is then inflated to create a cavity. Higher viscosity cement than is used in vertebroplasty is then placed into the void created by the balloon tamp and is less likely to leak from the vertebra. The balloon also theoretically aids in reducing the fracture by distracting the vertebral endplates relative to one another (Fig. 66-4)

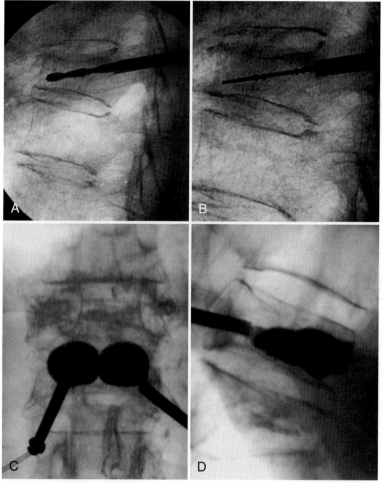

Figure 66-4. Balloon kyphoplasty, T12 vertebra. **A,** A 3-mm drill is directed through the anterior extent of the vertebral body after initial placement of 11-gauge needles and subsequent placement of a working cannula. **B,** Insertion of the inflatable balloon tamp before inflation. **C,** Inflation of the inflatable balloon tamp filled with sterile saline and radiocontrast dye, anteroposterior view. **D,** Deposition of bone cement following cavity creation and vertebral height restoration. (From Haaga J, Dogra V, Forsting M, et al. CT and MRI of the Whole Body. 5th ed. Philadelphia: Mosby; 2008.)

16. **Explain how to safely access the thoracic and lumbar spine with a Jamshidi needle to perform a vertebroplasty or kyphoplasty.**

The most common approach utilized is the transpedicular approach. Anteroposterior (AP) and lateral fluoroscopy is mandatory, and use of two C-arms is ideal, to permit simultaneous AP and lateral views of the target vertebra. The level of the fracture is localized on the AP view. The skin is marked at the lateral border of the pedicle on the AP view. A small incision is made and the needle is advanced to contact bone at the 10 o'clock position on the left pedicle and 2 o'clock position on the right pedicle on the AP view. Next, the lateral view is examined to guide needle trajectory in the sagittal plane. The needle is advanced into the vertebral body while monitoring its path on AP and lateral fluoroscopic images. To avoid violation of the medial pedicle wall and unintended entry into the spinal canal, *the needle should not cross the medial pedicle border on the AP fluoroscopic view until the needle has passed the posterior cortex of the vertebral body on the lateral view.*

In the thoracic spine, a modification of the standard approach, the lateral extrapedicular approach, may be used when the pedicles are small and difficult to cannulate. In the lumbar spine, a posterolateral extrapedicular approach is also an alternative to the standard transpedicular approach.

17. **When are vertebroplasty or kyphoplasty indicated for treatment of osteoporotic vertebral compression fractures?**

Minimally invasive vertebral augmentation procedures are indicated for the treatment of pain related to acute and subacute osteoporotic vertebral compression fractures following failure to control pain with medical management. No consensus exists regarding how long to wait to perform these procedures following an acute fracture. Early intervention can be considered after 1 to 2 weeks in patients who have become nonambulatory due to progressive vertebral body compression fractures. In ambulatory patients with adequate pain control, intervention can be deferred for 4 to 6 weeks. Certain fracture patterns are less likely to improve with standard medical management: burst fractures, wedge fractures with more than 30 degrees of kyphotic deformity, fractures at the thoracolumbar junction, fractures with intravertebral clefts, and fractures with progressive height loss on serial radiographs. Ideal candidates for vertebral augmentation report pain sufficiently severe to limit daily activities, demonstrate bone edema at the level of fracture on MRI, and have focal tenderness at the level of fracture on physical examination. In general, chronic vertebral compression fractures are not an indication for vertebral augmentation procedures.

18. **What are contraindications to minimally invasive vertebral augmentation?**

- Vertebral fractures associated with a high-velocity injury mechanism
- Vertebral fractures associated with retropulsed bone and/or discontinuity of the posterior vertebral body cortical margin
- Pain unrelated to vertebral body collapse
- Vertebral osteomyelitis in the vertebra considered for injection
- Severe vertebral collapse (vertebra plana) that makes injection technically impossible
- Patients with coagulopathy
- Severe cardiopulmonary difficulties
- Chronic fractures

19. **What complications have been reported in association with vertebroplasty and kyphoplasty?**

Significant complications include persistent pain, nerve root injury, spinal cord compression due to cement extravasation, cement embolism, infection, hypotension secondary to bone cement monomer, medical complications, and death. Rib fractures, pedicle fractures, and transverse process fractures may occur during the procedure. New vertebral fractures may occur following the procedure at adjacent levels, remote spinal levels, and previously treated vertebral levels. Although vertebral body cement augmentation procedures are usually well tolerated and associated with overall low complication rates, serious neurologic complications due to cement leakage may result in compression of adjacent neural structures and necessitate emergency decompressive surgery (Fig. 66-5). Cement injection into the paravertebral vessels may lead to pulmonary emboli with serious sequelae.

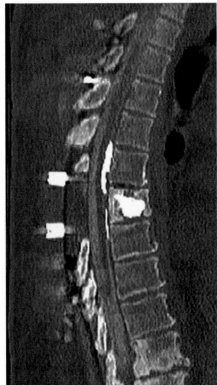

Figure 66-5. Sagittal computed tomography (CT) reconstruction demonstrating a clinically significant cement leak along the posterior longitudinal ligament. This reinforces the importance of careful fluoroscopic monitoring while injecting cement and ensuring that radiographic visualization of the target level is optimized.

20. Does kyphoplasty or vertebroplasty increase the risk of an adjacent level fracture?
This complication has been reviewed in multiple studies, and the data are conflicting as to whether or not placing cement in a vertebral body poses an independent increased risk of fracture in the adjacent bodies. Following kyphoplasty, the risk of adjacent-level fracture seems to be highest in the first 2 months following the procedure (Fig. 66-6). Evidence suggests that patients with steroid-induced osteoporosis are more likely to refracture than patients with primary osteoporosis. It is important to realize that certain adjacent level fractures may reflect the natural

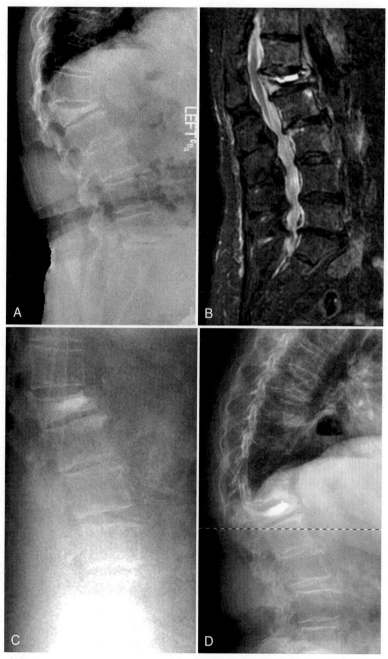

Figure 66-6. An 80-year-old woman with no antecedent trauma presented with 2 months of back pain, despite bracing and pain medication. **A,** Lateral radiograph demonstrating significant collapse of L1. **B,** T2 magnetic resonance imaging (MRI) of the same patient, with high signal intensity present at the L1 fracture. This is an intravertebral cleft, which implies dynamic mobility at fracture site. **C,** Radiograph immediately following kyphoplasty. Notice the adjacent vertebral body morphology. **D,** Radiograph at 6 weeks after kyphoplasty. Patient reported excellent pain relief immediately after surgery, but more pain at about week 5. Notice the deformity of the inferior endplate at T12, signifying acute adjacent-level vertebral fracture.

history of osteoporosis rather than the consequence of cement augmentation. In patients with osteoporotic compression fractures treated without kyphoplasty or vertebroplasty, the annual incidence of an additional vertebral compression fracture is approximately 20%. Appropriate medical therapy for osteoporosis can decrease this risk.

21. Is vertebral augmentation an effective treatment for osteoporotic compression fractures?

Multiple studies have reported that vertebral body augmentation with PMMA leads to rapid diminution of pain and improvement in quality of life measures that persist at least in the short and medium term in appropriately selected patients. There have been some trials directly comparing kyphoplasty and vertebroplasty, but the results of these investigations are mixed. In a meta-analysis of these techniques, adverse events were rare, but short-term adverse events were more common with vertebroplasty, specifically cement leakage. Publication of results from two randomized clinical trials in the *New England Journal of Medicine* in 2009 questioned the efficacy of vertebroplasty. A subsequent study (Vertos II) countered these arguments. The debate regarding effectiveness of vertebroplasty remains an area of controversy.

22. What other materials, beside PMMA, have been investigated for use in vertebral body augmentation?

Additional materials that have been investigated to augment vertebral bodies include calcium phosphate, calcium sulfate, and allograft bone. Unlike PMMA, calcium-based cements are biologically active. The osteoconductive nature of these products theoretically allows for the vertebral body to heal and integrate the cement, unlike PMMA.

23. When is spinal instrumentation and fusion considered for treatment of osteoporotic vertebral body compression fractures?

Major reconstructive spinal surgery consisting of instrumentation and fusion for osteoporotic spine fractures has a high rate of complications and is reserved for patients with significant neurologic deficits, spinal instability, or severe spinal deformities. Reconstructive spinal surgery is rarely indicated for patients with osteoporosis and multiple compression fractures in the absence of neurologic deficit.

24. What potential complications are associated with spinal instrumentation and fusion in the osteoporotic patient? Compare and contrast anterior, posterior, and circumferential surgical approaches.

Open treatment of osteoporotic spine fractures, although not common, remains a necessary procedure in some instances. General complications associated with spine surgery include blood loss, neurologic injury, dural tear, and infection, as well as perioperative anesthetic and medical complications. Problems specific to spinal instrumentation in osteoporotic bone include an increased risk of implant failure, loss of correction, and adjacent-level fractures.

- Anterior surgical approaches are often poorly tolerated in elderly patients. Anterior rods and screws provide poor purchase in osteoporotic bone. Anterior bone grafts and cages tend to subside and telescope into adjacent vertebral bodies leading to implant construct failure. It can be difficult to obtain and maintain correction of kyphotic deformities via an isolated anterior surgical approach.
- Isolated posterior spinal instrumentation and fusion procedures are insufficient for correction of kyphotic spinal deformity in patients with osteoporosis. Anterior spinal column load sharing is impaired in this setting, resulting in increased stress on posterior spinal implants. As posterior implants loosen and fail, kyphotic deformity recurs and the implant construct fails. An additional problem that can occur following posterior instrumentation and fusion in the osteoporotic patient is a fracture at the cranial or caudal fixation point or at the level above the construct, which leads to junctional kyphosis and the need for additional surgery.
- Circumferential surgical approaches provide a method for restoration of anterior column load sharing and improving arthrodesis rates, thereby decreasing the risk of implant construct failure. However, extensive anterior and posterior procedures are not well tolerated in elderly patients with osteoporotic compression fractures and are associated with significant morbidity.

25. What surgical procedure has developed as an alternative to a combined anterior and posterior procedure for treatment of patients with kyphotic deformities and neurologic deficits secondary to osteoporotic compression fractures?

A posterior closing wedge osteotomy procedure (pedicle subtraction osteotomy [PSO]) is an effective procedure in this setting and can be accomplished in a shorter operative time and with less morbidity than a combined anterior-posterior procedure. Pedicle screws are placed above and below the fractured vertebra and a wide laminectomy is performed. Under direct visualization, the pedicles and lateral vertebral body are removed. Next, the portion of the posterior vertebral body wall compressing the dural sac is removed. The kyphotic deformity is corrected by closing the osteotomy by connecting the screws to precontoured rods and by changing the patient's position on the operating table. Sagittal alignment and anterior spinal column load-sharing are restored through a single surgical approach.

26. What techniques can be considered to limit spinal instrumentation–related complications in osteoporotic bone?

- Use multiple points of fixation (segmental fixation) to distribute stress over many spine segments
- Use large-diameter screws that fill the pedicle

- Supplement screws with sublaminar wires or hooks
- Reinforce screws with PMMA (this indication for use is not approved by the United States Food and Drug Administration and represents "off-label" use)
- Use cross-links to connect rods on each side of the spine to increase stability of the implant construct
- Perform a supplemental anterior fusion to restore anterior column load sharing
- Accept fewer degrees of spinal deformity correction to decrease loads on spinal implants
- Avoid ending implant constructs at kyphotic spinal segments or at transitional areas of the spine
- Consider PMMA augmentation of vertebra at the proximal level of screw fixation and at the next adjacent vertebra to decrease the risk of fracture (this indication for use is not approved by the United States Food and Drug Administration and represents "off-label" use)

27. What are some emerging techniques for treatment of osteoporotic fractures?
Investigational techniques include use of bioactive cements and implantation of devices in combination with PMMA into the fractured vertebral body. Hybrid surgical procedures have been reported that combine vertebral body augmentation procedures with traditional open surgical techniques. In patients with spondylolisthesis or kyphotic deformity, posterior pedicle screw-rod fixation has been performed in combination with posterior surgical decompression and cement augmentation. Although compromise of the posterior vertebral body cortex was originally considered an absolute contraindication to vertebral augmentation due to risk of cement leakage into the spinal canal, intraoperative visualization of the posterior vertebral body wall during open surgical decompression combined with cement augmentation has been described in the treatment of patients with symptomatic neurologic compression related to fractures. This technique permits immediate detection and treatment of cement extravasation and allows for optimal cement placement, as well as immediate spinal canal decompression if a critical cement leak occurs. This technique has been applied to osteoporotic vertebral fractures, as well as vertebral defects resulting from metastatic tumors. Use of cement products not receiving United States Food and Drug Administration clearance specifically for vertebroplasty or kyphoplasty represents off-label use.

Key Points

1. Vertebral compression fractures are the most common type of fracture due to osteoporosis.
2. Kyphoplasty and vertebroplasty provide pain relief and improvement in quality of life measures in appropriately selected patients with acute and subacute osteoporotic vertebral body compression fractures.
3. When placing a needle into the vertebra during a kyphoplasty or vertebroplasty procedure, the needle should not cross the medial pedicle border on the AP fluoroscopic view until the needle has passed the posterior cortex of the vertebral body on the lateral view.
4. Major reconstructive spinal surgery for osteoporotic spine fractures has a high rate of complications and is reserved for patients with significant neurologic deficits, spinal instability, or severe spinal deformities.

Websites

1. Primer on compression fractures and kyphoplasty: http://www.kyphon.com/us/physician.aspx?contentid=83&siteid=1
2. Primer on compression fractures and vertebroplasty: http://www.vertebroplasty.com/
3. Treatments for compression fractures: kyphoplasty and vertebroplasty:
   http://www.spineuniverse.com/displayarticle.php/article1525.html

BIBLIOGRAPHY

1. Buchbinder R, Osborne RH, Ebeling PR et al. A randomized trial of vertebroplasty for painful osteoporotic vertebral fractures. N Engl J Med 2009;361(6):557–68.
2. Burval DJ, McLain RF, Milks R, et al. Primary pedicle screw augmentation in osteoporotic lumbar vertebrae. Spine 2007;32(10):1077–83.
3. Kallmes DF, Comstock BA, Heagerty PJ et al. A randomized trial of vertebroplasty for osteoporotic spinal fractures. N Engl J Med 2009;361(6):569–79.
4. Klazen CAH, Lohle PNM, deVries J, et al. Vertebroplasty versus conservative treatment in acute osteoporotic vertebral compression fractures (Vertos II): An open-label randomised trial. Lancet 2010; 376:1085–92.
5. Lee MJ, Dumonski M, Cahill P et al. Percutaneous treatment of vertebral compression fractures; a meta-analysis of complications. Spine 2009;34:1228–32.
6. Patel AA, Vaccaro AR, Martyak GG, et al. Neurologic deficit following percutaneous vertebral stabilization. Spine 2007;32:1728–34.
7. Singh K, Heller JG, Samartzis D, et al. Open vertebral cement augmentation combined with lumbar decompression for the operative management of thoracolumbar stenosis secondary to osteoporotic burst fractures. J Spinal Disord Tech 2005;18:413–9.
8. Suk S, Kim JH, Lee SM, et al. Anterior-posterior surgery versus posterior closing wedge osteotomy in posttraumatic kyphosis with neurologic compromised osteoporotic fracture. Spine 2003;28:2170–5.
9. Taylor RS, Taylor RJ, Fritzell P. Balloon kyphoplasty and vertebroplasty for vertebral compression fractures: A comparative systematic review of efficacy and safety. Spine 2007;31:2747–55.

67 SPINAL INFECTIONS

Vincent J. Devlin, MD, and John C. Steinmann, DO

1. How are spinal infections classified?
- **Host immune response:** Pyogenic versus granulomatous
- **Anatomic location:** Vertebral body, disc, epidural space, subdural space, facet joint, paraspinous soft tissue
- **Infectious route:** Hematogenous, local extension, direct inoculation
- **Host age:** Pediatric versus adult

PYOGENIC INFECTIONS

2. What are the three most frequent routes by which bacterial infection spreads to the spinal column?
The most common method for bacteria to spread to the spine is by the **hematogenous** route. Common sources of infection include infected catheters, urinary tract infection, dental caries, intravenous drug use, and skin infections.

The second most common route is **local extension** from an adjacent soft tissue infection or paravertebral abscess.

The third most common route is **direct inoculation** via trauma, puncture, or following spine surgery. The nucleus pulposus is relatively avascular, providing little or no immune response, and thus is rapidly destroyed by bacterial enzymes.

The disc is nearly always involved in pyogenic vertebral infections. In contrast, granulomatous infections typically do not involve the disc space.

3. Define risk factors for developing pyogenic vertebral osteomyelitis.
Pyogenic vertebral osteomyelitis is most common among adolescents, elderly patients, intravenous drug abusers, patients with diabetes or renal failure, and patients who have undergone spinal surgery. Patients with immune compromise, rheumatoid arthritis, and patients on chronic steroid therapy are also at increased risk.

4. Describe the clinical presentation of pyogenic vertebral osteomyelitis.
The most consistent symptom is back or neck pain, which is noted in 90% of patients. In contrast with pain due to degenerative spinal problems, pain is typically unrelated to activity. Fever is documented in approximately 50% of patients. Neurologic deficits are present in up to 17% of patients at presentation. Radicular pain occurs in 10% of patients. Weight loss is common and occurs over a period of weeks to months. Spinal deformity may be a late presenting finding. A delay in diagnosis is common, with 50% of patients reporting symptoms for more than 3 months before diagnosis. The lumbar region is the most common site of pyogenic vertebral osteomyelitis (48%), followed by the thoracic region (35%) and cervical region (17%).

5. What is the most common pyogenic organism responsible for osteomyelitis involving the spine?
Staphylococcus aureus is the most common organism and has been identified in over 50% of cases. However, infections due to a diverse group of gram-positive, gram-negative, and mixed pathogens may occur. Gram-negative organisms (*Escherichia coli, Pseudomonas* spp., *Proteus* spp.) are associated with spinal infections following genitourinary infections or procedures. Intravenous drug abusers have a high incidence of *Pseudomonas* infections. Anaerobic infections are common in diabetics and following penetrating trauma.

6. When pyogenic vertebral infection is suspected, what diagnostic tests are indicated?
An algorithm for evaluation of a suspected spinal infection includes:
- **Lab tests:** Complete blood count, erythrocyte sedimentation rate (ESR), C-reactive protein (CRP), blood cultures
- **Imaging studies:** Spinal radiographs, magnetic resonance imaging (MRI), technetium bone scan (only if MRI is unavailable or contraindicated)
- **Biopsy**

7. Discuss the relative value of different laboratory tests in the diagnosis of pyogenic vertebral infection.
The ESR is elevated in more than 90% of patients with infection but is nonspecific and may be normal in the presence of low virulence organisms. CRP is typically elevated in pyogenic infections and is considered more specific than ESR. The

leukocyte count is a less reliable indicator of spinal infection with elevation greater than 10,000 noted in less than half of cases. Blood cultures, although helpful if positive, yield the causative organism in only one quarter to one half of cases.

8. **Describe the role of the various imaging studies in the diagnosis of pyogenic vertebral infection.**

   Radiographs: Positive radiographic findings are not evident for at least 4 weeks after the onset of symptoms. The earlliest detectable radiographic finding is disc space narrowing, followed by localized osteopenia and finally destruction of the vertebral endplates. Radiographs remain valuable to rule out other noninfectious etiologies responsible for back pain symptoms

   MRI: This is the imaging modality of choice for diagnosis of vertebral infection. It provides detailed assessment of the vertebral body, disc space, spinal canal, and surrounding soft tissue not provided with any other single test. The typical findings associated with pyogenic vertebral infection are decreased signal in the vertebral body and adjacent discs on T1-weighted sequences and increased signal intensity noted in these structures on T2-weighted images. Paravertebral abscess, if present, also demonstrates increased uptake on T2-weighted images. Gadolinium contrast is a useful adjunct in diagnosing infection because the disc and involved regions of adjacent vertebral bodies typically enhance in the presence of contrast (Fig. 67-1A and B)

   Radionuclide studies: Technetium-99m bone scanning is valuable in the early diagnosis of pyogenic vertebral osteomyelitis because it demonstrates positive findings before the development of radiographically detectable changes. It serves as a good screening study but does not provide sufficiently detailed information to plan treatment.

   Computed tomography (CT): Plays a role in defining the extent of bony destruction and localization of lesions for biopsies

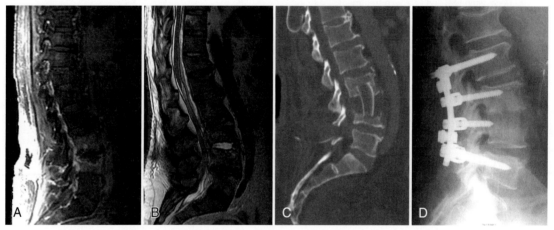

Figure 67-1. 60-year-old man with severe low back pain. T1-weighted magnetic resonance imaging (MRI) (**A**) and T2-weighted MRI (**B**) images reveal findings consistent with discitis/osteomyelitis at L3-L4. Treatment consisted of anterior debridement and fusion with iliac autograft (**C**) followed by posterior instrumentation and fusion (**D**).

9. **What is the role of biopsy in the diagnosis of pyogenic infections?**

   In the absence of positive blood cultures, biopsy of the site of presumed vertebral osteomyelitis or discitis is essential to provide a definitive diagnosis, identify the causative organism, and guide treatment. The biopsy ideally should be performed before initiation of antibiotics. If antibiotics have been given, they should be discontinued for 3 days before the biopsy. Computed tomography (CT)-guided, closed Craig needle biopsy is safe and effective and yields the etiologic organism in 70% of cases. If a closed biopsy is negative after two attempts, an open biopsy can be considered.

10. **What tests should be done on tissue samples from an open biopsy?**

    Tissue samples should be sent for Gram stain, acid-fast stain, aerobic and anaerobic cultures, and fungal and tuberculosis (TB) cultures. Bacterial cultures should be observed for at least 10 days to detect low-virulence organisms. TB cultures may take weeks to grow. Histology studies should also be performed to detect neoplastic processes and to differentiate acute versus chronic infection.

11. **What are the goals of treatment of pyogenic vertebral osteomyelitis?**

    The goals in treating vertebral osteomyelitis include early definitive diagnosis, eradication of infection, relief of axial pain, prevention or reversal of neurologic deficits, preservation of spinal stability, and correction of spinal deformity.

12. Describe the nonoperative treatment of pyogenic vertebral osteomyelitis.

Nonoperative treatment includes antibiotic administration, treatment of underlying disease processes, nutritional support, and spinal immobilization with an orthosis. Antibiotic selection is based on identification and sensitivity testing. Consultation with an infectious disease specialist is recommended. Intravenous antibiotics generally should be continued for 6 weeks, provided that satisfactory clinical results and reduction in ESR and CRP occur. In the setting of a broadly sensitive organism and rapid clinical resolution, intravenous antibiotics may be replaced with oral antibiotics at 4 weeks. Relapse of infection has been reported in up to 25% of patients who receive intravenous antibiotic treatment for less than 4 weeks.

13. What are the results of nonoperative treatment of pyogenic spinal infections?

Contemporary mortality rates resulting from pyogenic spinal infections range from 2% to 17%. Nonoperative treatment is reported as successful in up to 75% of appropriately treated patients when criteria for success focus on infection cure, infection recurrence, and neurologic status following treatment. Quality of life data suggest less favorable success rates with 31% of patients reporting unfavorable outcomes and only 14% of patients free of pain following treatment.

14. What factors suggest a successful outcome with nonoperative treatment?

The ideal patient for nonoperative treatment is a neurologically intact patient with primarily disc space involvement, minimal involvement of adjacent vertebrae, no kyphotic deformity, and who is not debilitated by systemic disease or immune suppression. The most consistent predictors of success for nonoperative treatment include:
- Patients younger than 60 years
- Patients who are immunocompetent
- Infections with *Staphylococcus aureus*
- Decreasing ESR and CRP with treatment

15. When is operative intervention indicated for the treatment of pyogenic vertebral osteomyelitis?
- Open biopsy (when closed biopsy is negative or considered unsafe)
- Failure of appropriate nonsurgical management as documented by persistently elevated ESR or CRP or refractory severe back pain
- Drainage of a clinically significant abscess (e.g. associated with sepsis)
- To treat neurologic deficit due to spinal cord, cauda equina, or nerve root compression
- To treat progressive spinal instability (e.g. secondary to extensive vertebral body destruction)
- Correction of progressive or unacceptable spinal deformity

16. What are the goals of surgical management in pyogenic vertebral osteomyelitis?

Surgery should achieve complete debridement of nonviable and infected tissue, decompression of neural elements, and long-term stability through fusion (use of autogenous graft material is gold standard). The surgical approach generally should include anterior debridement and grafting followed by a staged or simultaneous posterior spinal stabilization procedure (Fig. 67-1).

17. What principles guide the selection of the appropriate surgical approach for a spinal infection?

The *location of the infection, presence/absence of abscess, extent of bone destruction*, and *need for stabilization* are the critical decision-making factors. Spinal discitis/osteomyelitis is a disease process that predominantly affects the anterior spinal column. Anterior approaches or combined anterior and posterior approaches are indicated in the majority of spinal infections. Posterior approaches may be considered in special circumstances such as posterior epidural abscesses, disc space infections below the conus with satisfactory anterior column support, and in the absence of significant paravertebral abscess. Laminectomy alone is rarely advocated due to its destabilizing effect and association with deformity progression, worsening spinal instability, and neurologic deterioration (see Fig. 67-1).

18. Can posterior spinal instrumentation be utilized in the setting of an acute spinal infection without an increased rate of infection-related complications?

Experimental and clinical evidence supports the concept that bone infections are better controlled with antibiotics and bone stabilization than with antibiotics alone in an unstable osseous environment. In this setting, advantages of posterior spinal instrumentation include:
1. Preservation of spinal alignment and restoration of spinal stability following radical debridement
2. Increased fusion rates
3. Ability to correct kyphotic deformities
4. Avoidance of graft collapse or dislodgement
5. Rapid patient mobilization and early rehabilitation without the need for an external orthosis

Use of titanium alloys is preferable to stainless steel due to increased bacterial adherence to stainless steel implants.

19. **Are foreign bodies applied to the anterior spinal column such as structural allografts, cages, and anterior spinal instrumentation safe and effective in the setting of acute infection?**
    Case series report the use of structural allograft and titanium mesh cages in osteomyelitic vertebrae without adverse effect on eradication of infection. Successful use of anterior cervical plate fixation has been reported following anterior debridement of discitis/osteomyelitis. Use of anterior thoracic and lumbar spinal screw-rod instrumentation has been associated with complications including persistence of infection and sepsis.

20. **Are infection-related complications increased if combined anterior and posterior surgical procedures are performed under the same anesthetic versus performing the procedures in separate stages on different days?**
    Evidence does not support the superiority of staged anterior and posterior surgery versus single-stage (same day) surgery for pyogenic discitis/osteomyelitis. Decision making can be individualized based on patient-specific factors such as the presence/absence of systemic sepsis, patient response under anesthesia during the anterior procedure (hemodynamic stability), medical comorbidities, and inherent stability of the anterior spinal column construct following debridement.

21. **Describe the clinical presentation of an epidural abscess.**
    Epidural abscess can result from hematogenous spread, local extension, or direct inoculation. This condition is usually found in adults; risk factors include intravenous drug abuse, diabetes mellitus, prior spine trauma, renal failure, and pregnancy. The majority of cases are located in the thoracic spine. The initial presentation includes localized pain and fever with elevation of the ESR, CRP, and leukocyte count. Blood cultures are positive in 60% of patients. Without treatment, significant neurologic deficits occur and eventually paralysis may develop.

22. **What is the prognosis for neurologic recovery for a patient with an epidural abscess associated with neurologic deficit?**
    Significant neurologic recovery is observed in patients with mild neurologic deficits or paralysis of less than 36 hours' duration who undergo surgical intervention. Complete paralysis of greater than 36 to 48 hours' duration has not shown recovery. The death rate associated with epidural abscess has been reported as 12%.

23. **What operative approach is recommended for an epidural abscess?**
    The surgical approach is determined by the location of the epidural abscess. An abscess located posteriorly and extending over multiple levels is best treated by multiple-level laminotomies or laminectomy, taking care to preserve the facet joints. Alternatively, debridement of the spinal canal through fenestrations removing the ligamentum flavum and portions of adjacent lamina and use of catheters can be considered. An abscess located anteriorly and associated with vertebral osteomyelitis is most directly treated with an anterior surgical approach. If an abscess involves both the anterior and posterior epidural space, an anterior and posterior approach combined with spinal stabilization using posterior instrumentation is considered (Figs. 67-2 and 67-3).

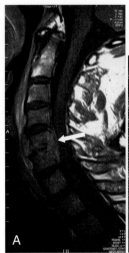
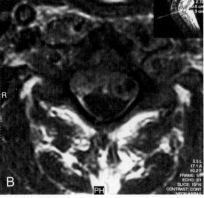

Figure 67-2. 61-year-old man with a C5–C6 disc space infection secondary to brucellosis extending into the anterior epidural space with anterior epidural abscess formation and prevertebral abscess. **A,** Sagittal image shows abscess *(arrow)* extending above and below the C5-C6 disc space. **B,** Axial image show abscess in anterior epidural space. (From Guzey FK, Emel E, Sel B, et al. Cervical spinal brucellosis causing epidural and prevertebral abscesses and spinal cord compression: A case report. Spine J 20007;7(2):240–4.)

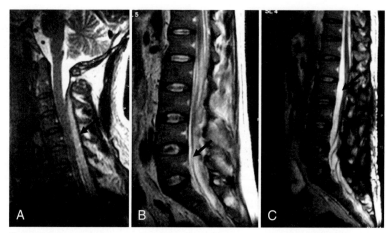

Figure 67-3. Epidural abscess in a 36-year-old man with a history of fever and severe neck pain due to infection with gram-positive coccus. The epidural abscess extended from C-2 to the sacral region. **A,** The epidural abscess *(arrow)* is located posterior to the spinal cord in the cervical region. **B, C,** The epidural abscess circumferentially surrounds the neural elements in the lumbar region. (From Urrutia J, Rojas C. Extensive epidural abscess with surgical treatment and long-term follow-up. Spine J 2007;7(6):708–11.)

24. Is nonoperative management of an epidural abscess ever indicated?

A symptomatic epidural abscess is considered a medical and surgical emergency. The combination of surgical and antibiotic treatment is required for a symptomatic epidural abscess. Nonoperative management is considered in patients who are extremely high-risk surgical candidates and in patients with an established complete neurologic deficit for greater than 72 hours. In addition, neurologically intact patients without sepsis can be considered for a trial of culture-specific antibiotic therapy under close clinical supervision.

25. Describe the presentation and management of a child with discitis.

The presentation of childhood discitis is highly variable. Spinal infection should be considered when children present with back pain, refusal to bear weight, or a flexed position of the spine. Children may also complain of nonspecific abdominal pain. Infants are more likely to become systemically ill, whereas nonspecific findings are more common in children older than 5 years. Less than 50% present with fever. After several weeks radiographs may demonstrate disc space narrowing, which is the earliest detectable radiographic finding. Endplate erosions, bony destruction, and paravertebral soft tissue swelling may occur later. The ESR is usually elevated. Blood cultures are usually negative, and the leukocyte count is usually normal. Initial treatment includes bedrest, immobilization, and administration of an antistaphylococcal antibiotic (initially parenteral but may be changed to oral medication after resolution of symptoms). Treatment failure or abscess formation requires biopsy and/or surgical intervention.

GRANULOMATOUS INFECTIONS

TUBERCULOSIS

26. Describe the presentation of a patient with a tuberculous spinal infection.

Tuberculosis is the most common granulomatous infection of the spine. The presentation is highly variable. Mild back pain is the most common symptom. Patients with tuberculous infections may present with malaise, fevers, night sweats, and weight loss. In addition, chronic infections may result in cutaneous sinuses, neurologic deficits (in up to 40% of patients), and kyphotic deformities.

27. What are the risk factors for contracting tuberculosis of the spine?

Certain factors define the high-risk population and should raise suspicion. Patients from countries with a high incidence of tuberculosis, such as Southeast Asia, South America, and Russia, are considered high risk. Patients who live in confinement with others, such as homeless centers and prisons, are also at risk. Elderly adults, chronic alcoholics, patients with AIDS, and patients with a family member or a household contact with tuberculosis are additional high-risk groups.

28. Discuss the value of laboratory tests in the diagnosis of tuberculous vertebral infection.

The leukocyte count may be normal or mildly elevated. The ESR is mildly elevated (typically <50) but may be normal in up to 25% of cases. Although the purified protein derivative (PPD) skin test may detect active infection or past exposure, this test is unreliable because false-negative results may occur in malnourished and immunocompromised patients. Anergy panel testing should be included for this reason. Urine cultures, sputum specimens, and gastric washings may be helpful for diagnosis if the primary source is unknown. The most reliable test for diagnosis is CT-guided biopsy. The characteristic finding on histology is a granuloma, which is described as a multinucleated giant-cell reaction surrounding a central region of caseating necrosis. Molecular detection of mycobacterium DNA or RNA is useful for rapid diagnosis and for determining drug resistance.

29. What is the value of imaging studies in the diagnosis of tuberculous vertebral infection?

Radiographs: A clue to diagnosis is the presence of extensive vertebral destruction out of proportion to the amount of pain. Typically, the intervertebral discs are preserved in the early stages of this disease. Chest radiographs can be useful in demonstrating pulmonary involvement

Radionuclide studies: Are not helpful because of the high false-negative rate in TB

MRI: The imaging modality of choice for diagnosis of spinal TB

CT: Plays a role in defining the extent of bony destruction and localization for biopsies

30. What are the three patterns of spinal involvement associated with tuberculosis?

The three patterns of spinal involvement are peridiscal, central, and anterior. The most common form, **peridiscal**, occurs adjacent to the vertebral endplate and spreads around a single intervertebral disc as the abscess material tracks beneath the anterior longitudinal ligament. The intervertebral disc is usually spared in distinct contrast to pyogenic infections. **Central** involvement occurs in the middle of the vertebral body and eventually leads to vertebral collapse and kyphotic deformity. This pattern of involvement can be mistaken for a tumor. **Anterior** infections begin beneath the anterior longitudinal ligament, causing scalloping of the anterior vertebral bodies, and extend over multiple levels.

31. Discuss the nonsurgical and surgical treatment of spinal tuberculosis.

Chemotherapy (four-drug regimen, for a minimum of 6-month duration, includes isoniazid, rifampin, pyrazinamide, and ethambutol) and brace immobilization are the initial treatment except in patients presenting with neurologic deficit or progressive deformity. The indications for surgery and the principles of surgical reconstruction are similar to those advised for pyogenic spinal infections.

NONTUBERCULOUS GRANULOMATOUS SPINAL INFECTIONS

32. Which organisms are associated with nontuberculous granulomatous spinal infections?

Atypical mycobacteria (*Actinomyces, Nocardia,* and *Brucella* spp.), as well as fungal infections (coccidioidomycosis, blastomycosis, cryptomycosis, candidiasis, aspergillosis), are potential pathogens. Immunocompromised patients are at high risk for developing infections with atypical mycobacteria. Fungal infections can occur following use of broad-spectrum antibiotics in combination with central venous catheters for parenteral nutrition. Sarcoidosis can involve the spine and cause lytic, granulomatous lesions and should be included in the differential diagnosis.

33. What treatment is advised for nontuberculous granulomatous spinal infections?

Basic principles of treatment include correction of host factors, antimicrobial drug therapy, and surgical treatment following the general principles for treatment of spinal infections.

34. Describe the presentation of coccidioidomycosis of the spine.

The patient with spinal coccidioidomycosis typically presents with a low-grade fever and an abscess with a draining sinus. Imaging findings include a paraspinal mass and multiple vertebral lesions with sparing of the disc spaces in combination with involvement of the ribs and posterior spinal elements.

Key Points

1. Spinal infection should be considered as a potential diagnosis when spinal pain is severe and unrelated to activity (e.g. present at rest or at night).
2. In general, antibiotic therapy should be withheld until cultures are obtained.
3. In general, antibiotic therapy should not be stopped before 6 weeks and/or until ESR and CRP normalize in order to decrease the risk of recurrent infection.
4. Spinal discitis/osteomyelitis is a disease process that predominantly affects the anterior spinal column, and surgical treatment most commonly requires anterior debridement and fusion.
5. Laminectomy for disc space infection associated with vertebral osteomyelitis is associated with a very high complication rate.
6. The disc is nearly always involved in pyogenic vertebral infections. In contrast, granulomatous infections typically do not involve the disc space.

Websites

1. Orthopaedic surgery articles, infection: http://emedicine.medscape.com/orthopedic_surgery#spine
2. Wheeless' Textbook of Orthopaedics, vertebral osteomyelitis:
   http://www.wheelessonline.com/ortho/vertebral_osteomyelitis
3. Spinal conditions:
   http://www.spine-health.com/conditions/pain/osteomyelitis-a-spinal-infection

BIBLIOGRAPHY

1. Butler JS, Shelly MJ, Timlin M, et al. Nontuberculous pyogenic spinal infection in adults: A 12-year experience from a tertiary referral center. Spine 2006;31:2695–2700.
2. Carragee EJ, Lezza A. Does acute placement of instrumentation in the treatment of vertebral osteomyelitis predispose to recurrent infection: Long-term follow-up in immune-suppressed patients. Spine 2008;33:2089–93.
3. Currier BL, Kim CW, Eismont FJ. Infections of the spine. In: Herkowitz HN, Garfin SR, Eismont FJ, et al, editors. The Spine. 5th ed. Philadelphia: Saunders; 2006. p. 1265–1316.
4. Dimar JR, Carreon Ly, Glassman SD, et al. Treatment of pyogenic vertebral osteomyelitis with anterior debridement and fusion followed by delayed posterior spinal fusion. Spine 2004;29:326–32.
5. Hadjipavlou AG, Mader JT, Necessary JT, et al. Hematogenous pyogenic spinal infections and their surgical management. Spine 2000;25:1668–79.
6. Kuklo TR, Potter BK, Bell RS, et al. Single-stage treatment of pyogenic spinal infection with titanium mesh cages. J Spinal Disord Tech 2006;19:376–82.
7. O'Shaughnessy BA, Kuklo TR, Ondra SL. Surgical treatment of vertebral osteomyelitis with recombinant human bone morphogenetic protein-2. Spine 2008;33:E132–E139.
8. Ruf M, Stoltze D, Merk HR, et al. Treatment of vertebral osteomyelitis by radical debridement and stabilization using titanium mesh cages. Spine 2007;32:E275–E280.
9. Tay BK, Deckey J, Hu SS. Spinal infections. J Am Acad Orthop Surg 2002;10:188–97.

RHEUMATOID ARTHRITIS

CHAPTER 68

Ronald Moskovich, MD, FRCS

1. What is rheumatoid arthritis?
Rheumatoid arthritis (RA) is a chronic, systemic inflammatory disorder of uncertain etiology. It is an immunologically mediated systemic disorder that affects articular and nonarticular organ systems. The articular involvement is a symmetrical peripheral joint disease affecting large and small joints. Axial involvement predominantly affects the cervical region, especially the upper cervical spine. The extra-articular involvement may affect the skin, eyes, and larynx, as well as the pulmonary, cardiovascular, hematologic, renal, neurologic, and lymphatic systems. Prevalence of RA is estimated to be 1% to 2% of the world's population. RA is the most common inflammatory disorder affecting the spine.

2. Describe the pathogenesis of RA.
According to current theories, an unknown antigen triggers the body to produce rheumatoid factor (RF), which is an IgM molecule directed against the Fc portion of immunoglobulin G (IgG). Antigen-activated CD4+ T cells amplify the immune response by stimulating monocytes, macrophages, and synovial fibroblasts to produce the proinflammatory cytokines interleukin-1, interleukin-6, and tumor necrosis factor α (TNF-α), as well as matrix metalloproteinases. Interleukin-1, interleukin-6, and TNF-α are the key cytokines that drive synovial inflammation. This synovial inflammation results in the production of synovial pannus, which is the major site of immune activation in RA. Synovial pannus has the capacity to invade and destroy the substructure of joints.

3. How does RA affect the cervical spine?
The cervical spine is composed of 32 synovial joints. The occiput–C1 and C1–C2 articulations rely on soft tissue integrity for stability. In the subaxial cervical spine, the facet joints are true synovial joints. Rheumatoid pannus produces enzymes that destroy cartilage, ligaments, tendons, and bone. This synovitis leads to spinal instability, subluxation, and spinal deformity. Secondarily, the discs in the subaxial spine degenerate, which may result in additional facet joint subluxation and/or ankylosis. Spinal cord and brainstem compression may develop secondary to static or dynamic spinal deformities or from direct pressure by synovial pannus.
Three types of cervical deformities develop secondary to rheumatoid disease:
1. **Atlantoaxial (C1–C2) Subluxation (AAS):** Most common type, responsible for 65% of deformities. The subluxation may be reducible or fixed.
2. **Atlantoaxial impaction (AAI):** Also termed superior migration of the odontoid, cranial settling, or pseudobasilar invagination. Second most common type, responsible for 20% of cervical rheumatoid deformities.
3. **Subaxial subluxation (SAS):** Responsible for 15% of deformities. May occur at multiple levels leading to a staircase deformity (Fig. 68-1, Fig. 68-2).

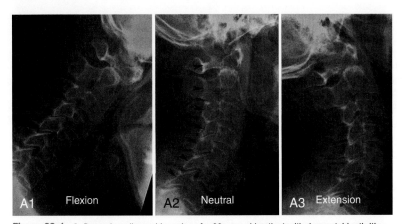

A1 Flexion   A2 Neutral   A3 Extension

Figure 68-1. A, Dynamic radiographic series of a 68-year-old patient with rheumatoid arthritis. The black arrows indicate the spinolaminar line. Anterior subluxation occurs in flexion, and slight posterior atlantoaxial subluxation is revealed in extension. Note the increased atlantodens interval (ADI), reduced space available for the cord (SAC), and broken spinolaminar line at C1–C2 in flexion. The subaxial spine is stable. *Continued*

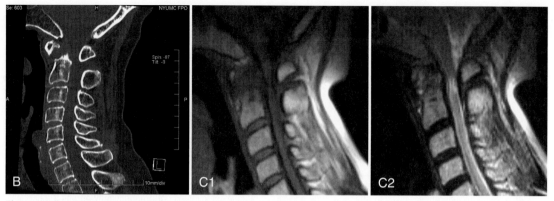

Figure 68-1, cont'd. B, Severe erosion of the dens is seen on the sagittal computed tomography (CT) reconstruction. **C,** T1 (1) and T2 (2) magnetic resonance imaging (MRI) sequences of the craniocervical junction. The florid pannus has eroded the dens and, combined with the subluxation, contributes to the degree of stenosis seen at the C1–C2 level. Abnormally increased signal in the spinal cord is evident in the T2 image.

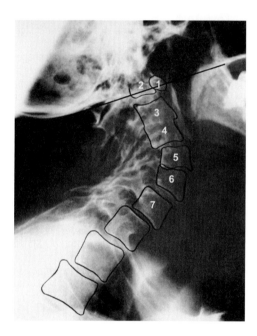

Figure 68-2. Lateral cervical radiograph of a rheumatoid patient (the cervical vertebrae are numbered). Note (1) atlantoaxial impaction (vertical atlantoaxial subluxation) with proximity of the base of the dens (C2) to McGregor's line and the paradoxically small atlantodens interval (ADI), the space between the anterior ring of C1 and the dens; (2) C3–C4 ankylosis; and (3) multilevel subluxations giving rise to the staircase appearance.

4. What is the differential diagnosis of RA of the cervical spine?

- **Seronegative spondyloarthropathies** (includes ankylosing spondylitis, psoriatic arthritis, reactive arthritis) may initially behave in a similar fashion to RA and can be distinguished by serologic testing and the radiographic pattern of osseous involvement. In seronegative spondyloarthropathies, the cervical abnormalities are associated with ligamentous calcification or new bone formation, which is not typical for RA.
- **Ankylosing spondylitis** results in progressive ankylosis of the entire spine associated with marked sacroiliac joint disease. The classic bamboo spine results from calcification of ligamentous attachments at the marginal areas of the vertebral body with maintenance of disc height and shape. Atlantoaxial subluxation (AAS) has been reported in up to 20% of patients.
- **Psoriatic spondyloarthritis** may present with calcification of the perivertebral structures and premature degenerative disc changes but is rarely associated with instability.
- **Reactive arthritis** and **enteropathic arthritis** rarely involve the cervical spine.
- **Systemic lupus erythematosus (SLE)**, a chronic, inflammatory autoimmune disorder, may involve the cervical region. However, most often the axial disease in SLE is secondary to the side effects of therapy, that is, vertebral collapse resulting from systemic use of corticosteroids due to osteoporosis.

5. How is RA diagnosed?

A comprehensive history and physical examination is performed. RA is a symmetrical, erosive polyarthritis of small and large joints along with involvement of the axial skeleton. The patient will complain of significant morning stiffness.

Rheumatoid nodules are common. Neck pain may or may not be present. Cervical radiographs are characterized by AAS, facet joint erosions without sclerosis, and disc space narrowing without osteophyte formation. Characteristic laboratory abnormalities include:

- Elevated erythrocyte sedimentation rate (ESR) and C-reactive protein (CRP)
- RF is present in 80% to 90% of patients but is a nonspecific finding
- Anti-CCP antibody may be present and is a less sensitive but more specific finding
- Antinuclear antibody (ANA) factor (positive in 30% of patients)
- Synovial fluid analysis is nonspecific or inflammatory
- Anemia and hypergammaglobulinemia may be present

6. What pharmacotherapy is recommended?

- Drug treatment should aim to accomplish remission
- Treatment is usually started with a traditional disease-modifying antirheumatic drug (DMARD), most commonly methotrexate. Nonsteroidal antiinflammatory agents and corticosteroids may also be considered
- In patients who continue to show high or moderate disease activity, adding or switching disease-modifying therapy, including addition of a TNF-α blocker (e.g. infliximab, etanercept, adalimumab), is considered
- Additional approaches to drug treatment include T-cell costimulatory blockade (abatacept), B-cell depletion (rituximab), and interleukin-1 antagonists (anakinra)
- It is highly advisable to manage the patient in concert with a rheumatologist

7. Is there evidence that cervical collars protect patients with cervical subluxation?

No. There is no evidence that cervical collars positively influence the natural history of rheumatoid cervical disease. An orthosis may be considered for patients with minor occipitocervical pain symptoms but is often poorly tolerated.

8. What symptoms and clinical findings may occur with rheumatoid involvement of the cervical spine?

- Pain (neck pain, occipital neuralgia, facial and ear pain)
- Lhermitte's sign (electric shock-like sensation in the limbs and trunk when the neck is flexed)
- Symptoms and signs of myelopathy or radiculopathy
- Symptoms of vertebrobasilar insufficiency (transient weakness, vertigo, visual disturbance, loss of equilibrium, dysphagia)

9. List typical symptoms and signs of myelopathy.

- Loss of endurance
- Gait disturbance
- Loss of dexterity
- Paresthesia
- Change in walking ability
- Bowel and bladder dysfunction
- Weakness
- Spasticity
- Loss of proprioception
- Brisk reflexes
- Babinski sign
- Hoffmann sign

10. What are some of the pitfalls in evaluating neurologic status in rheumatoid patients?

- Chronic polyarthritis and deformity interfere with motor and reflex testing. For example, the Babinski response may be absent in patients with severe forefoot deformity, hallux valgus, or ankylosis of the joints. Similarly, tendon reflexes and the Hoffmann reflex may be difficult to elicit
- Patients may have had operations to fuse joints, which interfere with muscle and reflex testing
- Muscle atrophy is common in chronic deforming arthritis and may not be due to neural compression
- Root symptoms may be confused with nerve entrapment and polyneuropathy

11. How is the American Rheumatologic Association (Steinbrocker) Classification of Functional Capacity scored?

- **Class I:** Complete ability to carry on all usual duties without handicap
- **Class II:** Adequate for normal activities despite a handicap of discomfort or limited motion at one or more joints
- **Class III:** Limited only to few or none of the duties of usual occupation or self-care
- **Class IV:** Incapacitated, largely or wholly bedridden, or confined to a wheelchair; little or no self-care

12. How is the Ranawat Class of Neurologic Function scored?

- **Class 1:** No neural deficit
- **Class 2:** Subjective weakness with hyperreflexia and dysesthesia
- **Class 3:** Objective findings of weakness and long-tract signs
- **Class 3A:** Able to walk
- **Class 3B:** Quadriparetic and not ambulatory

13. When are plain radiographs of the cervical spine indicated in patients with RA?

All patients with RA should be evaluated at initial presentation with cervical radiographs, because half of patients with radiographic instability are asymptomatic. Cervical radiographs are also advised prior to surgical procedures requiring endotracheal intubation. Additional indications for radiographs include new onset of cervical pain or neurologic signs or symptoms. Radiographs should include standard anteroposterior (AP) and lateral views, as well as lateral flexion and extension views. Radiographic findings that merit cervical magnetic resonance imaging (MRI) and referral to a spine surgeon include:

- AAS with a posterior atlantodens interval 14 mm or less
- SAS with a sagittal diameter of the spinal canal 14 mm or less
- Any degree of AAI

14. **Which radiologic measurements are useful to evaluate AAS?**
- **Anterior atlanto-dens interval (AADI) or atlantodens interval (ADI).** This is the distance from the posterior aspect of the anterior ring of the atlas to the anterior aspect of the odontoid. In normal adults, this distance should not exceed 3.5 mm.
- **Posterior atlantodental interval (PADI) and space available for the cord (SAC).** The PADI is measured from the posterior surface of the odontoid to the anterior aspect of the C1 lamina. This measurement represents the space available for the spinal cord defined by the osseous elements. The PADI has been demonstrated to be a more reliable predictor of neurologic symptoms than the AADI. PADI of 14 mm or less is associated with an increased risk of cord compression and myelopathy. The SAC as determined on MRI may actually be less than estimated on plain radiographs due to the presence of soft tissue pannus, causing a narrowing of the spinal canal.

15. **Which radiologic measurements are useful to evaluate AAI?**
Multiple radiographic measures have been proposed to assess AAI (Fig. 68-3):
- **Redlund-Johnell measurement.** This is the distance between McGregor's line (hard palate to base of occiput) and the lower endplate of the C2 vertebra. A distance less than 34 mm in men or 29 mm in women is defined as AAI. AAI may also be diagnosed by assessing when the top of the dens lies significantly above Chamberlin's line or when it is situated above the level of the foramen magnum (McRae's line). Visualization of these landmarks is often difficult due to the overlapping shadows and erosion of the dens. However, the landmarks used for the Redlund-Johnell measurement are usually easy to see.
- **Ranawat index:** On a lateral radiograph, the distance between the center of the C2 pedicle and a line connecting the anterior and posterior C1 arch is measured. A distance of less than 13 mm in females or less than 15 mm in males is abnormal
- **Station of the atlas:** The odontoid is divided into thirds on the lateral radiograph. Normally, the anterior ring of the atlas should lie adjacent to the upper third of the odontoid (station 1). If the anterior ring of the atlas lies at the middle third of the odontoid, mild AAI is present (station 2). If the anterior ring of the atlas lies at the lower third of the odontoid, severe AAI is present (station 3).

If the plain radiographic measurements or the clinical picture suggest AAI, advanced imaging with MRI or computed tomography (CT)-myelography is advised. The **cervicomedullary angle** is determined on the sagittal MRI by drawing a line along the anterior aspect of the cervical spinal cord and a second line along the brainstem longitudinally. This angle is normally between 135 and 175 degrees. An angle less than 135 degrees correlates with AAI as the odontoid migrates proximally and compresses the brainstem (see Figure 68-4).

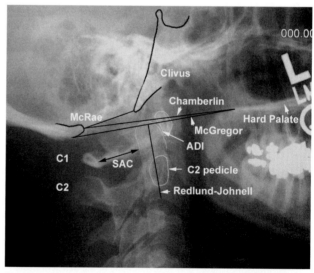

Figure 68-3. Radiologic landmarks and lines in the occipitocervical region.

16. **Which radiologic measurements are useful to evaluate SAS?**
On plain radiographs, subluxations greater than 20% or more than 4 mm are significant. The subaxial spinal canal diameter should be measured from the posterior aspect of the vertebral body to the ventral lamina. A sagittal canal diameter of 13 mm or less suggests a high risk of developing a neurologic deficit. MRI is indicated because the actual canal diameter may be less than suggested by osseous measurements due to the presence of pannus.

17. **What is the staircase phenomenon?**
Multiple SASs give the appearance of a staircase on a lateral radiograph of the cervical spine (see Figure 68-2).

18. **What neuroimaging techniques are used to evaluate the spine in RA?**
    - **Myelography and postmyelogram CT scan:** To evaluate the combined effects of bone and soft tissues on the neuraxis in flexion and extension
    - **MRI:** Noninvasive imaging with excellent visualization of soft tissues and neural structures, but dynamic studies are difficult to perform on conventional MRI scanners (Fig. 68-4)
    - **Dynamic MRI:** New technology that allows acquisition of flexion and extension views noninvasively

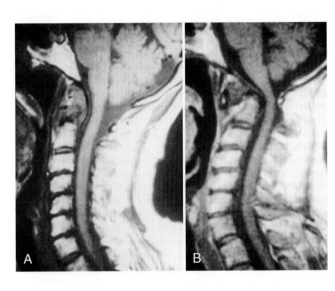

Figure 68-4. Extension **(A)** and flexion **(B)** sagittal magnetic resonance imagings (MRIs) demonstrating exuberant pannus with dens destruction and severe atlantoaxial instability. The high-grade subluxation and its effect on the craniocervical junction may have been missed if the flexion view had been omitted. These images were acquired using standard MRI equipment.

19. **What is the natural history of rheumatoid cervical disease?**
    Understanding of the natural history of rheumatoid cervical disease is incomplete. Neck pain is common and can be present in more than 80% of patients. AAS develops in 33% to 50% of patients within 5 years of diagnosing RA. However, up to half of patients with cervical radiographic instability are asymptomatic. The most common early instability pattern is AAS. Disease progression causes the AAS to become fixed. Erosion of the C1–C2 and occiput–C1 joints leads to superior migration of the odontoid (AAI) and can eventually cause brainstem compression. Two percent to 10% of patients with AAS develop myelopathy over the next 10 years. Once diagnosed with myelopathy, 50% die within a year. SAS is less common than the other deformity patterns and typically develops after AAI or following C1–C2 fusion or occipitocervical fusion.

20. **What are the indications for surgical treatment for RA involving the cervical spine?**
    Indications for surgical treatment include neck pain, neurologic dysfunction, or abnormal imaging parameters (instability). Often patients present with a combination of these factors:
    1. **Pain:** Neck pain or occipital pain has multiple etiologies. If pain is secondary to spinal instability or neurologic compression (e.g. radiculopathy, myelopathy), surgery is recommended
    2. **Neurologic dysfunction:** Cervical myelopathy is an indication for surgery to prevent neurologic deterioration and facilitate recovery
    3. **Abnormal imaging parameters:**
    A. **ATLANTOAXIAL SUBLUXATION (AAS)**
    - PADI 13 mm or less
    - AADI greater than 10 mm
    - Spinal cord diameter less than 6 mm in neutral or flexed position (MRI)
    - Spinal canal diameter less than 10 mm in flexed position (MRI)
    - Inflammatory tissue behind the dens greater than 10 mm
    B. **ATLANTOAXIAL IMPACTION (AAI)**
    - Cervicomedullary angle less than 135 degrees on sagittal MRI
    - Cranial migration distance less than 31 mm (Redlund-Johnell measurement)
    - Migration of odontoid greater than 5 mm above McGregor's line
    - Surgery is generally recommended following development of AAI due to risk of neurologic injury
    C. **SUBAXIAL SUBLUXATION (SAS)**
    - Subaxial canal diameter of 13 mm or less
    - SAS associated with neurologic deficit

21. What are the surgical treatment options for AAS?

Surgical treatment options are guided by whether AAS is **reducible** or **nonreducible**.

Options for reducible atlantoaxial subluxations include:

- Transarticular screw fixation with supplemental posterior wiring and autograft (Fig. 68-5)
- C1 lateral mass screws and C2 pedicle or translaminar screws and rods permit direct reduction and provide superior fixation for more complex cases; cancellous autograft bone should also be used
- Interlaminar (Halifax) clamps with structural autograft
- Posterior Brooks or Gallie wiring with autograft has a relatively high failure rate due to poor control of rotation and translation. Supplemental halo vest use may increase the success rate. More extensive procedures may be necessary if the bone quality is poor

Options for nonreducible atlantoaxial subluxations include:

- Posterior spinal fusion and posterior instrumentation (C1 lateral mass screws and C2 pedicle or translaminar screws and rods) combined with C1 laminectomy
- Occipitocervical fusion and posterior instrumentation combined with C1 laminectomy
- Transoral resection of the dens

22. What is the fate of rheumatoid pannus after atlantoaxial arthrodesis?

A solid posterior fusion usually results in reduction of pannus.

23. What are the surgical treatment options for AAI?

Preoperative halo traction is used to attempt to reduce the amount of AAI and avoid the need for posterior decompression of the foramen magnum or transoral dens resection. If adequate decompression is achieved with traction, the patient is treated with posterior occipitocervical fusion and instrumentation. If traction is unsuccessful, C1 laminectomy and posterior occipitocervical fusion and instrumentation or transoral odontoid resection, combined with posterior instrumentation and fusion, are options.

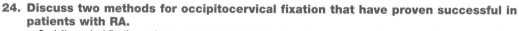

Figure 68-5. Posterior atlantoaxial fusion for rheumatoid atlantoaxial subluxation, 4 years postoperatively (63-year-old patient). Transarticular screws and modified Gallie wiring were used with autograft. The subaxial discs have progressively settled; the C7 to T1 spondylolisthesis has remained stable.

24. Discuss two methods for occipitocervical fixation that have proven successful in patients with RA.

- Occipitocervical fixation, using a contoured Hartshill-Ransford loop and sublaminar wires without bone grafting, is a well-validated technique with a high success rate and low morbidity. Sublaminar wires should not be placed in the setting of an irreducible C1–C2 subluxation or severely stenotic canal (Fig. 68-6)
- Occipitocervical fixation with plates and screws or rods and screws is another viable technique. Good bone stock for screw purchase and iliac crest bone harvest are required

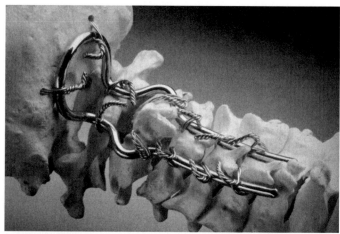
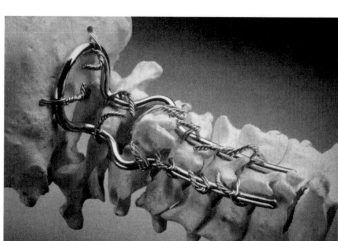

Figure 68-6. A Hartshill-Ransford loop wired into place on a skeleton model. The cranial loop is attached to the occiput using wires that pass through paired, full-thickness burr holes. The wires are not passed around the foramen magnum. The loop is prebent to conform to the posterior craniocervical angle and may be adjusted intraoperatively. The limbs of the loop are attached via sublaminar wires at each level. Note how the C2 laminar wires are tightened below the flare of the loop, which serves to maintain distraction between the occiput and the C2 vertebra. (From Moskovich R, Crockard HA, Shott S, et al. Occipitocervical stabilization for myelopathy in patients with rheumatoid arthritis: Implications of not bone grafting. J Bone Joint Surg 2000;82A:349–65, with permission.)

25. Under what circumstances is transoral resection of the dens considered?

- Fixed anterior neuraxial compression, especially with anterior osseous compression
- If satisfactory reduction of AAS cannot be obtained in a patient with a severe neurologic deficit
- Basilar invagination associated with the Chiari malformation

- Marked vertical subluxation (AAI) with cervicomedullary compression
- In select cases where the pannus itself results in severe cord compression

26. What airway management techniques are used when transoral surgery is performed on a rheumatoid patient?
- Nasotracheal intubation (commonly)
- Tracheostomy (rarely)
- Elective postoperative intubation for 24 to 48 hours to allow pharyngeal swelling to resolve

27. Describe the management of an elderly Ranawat IIIb patient who is bed-bound or has severe spinal cord atrophy.
The prognosis for surgical management is poor. Supportive management rather than an operation may be preferable.

28. List complications of bedrest and prolonged skull traction for rheumatoid vertical AAS.
- Pressure sores
- Deep venous thrombosis and pulmonary embolism
- Kidney stones and other problems of prolonged recumbency, such as osteoporosis and muscle wasting

29. What are the surgical treatment options for SAS?
- Anterior decompression (discectomy or corpectomy) and arthrodesis with anterior plate fixation. However, anterior grafts are prone to subsidence and pseudarthrosis, and anterior screw purchase is often poor. Concomitant posterior fixation should be strongly considered
- Posterior cervical arthrodesis with screw-rod fixation

Key Points

1. Three types of cervical deformities develop secondary to rheumatoid disease: atlantoaxial subluxation (AAS), atlantoaxial impaction (AAI), and subaxial subluxation (SAS).
2. Once patients with rheumatoid arthritis are diagnosed with cervical myelopathy, 50% die within 1 year if not treated.
3. Radiographic findings that merit cervical MRI and referral to a spine surgeon include atlantoaxial subluxation with a posterior atlantodens interval of 14 mm or less, subaxial subluxation with a sagittal diameter of the spinal canal of 14 mm or less, and any degree of atlantoaxial impaction.

Websites

Rheumatoid arthritis clinical presentation:
    http://www.hopkins-arthritis.org/arthritis-info/rheumatoid-arthritis/rheum_clin_pres.html
Rheumatoid arthritis: http://www.nlm.nih.gov/medlineplus/rheumatoidarthritis.html
Rheumatoid arthritis in the cervical spine: what you need to know:
    http://www.amjorthopedics.com/html/5points/archives/5points0807.pdf

BIBLIOGRAPHY

1. Boden SD, Dodge LD, Bohlman HH, et al. Rheumatoid arthritis of the cervical spine: A long term analysis with predictors of paralysis and recovery. J Bone Joint Surg 1993;75A:1282–97.
2. Casey A, Crockard HA, Bland JM, et al. Surgery on the rheumatoid cervical spine for the bed-bound, non-ambulant myelopathic patient—too much, too late? Lancet 1996;347:1004–7.
3. Crockard HA, Calder I, Ransford AO. One-stage transoral decompression and posterior fixation in rheumatoid atlanto-axial subluxation. J Bone Joint Surg 1990;72B:682–5.
4. Dvorak J, Grob D, Baumgartner H, et al. Functional evaluation of the spinal cord by magnetic resonance imaging in patients with rheumatoid arthritis and instability of upper cervical spine. Spine 1989;14:1057–64.
5. Kim DH, Hilibrand AS. Rheumatoid arthritis in the cervical spine. J Am Acad Orthop Surg 2005;13:463–74.
6. Moskovich R. Atlanto-axial Instability. Spine State Art Rev 1994;8:531–49.
7. Moskovich R, Crockard HA, Shott S, et al. Occipitocervical stabilization for myelopathy in patients with rheumatoid arthritis: Implications of not bone grafting. J Bone Joint Surg 2000;82A:349–65.
8. Olsen NJ, Stein CM. New drugs for rheumatoid arthritis. N Engl J Med 2004;26;351(9):937–8.
9. Riew KD, Palumbo MA, Sethi N, et al. Diagnosing basilar invagination in the rheumatoid patient: The reliability of radiographic criteria. J Bone Joint Surg 2001;83A:194–200.
10. Smolen JS, Aletaha D, Koeller M, et al. New therapies for treatment of rheumatoid arthritis. Lancet 2007;370:1861–74.

ANKYLOSING SPONDYLITIS

Edward D. Simmons, MD, MSc, FRCS(c), and Yinggang Zheng, MD

1. Define ankylosing spondylitis.

Ankylosing spondylitis (AS) is a seronegative inflammatory arthritis of the spine of unknown etiology. It presents in the early stages with an inflammatory arthritic pain that typically involves the sacroiliac joints initially and later the other spinal regions. The classic feature of AS is enthesopathy (inflammation at the attachments of ligaments, tendons, and joint capsules to bone). Initially, range of motion is normal or mildly limited. Disease progression leads to spinal ossification, osteoporosis, and altered spinal biomechanics. The spine may eventually fuse in a kyphotic position. The lack of spinal flexibility causes the spinal column to be vulnerable to fractures following minor trauma. AS may affect the lumbar, thoracic, and cervical spinal regions. Other skeletal manifestations include dactylitis (sausage-shaped digits), heel pain (Achilles tendon insertion), and hip arthritis. Extraskeletal manifestations occur and involve the eyes (anterior uveitis), as well as cardiac, pulmonary, renal, and neurologic systems Figure 69-1.

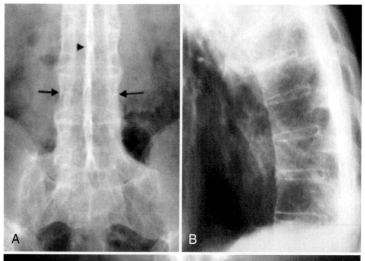
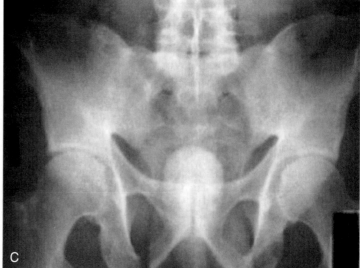

Figure 69-1. Ankylosis of the lumbar spine in a patient with ankylosing spondylitis. **A,** Anteroposterior radiograph of the lumbar spine demonstrates ossification of the interspinous ligament, known as the dagger sign *(arrowhead).* One can also see ankylosis of the facet joints resulting in the tram track sign *(arrows)* paralleling the dagger sign. **B,** Lateral radiograph of the thoracic spine in the same patient reveals the bamboo spine appearance owing to ossification of the outer fibers of the annulus fibrosus and resultant fusion of the thoracic spine. **C,** Grade 4 sacroiliitis (using the modified New York criteria) in a patient with ankylosing spondylitis. The radiograph readily demonstrates bilateral ankylosis of the sacroiliac joints. (From Bennett DL, Ohashi K, El-Khoury GY. Spondyloarthropathies: Ankylosing spondylitis and psoriatic arthritis. Radiol Clin North Am 2004;42(1).)

2. What is the incidence of AS?

AS affects about 0.2% to 0.3% of the U.S. population at any given time. It is more common in males than females.

3. What criteria are used to diagnose AS?

- Inflammatory pain and stiffness beginning in the sacroiliac joints with subsequent spread to the lumbar, thoracic, and cervical regions. Inflammatory back pain differs from mechanical back pain and is characterized by morning stiffness (>30 minutes), improvement with exercise, awakening in the second half of the night by pain, and alternating buttock pain
- Limitation of spinal motion in the coronal and sagittal planes
- Decreased chest expansion relative to normative values for age and sex
- Spinal deformity
- HLA-B27 antigen test positivity. This finding must be interpreted with caution. Although up to 90% of white patients with AS have HLA-B27, the gene is present in up to 8% of the white population, and less than 1% of persons in the United States develop AS
- Imaging studies. Arthritic changes in the sacroiliac joints have traditionally been considered the hallmark for diagnosis of AS. Additional radiographic findings include ossification of the spinal ligaments, squaring of the lumbar vertebrae and kyphotic spinal deformities. Recent studies have shown that evidence of sacroiliitis on plain radiographs is a late finding and occurs 5 to 10 years following disease onset. Evidence of sacroiliitis on magnetic resonance imaging (MRI) and thoracic MRI evidence of costovertebral joint inflammation are thought to represent the earliest detectable changes of AS on imaging studies. Figure 69-2

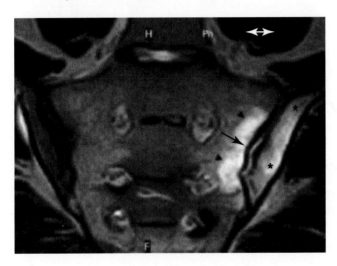

Figure 69-2. Coronal fat saturation FSE T2-weighted image shows increased periarticular signal about the left sacroiliac joint *(arrowheads and asterisks)* consistent with bone marrow edema and increased signal within the sacroiliac joint *(black and white arrows)*. These findings correlated with active left sacroiliitis in this patient with ankylosing spondylitis. (From Bennett DL, Ohashi K, El-Khoury GY. Spondyloarthropathies: Ankylosing spondylitis and psoriatic arthritis. Radiol Clin North Am 2004;42(1).)

4. What are the accepted therapies for patients with AS?

Treatment of AS is based on current disease manifestations and level of symptoms. Half of patients are able to control joint and spine pain/stiffness with a nonsteroidal antiinflammatory drug while half require stronger agents, such as a tumor necrosis factor α (TNF-α) inhibitor. Up to 30% of patients develop uveitis, which is treated with corticosteroid eye drops. Regular exercise and group physical therapy have been proven helpful. Total hip arthroplasty is considered for severe hip joint involvement. Spinal surgery is of value in select patients.

5. How is DISH different from AS?

DISH stands for diffuse idiopathic skeletal hyperostosis. It is also known as Forestier's disease. The disease affects the ligaments along the anterolateral aspect of the spine, which become ossified. DISH typically affects four or more vertebrae, is most common in the thoracic region, and typically spares the lumbar spine and sacroiliac joints. The radiographic hallmark of DISH is the presence of asymmetric nonmarginal syndesmophytes, which appear as flowing anterior ossification originating from the anterior longitudinal ligament. These syndesmophytes are more prominent on the right side of the spine and project horizontally from the vertebral column. The intervertebral discs and facet joints are typically not involved in DISH. In contrast, in AS the syndesmophytes are thin, vertically oriented, closely apposed to the spinal column and the facet joints, and disc spaces are typically involved.

DISH typically presents after age 50 and has a slight male predominance. It has a higher association with diabetes, hypertension, heart disease, and obesity. It is a seronegative disease and has no affiliation with HLA B-27 tissue type. There are no specific treatments for DISH other than use of antiinflammatory agents and physical therapy modalities for pain. Loss of spinal mobility leads to altered spinal biomechanics and predisposes to spine fractures following minor trauma. The long rigid lever arms of stiff spine segments above and below the level of injury increase instability and make fracture treatment challenging. Additional problems associated with DISH include dysphagia (secondary to cervical osteophytes), spinal stenosis, heterotopic ossification, and enthesopathy. Success following resection of anterior cervical osteophytes associated with severe dysphagia has been reported Figure 69-3.

Figure 69-3. Diffuse idiopathic skeletal hyperostosis (DISH) is seen in older individuals, predominantly, involving the thoracic spine with flowing anterior ossification (at least four levels) and associated with enthesophytes elsewhere (especially pelvis). Patients are at increased risk for heterotopic bone formation after joint replacement. Differentiated from ankylosing spondylitis by age (older); location (C, T spine > L spine, no sacroiliac involvement); and morphology (loosely flowing ossification on lateral view). **Left image,** lateral thoracic radiograph shows classic osteophyte pattern seen in DISH. **Upper right image,** anteroposterior pelvis radiograph shows pelvic enthesophyte. **Center image,** lateral cervical radiograph shows classic osteophyte pattern noted in DISH. **Lower right image,** lateral knee radiograph shows patella enthesophyte. (From Morrison W, Sanders T. Problem Solving in Musculoskeletal Imaging. 1st ed. Philadelphia: Mosby; 2008).

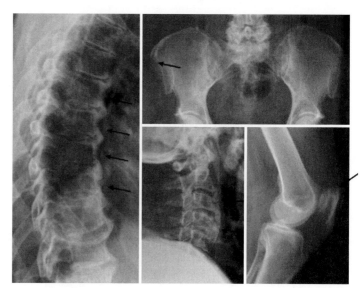

6. **What problems associated with AS should be considered in relation to patients undergoing surgical treatment?**
   The disease manifestations of AS involve multiple organ systems. Consideration must be given to a wide range of issues in patients undergoing surgical treatment including:
   - **Cardiac issues:** Valve insufficiency, aortitis, conduction abnormalities, ventricular dysfunction. Echocardiogram and cardiology consults are recommended
   - **Pulmonary issues:** Fibrobullous lung disease, decreased chest expansion, diaphragmatic contribution to ventilation (important in AS patients). Consider pulmonary function testing. Do not disrupt the diaphragm during an anterior surgical approach
   - **Airway issues:** Difficult intubation due to temporomandibular and cricoarytenoid arthritis, as well as cervical deformity. Awake intubation under fiberoptic visualization is recommended
   - **Positioning issues:** Kyphotic deformities and atlantoaxial instability require careful consideration to safely position patients for surgical treatment
   - **Renal issues:** Renal dysfunction may be present secondary to chronic use of nonsteroidal antiinflammatory medications or secondary to amyloidosis

7. **What spinal problems may require surgical treatment in AS patients?**
   - Atlantoaxial instability
   - Spondylodiscitis
   - Fractures
   - Sagittal plane spinal deformities

8. **How does instability of the cervical spine develop in patients with AS in the absence of a traumatic injury?**
   Despite the fact that AS results in ossification of the cervical region, spinal instability may still occur. Ossification occurs from the lumbar region and progresses proximally and may stiffen the lower cervical region while sparing the upper cervical region. This may result in increased stress concentration at the craniocervical junction and lead to instability. In addition, inflammation may result in attritional effects on the transverse ligament due to hyperemia at its bony attachments. As these changes progress, atlantoaxial subluxation and dislocation may occur.

9. **What is ankylosing spondylodiscitis?**
   The typical inflammatory process of AS results in erosion and sclerosis of bone adjacent to the sacroiliac joints. Occasionally, erosive sclerotic changes may involve the intervertebral disc and adjacent bone. This process is termed **spondylodiscitis**. It occurs in 5% to 23% of patients, most commonly in the lower thoracic spine. Spondylodiscitis is believed to arise from a stress fracture rather than from extension of a localized inflammatory process. Treatment consists of posterior spinal instrumentation and fusion. Supplemental anterior column bone grafting is sometimes necessary. Spinal stenosis may develop at the level of spondylodiscitis. When stenosis is present, spinal decompression is required in combination with spinal stabilization and fusion.

10. Discuss key points to consider in the initial assessment of a patient with AS following a traumatic spinal injury.

Spinal pain in the AS patient represents a spinal fracture until proven otherwise. A spine fracture in an AS patient is a high-risk injury with an associated mortality rate reported as high as 30%. These fractures are frequently three-column spinal injuries and are highly unstable due to the long, rigid lever arms created by fused spinal segments proximal and distal to the level of injury. Neurologic injury is common and may be due to initial fracture displacement, subsequent fracture displacement during transport or hospitalization, or as a result of associated epidural hematoma. Multiple noncontiguous spine fractures or skip fractures may be present. Special care must be taken during initial evaluation at the injury scene. Patients with kyphotic deformities are at risk of neurologic deterioration with supine positioning on a rigid spine board or application of a cervical collar. The spine-injured AS patient should be splinted in the position of injury with pillows and use of a scoop stretcher instead of a spine board. If a cervical collar does not fit the shape of the neck, immobilization can be achieved with blankets or sandbags. Supportive ventilation with adjuvants is recommended because intubation can be very challenging in this population and is best achieved with fiberoptic visualization in the emergency department setting. Figure 69-4

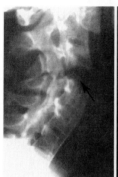
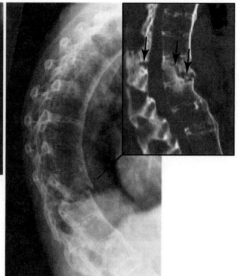

Figure 69-4. Fractures associated with ankylosing spondylitis typically involve the disc space and run obliquely through the fused segments. **Left image,** lateral cervical radiograph depicts an extension-distraction injury resulting in extreme cervical instability. **Center image,** lateral thoracic radiograph shows a three-column fracture typical for AS. **Right image,** magnified view depicting the three-column thoracic fracture. (From Morrison W, Sanders T. Problem Solving in Musculoskeletal Imaging. 1st ed. Philadelphia: Mosby; 2008).

11. What treatment is recommended for a cervical fracture in a patient with AS?

When such a fracture is recognized, a halo should be applied. Low-weight traction may be considered to restore the alignment of the head and the neck to its *prefracture position*. If the head was in a previously flexed position, realignment with traction into a neutral position may cause severe neurologic injury. When the appropriate alignment has been obtained, immobilization in a halo vest or a well-molded halo cast for 4 months is an option for injuries not associated with significant spinal instability or neurologic compromise. Unstable injuries (e.g. translational shear fractures, extension-distraction injuries) are highly unstable and are considered for combined anterior and posterior instrumented fusion.

12. Is a cervical spine fracture a common cause of flexion deformity in patients with AS?

Yes. Late flexion deformity of the cervical spine may result from a nondiagnosed fracture that heals in a displaced position. The site of injury is usually in the lower cervical spine or at the cervicothoracic junction. The fracture is generally a transversely oriented shear-type fracture. This injury may not be obvious on plain radiographs, and computed tomography (CT) scans and MRI are required for diagnosis. An epidural hematoma may occur and constitutes a surgical emergency in this population.

13. What treatment is recommended for a thoracic or lumbar fracture in a patient with AS?

Thoracic and lumbar fractures are most commonly treated with posterior spinal instrumentation and fusion. The goal is to stabilize the spine in its *preinjury alignment* and perform a posterior decompression if indicated. Supplemental anterior procedures are indicated when there is significant disruption of the anterior spinal column (e.g. burst fractures, distractive extension injuries) or when neurologic deficit is secondary to anterior compressive pathology. Attempts to improve on the preinjury sagittal spinal alignment (e.g. osteotomy) are not advised in the setting of an acute fracture.

14. What are the indications for spinal osteotomy in patients with AS?

Cervical spine osteotomy is indicated for fixed flexion deformity of the cervical region. In the most severe case, a chin-on-chest deformity is present. Cervical deformities impair the ability to maintain a forward gaze, cause difficulty with personal hygiene, and lead to swallowing difficulty. Because cervical osteotomy is a high-risk procedure, patients should have an earnest desire to accept the risks and rehabilitative measures required for surgical correction.

Kyphotic deformity of the thoracic spine in AS does not usually reach proportions that require surgical correction. Combined anterior and posterior approaches are necessary in rare cases that require surgical correction. The diaphragm must not be violated because patients breathe solely with the diaphragm due to absence of motion through the costovertebral joints.

Osteotomy of the lumbar spine is commonly done for AS patients with fixed flexion deformities due to lumbar hypolordosis or lumbar kyphosis.

Patients with fixed flexion deformities of the hip joints secondary to hip arthrosis should be considered for total hip replacement before a spinal osteotomy procedure is considered.

15. What are the advantages of spinal osteotomy in patients with AS?

Spinal osteotomy can be performed as a single-stage posterior procedure in the lumbar and cervical region. It allows a high degree of correction in a relatively safe manner. The results of spinal osteotomy procedures can be highly gratifying in terms of overall improvement in functional status and quality of life.

16. How does the surgeon determine how much correction is necessary when performing a cervical or lumbar osteotomy?

The angle between the chin-brow line and a vertical line (the chin-brow line to vertical angle) is measured. A long cassette lateral spinal radiograph is obtained with the patient standing with the hips and knees extended and the neck in its neutral or fixed position. Based on this angle, the size of the wedge removed during osteotomy is determined (Fig. 69-5).

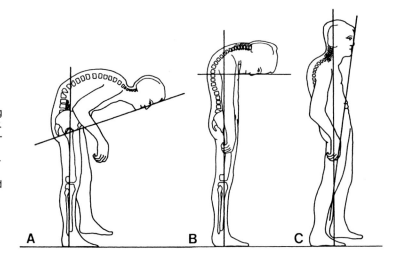

Figure 69-5. The chin-brow to vertical angle is used to measure the degree of flexion deformity of the spine in ankylosing spondylitis. **A,** For thoracolumbar deformity. **B,** For cervical deformity. **C,** For postoperative assessment. The chin-brow to vertical angle is the angle between a line connecting the brow to the chin and a vertical line with the patient standing with the hips and knees extended and the neck in a fixed or neutral position. (From Simmons ED Jr, Simmons EH. Ankylosing spondylitis. Spine State Art Rev 1994;8:589–604, with permission.)

17. What is the preferred level for a cervical osteotomy?

The osteotomy should be carried out at the C7–T1 level. The osteotomy should be centered over the posterior arch of C7. This site is below the entry point of the vertebral arteries, which typically enter at the foramen transversarium at C6. The spinal canal at C7–T1 is relatively capacious, and the cervical spinal cord and the eighth cervical nerve roots have reasonable flexibility. Injury to the C8 nerve root would cause less disability than injury to other cervical nerve roots.

18. Are the halo vest and skull traction useful during a cervical osteotomy procedure?

Yes. A halo vest is applied to the patient preoperatively, and a 9-pound traction weight is applied in direct line with the patient's neck to stabilize the head throughout the procedure.

19. What special considerations should be given to patient positioning and anesthesia for cervical osteotomy procedures in AS?

The operation is carried out under local anesthesia, with the patient awake in the sitting position using a dental chair. This protocol allows active spinal cord monitoring and immediate assessment of vital functions and neurologic status. Intravenous sedation may be used in conjunction with local anesthesia. Routine monitoring of vital signs, pulse oximetry, carbon dioxide, and systemic blood gases is performed. A Doppler device is fixed to the patient's chest to detect air embolism. The anesthetist may administer oxygen to the patient during the procedure by a face mask or nasal catheter. The patient is allowed to listen to music throughout the procedure and may converse with the anesthetist.

20. What is the extent of spinal decompression advised prior to completion of a cervical osteotomy?

The entire posterior arch of C7 with the inferior portion of C6 and the superior portion of T1 is removed. The eighth cervical nerve roots are identified at the C7–T1 neuroforamen and are widely decompressed through the lateral recess, removing the overlying bone at the foramen (Fig. 69-6). The cervical pedicles need to be undercut with Kerrison rongeurs to allow ample room for the eighth cervical nerve roots when the osteotomy site is closed. The amount of bone to be resected is carefully assessed preoperatively and intraoperatively to avoid compression of the nerve roots during closure of the osteotomy. The residual portions of the laminae of C6 and T1 must be carefully beveled and undercut to avoid any impingement or kinking of the spinal cord on closure of the osteotomy site.

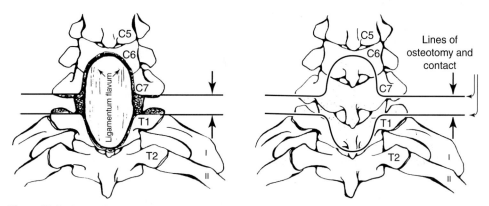

Figure 69-6. Outline of area of bony resection for a cervical osteotomy. The lines of resection of the laterally fused facet joints are beveled slightly away from each other, extending posteriorly so that the two surfaces will be parallel and in apposition following correction. The pedicles must be undercut to avoid impingement on the C8 nerve roots. The midline resection is beveled on its deep surface above and below to avoid impingement against the dura following extension correction. (From Simmons ED Jr, Simmons EH. Ankylosing spondylitis. Spine State Art Rev 1994;8:589–604, with permission.)

21. How is closure of a cervical osteotomy performed?

After adequate removal of bone, the osteotomy is completed (osteoclasis). The patient is given an intravenous dosage of short-acting barbiturate, usually Brevital sodium or sodium pentothal. The surgeon grasps the halo and brings the neck into an extended position. This maneuver closes the osteotomy posteriorly as osteoclasis occurs anteriorly. An audible snap and sensation of osteoclasis are noted. The lateral masses should be well approximated. With the surgeon holding the patient's head in the corrected position, the assistants attach the vest to the halo.

22. How is bone grafting of the cervicothoracic region performed after closure of the cervical osteotomy?

The posterior elements of the spine are decorticated at the C7–T1 area and autogenous bone graft is packed on each side over the decorticated areas. The local bone removed from the posterior decompression is used as bone graft.

23. Are there any secrets to facilitate closure of the posterior incision after cervical osteotomy?

Before closure of the osteotomy site, it is often helpful to place the deep sutures, which are somewhat difficult to insert after closure of the osteotomy. The wound is then closed in layers, and sterile dressings are applied. The posterior uprights are connected to the halo and secured.

24. What are the pitfalls and complications of a cervical osteotomy?

Potential pitfalls include osteotomy at the wrong level. If osteotomy is performed proximal to C7, injury to the vertebral arteries may occur. If osteotomy is performed below C7–T1, little or no correction is obtained. Radiographic confirmation is always necessary to prevent this pitfall. Other pitfalls include inadequate or excessive removal of bone, resulting in too little or too great correction.

Neurologic injuries may occur. The dura may infold in the region of the osteotomy and result in kinking of the spinal cord. If this problem is noted, the dura can be carefully opened to relieve compression. Most C8 nerve root problems resolve as long as they are partial. Some postoperative distraction through the halo vest can be carried out if C8 nerve root compression is noted.

Other potential complications include air embolism because surgery is performed in the sitting position. A Doppler monitor with sound amplification is fixed to the patient's chest preoperatively and monitored during the procedure. To prevent embolus, the wound should be filled with irrigation fluid and wet sponges.

25. Are there any alternative techniques for cervical osteotomy in AS?

The basic principles of cervical osteotomy have remained constant. However, in some spine centers, cervical osteotomy is performed with the patient under general anesthesia in the prone position using intraoperative neurophysiologic monitoring and internal fixation of the cervical and thoracic spine. An alternative osteotomy technique, C7 pedicle subtraction osteotomy, has been popularized in this setting.

26. What different types of lumbar osteotomies are used to treat spinal flexion deformities in patients with AS?

Two types of lumbar osteotomies may be used:
1. Smith-Petersen osteotomy: removal of a V-shaped wedge of bone from the posterior spinal column
2. Thomasen osteotomy: removal of bone from all three spinal columns through a posterior approach by a combination of laminectomy, pedicle resection, and posterior decancellation of the vertebral body (pedicle subtraction osteotomy)

27. What is the preferred level for performing a Smith-Petersen lumbar osteotomy?

The preferred level for Smith-Petersen osteotomy for AS deformity is the L3–L4 level. The posterior elements are removed with the apex of the osteotomy at the L3–L4 disc space. The L3–L4 level is located at the normal center of lumbar lordosis, below the termination of the conus medullaris. The spinal canal area is relatively capacious at this level. These factors decrease the neurologic risk of an osteotomy procedure at L3–L4, compared with osteotomy at proximal spinal levels, where the presence of the distal spinal cord and conus within the spinal canal increases the risk of neurologic injury. MRI and/or CT scans should be obtained to evaluate the spinal canal preoperatively and to assess for spinal stenosis.

28. How is the patient positioned during a lumbar osteotomy procedure?

The lumbar spine osteotomy is performed with the patient in the prone position. The patient must be carefully positioned on the operating table. Such patients have fixed ankylosed spines, and undue pressure in any one particular area must be avoided. The thoracic chest support must often be elevated considerably to accommodate patients on the operating table. The procedure is done under spinal cord monitoring. A wake-up test can also be used, if necessary.

29. How does the surgeon expose, decompress, and fixate the spine in preparation for a Smith-Petersen lumbar osteotomy?

- **Exposure:** Radiographic confirmation of the level of osteotomy is necessary because the posterior bony landmarks are indistinct. Because the interspinous ligaments are usually ossified, the osteotomy can be initiated with a large bone cutter. Bone and spinous processes are removed in a V-shaped fashion. The laminae are thinned out with Leksell rongeurs, and the bone is saved for use as autogenous bone graft. A high-powered burr can also be used. However, exclusive use of a burr decreases the amount of bone that can be saved for subsequent grafting
- **Decompression:** The precise amount of bone requiring removal posteriorly is calculated to arrive at the amount of correction desired. The entire L4 lamina is removed along with a portion of the L3 and L5 laminae. The laminae are undercut to bevel their undersurfaces and prevent impingement during closure of the osteotomy. It is necessary to remove the entire superior L4 facet and widely expose and undercut the L3–L4 neuroforamina to prevent neural impingement during closure of the osteotomy (Fig. 69-7). The pedicles also must be undercut, removing the superior

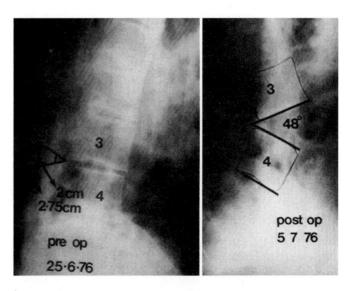

Figure 69-7. **A,** Lateral preoperative lumbar radiograph showing the angle of correction and amount of bone to be resected. Removal of 2 cm of bone is required on each side at the level of the fused posterior joints, 2.5 cm at the level of the laminae, and 5 cm at the level of the tips of the fused spinous processes. **B,** Postoperative lateral radiograph showing angle of correction obtained after closure of resected defect posteriorly with anterior osteoclasis through the L3–L4 disc space. (From Simmons ED Jr, Simmons EH. Ankylosing spondylitis. Spine State Art Rev 1994;8:589–604, with permission.)

edge of the L4 pedicle and inferior edge of the L3 pedicle, again to allow adequate room for the nerve roots during the extension correction of the spine. On closure of the osteotomy by osteoclasis of the spine anteriorly, the lateral masses should meet with good bone surface contact

- **Fixation:** Pedicle screw fixation is the preferred method of fixation after osteotomy because pedicle screws permit control of all three spinal columns. After decompression, pedicle screws should be inserted in L1, L2, L3, L5, and S1. It is not usually possible to have screws in L4 because they will impinge on the L3 screws after closure of the osteotomy

30. How is closure (osteoclasis) of a Smith-Petersen lumbar osteotomy performed?

Osteoclasis is carried out by extending the foot-end of the operating table, thereby bringing the hips and thighs into an extended position. Additional pressure can also be applied manually by pushing downwards at the L3–L4 level and creating a fulcrum around which osteoclasis may occur. As the anterior spinal column is disrupted, the lateral edges of the posterior column osteotomy come together in extension. Anterior column disruption can be detected by manual palpation and may be accompanied by an audible snap. The lower extremities and hips are kept in an extended position, preferably with the knees flexed to avoid tension on the lumbar nerve roots. Rods are then cut and contoured to the appropriate length and shape and connected to the pedicle screws.

31. What are the potential complications of a Smith-Petersen lumbar osteotomy?

Potential complications specific to this procedure include:

- Neurologic injury may result from neural impingement during osteotomy closure or intraspinal hematoma
- Instrumentation-related problems may result from poor screw purchase in osteopenic bone or difficulty with implant insertion due to distortion of normal anatomic landmarks
- Removal of too little or too much bone posteriorly can result in too little or too great a correction. Asymmetric bone removal may lead to postoperative imbalance in the coronal plane. Careful preoperative planning is necessary to determine the amount of correction desired and the appropriate amount of bone removal
- Gastrointestinal difficulties can be minimized by leaving a nasogastric tube in place for several days until intestinal motility has returned. Failure to do so may result in emesis and aspiration due to the patient's inability to rotate the neck and clear the airway

Key Points

1. The classic feature of ankylosing spondylitis is inflammation at the attachments of ligaments, tendons, and joint capsules to bone and is termed enthesopathy.
2. Acute spinal pain in the ankylosing spondylitis patient following minor trauma represents a spinal fracture until proven otherwise.
3. Surgical intervention in ankylosing spondylitis patients may be required for atlantoaxial instability, spondylodiscitis, fractures, and sagittal plane spinal deformities.

Websites

Ankylosing spondylitis: http://emedicine.medscape.com/article/386639-overview
Ankylosing spondylitis: managing patients in an emergency setting— a primer for first responders: http://www.spondylitis.org/physician_resources/ems_video.aspx
Diffuse idiopathic skeletal hyperostosis: http://emedicine.medscape.com/article/388973-overview
Medical and surgical approach to spine disease and spine deformity in ankylosing spondylitis: http://www.spondylitis.org/physician_resources/cedars_cme2.aspx

BIBLIOGRAPHY

1. Belanger TA, Rowe DE. Diffuse idiopathic skeletal hyperostosis: Musculoskeletal manifestations. J Am Acad Orthop Surg 2001;9:258–67.
2. Chang KW, Tu MY, Huang HH, et al. Posterior correction and fixation without anterior fusion for pseudarthrosis with kyphotic deformity in ankylosing spondylitis. Spine 2006;31:E408–E413.
3. Chang KW, Chan YY, Lin CC, et al. Closing wedge osteotomy versus opening wedge osteotomy in ankylosing spondylitis with thoracolumbar kyphotic deformity. Spine 2005;30:1584–93.
4. Chin KR, Ahn J. Controlled cervical extension osteotomy for ankylosing spondylitis utilizing the Jackson operating table—technical note. Spine 2007;32:1926–9.
5. Etame AB, Than KD, Wang AC, et al. Surgical management of symptomatic cervical or cervicothoracic kyphosis due to ankylosing spondylitis. Spine 2008;33:E559–E564.
6. Kubiak EN, Moskovich R, Errico TJ. Orthopaedic management of ankylosing spondylitis. J Am Acad Orthop Surg 2005;13:267–78.
7. Rudwaleit M, van der Heijde D, Landewe R, et al. The development of assessment of spondyloarthritis international society classification criteria for axial spondyloarthritis (part II): Validation and final selection. Ann Rheum Dis 2009;68:777–83.

8. Simmons ED, DiStefano RJ, Zheng Y, et al. Thirty-six years experience of cervical extension osteotomy in ankylosing spondylitis. Spine 2006;26:3006–12.
9. Simmons ED, Simmons EH. Ankylosing spondylitis. In: Farcy JPC, editor. Complex Spinal Deformities. Philadelphia: Hanley & Belfus; 1994. p. 589–603.
10. Simmons EH. Kyphotic deformity of the spine in ankylosing spondylitis. Clin Orthop 1977;128:65.
11. Whang PG, Goldberg G, Lawrence JP, et al. The management of spinal injuries in patients with ankylosing spondylitis or diffuse idiopathic skeletal hyperostosis. J Spinal Disord Tech 2009;22:77–85.

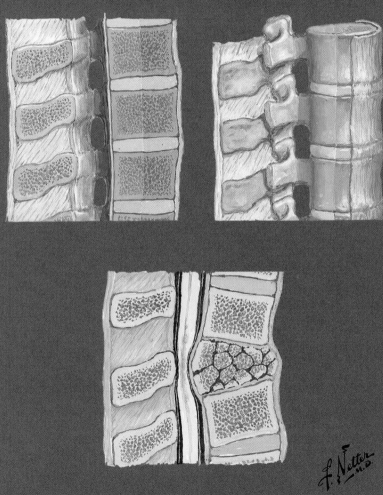

MINIMALLY INVASIVE SPINE SURGERY

Vincent J. Devlin, MD

1. What is minimally invasive spine (MIS) surgery?

Minimally invasive spine (MIS) surgery is a surgical approach or technique intended to provide equivalent or superior outcomes compared with conventional open spine surgery as a result of limiting approach-related surgical morbidity. In spine surgery, as with most other invasive procedures, less is more as long as surgical goals are fully met. Principles shared by MIS procedures include:

- Small surgical incisions
- Minimal disruption of musculature compared with standard open approaches
- Requirement for specialized equipment, retractor systems, and implants
- Dependence on intraoperative neurophysiologic monitoring and intraoperative imaging modalities including fluoroscopy and computerized navigation technologies

2. Have MIS procedures been proven safer or more effective than traditional open spine procedures?

No. Despite the fact that MIS procedures are performed through smaller skin incisions, the potential for serious and life-threatening complications is not eliminated. All spine procedures are maximally invasive because neural, visceral, and vascular structures remain at risk for serious injury. Claims that MIS procedures are more effective than traditional spine procedures remain unproven in the current medical literature. This may change in the future depending on technologic advances, surgeon education, and changing practice patterns.

3. Name four different pathways through which MIS procedures have evolved. Give examples of each.

- Development of techniques intended to limit exposure-related tissue trauma
  Example: Tubular retractor systems
- Improvement upon existing surgical spine techniques
  Example: Mini-open laparotomy retroperitoneal exposure of the anterior lumbar spine
  Example: Percutaneous pedicle screw placement
- Introduction of new surgical procedures
  Example: Vertebroplasty and kyphoplasty
  Example: Interspinous spacer technologies
- Application of established techniques from other medical specialties to spine pathology
  Example: Endoscopy, laparoscopy, and thoracoscopy

4. Are the goals of MIS procedures different from standard open procedures?

No. The surgeon must be able to achieve the same surgical goals with MIS techniques as with standard open surgical procedures:

- Adequate neural decompression
- Stabilization and arthrodesis
- Balanced correction of spinal deformity
- Relief of axial and/or radicular pain

5. What are reasonable steps for a surgeon to take in order to overcome the learning curve and maximize patient safety when learning MIS techniques?

- Attend technique-specific courses
- Study the anatomy, indications, and potential complications of MIS surgery
- Rehearse surgical techniques through practice in animal and cadaver laboratory models
- Visit experienced surgeons currently performing these procedures
- Perform initial cases in conjunction with an experienced surgeon
- Develop a game plan for addressing intraoperative problems
- Maintain competence in MIS techniques through adequate surgical case volume
- Perform a critical analysis of personal surgical outcomes

MINIMALLY INVASIVE LUMBAR SPINE SURGERY

6. List common current applications of MIS techniques for lumbar spine pathology

POSTERIOR-BASED APPROACHES

- Tubular microdiscectomy
- Tubular decompression for spinal stenosis
- Transforaminal lumbar interbody fusion via unilateral MIS approach
- Lumbar intertransverse fusion via MIS approach
- Percutaneous pedicle screw-rod placement
- Percutaneous presacral approach

ANTERIOR-BASED APPROACHES

- Mini-open laparotomy retroperitoneal approach

LATERAL-BASED APPROACHES

- Lateral transpsoas approach

7. What are the key steps in tubular microdiscectomy?

Using fluoroscopic guidance, a guidewire is inserted through the skin and paraspinous muscles to dock at the spinolaminar junction at the spinal level to be decompressed. A 2.5 cm skin incision is made to permit placement of dilators with sequentially increasing diameter. The tubular retractor is placed over the last dilator. Next, the dilator is removed and the retractor remains in place and is stabilized by attachment to a flexible arm assembly. A laminotomy is created with conventional tools (motorized burr, Kerrison rongeur), and the disc fragment is removed under microscopic or endoscopic visualization. Radiographic confirmation of exposure of the correct surgical level is critical. A tubular microdiscectomy approach is also possible for treatment of disc pathology located lateral to the pedicle. This region is accessed through a more lateral approach to the disc space using the intertransverse window. See Figure 70-1.

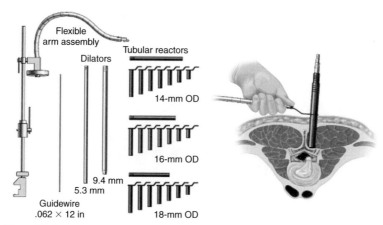

Figure 70-1. Tubular microdiscectomy. METRx sequential dilator system (Medtronic Sofamor, Danek) for minimally invasive lumbar surgery. (Adapted from Medtronic Sofamor, Danek. From Shen FH, Shaffrey CI. Arthritis and Arthroplasty: The Spine. Philadelphia: Saunders; 2010.)

8. How is the MIS technique modified for treatment of lumbar spinal stenosis?

The tubular retractor may be angulated (wanded) to provide the enhanced visualization required to perform a bilateral decompression from a unilateral approach. A laminoplasty technique in which contralateral and ipsilateral hemilaminectomies and foraminotomies are performed using a high-speed burr and Kerrison rongeurs has been popularized. Appropriate angulation of the tubular retractor and tilting of the operating room table is used to facilitate contralateral and ipsilateral decompression of the spinal canal.

9. Explain the principles involved in placement of percutaneous lumbar pedicle screws and rods.

The percutaneous technique is dependent on ability to accurately visualize pedicle anatomy with fluoroscopy or surgical navigation technology. A Jamshidi needle is placed with its tip at the lateral border of the pedicle on a true anteroposterior (AP) view of the vertebra to be instrumented. The depth from the entry point of the needle into bone to the pedicle/vertebral body junction is approximately 20 mm (Fig. 70-2A). Therefore, if at an insertion depth of 20 mm the tip of the needle remains lateral to the medial border of the pedicle, the needle is traversing the pedicle and entering the vertebral body without entering the spinal canal. Next, a guidewire is inserted through the Jamshidi needle into the vertebral body and the Jamshidi needle is removed (Fig. 70-2B). A cannulated tap is placed over the guidewire and used to create a screw channel for placement of a cannulated pedicle screw. Electromyography (EMG) is used to test the tap and/or screw to detect a critical violation of the pedicle wall. After placement of screws, rods are introduced into the screws and secured to complete the construct (Fig. 70-2C). A myriad of innovative techniques have been devised to facilitate percutaneous rod passage and subsequent linkage to pedicle screws.

An alternative mini-open technique has evolved aided by development of expandable tubular retractors. The retractor is placed over the pedicle access site, and screws are placed using the identical technique utilized for conventional open pedicle screw placement.

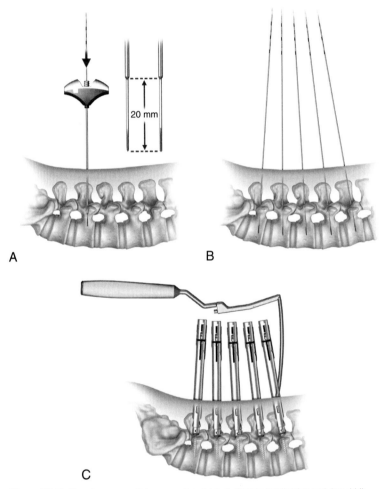

20 mm

A

B

C

Figure 70-2. Percutaneous pedicle screw placement. **A,** Pedicle localization and Jamshidi needle placement. **B,** Guidewire placement is followed by use of a cannulated tap and screw placement. **C,** Percutaneous rod placement is facilitated by extensions that attach to the top of the pedicle screws. (Courtesy of DePuy Spine, Inc. All rights reserved.)

10. What are the key steps involved in minimally invasive interbody fusion from a posterior approach.

The most common technique is to perform a unilateral transforaminal lumbar interbody fusion (TLIF) applying the basic principles of MIS surgery. An expandable tubular retractor is placed over the pedicle region on the side selected for the interbody approach. The facet complex is removed to provide access to the disc space lateral to the traversing nerve root. Disc space preparation is carried out in a similar fashion as for a conventional TLIF. The disc space is packed with

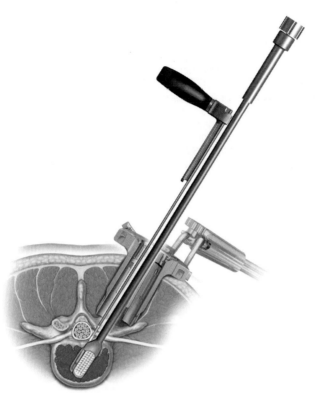

Figure 70-3. Minimally invasive transforaminal lumbar interbody fusion using an expandable tubular retractor. (Courtesy of DePuy Spine, Inc. All rights reserved.)

bone graft and a structural intervertebral spacer is placed. Pedicle screws are placed on the side of the approach under direct visualization. Pedicle screws on the contralateral side may be placed percutaneously or following placement of a tubular retractor on the opposite side. Finally, rods are placed bilaterally and compression forces are applied across the disc space to interlock the structural spaced between the adjacent vertebral endplates. See Figure 70-3.

11. What is the lateral transpsoas approach?

The approach is performed from the left side with the patient positioned in the right lateral decubitus position. Fluoroscopy is used to mark a small skin incision over the anterior third of the target disc space at the posterior border of the paraspinous muscles. The layers of the lateral abdominal wall are bluntly dissected to enter the retroperitoneal space. The peritoneum is mobilized anteriorly and the psoas muscle is identified. The psoas is dissected, mobilized, and retracted to expose the disc space. Palpation, direct visualization, and neurophysiologic monitoring are used to facilitate safe placement of a specialized expandable tubular retractor. While working through the retractor, the disc space is prepared for fusion and a transversely oriented structural interbody spacer containing graft material is inserted.

The lateral transpsoas approach was developed as a less invasive option for achieving anterior fusion from L1 to L5. This approach avoids the need to mobilize the iliac vessels or sympathetic plexus. However, the genitofemoral nerve, lateral femoral cutaneous nerve, and femoral nerve are placed at risk due to their intimate relationship with the psoas muscle. The approach is not feasible at L5–S1 due to the location of the iliac vessels. The approach is challenging at L4–L5 and may not be possible due to obstruction by the iliac crest or due to the relationship of the lumbosacral plexus to the lateral aspect of the disc space. See Figure 70-4.

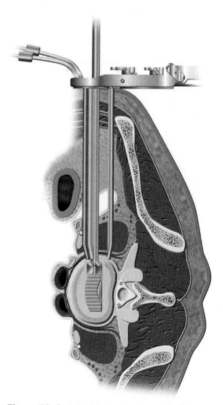

Figure 70-4. Lateral transpsoas approach. (From Kim DK, Henn JS, Vaccaro AR, et al. Surgical Anatomy and Techniques to the Spine. Philadelphia: Saunders; 2006.)

12. Explain the presacral surgical approach to the lumbosacral junction and its rationale.
With the patient in the prone position, a small incision is made lateral to the coccyx. A blunt trocar is inserted under biplanar fluoroscopic guidance and advanced into the presacral space while maintaining contact with the anterior surface of the sacrum. A midline position is maintained and a guide pin is inserted into the sacrum at the S1–S2 level and advanced across the L5–S1 disc space into the L5 vertebral body. A series of dilators are used to create an intraosseous working channel. Using specialized instruments, the disc material is removed and the disc prepared for fusion. Finally an axial rod (AxiaLIF, TranS1, Wilmington, NC) is inserted to stabilize the disc space, and bone graft material is injected.

The presacral approach is intended to provide an option for minimally invasive surgical access to the lumbosacral junction that does not require mobilization of the iliac vessels, limits muscle dissection, and avoids disruption of the autonomic nerves overlying the lumbosacral disc. Potential complications associated with this approach include wound dehiscence, infection, bowel injury, vascular injury, and pseudarthrosis. See Figure 70-5.

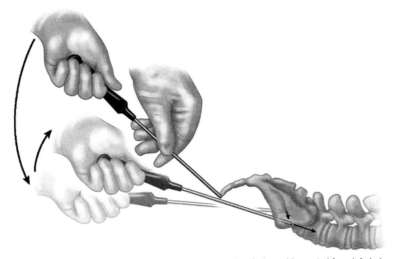

Figure 70-5. Presacral approach to the lumbosacral spine. A channel is created from inferiorly in the sacrum to allow access to the center of the L5–S1 disc. Discectomy and bone grafting are then performed through this channel. (From Shen FH, Shaffrey CI. Arthritis and Arthroplasty: The Spine. Philadelphia: Saunders; 2010.)

13. Why are mini-open laparotomy approaches preferred by many surgeons for lumbar interbody fusion?
Mini-open laparotomy approaches offer many advantages compared with alternative minimally invasive techniques while avoiding many of their challenges. Mini-open techniques are routinely accomplished through a single small incision and generally require shorter operative times. Extensile exposure of the lumbar spine from L2 to sacrum can be achieved. Complete removal of disc material and meticulous endplate preparation are facilitated by direct visualization of the entire disc space. The approach is associated with a low complication rate and allows relatively rapid patient recovery.

MINIMALLY INVASIVE THORACIC SPINE SURGERY

14. List common applications of MIS techniques for thoracic spine pathology.

POSTERIOR-BASED APPROACHES

- Tubular microdiscectomy
- Percutaneous pedicle screw-rod placement and thoracic posterior fusion via MIS approach

ANTERIOR-BASED APPROACHES

- Thoracoscopic discectomy and corpectomy
- Mini-open thoracoscopic-assisted discectomy and corpectomy
- Anterior instrumentation and fusion for spinal instabilities
- Video-assisted spinal instrumentation and fusion for idiopathic scoliosis

15. What neural structures may be encountered in the thoracoscopic operative field?
- Sympathetic chain
- Greater and lesser splanchnic nerves

- Vagus nerve
- Phrenic nerve
- Intercostals nerves

16. List potential complications of thoracoscopic spinal decompression, fusion, and instrumentation.
- Dural tear
- Direct spinal cord injury
- Pulmonary complications (pneumothorax, hemothorax, mucous plug, pneumonia)
- Intercostal neuralgia
- Vessel injury (segmental artery and vein, azygous vein, aorta, vena cava)
- Pseudarthrosis
- Implant misplacement

17. What are the potential advantages of video-assisted thoracoscopic spinal fusion and instrumentation compared with traditional open thoracotomy approaches for treatment of idiopathic scoliosis?
- Reduced blood loss
- Decreased postoperative pain
- Improved cosmesis due to small incisions
- Diminished length of hospital stay

18. How does video-assisted thoracoscopic spinal instrumentation and fusion compare with posterior spinal instrumentation and fusion using pedicle fixation for treatment of adolescent idiopathic scoliosis?
Similar patient outcomes and complication rates are observed in adolescent idiopathic scoliosis patients with single thoracic curves less than 70° treated with either video-assisted thoracoscopic spinal instrumentation and fusion or posterior pedicle instrumentation and fusion. Thoracoscopic surgery is associated with reduced blood loss but has a significant learning curve and requires specialized equipment. Posterior fusion with pedicle fixation techniques are applicable to all curve types, provide greater curve correction, and require less operative time.

MINIMALLY INVASIVE CERVICAL SPINE SURGERY

19. List common applications of MIS techniques for cervical spine pathology.

POSTERIOR-BASED APPROACHES

- Tubular laminoforaminotomy
- Posterior screw-rod fixation (lateral mass screws) and fusion

ANTERIOR-BASED APPROACHES

- Endoscopic approaches to the upper cervical spine and craniovertebral junction
- Anterior cervical foraminotomy

Key Points

1. Minimally invasive spine procedures intend to limit approach-related surgical morbidity through use of smaller skin incisions and targeted muscle dissection but do not eliminate the potential for serious and life-threatening complications.
2. Use of minimally invasive spine techniques is widespread but claims that MIS procedures are more effective than traditional spine procedures await validation in the current medical literature.

Websites

Society for minimally invasive spine surgery: http://www.smiss.org/
Lumbar lateral transpsoas approach: http://www.medscape.com/viewarticle/487929

BIBLIOGRAPHY

1. Arts MP, Brand R, van den Akker ME, et al. Tubular diskectomy vs. conventional microdiskectomy for sciatica: A randomized controlled trial. JAMA 2009;302:149–58.
2. Bergey DL, Villavicencio AT, Goldstein T, et al. Endoscopic lateral transpsoas approach to the lumbar spine. Spine 2004;29:1681–8.
3. Brau SA. Mini-open approach to the spine for anterior lumbar interbody fusion: Description of the procedure, results and complications. Spine J 2002;2:216–23.
4. Cragg A, Carl A, Casteneda F, et al. New percutaneous access method for minimally invasive anterior lumbosacral surgery. J Spinal Disord Tech 2004;17:21–8.
5. Eck JC, Hodges S, Humphreys SC. Minimally invasive lumbar spinal fusion. J Am Acad Orthop Surg 2007;15:321–9.
6. Fourney DR, Dettori JR, Norvell DC, et al. Does minimal access tubular assisted spine surgery increase or decrease complications in spinal decompression or fusion? Spine 2010;35:S57–S65.
7. Lonner BS, Auerbach JD, Estreicher M, et al. Video-assisted thoracoscopic spinal fusion compared with posterior spinal fusion with thoracic pedicle screws for thoracic adolescent idiopathic scoliosis. J Bone Joint Surg 2009;91A:398–408.
8. Newton PO, Shea KG, Granlund KF. Defining the pediatric spinal thoracoscopy learning curve: Sixty-five consecutive cases. Spine 2000;25:1028–35.
9. Osgur BM, Aryan HE, Pimenta L, et al. Extreme lateral interbody fusion (XLIF): A novel surgical technique for anterior lumbar interbody fusion. Spine J 2006;6:435–43.

ARTIFICIAL DISC REPLACEMENT

Brian W. Su, MD, Adam L. Shimer, MD, and Alexander R. Vaccaro, MD, PhD

CHAPTER 71

1. **Discuss limitations associated with traditional surgical treatment options for degenerative spinal problems.**
Procedures for neural decompression violate the structural integrity of the spine and may lead to segmental spinal instability unless fusion is performed. Spinal fusion procedures increase stress at adjacent spinal levels and may accelerate the degenerative process leading to adjacent level degeneration, instability, and spinal stenosis. An initial fusion procedure may generate the need for further procedures, such as implant removal or pseudarthrosis repair. In addition, bone graft harvest for fusion procedures is accompanied by a myriad of problems, including chronic bone graft donor site pain. When the indication for fusion is axial pain without associated neural compression, pain relief is often unpredictable despite achievement of a radiographically healed fusion.

LUMBAR TOTAL DISC ARTHROPLASTY

2. **What is the rationale for lumbar total disc arthroplasty?**
Lumbar fusion for axial pain is an option for treatment of symptomatic degenerative disease refractory to nonsurgical treatments. Results following fusion surgery may be unsatisfactory due to persistent pain despite achievement of a radiographically healed fusion or as a result of procedure-related complications. The rationale for development of lumbar total disc replacement (TDR) as an alternative surgical procedure was based on the following principles:
   - Avoid the negative effects associated with lumbar fusion (e.g. pseudarthrosis, need for additional procedures for implant removal, bone graft donor site problems, adjacent segment problems)
   - Protect adjacent levels from iatrogenically accelerated degeneration
   - Provide improved treatment outcomes with respect to relief of low back pain
   - Enhance postoperative recovery (earlier return to work and activity, avoid use of spinal orthoses)

3. **Discuss the problem of adjacent-level degeneration following lumbar fusion.**
Lumbar fusion results in load transfer to unfused proximal and distal spinal segments resulting in increased intradiscal pressure and increased intersegmental motion at neighboring spinal segments. This may result in radiographic degenerative changes in the adjacent spinal segments (adjacent segment degeneration) and symptoms requiring additional surgical intervention (adjacent segment disease). It has been estimated that the rate of adjacent segment disease (development of symptoms sufficiently severe to require additional surgery for decompression or arthrodesis) is 4% per year for the first 10 years following a lumbar arthrodesis procedure. Whether the radiographic and clinical findings are a result of the iatrogenically created rigid spinal segment or progression of the natural history of an underlying degenerative process remains controversial.

4. **What is the currently accepted indication for performing lumbar TDR?**
In the United States, lumbar TDR has received Food and Drug Administration (FDA) approval for treatment of isolated, single level (L3 through S1) discogenic back pain without instability. Objective evidence of disease should be displayed on computed tomography (CT) or magnetic resonance imaging (MRI). Provocative discography is a potential tool for confirmation of a symptomatic lumbar level and to verify that adjacent segments are normal and pain free. Surgery should be reserved for patients who have failed at least 6 months of conservative therapy.

5. **What are the contraindications for performing lumbar TDR?**
Contraindications to lumbar TDR have been divided into four main groups:
   - **Painful lumbar spinal pathology unrelated to the intervertebral disc:** Pain related to facet joint degeneration, radiculopathy due to disc herniation or spinal stenosis, and poorly defined pain syndromes will not respond favorably to treatment with lumbar TDR
   - **Conditions that potentially compromise stability of a lumbar disc prosthesis:** Examples include osteoporosis, spinal instability (spondylolysis, spondylolisthesis, prior laminectomy), and spinal deformities
   - **Limited or absent segmental motion at the operative level:** Severe spondylosis, prior lumbar fusion
   - **Patient-specific factors:** Metal allergy, systemic disease (e.g. diabetes mellitus), malignancy, active infection, morbid obesity, chronic steroid use, females who desire to become pregnant
   Studies investigating the prevalence of contraindications in the population of patients presenting to spine surgeons for surgical treatment of lumbar degenerative pathology have demonstrated that only a small percentage of patients are appropriate candidates for lumbar TDR.

6. What lumbar total disc replacements are currently FDA approved for use in the United States?

The Charité® artificial disc (DePuy Spine, Inc.) was the first implant to receive FDA approval for lumbar total disc replacement. It possesses an unconstrained three-part anatomic design. It is an articulating metal on polyethylene implant. It has a mobile core composed of moderately cross-linked ultrahigh molecular weight polyethylene. The core is free to move between the two cobalt-chromium-molybdenum alloy endplates. Teeth on the undersurface of the endplates provide anchorage to the vertebrae. A metal wire surrounds the core to aid in imaging (Fig. 71-1).

The ProDisc®-L (Synthes Spine) was the second lumbar TDR to receive FDA approval. It is a semiconstrained articulating metal on polyethylene implant composed of two cobalt-chromium-molybdenum alloy endplates and an ultrahigh-molecular-weight polyethylene core. The polyethylene core locks into the lower endplate and prevents core extrusion. Small keels and a titanium, plasma-sprayed finish on the device endplates provide for both immediate fixation and long-term fixation by osseous ingrowth (Fig. 71-2).

Many alternative lumbar disc replacement designs are currently under study both in the United States and internationally.

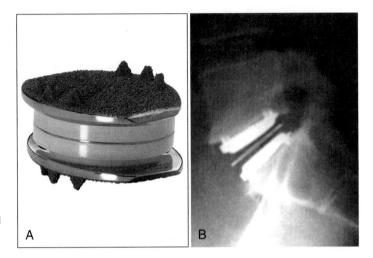

Figure 71-1. **A** and **B,** The Charité III artificial disc. (Courtesy of DePuy Spine, Inc. All rights reserved.) A   B

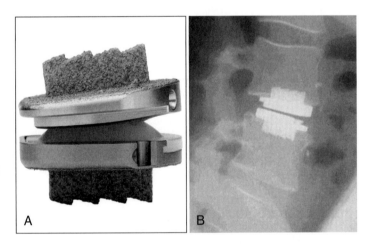

Figure 71-2. **A** and **B,** The ProDisc-L artificial disc (Synthes Spine). (**A** from Yue JJ, Bertagnoli R, McAfee PC, et al. Motion Preservation of the Spine. Philadelphia: Saunders; 2008. **B** from Zigler JE. Lumbar spine arthroplasty using the ProDisc II. Spine J 2004;4:231S–238S.) A   B

7. What particular considerations regarding patient positioning, setup, and surgical technique are important when performing a lumbar TDR compared with an anterior lumbar interbody fusion (ALIF)?

Patient positioning for a lumbar TDR is similar to an ALIF. An inflatable bolster may be placed under the sacrum to extend the L5–S1 disc space and to allow adjustment of lumbar lordosis. Placement of the bolster directly behind the lumbar spine should be avoided because it tends to *fish-mouth* the disc space, making critical parallel distraction more difficult. Incision options include a Pfannenstiel incision or midline vertical incision (rectus-splitting) for the L5–S1 disc level. Either a midline (rectus splitting) approach or paramidline (lateral to rectus) approach is used for the L3–L4 and L4–L5 disc levels. A retroperitoneal approach is preferred over a transperitoneal approach. As in an ALIF approach, careful identification and retraction of the ureter, peritoneum, sympathetic plexus, and blood vessels are required. Lower extremity pulse oximetry is useful to ensure adequate lower extremity perfusion during and following vessel retraction. Thorough discectomy and accurate midline localization are critical to ensure a technically well-placed lumbar TDR. The anterior, posterior, and lateral margins of the disc space should be clearly delineated. The midline is marked using an intraoperative fluoroscopic Ferguson view. A lateral fluoroscopic view is helpful to confirm parallel disc distraction. The lumbar TDR should only recreate the native disc height because *overstuffing* may lead to posterior structure (facet capsule) tension and pain. The center of rotation of the implant should be approximately 3 mm posterior to the midaxis of the vertebral bodies. The bony endplate should be preserved to minimize risk of subsidence or bridging ossification.

8. **What complications have been reported in association with lumbar total disc arthroplasty?**
Complications following lumbar TDR may be a result of:
- **Improper surgical indications:** Poor patient selection (e.g. nonorganic pain syndrome), segmental instability, osteoporotic patients, patients with facet arthropathy
- **Complications related to the surgical approach:** Vascular injury, dural tear, neurologic injury, ureteral injury, visceral injury, deep vein thrombosis, heterotopic ossification
- **Complications related to the implant:** Migration, dislocation, subsidence, vertebral body endplate fracture, polyethylene and metal wear
- **Miscellaneous complications:** Heterotopic ossification

9. **How do the results of lumbar total disc arthroplasty compare with lumbar fusion?**
The United States FDA Investigational Device Exemption (IDE) study for the Charité artificial disc supported the conclusion that the Charité disc was not inferior to anterior lumbar interbody fusion with BAK threaded titanium cages augmented with iliac crest autograft. The IDE study for the ProDisc-L compared total disc arthroplasty with circumferential fusion using anterior femoral ring allograft and instrumented posterolateral fusion with iliac autograft and showed statistically similar improvement over preoperative status in both patient groups.

10. **Describe the workup of a patient with persistent low back pain following lumbar total disc arthroplasty?**
A variety of diagnoses are considered in the patient who presents with continued or new-onset symptoms following lumbar total disc arthroplasty:
- Implant malposition, migration, subsidence, or instability
- Pain due to posterior facet joint arthrosis
- Pain due to neural impingement or excessive elevation of disc space height
- Symptomatic adjacent level pathology
- Infection
- Pain of unknown etiology

After a detailed history and physical examination are completed, imaging is initiated with plain radiography including standing anteroposterior (AP) and lateral views and flexion-extension views. Fluoroscopy may be valuable to assess the operative level under dynamic loading conditions. CT imaging including axial, sagittal, and coronal views can add information. If neurologic compression is a concern, CT-myelography is indicated because MRI evaluation of currently approved lumbar TDRs is compromised by metal artifact. Injection studies including facet blocks, adjacent level discography, and periprosthetic anesthetic injection may be of value in diagnosis of facet-mediated pain, symptomatic adjacent level disc degeneration, and determining whether the surgical level is the source of pain. Angiography and venography are considered when vessel impingement by displaced prosthetic components is suspected. Periprosthetic infection can be challenging to diagnose, and potentially useful imaging studies include technetium radionuclide scans or positron emission tomography (PET)-CT scans in combination with laboratory studies (complete blood count [CBC], erythrocyte sedimentation rate [ESR], C-reactive protein).

11. **What treatment options and challenges are associated with revision of a failed lumbar disc arthroplasty?**
Surgical options to treat a failed lumbar total disc arthroplasty include:
- Posterior foraminotomy
- Posterior instrumentation and fusion
- Replacement of the prosthesis with a new arthroplasty device
- Device removal, anterior interbody fusion, and posterior spinal instrumentation and fusion

Posterior foraminotomy is considered in the patient with a well-positioned prosthesis who presents with new-onset radiculopathy due to retropulsed disc or endplate material following lumbar TDR. Posterior fusion and pedicle fixation is a surgical option to address continued low back pain attributed to the operative level in the absence of gross instability, prosthesis displacement, or infection. Posterior dynamic stabilization has also been suggested as an alternative treatment in this setting, but is an "off-label" use of this technology in the United States. However, long-term results of this approach are not known and use of dynamic stabilization systems have received United States Food and Drug Administration clearance for marketing only in relation to fusion indications. An anterior approach for prosthesis revision or conversion to a fusion is a more complex and challenging procedure. Within the first 2 weeks following the index procedure, the difficulty of a revision anterior approach is similar to a primary approach. After this time period, the risk of iatrogenic injury due to scarring around retroperitoneal, vascular, and visceral structures is extremely high and may lead to life-threatening complications during a revision anterior surgical exposure. Suggested measures to minimize complications include placement of ureteral stents to aid in identification and protection of the ureters, placement of balloon catheters in the iliac vessels as an aid to limiting intraoperative blood loss in anticipation of major vessel injury, and use of an alternative approach for surgical exposure. Use of the direct lateral (transpsoas) retroperitoneal approach or use of a contralateral retroperitoneal approach has been suggested.

CERVICAL DISC ARTHROPLASTY

12. What is the rationale for cervical total disc arthroplasty?

Anterior cervical discectomy and fusion (ACDF) for radiculopathy or myelopathy remains one of the most successful procedures in spine surgery. The rationale for development of cervical TDR as an alternative procedure was based on the following principles:

- Avoid the negative effects associated with ACDF (e.g. pseudarthrosis, plate-related complications, adjacent segment degeneration, and adjacent segment disease)
- Favorably alter the natural history of motion segments adjacent to the operative level
- Enhance postoperative recovery (e.g. avoid brace immobilization, permit earlier return to unrestricted activity)

13. Discuss the issue of adjacent-level problems in the cervical spine following nonfusion and fusion procedures.

Adjacent segment degeneration and adjacent segment disease are common findings when patients are evaluated over time following cervical spine surgery. The annual incidence of adjacent segment disease requiring additional cervical surgery following an initial cervical spine procedure (ACDF or a posterior cervical foraminotomy) is 3% per year. Because the rates of adjacent segment problems are similar following fusion and nonfusion procedures, it remains uncertain whether adjacent segment degeneration (radiographic degenerative changes) and adjacent segment disease (symptoms requiring additional surgical intervention) reflect a natural progression of cervical spondylosis or a consequence of arthrodesis.

14. What is the currently accepted indication for performing cervical TDR?

The current FDA-approved indication for cervical disc arthroplasty is the treatment of radiculopathy and/or myelopathy due to neural compression caused by a disc herniation or spondylotic changes from degenerative disc disease (DDD) at a single level between C3 and C7 refractory to 6 weeks of nonoperative treatment.

15. What are the contraindications to performing cervical TDR?

Contraindications to cervical TDR include:

- **Coexistent spinal pathology unrelated to the intervertebral disc:** Pain related to facet joint degeneration, cervical or radicular arm pain of unknown etiology
- **Conditions that potentially compromise stability of a cervical disc prosthesis:** Spinal instability, vertebral body deficiency, or deformity (post-trauma, kyphosis)
- **Limited or absent segmental motion at the operative level:** Severe spondylosis, prior anterior cervical fusion
- **Patient-specific factors:** Malignancy, active infection, spondyloarthropathy, metal allergy, chronic steroid use, systemic diseases (e.g. insulin-dependent diabetes), females who desire to become pregnant

Studies investigating the prevalence of contraindications in the population presenting to spine surgeons for surgical treatment of cervical degenerative disorders have documented that the percentage of patients who are appropriate candidates for cervical TDR ranges between 40% and 50%. This is a significantly greater number of patients than the proportion of lumbar surgery candidates who qualify for lumbar TDR.

16. What cervical total disc replacements are currently FDA approved for use in the United States?

Current FDA-approved cervical total disc replacements include:

- Prestige® ST (Medtronic Sofamor Danek)
- Bryan® (Medtronic Sofamor Danek)
- ProDisc-C® (Synthes Spine)

The Prestige ST was the first cervical TDR approved by the FDA for use in the United States. This device is composed of two stainless steel articulating components that attach to the adjacent cervical vertebrae with locking screws. The convex superior component moves in a relatively unconstrained manner in the groove located on the inferior component (Fig. 71-3).

The Bryan disc is a relatively unconstrained single-piece device consisting of porous, coated titanium endplates and a polyurethane core. The polyurethane nucleus between the endplates is surrounded by a polyurethane sheath that contains wear debris. Saline is injected into the sheath to provide lubrication and a dampening effect to resist axial loads (Fig. 71-4).

The ProDisc-C is similar to the lumbar version consisting of an articulating metal on ultra high-molecular-weight polyethylene ball and socket device. The endplates are cobalt-chromium-molybdenum alloy with a midline keel for fixation and a titanium plasma spray coating for bony ingrowth (Fig. 71-5).

Many alternative cervical disc replacement designs are currently under study both in the United States and internationally.

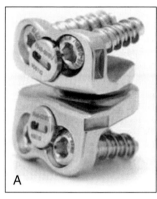
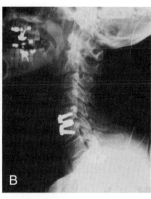

Figure 71-3. **A** and **B,** The Prestige ST cervical disc (Medtronic Sofamor Danek). (From Singh K, Vaccaro AR, Albert TJ. Assessing the potential impact of total disc arthroplasty on surgeon practice patterns in North America. Spine J 2004;4:195S–201S.)

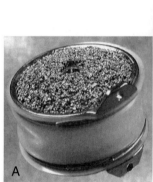
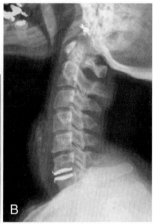

Figure 71-4. **A** and **B,** The Bryan cervical disc (Medtronic Sofamor Danek). (From Singh K, Vaccaro AR, Albert TJ. Assessing the potential impact of total disc arthroplasty on surgeon practice patterns in North America. Spine J 2004;4:195S–201S.)

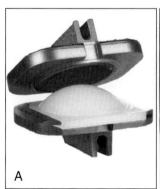
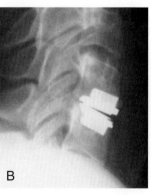

Figure 71-5. **A** and **B,** The ProDisc-C artificial disc (Synthes Spine). (From Slipman CW, Derby R, Simeone FA, et al. Interventional Spine: An Algorithmic Approach. Edinburgh: Saunders; 2007.)

17. **What considerations regarding patient positioning, setup, and surgical technique are important when performing a cervical TDR compared with an anterior cervical discectomy and fusion (ACDF)?**
Patient positioning for ACDF and cervical TDR is identical with the exception of routine use of the C-arm for a cervical TDR. One may consider turning the operating room table 180° to facilitate use of the C-arm and navigation around anesthesia equipment and personnel. Using cloth tape to pull the shoulders inferiorly is particularly important to allow for adequate visualization of the lower cervical levels, particularly at the C6–C7 level. Prior to prepping, it is important to check that the operative level is easily visualized using the C-arm. One should always be prepared to convert the procedure to an ACDF. The position of the neck should be similar to the preoperative neutral lateral radiograph and remain fixed throughout the procedure to avoid improper sagittal alignment of the spine.

Fluoroscopy may be used to select the appropriate incision location. The surgical approach is identical to an ACDF. However, because a plate is not used, less of each vertebral body needs to be exposed and dissection can be limited to the disc space itself. It is critical that the midline is established early in the procedure using the uncovertebral joints, as well as with fluoroscopy. It is critical to ensure that the head is positioned straight up and down and that the fluoroscopic views obtained are true AP and lateral views of the cervical spine. Once midline is established and dissection of the uncovertebral joints is completed, distraction pins are placed in the midline. Distraction pins are typically placed under fluoroscopic guidance on the lateral view. It is critical that the pins are placed at the center of the vertebral body and parallel to the disc at the operative level because parallel distraction is important for appropriate placement of the cervical TDR. Complete discectomy and foraminotomy with removal of all osteophytes is critical prior to prosthesis insertion.

18. **What complications have been reported in association with cervical total disc arthroplasty?**
Complications following cervical TDR may be a result of:
- **Improper surgical indications:** Poor patient selection (e.g. axial pain syndromes, nonorganic pain syndromes), segmental instability, osteoporotic patients, patients with facet arthropathy
- **Complications related to the surgical approach:** Dysphagia, recurrent laryngeal nerve injury, vertebral artery injury, esophageal injury
- **Complications related to the implant:** Migration, subsidence, vertebral body endplate fracture, polyethylene or metal wear, kyphotic deformity
- **Complications related to decompression of the spinal canal:** Inadequate foraminal decompression leading to radiculopathy, dural tear, neurologic injury
- **Miscellaneous:** Heterotopic ossification

19. **What is the major determinant of MRI clarity of a cervical TDR device following implantation?**
The material composition of the device is the most important determinant of its imaging properties. Titanium devices allow satisfactory visualization of neural structures at the index and adjacent levels on postoperative MRI scans. Cobalt-chrome metal alloys and stainless steel cause significant deterioration of MR image quality, and CT-myelography is recommended for evaluation of the neural elements with these devices.

20. **Compare the results of cervical TDR and anterior cervical discectomy and fusion (ACDF).**
Current FDA-approved cervical total disc replacements (Prestige ST, Bryan and ProDisc-C) have completed 2-year clinical trials in which the cervical TDR patients were compared with patients treated with ACDF using allograft and an anterior cervical plate. Cervical TDR demonstrated comparable safety and efficacy in terms of neural decompression and pain relief as ACDF. Cervical TDR was associated with a low rate of complications. Cervical TDR was shown to be safe and effective in treating cervical spondylotic disorders.

21. **Are there any specific challenges associated with revision of a cervical TDR to ACDF?**
The challenges associated with revision surgery for failed cervical TDR are similar in scope and magnitude to those associated with revision surgery for a failed ACDF. It is important to have device-specific instruments to facilitate removal of cervical total disc components. The options for revision of a patient with persistent or new-onset symptoms following cervical TDR include:
- Posterior cervical foraminotomy
- Removal of the device in combination with anterior cervical fusion with plate fixation
- Revision with placement of a new cervical TDR

22. **What are the outcomes of cervical TDR when placed adjacent to a prior fusion when compared with a primary cervical TDR?**
Early studies have indicated that a cervical TDR placed adjacent to a fusion leads to similar clinical outcomes compared with a primary cervical total disc replacement.
Extending a fusion for adjacent-level disease typically requires removal of an anterior cervical plate with bone grafting and reapplication of an anterior cervical plate at the adjacent level. These steps can be avoided by using a cervical TDR adjacent to the prior fusion.

23. **When is cervical TDR an appropriate option for treatment of cervical myelopathy?**
Cervical total disc arthroplasty has been shown to be successful for treatment of select patients with cervical myelopathy in whom spinal cord compression is localized to the level of the disc space (retrodiscal). This procedure is not appropriate for patients with severe facet joint degenerative changes at the operative level, severe loss of disc space height, myelopathy due to congenital spinal canal narrowing, and cervical stenosis due to retrovertebral cord compression (e.g. ossification of the posterior longitudinal ligament).

Key Points

1. Cervical total disc arthroplasty is an option for treatment of radiculopathy and/or myelopathy due to neural compression caused by a disc herniation or spondylotic changes between C3 and C7 that are refractory to nonoperative treatment.
2. Lumbar total disc arthroplasty is an option for treatment of isolated discogenic low back pain (usually without radiculopathy) caused by degenerative disc disease between L3 and S1 without associated instability that is refractory to nonoperative treatment.
3. Explantation of a failed lumbar total disc arthroplasty is a complex and high-risk procedure in comparison with revision surgery for a failed cervical total disc arthroplasty.

Websites

Cervical total disc arthroplasty: http://www.ncbi.nlm.nih.gov/pmc/articles/PMC2684211/
Lumbar total disc arthroplasty: http://www.ncbi.nlm.nih.gov/pmc/articles/PMC2335389/

BIBLIOGRAPHY

1. Blumenthal S, McAfee PC, Guyer RD, et al. A prospective, randomized, multicenter Food and Drug Administration investigational device exemptions study of lumbar total disc replacement with the CHARITE artificial disc versus lumbar fusion: Part I: Evaluation of clinical outcomes. Spine 2005;30:1565–75.
2. Guyer RD, McAfee PC, Banco RJ, et al. Prospective, randomized, multicenter Food and Drug Administration investigational device exemption study of lumbar total disc replacement with the CHARITE artificial disc versus lumbar fusion: Five-year follow-up. Spine J 2009;9:374–86.
3. Heller JG, Sasso RC, Papadopoulos SM, et al. Comparison of BRYAN cervical disc arthroplasty with anterior cervical decompression and fusion: Clinical and radiographic results of a randomized, controlled, clinical trial. Spine 2009;34:101–7.
4. Hilibrand AS, Carlson GD, Palumbo MA, et al. Radiculopathy and myelopathy at segments adjacent to the site of a previous anterior cervical arthrodesis. J Bone Joint Surg 1999;81A:519–28.
5. Mummaneni PV, Burkus JK, Haid RW, et al. Clinical and radiographic analysis of cervical disc arthroplasty compared with allograft fusion: A randomized controlled clinical trial. J Neurosurg Spine 2007;6:198–209.
6. Murrey D, Janssen M, Delamarter R, et al. Results of the prospective, randomized, controlled multicenter Food and Drug Administration investigational device exemption study of the ProDisc-C total disc replacement versus anterior discectomy and fusion for the treatment of 1-level symptomatic cervical disc disease. Spine J 2009;9:275–86.
7. Phillips FM, Allen TR, Regan JJ, et al. Cervical disc replacement in patients with and without previous adjacent level fusion surgery: A prospective study. Spine 2009;34:556–65.
8. Pimenta L, McAfee PC, Cappuccino A, et al. Superiority of multilevel cervical arthroplasty outcomes versus single-level outcomes: 229 consecutive PCM prostheses. Spine 2007;32:1337–44.
9. Riew KD, Buchowski JM, Sasso R, et al. Cervical disc arthroplasty compared with arthrodesis for the treatment of myelopathy. J Bone Joint Surg 2008;90A:2354–64.
10. Zigler J, Delamarter R, Spivak JM, et al. Results of the prospective, randomized, multicenter Food and Drug Administration investigational device exemption study of the ProDisc-L total disc replacement versus circumferential fusion for the treatment of 1-level degenerative disc disease. Spine 2007;32:1155–62.

72 CHAPTER

BONE GRAFTS, BONE GRAFT SUBSTITUTES, AND BIOLOGICS

Munish C. Gupta, MD, and Vincent J. Devlin, MD

1. What graft materials are currently available for use in spinal fusion procedures?

- Autograft
- Allograft
- Demineralized bone matrix (DBM)
- Ceramics
- Composite grafts (synthetic scaffold combined with biologic elements to stimulate fusion)
- Bone morphogenetic proteins (BMPs)

2. How are graft materials classified?

Autograft bone has been considered the gold reference standard for bone graft materials for spinal fusion. Alternative graft materials may be classified according to their intended use:

- **Extender:** This type of graft material is indicated for use in combination with autograft bone. The material permits use of a lesser volume of autograft without compromising fusion rates. Alternatively, the material may permit a finite amount of autograft to be utilized over a greater number of spinal segments without compromise of the fusion rate
- **Enhancer:** This type of graft material is used in conjunction with autograft bone to increase the rate of successful arthrodesis
- **Substitute:** This type of graft material is used as an alternative to autograft bone and is intended to provide equivalent or superior fusion success

3. Define autograft, allograft, and xenograft.

- **Autograft:** Bone harvested from the patient undergoing the spinal fusion
- **Allograft:** Bone harvested in a sterile manner from cadaver donors. This bone is preserved and processed for use in other patients
- **Xenograft:** Bone or other graft material derived from different species such as cows or pigs

4. What three properties should be provided by the ideal bone graft material for spinal fusion?

1. **Osteoinduction:** The graft should contain growth factors (noncollagenous bone matrix proteins) that can induce osteoblast precursors to differentiate into mature bone-forming cells
2. **Osteoconduction:** The graft should provide a framework or scaffold (bone mineral and collagen) onto which new bone can form
3. **Osteogenesis:** The graft should contain viable progenitor stem cells that can form new bone matrix and remodel bone as needed

5. Compare the properties of current bone graft materials in relation to an ideal bone graft material.

See Table 72-1.

Table 72-1. Properties of Current Bone Graft Materials

GRAFT	PROPERTIES	EXAMPLES
Autograft	Osteogenic, osteoconductive, osteoinductive	Iliac crest, fibula, rib
Allograft	Osteoconductive, weakly osteoinductive	Structural: femur, fibula Nonstructural: morselized femoral head
Demineralized bone matrix	Osteoinductive, osteoconductive	Grafton, Opteform, Dynagraft, Osteofil, DBX
Ceramics	Osteoconductive	Hydroxyapatite, tricalcium phosphate
Composite grafts	Osteoinductive, osteoconductive	Ultraporous beta-tricalcium phosphate (Vitoss) combined with bone marrow aspirate
Bone morphogenetic proteins	Osteoinductive	rhBMP-2, rhBMP-7

6. **How does the location and site of spinal fusion influence the choice of graft material?**

Biologic factors and **biomechanical factors** are different in the anterior and posterior spinal columns. Bone graft placed in the anterior column is subject to compressive loading, which promotes fusion. In the anterior spinal column, the wide bony surface area combined with the excellent vascularity of the fusion bed creates a superior biologic milieu for fusion. Extremely high fusion rates are typical whether a surgeon uses autograft or allograft bone. In contrast, bone graft placed in the posterior column is subjected to tensile forces, which provides a less favorable healing environment. In the posterior spinal column, fusion is more dependent on biologic factors such as the presence of osteogenic cells, osteoinductive factors, and the quality of the soft tissue and osseous bed into which the graft material is placed. In view of this more challenging healing environment, autogenous iliac bone graft has traditionally been the gold standard for achieving posterior spinal fusion. **Regional differences** along the spinal column influence healing of posterior fusions with the highest fusion rates associated with cervical and thoracic fusions and the lowest rates with posterolateral lumbar fusions.

7. **Do patient age and medical history play a role in selection of the appropriate graft material?**

Yes. The bone of skeletally immature patients has an inherent osteogenic potential, and high rates of arthrodesis are reported regardless of whether the autograft, allograft, composite grafts, or ceramics are utilized. Lower fusion rates are encountered in the adult population and healing rates have been shown to decline with increasing age. Additional factors that negatively impact fusion rates in adults include endocrine disorders (e.g. diabetes), medications (e.g. corticosteroids), and tobacco use.

8. **What properties make autograft bone an ideal choice for spinal fusion?**

Autograft bone has all of the necessary properties for achieving a spinal fusion; it is osteoinductive, osteoconductive, and osteogenic.

9. **What are the drawbacks of using autograft bone for spinal fusions?**

- Supply of autograft is limited. This is a problem in revision spinal surgery after prior bone graft harvest or when fusion of multiple levels is necessary.
- Increased operative time and a second incision are required to obtain bone graft.
- Iatrogenic complications can occur secondary to graft procurement. Bone graft site pain, infection, hematoma, lumbar hernia, sciatic nerve injury, pelvic fracture, and superior gluteal artery injury are a few examples of graft-related complications associated with harvest of iliac crest autograft.

10. **What are the two available methods for preserving allograft bone grafts?**

Allograft bone is harvested under sterile conditions and preserved by freezing or freeze-drying. These methods reduce immunogenicity and permit extended storage. Allograft bone is available either as a nonstructural graft (e.g. corticocancellous or cancellous chips) or as a structural graft (e.g. femoral rings, tricortical wedges, fibular shaft, tibial or femoral shaft, machine-contoured ramps or threaded dowels). See Figures 72-1 and 72-2.

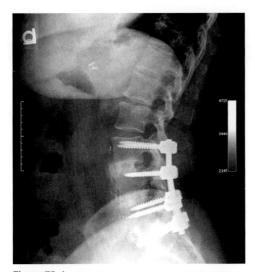

Figure 72-1. Allograft femoral rings packed with various graft materials are used with a high rate of success for anterior lumbar interbody fusion.

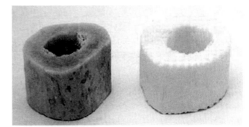

Figure 72-2. Examples of femoral allograft rings. (Kim DH, Chang UK, Kim SH, et al. Tumors of the Spine. Philadelphia: Saunders; 2008.)

11. What is the risk of disease transmission with allograft bone graft?

The risk of disease transmission with allograft bone is extremely low. Donors are screened for a history of medical problems, and serologic tests are performed to identify HIV, hepatitis B, and hepatitis C. The incidence of HIV transmission from allograft bone is estimated as 1 in 1.6 million. Bone allografts have a much lower incidence of disease transmission than blood transfusions.

12. Compare advantages and disadvantages of freeze-dried and fresh-frozen allograft bone.

- Freeze-dried allograft bone can be stored at room temperature, whereas fresh frozen grafts require storage in a −70° C freezer.
- As a result of processing, fresh-frozen allograft bone contains more viable osteoinductive factors than freeze-dried allograft.
- Freeze-dried bone is brittle if not hydrated adequately. Fresh-frozen bone must be thawed to body temperature and consequently requires more preparation time but has better mechanical properties and higher fusion rates than freeze-dried bone.

13. Give three examples of how allograft is used successfully in spinal fusion procedures. See Figure 72-3.

1. Structural allograft (fibular allograft) used to reconstruct the anterior spinal column after cervical corpectomy
2. Structural allograft (femoral ring allograft) used for anterior lumbar interbody fusions. The medullary canal may be filled with a variety of graft materials
3. Nonstructural allograft (corticocancellous chips) used in multilevel instrumented posterior spinal fusions for pediatric neuromuscular scoliosis

14. How does allograft incorporate into a spinal fusion mass?

The method of incorporation into a fusion mass depends on the type of allograft bone graft. Allograft cortical bone can take years to incorporate fully because it is remodeled by creeping substitution. Osteoclasts resorb the allograft, and osteoblasts form new bone as the graft is revascularized. Corticocancellous allograft bone is incorporated more rapidly because bone apposition on existing bony trabeculae is the primary mode of incorporation.

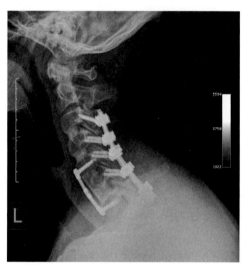

Figure 72-3. Fibula strut graft and anterior plate (lower levels); machine-prepared structural interbody allografts (upper levels).

15. What are the advantages of allograft bone in spinal fusion procedures?

Nonstructural allograft can supplement autograft in posterior fusion surgery when the volume of autograft available is insufficient. Structural allograft (e.g. fibula, femoral cortical shaft) can be used to fill anterior column defects following discectomies and corpectomies. Structural allograft provides superior mechanical strength compared with autograft iliac crest wedges or rib grafts and avoids the morbidity associated with graft harvest.

16. What are the disadvantages of allograft bone in spinal fusion procedures?

Allograft bone weakens as it undergoes remodeling. Allograft, in rare instances, can transmit infections. In some countries allograft bone is not allowed to be used based on cultural, religious, or ethical grounds. Lastly, the expense involved in processing, preserving, and storing allograft can make it difficult to obtain.

17. What is demineralized bone matrix (DBM)?

DBM is an osteoconductive scaffold produced by acid extraction of banked bone. It lacks structural mechanical properties. Its constituents include noncollagenous proteins, osteoinductive growth factors, and type 1 collagen. DBM is more osteoinductive than allograft bone because the demineralization process makes growth factors (BMPs) more accessible. Clinical data support the use of DBM as a bone graft extender or enhancer in posterior spinal fusion procedures performed with autograft bone. It is not intended to be used in isolation as a bone graft substitute. Few studies address its efficacy in anterior spinal fusion procedures. Significant variation in the biologic activity of DBM preparations has been documented. Bioassays are available to assess osteoinductivity, although no accepted standards exist.

18. What is the role of ceramics in spinal fusion procedures?

Ceramic materials (beta tricalcium phosphate, hydroxyapatite, calcium sulfate, natural coral ceramics, bioactive glass) have been evaluated for spinal fusion applications. Data support the role of ceramics in osteoconduction. Ceramics are recommended for use as bone graft extenders in combination with osteoinductive materials but not for use as bone graft substitutes. Ceramics also play a role as part of a composite graft composed of a ceramic delivery vehicle and osteoinductive bone growth factors or osteoprogenitor cells.

19. **Explain what is meant by a composite graft and provide an example of this class of graft material.**
A composite graft consists of a synthetic scaffold that is combined with biologic elements to stimulate fusion. Healos (DePuy) is a matrix of bovine type I collagen fibers that are circumferentially coated with hydroxyapatite. This matrix is combined at the time of surgery with autogenous bone marrow and heparin to create a bone graft substitute intended to remodel into bone. This graft material may also be used as a bone graft extender in conjunction with autograft bone. Matrices composed of a mixture of hydroxyapatite and tricalcium phosphate with bovine type I collagen have been investigated in combination with bone marrow aspirate, autograft, or BMPs.

20. **What are bone morphogenetic proteins (BMPs)?**
BMPs are part of a larger transforming growth factor beta superfamily that contains 30 such related proteins. These proteins are cytokines that can induce bone formation. They were first identified as the active osteoinductive fraction of DBM. Molecular cloning techniques permitted subsequent identification and characterization of these proteins. Using genetically modified cell lines, recombinant BMP has been produced. Currently only one BMP, recombinant human bone morphogenetic protein-2 (rhBMP-2), is approved for clinical use. The U.S. Food and Drug Administration (FDA) approved rhBMP-2 (Infuse®) for single-level anterior interbody fusion with an LT-Cage (lordotic tapered titanium cage). Use at other spinal regions (e.g. cervical spine) and for other types of fusion procedures (e.g. posterolateral lumbar fusion) are currently considered off-label use.

21. **How do BMPs signal for bone formation on a cellular level?**
BMPs bind to BMP receptors on the cell surface. There are five type I and seven type II receptors. These receptors are serine/threonine protein kinases that phosphorylate and activate proteins called Smads (term derived from merging Sma and Mad, which are cytoplasmic proteins activated by BMP in different species).

22. **Describe the potential advantages of using rhBMP-2 for spinal fusion.**
   - Obviates the need for autograft
   - Provides a high rate of successful fusion
   - Accelerates the fusion process (e.g. a structural bone graft such as allograft bone dowel or femoral ring is incorporated more quickly)

23. **Describe some potential disadvantages or concerns with use of rhBMP-2 for spinal fusions.**
   - Possibility of bone formation in ectopic sites separate from the area of intended fusion (e.g. within the spinal canal following transforaminal lumbar interbody fusion)
   - High cost
   - Incomplete knowledge about optimal dose, carrier, and long-term follow-up of the procedure in humans
   - Tissue swelling and edema (multiple reports regarding problems associated with use in anterior cervical spine due to delayed postoperative swelling and airway problems)
   - Vertebral osteolysis and vertebral edema (may lead to misdiagnosis as infection or lead to cage/graft subsidence)
   - Postoperative radiculitis without evidence of neural compression

24. **In what form is rhBMP-2 used in spinal fusions?**
RhBMP-2 is used in combination with a carrier. A carrier is a substance that serves as a delivery vehicle for the osteoinductive protein. A variety of carriers have been investigated as delivery vehicles for rhBMP-2 including:
   - Collagen: Sponge or putty form
   - Polymers: Polylactic acid and polyglycolic acid
   - Organic matrices: Cortical allograft and DBM
   - Inorganic matrices: Tricalcium phosphate or hydroxyapatite

25. **Are carriers equally effective when used for anterior and posterior fusion procedures?**
No. Certain carriers are optimal for use in anterior compared with posterior fusion sites. Anterior interbody fusion can be successfully achieved with a compressible collagen sponge protected by a structural support such as a bone dowel or titanium cage. In a posterolateral spinal fusion, a noncompressible matrix such as a combination of tricalcium phosphate and hydroxyapatite is more effective.

26. **What are the two major methods of gene therapy used to enhance spinal fusion in experimental studies?**
   1. In vivo: The vector carrying the genetic material is placed in the site of fusion.
   2. Ex vivo: The marrow cells or other cells are transfected in a culture and introduced into the spine fusion site.

27. What are the potential advantages and disadvantages of gene therapy over rhBMP for spinal fusions?

- Advantage: Gene therapy has the potential to deliver a sustained production of osteoinductive proteins compared with a one-time dose of rhBMP, which disappears from the surgical site within 72 hours.
- Disadvantage: An immune response from the host may block any therapeutic benefit. Ineffective transfer of genetic material and insufficient production of osteoinductive factors may occur.

Key Points

1. The ideal graft material for spine fusion is cost-effective, osteoinductive, osteoconductive, osteogenic, biocompatible and has favorable structural properties analogous to autogenous bone.
2. Graft materials may function as extenders, enhancers, or bone graft substitutes.

Websites

Bone graft substitute materials: http://emedicine.medscape.com/article/1230616-overview
Bone grafting: http://www.medscape.com/viewarticle/449880

BIBLIOGRAPHY

1. An HS, Lynch K, Toth J. Prospective comparison of autograft vs. allograft for adult posterolateral lumbar spine fusion: Differences among freeze-dried, frozen, and mixed grafts. J Spin Disord 1995;8:131–5.
2. Dimar JR, Glassman SD, Burkus KJ, et al. Clinical outcomes and fusion success at 2 years of single-level instrumented posterolateral fusions with recombinant human bone morphogenetic protein-2/compression resistant matrix versus iliac crest bone graft. Spine 2006;31:2534–9.
3. Hidaka C, Goshi K, Rawlins B, et al. Enhancement of spine fusion using combined gene therapy and tissue engineering BMP-7 expressing bone marrow cells and allograft bone. Spine 2003;28:2049–57.
4. Louis-Ugbo J, Boden SD. Biology of spinal fusion. In: Bona CM, Garfin SR, editors. Orthopaedic Essentials–Spine. Philadelphia: Lippincott; 2004. p. 297–324.
5. Luhmann SJ, Bridwell KH, Cheng I, et al. Use of bone morphogenetic protein-2 for adult spinal deformity. Spine 2005;30:S110–S117.
6. Mroz TE, Joyce MJ, Steinmetz MP, et al. Musculoskeletal allograft risks and recalls in the United States. J Am Acad Orthop Surg 2008;16:559–65.
7. Peterson B, Whang PG, Iglesias R, et al. Osteoinductivity of commercially available demineralized bone matrix preparations in a spine fusion model. J Bone Joint Surg 2004;86:2243–50.
8. Reddi AH. Bone morphogenetic proteins: from basic science to clinical applications. J Bone Joint Surg 2001;83A(Suppl. 1–1):S1–S6.
9. Slosar PJ, Josey R, Reynolds J. Accelerating lumbar fusions by combining rhBMP-2 with allograft bone: A prospective analysis of interbody fusion rates and clinical outcomes. Spine J 2007;7:301–7.
10. Stambough JL, Clouse EK, Stambough JB. Instrumented one and two level posterolateral fusions with recombinant human bone morphogenetic protein-2 and allograft: A computed tomography study. Spine 2010;35:124–9.
11. Thalgott JS, Fogarty ME, Giuffre JM, et al. A prospective, randomized, blinded, single-site study to evaluate the clinical and radiographic differences between frozen and freeze-dried allograft when used as part of a circumferential anterior lumbar interbody fusion procedure. Spine 2009;34:1251–6.

INDEX

Note: Page numbers followed by *f* indicate figures. Page numbers followed by *t* indicate tables. Page numbers in **boldface type** windicate complete chapters.

Bone scan *(Continued)*
 for presurgical patient evaluation, 238
 in spondylolisthesis, 263
 in spondylolysis, 98, 98f, 263
 superscan phenomenon, 99
 technetium
  accuracy improvement, 98
  in adult patients with back pain, 98
  normal, 97f
  in osteoporotic compression fractures, 99, 99f
  in pediatric patients with back pain, 98
  performance of scan, 97
  in sacral insufficiency fracture, 99, 99f
  of spinal neoplasms, 99
  of spine infections, 98
 three-phase, 97
 when to order, 68-69
Bone tumors. *See* Tumors, primary spine
Boston brace, 143, 143f
Bow-tie sign, 382
Braces
 for adolescent idiopathic scoliosis, 273
 for congenital kyphosis, 281
 for congenital scoliosis, 293
Brooks technique, 200, 200f, 372
Brown-Séquard syndrome, 49, 405
Bulbocavernosus reflex, significance of, 47
Bulges, of discs, 84, 85-86f, 85f, 333
Burner, 412-413
Burst fracture
 compression fracture distinguished from, 390
 lower cervical, 379, 379-380f, 380-381
 in pediatric patients, 307-308
 thoracic and lumbar, 93f, 169, 307-308
  stable, 389-390, 390f
  unstable, 391-392f, 391-394, 393f, 394f
Buttress plates, 204, 204f

C
C1 screw placement, 196-197, 197f
C1–C2 screw-rod fixation, 372-373
C1–C2 transarticular screw, 198-199, 199f, 372-373
C1–C2 wire techniques
 Brooks technique, 200, 200f, 372
 Gallie technique, 199, 200f, 372
C2 pars screw, 197, 197f
C2 pedicle screw, 197, 198f
C2 translaminar screw, 198, 198f
Cage devices, 212
Calcitonin, for osteoporosis, 453
Calcium, daily requirements for, 452, 452t
Capsaicin, 118
Cardiac risk stratification, 161-162
CARF (Commission on Accreditation of Rehabilitation
  Facilities), 104
CASH (cruciform anterior spinal hyperextension) orthosis,
  139, 140f
Catheter, implanted spinal, 246
Cauda equina
 anatomy of, 21-22, 29
 tumors, 427
Cauda equina syndrome, 44, 231, 332, 405
Cell saver, 227

Central cord syndrome, 49, 384, 405
Ceramics, role in spinal fusion, 506-507
Cerebral palsy, scoliosis secondary to, 288
Certified Clinical Competence-Audiology (CCC-A), 220
Certified neurologic intraoperative monitoring technologist,
  220
Cervical anomalies, 257-260
Cervical collar, 475
Cervical cord neurapraxia, 413
Cervical disc arthroplasty, 491
Cervical myelopathy, 320-321, 321-322f, 323-324
 assessment of reflexes and signs, 37-38
 magnetic resonance imaging (MRI), 86
 presentation of, 36-37
 total disc replacement for, 502
Cervical orthoses, 134-135
Cervical osteotomy, 484-485, 485f
Cervical radiculopathy
 computed tomography, 93
 described, 36
 disc replacement, 320
 electrodiagnosis, 132
 magnetic resonance imaging (MRI), 86, 93
 natural history of, 104
 nonsurgical treatment plan for, 105
 provocative maneuvers for evaluation, 36
 surgery indications, 153
Cervical spine
 anatomy, **9-18**
  articulations, ligaments, and disks, 12-14
  fascia and musculature, 17
  magnetic resonance imaging (MRI), 82f
  neural, 14-15
  osteology, 10-12, 10f, 11f
  vascular, 16, 16f
 corpectomy, 174
 disorder evaluation, **33-39**
  Adson's test, 36
  axial cervical compression test, 36
  Babinski's test, 37, 38f
  cervical myelopathy, 36-37
  clonus, 38
  disc herniation symptoms, 36
  finger escape sign (finger adduction test), 38
  grading motor strength and reflexes, 35t
  Hoffmann's sign, 37, 38f
  inverted radial reflex, 38
  Lhermitte's sign, 38
  nerve root testing, 36t
  neural pathway testing, 35
  overall approach, 35
  palpation, 34-35
  radiculopathy, 36
  range of motion, 35
  scapulohumeral reflex, 38
  sensation assessment, 35
  shoulder adduction test, 36, 37f
  testing sensory, motor, and reflex function, 35t
  Valsalva maneuver, 36
 disorders
  degenerative, **316-324**
  evaluation of, **33-39**
  in pediatric patients, **256-260**
  rehabilitation medicine, 104-105

Sinuvertebral nerve, 15
Slip angle, 263, 263f
Slipped vertebral apophysis, 254
Smith-Petersen osteotomy, 357, 349, 349f, 357f, 486-487
Smith-Robinson approach, 181, 181f
Smoking, interference with spinal fusion, 171
Social Security Administration
    disability definition, 60
    filling out forms for, 62-63
Social Security Disability (SSD), 60
Social Security Disability Insurance (SSDI), 60
Soft collar, 134, 134f
Somatic dysfunction, 146
Somatosensory-evoked potentials, 221
SOMI (sternal occipital mandibular immobilizer) cervicotho-
    racic orthosis, 136, 136f
Space available for the cord, 476
Spasticity, 409
Spear tackler's spine, 412
Spina bifida
    clinical features, 430
    congenital lumbar kyphosis and, 289
    defined, 429-430, 429f
Spinal balance, 77
Spinal construct, 208-209
Spinal cord
    anatomy
        cervical, 14, 14f
        thoracic, 21-22, 21f
    blood supply
        cervical, 16
        critical supply zone, 15
        thoracic, 14
        watershed region, 15
    decompression procedures for, **165-170**
    monitoring function, 221
    stimulation and implantable drug delivery systems, **243-248**
Spinal cord disorders, **423-433**
    amyotrophic lateral sclerosis (ALS), 432-433
    Chiari malformation, 428-429, 429f
    multiple sclerosis, 432
    myelopathy, 432
    spinal dysraphism, 429-432, 429f
    syringohydromyelia, 428-429
    tumors, 424-427
        extradural, 424-425, 425f, 425t
        intradural-extramedullary, 424, 426, 426f, 426t
        intramedullary, 424, 427, 427f, 427t
        location, 424, 424f
Spinal cord injury, **404-410**
    complete, 377, 405
    evaluation of, **46-51**
        ASIA Impairment Scale, 49
        bulbocavernosus reflex, significance of, 47
        elements of exam, 41f, 47
        Frankel classification, 49
        imaging studies, initial, 50
        MRI, 50
        osteoligamentous injury, 47-49
        radiograph, cervical flexion-extension views, 50
        radiograph, lateral cervical, 50
        sacral sparing, 47
        spinal shock, 47
        tract assessment, 49

Spinal cord injury *(Continued)*
        transient neurologic deficit, 47
    functional outcomes
        C1 to C5 injuries, 408t
        C6 to L1 injuries, 408t
    hypotension in, 46-47
    incidence and causes of, 46
    incomplete, 377, 405
    pediatric spinal trauma, **304-310**
    spinal deformity risk with, 288-289
    syndromes, 49
        anterior cord syndrome, 49
        Brown-Séquard syndrome, 49
        central cord syndrome, 49
        posterior cord syndrome, 49
        SCIWORA (spinal cord injury without radiographic
            abnormality), 50
    treatment
        goals of, 46
        steroids, 46
Spinal cord stimulation, **243-248**
Spinal decompression. *See* Decompression
Spinal deformities. *See also* Kyphosis; Scoliosis
    congenital, 56, **291-297**
    evaluation of, **52-58**
    neuromuscular, **284-290**
    radiographic assessment, 75-79
        Cobb method, 76
        flatback syndrome, 79
        measurement of scoliosis/kyphosis, 77f
        normal values for sagittal curves, 77
        sacral parameters, 78, 78f
        sagittal curves, 78f
        specialized radiographs, 76, 76f
        spinal balance, 77
        standard radiographs, 75, 75f
        when to order, 76
    revision surgery for, 241
    sagittal plane deformities
        in adults, **354-358**
        in pediatric patients, **278-283**
    secondary to neuromuscular disease, 56-58, 57f
Spinal disorders
    degenerative, pathophysiology and pathoanatomy of,
        311-315
    electrodiagnosis in, **128-133**
    imaging strategies for, **65-69**
    nuclear imaging and, **97-100**
    rehabilitation medicine approaches to, **101-111**
    surgery
        indications for, **151-156**
        when not to operate, **157-159**
    tumors
        metastatic, **443-449**
        primary, **434-442**
Spinal fusion, 171-176. *See also* Arthrodesis
    for adolescent idiopathic scoliosis, 274, 274f, 275-276,
        275f, 276f
    for adult scoliosis, 350-351, 352
    after thoracic discectomy, 327
    anterior cervical discectomy and fusion, 495
    anterior technique, 173, 173f, 275-276, 276f
    in athletes, 420
    for cervical disc herniation, 318-319, 319t